Geriatric Cardiology

Geriatric Cardiology
Principles and Practice

Edited by

ANTHONY MARTIN MD FRCP(Edin) MHSM

Crawley and Jersey Research Unit, Crawley, Sussex and The General Hospital, Jersey, Channel Islands, UK

and

A. JOHN CAMM MD FRCP FESC FACC

St George's Hospital Medical School, London, UK

JOHN WILEY & SONS LTD

Chichester · New York · Brisbane · Toronto · Singapore

Other Wiley Editorial Offices

John Wiley & Sons, Inc., 605 Third Avenue,
New York, NY 10158-0012, USA

Jacaranda Wiley Ltd, 33 Park Road, Milton,
Queensland 4064, Australia

John Wiley & Sons (Canada) Ltd, 22 Worcester Road,
Rexdale, Ontario M9W 1L1, Canada

John Wiley & Sons (SEA) Pte Ltd, 37 Jalan Pemimpin #05-04,
Block B, Union Industrial Building, Singapore 2057

Library of Congress Cataloging-in-Publication Data

Clinical heart disease in old age / edited by Anthony Martin and A. John Camm.
p. cm.
Includes bibiographical references and index.
ISBN 0 471 94064 X
1. Geriatric cardiology. I. Martin, Anthony, MD. II. Camm, A. John.
[DNLM: 1. Heart Diseases—in old age. 2. Aging—physiology.
3. Heart—physiopathology. WG 200 C6405 1993]
RC682.C57 1993
618.97′612—dc20
DNLM/DLC
for Library of Congress   93-40107
CIP

British Library Cataloguing in Publication Data

A catalogue record for this book is available from the British Library

ISBN 0 471 94064 X

Typeset in 10/12pt Times by Vision Typesetting, Manchester
Printed and bound in Great Britain by Biddles Ltd, Guildford, Surrey

Contents

III PATHOPHYSIOLOGY OF AGEING

IV SYSTEMATIC DISEASES

V SYNDROMES

List of Contributors

Yaver Bashir MA MRCP
Research Fellow, Department of Cardiological Sciences, St George's Hospital Medical School, Cranmer Terrace, London SW17 0RE, UK

David G. Benditt MD
Professor of Medicine, Director, Cardiac Arrhythmia Service, University of Minnesota Hospital, Box 341 UMHC, Minneapolis, Minnesota 55455, USA

Nick Bosanquet BA MSc
Professor of Health Policy, Health Policy Unit, Department of General Practice, Lisson Grove Health Centre, Gateforth Street, London NW8 8EG, UK

Stephen J. D. Brecker BSc MRCP
British Heart Foundation Junior Research Fellow, Cardiac Department, The Royal Brompton National Heart and Lung Hospital, Sydney Street, London SW3 6NP, UK

A. John Camm MD FRCP FESC FACC
Professor of Clinical Cardiology, Department of Cardiological Sciences, St George's Hospital Medical School, Cranmer Terrace, London SW17 0RE, UK

Andrew J.S. Coats MA MRCP FRACP
Senior Lecturer and Honorary Consultant Cardiologist, The Royal Brompton National Heart and Lung Institute, Dovehouse Street, London SW3 6LY, UK

Michael J. Davies MD FRCPath FACC
St George's Hospital Medical School, Cranmer Terrace, London SW17 0RE, UK

David J. Delany MA MB BChir FRCR
Consultant Cardiothoracic Radiologist, Wessex Cardiothoracic Centre, Southampton University Hospital, Tremona Road, Southampton SO9 4XY, UK

Andrew T. Elder MRCP
Lecturer in Geriatric Medicine, University Department of Geriatric Medicine, City Hospital, Greenbank Drive, Edinburgh EH10 5SB, UK

Jerome L. Fleg MD
Senior Investigator, Laboratory of Cardiovascular Science, Gerontology Research Center, National Institute on Ageing, Associate Professor of Medicine, Johns Hopkins Medical Institutions, Baltimore; Gerontology Research Center, 4940 Eastern Avenue, Baltimore, MD 21224, USA

Martin D. Fotherby BSc MB ChB MRCP
British Heart Foundation Research Fellow, University of Leicester, Department of Medicine for the Elderly, Leicester General Hospital, Gwendolen Road, Leicester LE5 4PW, UK

Keith A. A. Fox FRCP FESC
Duke of Edinburgh Professor of Cardiology, Department of Cardiology, Royal Infirmary, Lauriston Place, Edinburgh EH3 9YW, UK

Charles F. George BSc MD FRCP
Clinical Pharmacology Group, Biomedical Sciences Building, University of Southampton, Bassett Crescent East, Southampton SO9 3TU, UK

Bernard J. Gersh MB ChB DPhil
Consultant in Cardiovascular Disease, Mayo Clinic; Professor of Medicine, Mayo Medical School, 200 First Street SW, Rochester, MN 55905; Georgetown University School of Medicine, Washington D.C., USA

Ian R. Hastie MBBS FRCP
Consultant and Senior Lecturer in Geriatric Medicine, St George's Hospital Medical School, Level 01, Jenner Wing G2, Cranmer Terrace, London SW17 0RE, UK

David L. Hayes MD
Consultant, Division of Cardiovascular Diseases and Internal Medicine, Mayo Clinic and Mayo Foundation; Associate Professor Medicine, Mayo Medical School; c/o Section of Publications, Mayo Clinic, Rochester, MN 55905, USA

John Herbetko MB MRCP FRCR
Senior Registrar in Radiology, Southampton University Hospital, Tremona Road, Southampton SO9 4XY, UK

R. M. Jones MD FCAnaes
Academic Department of Anaesthetics, St Mary's Hospital Medical School, Praed Street, Paddington, London W2 1NY, UK

Demosthenes Katritsis MD PhD
Lecturer, Department of Cardiological Sciences, St George's Hospital Medical School, Cranmer Terrace, London SW17 0RE, UK

P. J. Keeling BSc MRCP
BHF Research Registrar, St George's Hospital Medical School, Cranmer Terrace, London SW17 0RE, UK

Yoichi Kobayashi MD
Visiting Fellow in Cardiac Electrophysiology, University of Minnesota Hospital, Minneapolis, MN, USA; Associate Professor of Medicine, Showa University Medical School, Tokyo, Japan

Edward G. Lakatta MD
Chief, Laboratory of Cardiovascular Science, Gerontology Research Center, National Institute on Aging; Professor of Medicine, Johns Hopkins School of Medicine; Professor of Physiology, University of Maryland, School of Medicine, 4940 Eastern Avenue, Baltimore, MD 21224, USA

Aubrey Leatham MD   FRCP
45 Wimpole Street, London S1M 7DG, UK

Keith G. Lurie MD
Assistant Professor of Medicine, Co-Director, Minnesota Syncope Center, University of Minnesota, Box 508 UMHC, 420 Delaware Street SE, Minneapolis, MN 55455, USA

Jean R. McEwan PhD MRCP
Departments of Clinical Cardiology and Medicine, Hammersmith Hospital and The Royal Postgraduate Medical School, Du Cane Road, London W12 0NN, UK

Henry D. McIntosh MD FACP FACC
Clinical Professor of Medicine, University of Florida School of Medicine, Gainesville, Florida and the University of South Florida School of Medicine, Tampa, Florida; St Joseph's Heart Institute, 3003 West Martin Luther King Junior Boulevard, PO Box 4227, Tampa, FL 33677-4227, USA

William J. McKenna MD
Honorary Consultant Cardiologist, Department of Cardiological Sciences, St. George's Hospital Medical School, Cranmer Terrace, London SW17 0RE, UK

Jessica M. Mann MD
Lecturer, Cardiovascular Pathology, Department of Cardiological Sciences, St George's Hospital Medical School, Cranmer Terrace, London SW17 0RE, UK

Anthony Martin MD FRCP(Edin) MHSM
Consultant Physician, Crawley and Jersey Research Unit, West Green Drive, Crawley, West Sussex RH11 7DH, UK

John M. Morgan MD MRCP
Wessex Cardiac Centre, Southampton General Hospital, Tremona Road, Southampton SO9 4XY, UK

Francis D. Murgatroyd MA MRCP
Research Fellow, Department of Cardiological Sciences, St George's Hospital Medical School, Cranmer Terrace, London SW17 0RE, UK

Celia M. Oakley MD FRCP FACC FESC
Professor of Clinical Cardiology, Departments of Clinical Pharmacology and Medicine (Clinical Cardiology), Hammersmith Hospital and The Royal Postgraduate Medical School, Du Cane Road, London W12 0NN, UK

Paul J. Oldershaw MD FRCP
Consultant Cardiologist, Cardiac Department, The Royal Brompton National Heart and Lung Hospital, Sydney Street, London SW3 6NP, UK

Lionel H. Opie MD DPhil FRCP
Heart Research Unit and Hypertension Clinic, University of Cape Town, Observatory 7925, Cape Town, South Africa

Michael W. Platt FCAnaes FRCA
Academic Department of Anaesthetics, St Mary's Hospital Medical School, Praed Street, Paddington, London W2 1NY, UK

Philip A. Poole-Wilson
Department of Cardiac Medicine, The Royal Brompton National Heart and Lung Institute, Dovehouse Street, London SW3 6LY, UK

John F. Potter BMedSci DM FRCP
Senior Lecturer and Honorary Consultant Physician, University of Leicester, Department of Medicine for the Elderly, Leicester General Hospital, Gwendolen Road, Leicester LE5 4PW, UK

Colin Powell MB FRCP(Edin.) FRCP(Glas.)
Professor and Head, Section of Geriatric Medicine, St Boniface General Hospital, 409 Taché Avenue, Winnipeg, Manitoba, R2H 2A6, Canada

John Reckless
Bath University School of Postgraduate Medicine, Royal United Hospital, Bath, UK

Stephen Remole MD
Associate Professor of Medicine, University of Minnesota Hospital, Box 341 UMHC, Minneapolis, MN 55455, USA

Janice B. Schwartz MD
Associate Professor of Medicine and Pharmacy; Associate Staff, Cardiovascular Research Institute, University of California at San Francisco, Moffitt Hospital, Room 10086, 505 Parnassus Avenue, San Francisco, CA 94143-0124, USA

Carol A. Seymour MA MSc PhD FRCP
Professor of Clinical Biochemistry and Metabolism, Department of Clinical Biochemistry, St George's Hospital Medical School, Jenner Wing, Cranmer Terrace, London SW17 0RE, UK

David P. Taggart MD FRCS
Senior Registrar, Department of Cardiothoracic Surgery, The Royal Brompton National Heart and Lung Hospital, Sydney Street, London SW3 6NP, UK

John J. Taylor MB BS(Lond) FRCPath, DMJ
Director, States Laboratory, St Helier, Jersey, Channel Islands

Ann C. Tweddel
Department of Medical Cardiology, Glasgow Royal Infirmary, 10 Alexandra Parade, Glasgow G31 2ER, UK

Angus Turner
91A Gilbey Road, Tooting, London SW17 0QH, UK

Derek Waller
Clinical Pharmacology Group, Biomedical Sciences Building, University of Southampton, Bassett Crescent East, Southampton SO9 3TU, UK

David E. Ward MD FRCP FACC FESC
Consultant Cardiologist, Regional Cardiothoracic Unit, St George's Hospital, Blackshaw Road, London SW17 0QT, UK

Nanett K. Wenger MD
Professor of Medicine, Department of Medicine, Division of Cardiology, Emory University School of Medicine; Director, Cardiac Clinics, Grady Memorial Hospital, Thomas K. Glenn Memorial Building, 69 Butler Street SE, Atlanta, GA 30303, USA

David J. Wheatley MD ChM FRCS
British Heart Foundation Professor of Cardiac Surgery and Honorary Consultant Cardiothoracic Surgeon, University of Glasgow, Royal Infirmary, 10 Alexandra Place, Glasgow G31 2ER, UK

Brian O. Williams MD FRCP(Glas) FRCP(London) FRCP(Edin)
Consultant in Administrative Charge, W Glasgow Geriatric Medical Service, Gartnavel General Hospital, 1053 Great Western Road, Glasgow G12 0YN, UK

Alan G. Wilson FRCR FRCP
Consultant Radiologist, St James' Wing, St George's Hospital, Blackshaw Road, London SW17 0QT, UK

Anna Zajdler
Research Worker, Health Policy Unit, Department of General Practice, Lisson Grove Health Centre, Gateforth Street, London NW8 8EG, UK

Preface

The population of all westernized countries is growing older and aged people now constitute over 15% of the total population and this figure is likely to rise to over 20% by the end of the century. Thus the importance of cardiovascular disease and its management cannot be over-emphasized.

Fortunately the increase in the numbers of people who are past retiring age has been matched by greater understanding of the ageing processes and by improvements in investigational techniques and pharmacological and surgical procedures.

Such changes have now made it possible to be more critical in our evaluation of the management of older people with cardiovascular disease. Recent initiatives have led to a much greater emphasis on the prevention of disease, quality of life aspects of management and, inevitably, the costs that prevention and treatment incur. Because of the increasing size of the elderly population and the relatively smaller proportion of wage-earning people it must be right that cost-effectiveness of management is put into the equation of health care economics from a national point of view.

We have structured this book to be a comprehensive review of the subject and have been fortunate in obtaining the help of authors of international repute. We are aware that there are differences, although often subtle, in approaches to the management of heart disease in older people between continents and countries. As far as possible we have tried to cater for an international readership by representing alternative views of the same subject, for example on ethical considerations.

Since we last published a book on heart disease (1) there have, as we anticipated, been major changes in attitudes to the management of elderly people, partly as a result of the development of non-invasive assessment and treatment measures. We would expect that these developments will continue further. However, there have also been significant changes in social attitudes to older people with a reaffirmation of the view that elderly people have an important and continuing role in positively developing and contributing to our society. For example, the term 'third age' (or the 'age of living'), is often used to describe the life phase following that of active paid employment, and for a few people there is a 'fourth age', the age of dependence, which may follow the age of living. We do not suggest that numerical age is totally irrelevant as far as ageing processes are concerned, but we do believe that the quality of life for those with heart disease in the 'third age' can be greatly enhanced by appropriate aggressive management whatever their numerical age may be.

REFERENCE

1. Martin A, Camm AJ (1984) *Heart Disease in the Elderly*. Wiley, Chichester.

Part I

FUNDAMENTALS OF AGEING

1 Demography

ANTHONY MARTIN
The General Hospital, Jersey, Channel Islands

The end of the twentieth century has seen the phenomenon of greatly increased numbers of elderly people in almost all Western countries and this will be repeated in other countries in the next decades. The socio-economic implications of this are obvious when it is realized that the enlarged cohort of people over 65 years is accompanied by a diminution in the number and proportion of people in paid employment. The situation is exacerbated by the fact that it is not only the total population over 65 years that is growing, but that the numbers of people aged 80 years and over are growing at a disproportionately faster rate, especially in the UK.

The reasons for these demographic changes are chiefly due to a fall in the birth rate and a decrease in the death rate in the last 20 years, which are inversely related to the situation in the first decades of the twentieth century, where there was a high birth rate, a falling perinatal mortality rate and a high death rate. This is well illustrated in Great Britain, where there has been a reduction in the death rates in all age groups below 65 years for several decades, especially in the first year of life. In 1851 the infant mortality rate was 153 per 1000 live births in England and Wales. The impact of public health measures, such as the Sewage and Sanitation Act and the Smallpox Vaccination Act at the end of the last century, resulted in a great reduction in infant mortality so that by 1941 the mortality rate in the first year of life had fallen to 58 per 1000 live births and by the present time to just over eight per 1000 live births. The number of live births fell appreciably during the 1970s and in the 1980s has risen slightly, although in 1988 the birth rate was still 13% lower than in 1971 (1). The net result of these changes is that the population of Great Britain is now 57.5 million, with 19% under 15 years and 8 million or 16% over 65 years (1). Apart from Sweden and Denmark (18%), Great Britain has the highest percentage of the population over 65 years in the world.

A similar picture is seen in Europe and North America as a whole (see Table 1). The proportion of elderly people is high in these continents and the birth rate is low. In contradistinction, the situation in less developed countries is different, with a high birth rate, large numbers of people under 15 years and a small percentage of the population over the age of 65 years.

Geriatric Cardiology. Principles and Practice.   Edited by A. Martin and A. J. Camm
© 1994 John Wiley & Sons Ltd

Table 1. Mid-1991 population estimates, birth rate and proportion of people under 15 and over 65 years

Continent	Population (millions)	Birth rate/ 1000 pop.	% under 15 yr of pop.	% over 65 yr of pop.
Europe	502	13	20	13
N. America	280	16	22	12
Africa	677	44	45	3
Asia	2003	27	33	5
L. America	451	28	36	5

Adapted from Population Concern (1991).

Current statistics from Asian countries conceal some major anomalies, however. In Japan there has been a precipitous fall in the birth rate since 1950 and it now has the lowest birth rate in the world. This fall in the birth rate, allied to much improved standards of health care, has already contributed to the start of a very steep rise in the numbers and proportion of elderly people in that country, probably the greatest rise in an elderly age group that the world has ever seen (see Table 2).

The demography of the ageing population is important since there is a progressive amount of physical disability with advancing years (2). This is particularly noticeable in those aged 75 years and over. Late age sees the arrival of the major diseases of middle life, such as ischaemic heart disease, with much greater frequency. Degenerative disease, such as disintegration of the heart's conducting system and senile cardiac amyloidosis, rarely occur before the advent of late life (3,4). The impact of such diseases is much greater on old people than on the young and middle-aged, since elderly people suffer from multi-system degenerative changes. Thus relatively minor degrees of cardiovascular malfunction may have devastating effects on cerebral, renal, pulmonary and gastrointestinal function.

Table 2. Rise in the elderly populations in the USA and Japan 1991–2030

	1991	2010	2025	2030
USA				
Population (millions)	252.8	299.0		333.7
% under 15 yr	22.0			
% over 65 yr	12.0	13.8		21.2
Japan				
Population (millions)	123.8	135.8	134.6	
% under 15 yr	18.0			
% over 65 yr	12.0	20.0	23.4	

Adapted from Population Concern (1991).

Heart disease in itself is not only likely to contribute to increased morbidity in elderly people but is a significant factor in limiting the recovery of patients with other medical and surgical problems. The lessons that have already been learnt in developed Western nations with large cohorts of elderly people will have to be applied to the nations with a prospective increase in their elderly folk. There is much still to learn, but at least there is the opportunity to be forewarned and for developing nations to prepare for the almost inevitable growth of their elderly population.

REFERENCES

1. Population Concern (1991) *1991 World Population Data Sheet*. Population Concern, London.
2. Sheldon JH (1948) *The Social Medicine of Old Age: Report of an Inquiry in Wolverhampton*. Oxford University Press, London.
3. Pomerance A (1965) Senile cardiac amyloidosis. *Brit. Heart J* **27**: 711–714.
4. Davies MJ (1971) *Pathology of the Conducting System of the Heart*. Butterworth, London.

2 Epidemiology

COLIN POWELL
St Boniface General Hospital, Manitoba, Canada

The biological characteristics of ageing are of a process which is irreversible, universal and detrimental. However, this process is not random. In human biology death is more likely after a certain age; subjects die from causes which would not have killed them at a younger age—the force of mortality increases with age. Ageing is thus the loss of adaptability and consequent increase in vulnerability over time. Happily, there is more to ageing than biology.

An ageing population means an increased survival to older ages producing the phenomenon of 'rectangularization of the survival curve' (1); Figure 1). A major current gerontological controversy is whether rectangularization of the survival curve is accompanied by 'compression of morbidity' (2). Does prolongation of life expectancy result in a proportionately longer period of antemortem morbidity, or the same, or less? Advocates of compression of morbidity argue that with control and diminution of chronic diseases such as ischaemic heart disease, osteoarthritis and strokes then old age will mean longer and fitter lives. An implication is that of lessened necessity for supportive services for the 'frail' elderly, of whom there will be fewer. At present there is no unequivocal evidence to support or refute this proposition. Even less certain is the related matter of whether prolongation of lifespan is occurring *pari passu* with the increase in life expectancy. Life expectancy is the average number of years an individual can be expected to live from a given point (e.g. from birth, from age 65). Lifespan is the life expectancy of a species from birth under optimum conditions.

Much energy is expended in gerontological investigations in attempting to distinguish between normal or healthy, ageing and abnormal or pathological ageing (3). Such a simple dichotomy fails to recognize the confounding nuances which moderate differences apparently attributable solely to the passage of time. A further practical problem is that when faced with an elderly patient it is usually impossible to isolate and define the facets of illness which might be considered as resulting from ageing, and hence be irreversible, and those arising from disease, and hence be amenable to cure, control or even spontaneous recovery. Although age *per se* is of value in predicting morbidity and mortality in population terms, it is less useful when an individual is considered; indeed, consideration of age alone

Geriatric Cardiology. Principles and Practice. Edited by A. Martin and A. J. Camm
© 1994 John Wiley & Sons Ltd

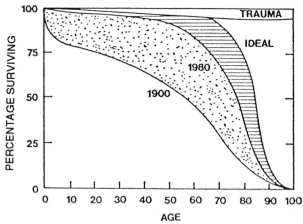

Figure 1. The human survival curve. Reproduced from Bromley *et al.* (1) with permission from Cambridge University Press

may thwart appropriate intervention. There is more to assessment of an older patient than mere examination of the birth certificate!

Evans (4) helpfully observes that not all changes over time result from ageing processes (Figure 2). In false ageing the differences between old and young are *not* due to age. A *cohort effect* is that today's 20-year-olds will be different when they are 80 from today's 80-year-olds as a result of different environmental and other experiences (this is strictly a cohort–period effect). Unfortunately cross-sectional studies—still the easiest gerontological investigations to perform—fail to identify cohort effects. This readily leads to ageist interpretations of data. As a general rule, longitudinal studies show smaller reductions in parameters with age compared with cross-sectional studies. A further confounding factor is that of *selective survival* whereby older subjects reflect survival of the fittest; thus in longitudinal studies these subjects no longer typify the original population which entered the study. A third factor is that of *aggravated ageing*. By this Evans suggests that differences between age groups result from unequal challenges facing old and young, thus enabling the young to perform more easily and better than the old. An example from health care delivery showed that older people receive significantly shorter consultation time with their doctors than younger people (5).

A further characteristic of most comparisons of the old with the young is that

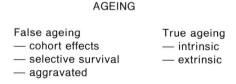

Figure 2. Ageing processes

there is increased variability with age. Thus some elderly subjects are healthier or perform more successfully, depending on the parameter being measured, than some younger subjects even though the overall mean shows decline with age.

Evans considers that true ageing (Figure 2) results from the interaction of intrinsic and extrinsic ageing. *Intrinsic ageing* is that solely resulting from genetic processes and in humans this largely arises through immunosenescence. By *extrinsic ageing* is meant change derived from those long-term environmental factors which modulate intrinsic ageing. This analysis indicates that some aspects of ageing are, currently, irreversible (*viz.* intrinsic) and some are potentially reversible or controllable (*viz.* extrinsic). It also emphasizes that the study of ageing is not just the study of the elderly; what happens in old age usually results from factors at work over a much longer period of the lifespan.

Extrapolating data from middle-aged populations to older people may be unwise. Ischaemic heart disease may present atypically in old age, given physical signs or history may have different prognoses from that in younger groups, and co-morbidity may greatly modify the clear-cut implications of established ischaemic heart disease at an earlier age. Differences in outcomes at different ages may reflect differences in patient selection and management rather than age *per se.* Elderly people, so readily defined as the over 65s, are commonly regarded as a homogeneous group.This is biological, psychological and sociological nonsense.

Early cross-sectional studies purporting to identify differences in age groups introduced additional confounding by comparing the well young—usually fit undergraduates of the investigator's discipline—with the old ill—readily found in nearby long-term institutional care. Occasionally, this still occurs (6). A further consideration arises from the numbers of subjects in different age groups that might be benefited by a medical intervention—whether preventive or curative. A relative 'marginal' improvement can be magnified by the larger numbers of older subjects, who might be helped, into worthwhile overall improvement.

ISCHAEMIC HEART DISEASE: RISK FACTORS

Ischaemic heart disease is common in old age. About 30% of 70-year-olds have evidence of coronary heart disease (7). The following risk factors will be considered: raised arterial pressures, smoking, exercise, gender, sex hormones and lipids.

Some definitions

Risk generally means the likelihood of some untoward event occurring. A *risk factor* is one associated with the development of a disease. Risk factors may be genetic, environmental, behavioural or social. Risk factors, while statistically associated with the development of a disease, are not necessarily causal for its development.

Exposure is the time of contact a person (or population) has with a risk factor; usually, the longer the exposure the greater the likelihood of occurrence of the disease. Several problems arise when trying to link a given risk factor with a particular disease. *Latency* is the time between exposure and the onset of the disease: a long latency obscures the relation between risk factor and disease. Commonly, there are several risk factors associated with a disease, making it difficult to assign to any one factor its specific role in aetiology or to identify a hitherto unrecognized factor. Mere presence of a factor does not inevitably lead to the development of the disease.

Risk is a useful concept: (a) it can be used to predict the development of disease; (b) it may indicate aetiology; although a risk factor, while not being causative, may be associated with a common precursor causative both for the risk factor and the disease; (c) a risk factor can be of diagnostic help in that its presence makes the diagnosis more likely; and (d) the removal or amelioration of a risk factor is a primary preventive measure (Figure 3). Essential characteristics of effective prevention are that interventions are feasible and that as a result the underlying pathology is reversible or, at least, can be retarded.

A further useful manoeuvre is to compare risks between individuals (or populations) which may have different exposures to a possible risk factor. *Attributable risk* (risk difference) compares those exposed to the risk factor with those who are not exposed by subtracting the incidence of the disease in those not exposed from the incidence of the disease in those exposed to the risk factor. This attempts to isolate the effect of the risk factor from the background incidence of the disease and thus define the excess incidence of the disease attributable to the risk factor. This implies the risk factor is truly causative.

Relative risk (risk ratio) expresses the increased likelihood of those exposed to the risk factor getting the disease compared with those not exposed, by taking the ratio of the incidence in the exposed to the incidence in the non-exposed. It helps establish the degree of association between disease and risk factor. A high relative risk may be of little practical import in a rare disease where the

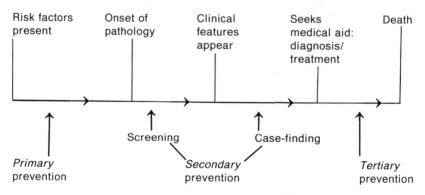

Figure 3. Prevention

attributable risk is small. A further consideration is that of how common is the risk factor. If a relative risk is small but the risk factor is very common then the overall effect of the risk factor may be greater than a larger relative risk in a population with much less exposure to the risk factor.

In the perennial debate concerning the relative merits of nature and nurture in biology, Barker and his colleagues in analysing a unique data set derived from adult men, together with their antenatal and infancy information, have concluded that early childhood influences are important ingredients in adult cardiovascular risk factors (e.g. 8). These views are not undisputed (9, 10) but they point to a wider view of risk factors than hitherto assumed. Lever and Harrap (11) consider that adult hypertension reflects a childhood pressor mechanism which later continues into adulthood.

BLOOD PRESSURE

Age and blood pressure are continuous variables, with no detectable biological or pathological point where morbidity or mortality dramatically increases. Nevertheless, 'whether systolic or diastolic, labile or fixed, at any age in either sex, hypertension is dangerous'—so comments Kannel, reviewing the Framingham experience (12). The risk attributable to raised arterial pressures is independent of other risk factors but is related to them. For example, in some parts of eastern Europe high blood pressure may be common, but in association with a low-cholesterol diet coronary heart disease is lower than would be expected in those societies with both hypertension and high-cholesterol diets (13). Nevertheless, hypertension emerges as the dominant risk factor for cardiovascular disease in older persons, with systolic blood pressure being the more consistent predictor of cardiovascular disease (14).

The traditional resource of epidemiology to study vital statistics gleaned from death certificates is potentially suspect when considering hypertensive and cardiovascular deaths in that when doctors know of a patient's hypertension they may be more likely to record a cardiovascular cause of death. Stehbens (15), in an exhaustive review of *postmortem* findings and death certificates, found that diagnostic errors in death certificates, both for all-cause mortality and for coronary heart disease mortality, meant that vital statistics were too unreliable for determining secular changes in the incidence of coronary heart disease. These errors increased with the age of the decedent. Stehbens has also questioned the assumption that clinical coronary heart disease accurately reflects coronary atheroma, claiming that coronary heart disease relates to risk factors operating in middle age whereas coronary atheroma begins in childhood (16).

Until latterly, the prevalence and effect of raised arterial pressures in old age were largely deduced from extrapolation of actuarial and other data derived from males aged under 65 years. It was also believed that hypertension in old age was not as clinically harmful as in younger people and, indeed, that raised blood pressure might be necessary to ensure organ (particularly brain) perfusion (17).

Several major placebo-controlled treatment studies have shown that in urban Westernized societies raised blood pressure in old age is harmful. It is less clear whether raised arterial pressures remain a risk factor after the age of 85 years (18).

The STOP randomized controlled trial (19), which studied diastolic hypertension in 1627 men and women aged 70–84 years (excluding subjects with isolated systolic hypertension), found that active treatment significantly reduced the trial's primary endpoints of stroke, non-myocardial infarction cardiovascular deaths and total mortality. The reduction of myocardial infarction in the treated group did not reach statistical significance. The SHEP Study (20) of isolated systolic hypertension examined 4736 subjects (being 1% of those screened) aged over 60 years (14% aged over 80 years) and showed that hypotensive treatment significantly reduced the risk of non-fatal stroke, myocardial infarction and left ventricular failure. The Medical Research Council trial (21), reporting on 4396 subjects aged 65–74 years with systolic and diastolic hypertension, showed significant reduction in coronary events, cardiovascular events and strokes in those treated with diuretics (but not β-blockers). Happily, the Framingham and SHEP studies found no drug-induced cognitive impairment or depression (22,23). The STOP Study indicated that 14 elderly patients with diastolic hypertension would have to be treated for 5 years in order to prevent one stroke and one death; the SHEP Study indicated that treating 33 elderly patients with isolated systolic hypertension for 5 years would be expected to prevent one stroke or two major cardiovascular events (24).

Isolated systolic hypertension

In the last decade it has become clear that systolic blood pressure is at least as important a predictor of untoward cardiovascular events as diastolic pressure. The phenomenon of isolated systolic hypertension has been recognized as a risk factor for cardiovascular and cerebrovascular events. Isolated systolic hypertension is most often defined as a systolic pressure over 160 mmHg and a diastolic pressure of under 90 mmHg. It is said to be commoner in women and black subjects (25). Staessen *et al.* (26) in a meta-analysis of 11 studies reported that the prevalence of isolated systolic hypertension at the age of 60 years was 5%, at 70 years was 12.6% and at 80 years was 24%.

The J-shaped curve

Controversy surrounds the existence and explanation of a J-shaped curve expressing the relationship between cardiovascular mortality and blood pressure, *i.e.* is there a level of blood pressure below which cardiovascular mortality increases (24,27)? Most authorities agree that in subjects with established coronary heart disease there is a level of diastolic blood pressure (whether spontaneous or drug-induced) below which coronary events are more likely to occur (28). Staesen *et al.* (29) found similar relationships important for elderly people with systolic and diastolic hypertension. Explanations for harmful lower arterial pressures include the effect of 'white coat hypertension' at assessment with consequent over-treatment in 'non-white coat' situations and lowering of diastolic blood pressure as a prodromal premorbid event (30). Fletcher and Bulpitt (31) interestingly suggest that the phenomenon is a consequence rather than a cause of ischaemic heart disease. There is little evidence concerning the occurrence and relevance of the J curve in those aged over 70 but it may well constitute another hazardous cause of hypotension in old age (32).

Left ventricular hypertrophy

Aronow (33) has recently reviewed the epidemiology of left ventricular hypertrophy. Left ventricular mass increases with age (at least in subjects from urbanized societies), hypertension, obesity and following myocardial infarction.

Geographical variation

A rise in blood pressure is not invariably associated with ageing. Geographical variation in blood pressure suggests that blood pressure does not rise with age in societies which are isolated from industrialized, urbanized cultures. There is no evidence that in these non-urban societies selective mortality operates to remove those individuals who would have had raised arterial pressures, through those causes of death (usually infective or traumatic) effective in young adulthood.

Unfortunately, cross-cultural studies are hampered by differences in sample selection and measurements of blood pressure and other variables. The cross-sectional Cook Island Study (34) showed that isolated islanders remote from the administrative capital had lower mean blood pressure and there was less rise with age, whereas in those more urbanized islanders there was a higher mean blood pressure and a significant rise with age, particularly of systolic blood pressure. This 'urban factor' has been studied by examining groups as they become urbanized, by comparing similar racial groups under different degrees of urbanization and by following migrants as they move from rural to urban settings and comparing them with their non-migrant confrères (e.g. 35). In general, there is support for the concept of an urban factor(s) but there are conflicting results (36) *e.g.* in Japan, where some rural populations may have higher blood pressures than urban groups; here sodium intake and dietary factors may confound the issue.

SMOKING

The control of multiple risk factors, of which smoking is one, is well-recognized primary prevention for cardiovascular disease in younger adults (37). Predictions of the effect of stopping smoking upon the US male population have been made by Tosteson *et al.* (38). However, with respect to elderly males, reduction in deaths from 'non-coronary smoking-related' conditions will conceivably increase the number of older men available to suffer from ischaemic heart disease, thus they suggest there will be a lag time before benefits from stopping smoking are apparent. Psaty *et al.* (39), in analysing published studies, treated the three major risk factors (hypertension, smoking and raised cholesterol) separately in additive and multiplicative statistical models. An additive model suggests that the combined effect of two risk factors is the sum of their independent effects, and a multiplicative model best describes the combined effect as the product of their effects. They concluded that smoking and cholesterol levels are less important risk factors for coronary heart disease in old age, being best described by an additive model, whereas in younger age groups these risk factors are considered multiplicative.

LaCroix *et al.* (40) studied 7178 subjects aged over 65 years. They found that mortality from any cause in current smokers was approximately twice (males: 2.1; females: 1.8) those who had never smoked, with a similar increased risk for cardiovascular mortality (males: 2.0; females: 1.6), whereas former smokers ('quitters') had cardiovascular mortality similar to those who had never smoked (rates for cancers remained elevated in the quitters). They concluded that cessation will continue to improve life expectancy in older people.

Mariotti *et al.* (41), in reporting the European samples of the Seven Countries Study (which followed two cohorts of 12 763 men for 15 years), found that the relative risk of death from coronary heart disease from smoking fell with age but this was complicated by a period effect whereby smoking was more harmful in 1970–75 than in 1960–65. These two effects tended to cancel each other out. They noted a dramatic shift in the type of tobacco used in southern Europe during these time periods and thought this might account for their findings. A comprehensive review of the literature concerning smoking and older adults is found in LaCroix and Omenn (42).

EXERCISE

The relation of exercise to ischaemic heart disease has been studied by comparing subjects' histories of (a) leisure time physical activity and (b) physical fitness, with the prevalence of coronary heart disease (as would be expected, reported physical activity and ergometrically measured physical fitness correlate well). Three studies of male middle-aged British civil servants (43), Harvard graduates (44), middle-aged men considered to be at relatively high risk of developing ischaemic heart disease (45), have shown that the more the regular vigorous exercise the less the chance of developing coronary heart disease. Even 80-year-old regularly exercising Harvard graduates had half the relative risk of death of their non-exercising confrères. Comparable results were found with physical fitness and ischaemic heart disease (e.g. 46,47). Master older athletes (aged 52–66 who had recently won a marathon or triathlon) had cardiovascular variables resembling younger healthy adults, implying that the expected deterioration with age (found in age-matched controls) had not occurred (48). Nevertheless, Siconolfi *et al.* (49), in considering the triad fitness, blood pressure and age, warned against accepting that physical fitness was strongly inversely correlated with arterial pressures without allowing for the confounding by age.

Information is also available about physical exercise begun in old age. Morey *et al.* (50) showed that a 2-year supervised exercise programme for men aged 65–74 years significantly improved cardiovascular variables. Intensive endurance exercise has been shown to decrease abdominal fat in older men (51) and thus reduce a risk factor (52). Posner *et al.* (53) carried out a randomized controlled trial on the effect of exercise in older subjects and showed that those who exercised had significantly delayed onset of cardiovascular disease. Hagberg *et al.* (54) showed that in septuagenarians prolonged endurance exercise diminished other expected cardiovascular changes associated with age, whereas resistance training had no effect on cardiovascular response to exercise. Exercise training in patients with controlled congestive cardiac failure has a beneficial effect on exercise tolerance and symptoms (55–57).

SEX, HORMONES AND CORONARY HEART DISEASE

Sex differences in ischaemic heart disease

Given the increase in life expectancy in developed countries, most women can expect to spend at least a third of their lives in a postmenopausal state. It is widely accepted that the menopause is associated with an abrupt increase in the risk of ischaemic heart disease. However, some epidemiological opinion finds no evidence of this by considering mortality data, which show that the much-quoted decline in the male/female ratio of death rates in middle age is more due to a relative decline in the age-associated increase in risk among males than to an unprecedented increase among females (58,59). One cohort study suggested that risk for myocardial infarction was five times higher in demented women. No association was found in men of cardiovascular disease and dementia (60). There are other unexplained sex differences in ischaemic heart disease. For example, angina is commoner in women whereas electrocardiograms (ECGs) compatible with ischaemic heart disease are commoner in men.

Lipoproteins and sex hormones

A suggested mechanism to explain the difference in prevalence of ischaemic heart disease both between the sexes and before and after the menopause invokes differences in plasma lipoproteins, of which very-low-density (VLDL), low-density (LDL) and high-density (HDL) lipoproteins are the most relevant (61,62). In general, exogenous oestrogen increases HDL, VLDL and possibly triglycerides, and decreases LDL, giving a 'preferred coronary heart disease profile'. Matthews *et al.* (63) suggest that the menopause has an unfavourable effect on lipid metabolism and that hormone replacement therapy may alleviate these changes. When a progestogen is added cyclically this advantage may be lost, particularly the more androgenic the progestogen (although Farish *et al.* (64) found some improvement in lipoprotein pattern). Studies in this domain are handicapped by inadequate numbers, being of relatively limited duration, using different doses and routes of administration, in timing of blood samples in the oestrogen/progestogen cycle and by the general assumption that cessation of menses indicates concomitant total ovarian failure. The issue is also complicated by possible changes in risk factor status occurring about the time of the menopause, *e.g.* perimenopausal weight gain (65). There is some evidence that increased risk of ischaemic heart disease begins *before* the onset of the menopause (66). Oestrogen affects more than lipoproteins. Direct effects on arterial wall and vasomotor control may be as important, although less easily measured (67).

Change in sex hormones in males with respect to cardiovascular disease has been studied. A cohort study of men aged 40–70 years (mean age: 63 years) and followed for 12 years found no sex hormone was significantly associated with cardiovascular morbidity or mortality (68). Duell and Bierman (69) found no correlation between HDL levels and sex hormones in healthy males; most of the variation in HDL levels could be accounted for by strenuous exercise, age and alcohol intake.

Atheroma and oestrogen

Attempts have been made to visualize the degree of perimenopausal atheroma. Witteman *et al.* (70) measured the radiographic size of calcific depositions in the abdominal aorta (considering this to reflect intimal atheroma) in a community study of female volunteers aged 45–55 years without cardiovascular disease. Three per cent of the premenopausal and 13% of the postmenopausal subjects showed calcification and they concluded 'after adjustments for age and other indicators of cardiovascular risk' that there was thrice the risk of aortic calcification for women undergoing a natural menopause and five times the risk for those having an artificial menopause. Only 10% of their general female population (Netherlands) use hormone replacement therapy and no conclusions were drawn about its effect in this sample.

Several authors (71,72,73) have studied the highly selected population of postmenopausal women who have undergone coronary arteriography (see Table 1 for comparisons and conclusions).

Hormone replacement therapy and cardiovascular disease

In a review of 10 cohort and eight case–control studies reporting on the use of oestrogen in the 1970s (*i.e.* without currently prescribed combined oestrogen/

Table 1. Oestrogen and coronary angiography

	Gruchow (71)	McFarland (72)	Sullivan (73)
n	933 (with complete information)	345 (consented to questionnaire)	2268 (+570 incomplete)
Years of study	1972–1985	2-year period	1972–1985
Age	50–75	35–59	≤55 (or surgical MP or referred as MP)
Menopausal indications	All Angina (2/3) Unexplained SOB/pain	283 Suspected coronary disease	All Symptoms related to the chest
HRT history	Pre-angio. history	Post-angio. mail/phone questionnaire	Pre-angio. history
Angio. report	Blinded (scoring system given)	Cardiologist's report of % occlusion (random) sample validated)	Blinded (% occlusion)
No. without occlusion detected	?	208	446
HRT	<3/12 pre-angio.	For 6/12	Current at angio. or FU
(No study records information about dose of oestrogen or use of progestogen)			
Conclusion	HRT protects after natural and surgical MP	HRT protects after surgical MP	HRT prolongs 10-year survival[a] in CHD group

HRT, hormone replacement therapy; CHD, coronary heart disease; MP, menopause/menopausal; FU, follow-up; SOB, shortness of breath.
[a]No information about cause of death.

progestogen), Barrett-Connor and Bush (74) conclude that oestrogen replacement therapy in the postmenopausal woman is beneficial and 'protective' for heart disease. The principal exception to this conclusion was found in the Framingham Study (75). Here 1234 women aged 50–84 years (291 aged over 70 years) were followed for 8 years and showed an increased risk for cardiovascular morbidity (of 50%) and cerebrovascular disease (of 200%). Initial criticism was that the study included all cardiovascular events (*e.g.* the less reliable endpoint of angina) rather than definite myocardial infarction, perhaps forgetting the Framingham Study's undoubted ability to identify and quantify the presence of 'silent' infarction. Barrett-Connor and Bush (74), reviewing the Framingham data, claim that 'a re-analysis of the data . . . on women aged 50–60 using specific endpoints and 10-year incidence rates, and not adjusting for the cholesterol and lipoprotein ratio, has shown that the overall risk of coronary heart disease in oestrogen users was approximately half that of non-users'; unfortunately, no details of this re-analysis are given, although it is alluded to be Stampfer *et al.* (76). One of the Framingham authors has emphasized the importance of the study with respect to cerebrovascular disease and apparently concedes that 'the Framingham data do not show a serious adverse effect of oestrogen use for cardiovascular disease' (77).

The Nurses' Health Study (78) followed for 10 years a cohort of 48 470 volunteer postmenopausal women aged 30–63 years who were initially free of cancer and cardiovascular disease. One-quarter continued with hormone replacement therapy, one-quarter had formerly used hormone replacement therapy and the rest had never used hormone replacement therapy. They reported on those who had used conjugated oestrogen unopposed by progestogen. For those who continued to take oestrogen, the risk of 'major coronary disease' (*viz.* non-fatal myocardial infarction, fatal cardiovascular disease, coronery artery bypass grafting or angioplasty) was half that of those who had never taken hormone replacement therapy. Considering former and current users together, the risk was three-quarters of those who had never taken oestrogen. There was no reduction in the risk of stroke. However, for the former users, the confidence intervals for the risk of major coronary disease and fatal cardiovascular disease included unity and there was no reduction in coronary artery surgery. The time since stopping oestrogen was not related to the cardiovascular risk. The users were considered 'slightly healthier' than the non-users and were described as less likely to be diabetic, to be leaner and to engage in regular vigorous exercise. For the very few nurses using high doses of oestrogen (over 1.25 mg daily) there was no advantage in cardiovascular risk. An accompanying editorial (79), echoed in the *Lancet* (80), strongly urged use of hormone replacement therapy to reduce coronary heart disease in women, although conceded that only a random controlled trial can elucidate whether women who use hormone replacement therapy have other characteristics which diminish their risk of cardiovascular disease.

Ross *et al.* (81) observed that 10 years of hormone replacement therapy reduced stroke mortality by 50% and, taking hip fracture, breast and uterine cancer and ischaemic heart disease into account, calculated a reduced annual mortality for women aged 65–74 years of 302 per 100 000 non-hysterectomized women. These researchers have reported a lower mortality, including cardiovascular deaths, in users of hormone replacement therapy (82). Nevertheless, in attempting to improve the quality of life in the postmenstrual woman, a randomized placebo-controlled trial of hormone replacement therapy is still awaited (83).

In these relatively short studies (of up to 10 years beginning at or near the menopause) risk factors operating at an earlier age are unlikely to be identified and elucidated (84). The increasing variability associated with age may also account for apparently conflicting findings.

Where recorded it is clear that smoking continues to be the overwhelming greatest risk factor, and any possible beneficial effect of hormone replacement therapy may be negated if the subject continues to smoke. Most studies indicate that users of hormone replacement therapy are more likely to be smokers and that smoking is associated with an earlier menopause. Criqui *et al.* (85) showed that postmenstrual oestrogen use was 'strongly protective' in current smokers but was associated with increased risk in past smokers.

CHOLESTEROL, CORONARY HEART DISEASE AND OLD AGE

The late J. R. A. Mitchell (86), in his perceptive, disturbing manner, challenged the widespread assumptions about the aetiology of coronary heart disease, the role of plasma lipids and the relevance of dietary manipulation. He noted that there is more to ischaemic heart disease than atheroma—the fatty deposition in arterial walls; disruption of the arterial plaque and consequent thrombosis are also necessary. Smoking and high blood pressure are far better predictors of ischaemic heart disease than raised serum cholesterol.

Nevertheless, the predictive relation of serum lipids to coronary heart disease is generally accepted; problems arise when the different components of lipids are considered and whether attempts to change the proportion of these components by diet or drugs are of benefit. Given that most of the evidence for the cholesterol/coronary heart disease relation is derived from studies of white middle-aged males from Western industrialized societies, the extrapolation to old people in general is questionable; the same was once said of hypertension.

Earlier reports from the Framingham Study (87) suggested that raised cholesterol in old age was less predictive of coronary heart disease than in younger people. Later data from the same study seem to suggest the opposite (88). It was noted that changes in lipids in old age are partially explained by age and weight loss. The Whitehall Civil Servant Study (of 18 296 men aged 40–69 years and free of ischaemic heart disease at recruitment, being followed for 18 years) found that raised cholesterol was predictive of coronary heart disease but this association declined with age. The earlier the raised cholesterol was identified the better the prediction of coronary heart disease (89). The Honolulu Heart Program (90) studied 1480 men, aged 65 or over, of Japanese ancestry who were initially free of ischaemic heart disease, for an average of 12 years and found that cholesterol remained an independent predictor of coronary heart disease little different from that in younger men (relative risk of coronary heart disease among men aged 65–74 years was 1.68, and in men aged 52–59 years it was 1.71). The Lipid Research Clinics Follow-up Study of 923 men and women aged over 65 and followed for 15 years also found that cholesterol was significantly predictive of coronary heart disease (91). Rubin *et al.* (92), studying 2746 male members of a health maintenance organization aged over 60 years and initially without coronary heart disease, found the relative risk of death from ischaemic heart disease predicted by serum cholesterol in those aged 60–64 years was 1.4, and was 1.7 in those aged 75–79 years. Because mortality from ischaemic heart disease increases with age, the excess risk of death from ischaemic heart disease attributable to raised cholesterol was five-fold.

A J-curve relation between cholesterol and total mortality has been described (93). This has been ascribed to cancer with its consequent regression of atheroma but Forette *et al.* (94) studying institutionalized women aged over 60 years found that the relation between low cholesterol and death was independent of the incidence of cancer.

Important questions remain. We do not know if hyperlipidaemia of recent onset in old age occurs and what the characteristics are of those who survive into old age with raised lipids (95). The financial cost of screening asymptomatic old people for raised lipids is astronomical and its clinical efficacy unknown (96).

COMBINATIONS OF RISK FACTORS

The Framingham Study (97) examined 2501 subjects surviving to 65 years without evidence of coronary heart disease and found the following relative risks of developing coronary heart disease when associated with the respective risk factors: being male, 1.7; left ventricular hypertrophy, 2.4; raised systolic blood pressure, 2.2; raised blood glucose, 2.2; increased weight, 1.3; raised cholesterol, 1.8; and smoking, 1.2. Mathematical models (e.g. 39,98) have been developed to describe the cumulative predictive effect of several independent factors. Pryor *et al.* (99) have constructed a nomogram for estimating the likelihood of severe coronary heart disease in men and women. This enables physicians not to overlook high-risk candidates with multiple marginal abnormalities (100) and prompts them to attempt to control all risk factors rather than focus solely on one.

ISCHAEMIC HEART DISEASE AS 'PREMATURE' AGEING

The earlier view that raised arterial pressures, smoking and unfavourable lipid profiles were less predictive of ischaemic heart disease in old age led to the conclusion that ischaemic heart disease was a form of premature or accelerated ageing. Hence preventive measures would be of less value in older people. It is becoming clearer that this view is wrong and modification of risk factors is beneficial at any age.

CONTROLLING RISK FACTORS

As risk factors are increasingly controlled, one could expect a fall in cardiovascular mortality but an increase in other causes of death (and of interventions more harmful to the elderly). Rose and Shipley (101) show this is too simple a view. Control of risk factors reduces age-specific risk, thus increasing longevity and hence increasing exposure to risk of death from coronary heart disease. For example, reduction in smoking has diminished deaths from cancer but increased the lifelong probability of fatal coronary heart disease and, importantly, increased the age at which death from coronary heart disease might be expected.

CONGENITAL HEART DISEASE

Serious congenital heart disease is not compatible with old age. Hallgrimsson and Tulinus (102) estimated, from an autopsy series, congenital bicuspid aortic valves in 25 per 1000 men aged over 65 years and five per 1000 women aged over 65 years. Clearly, this sample is highly selected and finding a lesion *post mortem* does not necessarily imply haemodynamic significance during life. With atrial septal defect (ASD) only 10% survive beyond 60 years (103); however, there are a few case reports of ASD being fortuitously discovered in old people during investigation of other cardiorespiratory disease (104).

RHEUMATIC HEART DISEASE

The prevalence of rheumatic fever was steadily declining this century in industrialized developed countries before the advent of antistreptococcal antibiotics and valve replacements, and probably reflects changes in the virulence of the organism interacting with improved social conditions, diminishing opportunities for infection (105). Thus rheumatic heart disease in the elderly represents 'a mere medicohistorical remnant' of widespread streptococcal infection earlier this century (106). These elderly subjects illustrate selective survival in that the more seriously afflicted of their cohort have not survived into old age. It remains to be seen if the present outbreaks of rheumatic fever in 'Westernized' countries, albeit largely among the poor although there are reports of outbreaks in military personnel, will eventually result in rheumatic heart disease in these subjects when older. Older subjects, particularly if institutionalized, are not immune from other streptococcal infections.

The prevalence of rheumatic heart disease in the elderly is unknown. Kennedy *et al.* (107) found 4% of the over-65s living at home had valvular heart disease but did not indicate what was rheumatic. Sherrid *et al.* (108) found 12% of a consecutive series of subjects undergoing echocardiography had clinically unsuspected mitral stenosis, half of whom had moderate to very severe stenosis. The median age of the newly discovered cases was 72 years and one-third underwent significant changes of management, reflecting the haemodynamic consequence of the stenosis. Unsuspected cases were significantly older by 7 years and more likely to have coexisting cardiac disease masking the rheumatic condition.

Infective endocarditis

'The proportion of elderly patients contracting infective endocarditis is increasing. The prognosis is poor'—thus a recent WHO book introduces infective endocarditis in old age (109). The incidence for elderly subjects in Western societies is unknown. King *et al.* (110) in developing a reporting system to study infective endocarditis in Louisiana found an annual incidence of 1.7 per 100 000 persons of all ages. Young (111), reviewing several British epidemiological databases, reported an annual incidence of two per 100 000 of the general population, about a third of whom are aged over 65 years. Infective endocarditis deaths were more likely in the elderly (≥ 65 years: 1.4 deaths annually per 100 000; 20–44 years: 0.13 deaths annually per 100 000).

In a thorough retrospective analysis of 102 episodes (98 patients) of infective endocarditis presenting to a general hospital, Wells *et al.* (112) found that the in-hospital mortality was almost a third, being greater in those over 60 years. The 3-year mortality of the entire group was 43.5% (21% for those surviving their first admission, 44% of the over-60s surviving their first admission).

Steckelberg *et al.* (113) helpfully points out that different sources of subjects will produce different estimates of a disease. They retrospectively compared a population-based series of cases with a series of referred cases (Mayo Clinic) presenting from 1970 to 1987. Episodes in elderly patients were under-represented in the referral practice, perhaps reflecting the selection bias which discriminates against older subjects being seen in tertiary care centres.

MITRAL VALVE PROLAPSE

There are few studies of the prevalence of mitral valve prolapse in elderly people. The variation in reported prevalence reflects different populations being studied and different methods of study. In a community study, Hickey *et al.* (114) found mitral valve prolapse in 4% of subjects aged under 80 years. Knight and Ballantyne (115) retrospectively surveyed 43 elderly patients who had undergone echocardiography and found one patient (2.4%) with unequivocal idiopathic mitral valve prolapse (they excluded those with connective tissue disorders, congenital, ischaemic or rheumatic heart disease, or cardiomyopathy), whereas Taylor and Rodger (116), with less rigid exclusion criteria, found mitral valve prolapse in 17 out of 415 (4%) patients aged over 65 having echocardiography. Sainsbury *et al.* (117) found 10 patients with abnormal movements of the mitral valve out of 49 elderly patients currently not in heart failure and undergoing echocardiography. Mills *et al.* (118) reviewed 53 patients (aged 17–78) at least 10 years after an initial diagnostic phonocardiograph and found that when mitral valve prolapse was an isolated abnormality then there was little risk of an untoward subsequent event.

ALCOHOL, AGE AND ISCHAEMIC HEART DISEASE

Alcohol dependency declines with age. Partly this reflects death from cirrhosis, cardiomyopathy, trauma and nervous system damage. Dependency may be less recognized in older subjects and may be less socially catastrophic (*e.g.* loss of a job is irrelevant to the retired person). Collusion by relatives and friends is more likely ('he has so few pleasures at his age'). Alcohol dependency is commoner among men although there are suggestions that as drinking becomes more socially acceptable for older women this will change (119). About two-thirds of subjects have been dependent since early adulthood. In many of the one-third (late-onset) group, dependency will be a presenting feature of depression.

Little is known about the role of alcohol in the epidemiology of cardiovascular pathology of old people. In a recent comprehensive review, Moushmoush and Abi-Mansour (120) made no comment on advanced age *per se*. Manolio *et al.* (121), in Framingham Study subjects aged 17–90 years, showed that after adjustments for other risk factors overall alcohol intake was positively associated with left ventricular mass (measured echocardiographically) in men only; however, the association in both sexes varied with the type of alcoholic beverage ingested.

Alcohol and the U-shaped curve

The relation of mortality and alcohol intake has been likened to a U- (or J-) shaped curve, *i.e.* light alcohol drinkers having a lower total and cardiovascular mortality than non-drinkers and heavy drinkers. Anderson (122), in reviewing five longitudinal studies to devise an estimate of deaths due to alcohol using techniques comparable with those used to estimate deaths from smoking, endorsed the U-shaped phenomenon. (Only one study (123) dealt with older subjects where the relation of alcohol use to mortality was 'relatively weak'.) However, Shaper *et al.* (124) challenged acceptance of the U-shaped curve, pointing out that the category of non-drinker includes both life-long abstainers and former drinkers. This latter group are often former heavy drinkers, weigh more, are more hypertensive, and are more likely to be smokers than teetotallers (so called 'sick quitters'). An accompanying *Lancet* annotation (125) commented 'it seems likely that a substantial proportion of them had given up drinking because of ill-health'. Shaper concludes 'evidence that alcohol is positively of benefit to health, *i.e.* protective against disease, has not been produced' (126). This continues to be disputed (127). Marmot and Brunner (128) argue strongly from ecological, cohort and case–control studies that there is a 'protective' effect of alcohol. They conclude by wisely warning against recommending public advertisement of this effect of light drinking given the inevitable consequence of increased heavy drinking, with its ensuing biological and social catastrophes.

Few of the studies purporting to study the U-shaped curve consider the over-65s. Rimm *et al.* (129) studied health professionals (*e.g.* dentists, pharmacists, veterinary surgeons) aged 40–75 years (mean age 53 years) but give no information specifically on the older subjects. Razay *et al.* (130) studied a random sample (70% response rate) of 1048 women aged 25–69 years (83 subjects aged 60–69 years) and confirmed the 'protective coronary heart disease lipid profile' but reported nothing specifically on the older women.

CARDIOMYOPATHY

Hypertrophic cardiomyopathy in the elderly has been increasingly recognized with the widespread use of echocardiography; however, there is little information concerning its prevalence. McKenna *et al.* (131) found seven (3%) patients aged over 60 years out of 254 patients with hypertrophic cardiomyopathy. Koch *et al.* (132), in 20 years, operated on 276 patients with hypertrophic cardiomyopathy of whom 21 (8%) were over 65 years, whereas Krasnow and Stein (133) found 15 (65%) aged over 60 years out of 23 patients. All these papers came from tertiary care referral units, and both the non-surgical papers agreed that older patients had a better prognosis than younger patients. Aronow and Kronzon (134) reported a prevalence of 4% (detected by Doppler echocardiography) among 379 long-stay patients (mean age 85 years). They also noted that mitral annular calcification was commoner among patients with hypertrophic cardiomyopathy. An autopsy study of the over-60s from Japan found a prevalence of 1.4% of non-ischaemic cardiomyopathy (135).

Coughlin *et al.* (136) studied idiopathic dilated cardiomyopathy by comparing newly diagnosed cases (aged 16–80, mean age 52) ascertained in four Baltimore hospitals with age- and sex-matched neighbourhood controls and found a predominance of blacks not explained by income, alcohol consumption, cigarette usage, body mass index, hypertension or asthma. They did not comment on differences associated with age. A Mayo Clinic study of dilated cardiomyopathy reported that one-fifth of cases were familial (age range 1–70, mean 45 years). No age differences were found between familial and non-familial cases (137).

CONGESTIVE CARDIAC FAILURE

Defining the epidemiology of congestive cardiac failure has been difficult because of problems with diagnostic criteria and the unreliability of routine death certificates (138). The incidence of congestive cardiac failure in the general population has been variously reported as 3–10 cases per 1000 (139). The Framingham data suggest that the annual incidence for those aged 65–94 is 10 per 1000 men and eight per 1000 women (140). Smith (141) notes that the rate doubles for each decade and that 90% of those Framingham subjects with congestive cardiac failure had pre-existing hypertension or coronary heart disease or both. Hypertension (systolic or diastolic) was an independent predictor of congestive cardiac failure, as was diabetes (the relative risk of coronary heart disease in diabetics aged 45–74 years was 2.36 for men and 5.14 for women compared with non-diabetics). Congestive cardiac failure has a poor prognosis. Of 94 male veterans aged over 75 years, 28% died within 1 year of the onset of heart failure and 60% within 5 years (142).

REFERENCES

1. Bromley D, Isaacs B, Bytheway B (1982) Ageing and the rectangular curve. *Ageing Soc* **2**: 383–392.
2. Fries JF (1980) Aging, natural death, and the compression of morbidity. *N Engl J Med* **303**: 130–136.
3. Forbes WF, Thompson ME (1990) Age-related diseases and normal aging: the nature of the relationship. *J Clin Epidemiol* **43**: 191–193.
4. Evans JG (1981) The biology of human ageing. In *Recent Advances in Medicine: 18*, Dawson AM, Compston N, Besser GM (eds). Churchill Livingstone, Edinburgh, pp 20–22.
5. Keeler EM, Solomon DH, Beck JC, Mendenhall RC, Kane RL (1982) Effect of patient age on duration of medical encounters with physicians. *Med Care* **20**; 1101–1108.
6. Powell C (1983) Postprandial reduction in blood pressure in the elderly. *N Engl J Med* **309**: 1255.
7. Lernfelt B, Landahl S, Svanborg A (1990) Coronary heart disease at 70, 75 and 79 years of age: a longitudinal study with special reference to sex differences and mortality. *Age Ageing* **19**: 297–303.
8. Fall, CHD, Barker DJP, Osmond D, Winter PD, Clark PMS, Hales CN (1992) Relation of infant feeding to adult serum cholesterol concentration and death from ischaemic heart disease. *Br Med J* **304**: 801–805.
9. Elford J, Whincup P, Shaper AG (1992) Early life experience and adult cardiovascular disease: longitudinal and case–control studies. *Int J Epidemiol* **20**: 833–844.
10. Robinson RJ (1992) Is the child the father of the man? *Br Med J* **304**: 789–790.
11. Lever AF, Harrap SB (1992) Essential hypertension: a disorder of growth with origins in childhood? *J Hypertens* **10**; 101–120.
12. Kannel WB (1987) Hypertension and other risk factors in coronary heart disease. *Am Heart J* **114** (Pt 2): 918–925.
13. Leren P (1990) Hypertension: the coronary heart disease dilemma. *Atherosclerosis Rev* **21**: 195–200.
14. Vokonas PS, Kannel WB, Cupples LA (1988) Epidemiology and risk of hypertension in the elderly: the Framingham Study. *J Hypertens* **6**: S3–9.
15. Stehbens WE (1987) An appraisal of the epidemic rise of coronary heart disease and its decline. *Lancet* **i**: 606–611.
16. Stehbens WE (1991) Imprecision of the clinical diagnosis of coronary heart disease in epidemiological studies and atherogenesis. *J Clin Epidemiol* **44**: 999–1006.
17. Smith WM (1988) Epidemiology of hypertension in older patients. *Am J Med* **85** (3B): 2–6.
18. Mattila K, Haavisto M, Rajala S, Heikinheimo R (1988) Blood pressure and five year survival in the very old. *Br Med J* **296**: 887–889.
19. Dahlöf B, Lindholm LH, Hansson L *et al.* (1991) Morbidity and mortality in the Swedish Trial in Old Patients with hypertension (STOP–Hypertension). *Lancet* **338**: 1281–1285.
20. SHEP Cooperative Research Group (1991) Prevention of stroke by antihypertensive drug treatment in older persons with isolated systolic hypertension. *JAMA* **265**: 3255–3264.
21. MRC Working Party (1992) Medical Research Council trial of treatment of hypertension in older adults: principal results. *Br Med J* **304**: 405–412.
22. Farmer ME, Kittner SJ, Abbott RD *et al.*(1990) Longitudinally measured blood pressure, antihypertensive medication use, and cognitive performance: the Framingham Study. *J Clin Epidemiol* **43**: 475–480.

23. Gurland BJ, Teresi J, McFate Smith W *et al.* (1988) Effects of treatment for isolated systolic hypertension on cognitive status and depression in the elderly. *J Am Geriatr Soc* **36**: 1015–1022.

24. Editorial (1991) New trials in older hypertensives. *Lancet* **338**: 1299–1300.

25. Curb J, Borhani NO, Entwhistle G. *et al.* (1985) Isolated systolic hypertension in 14 communities. *Am J Epidemiol* **121**: 362–370.

26. Staessen J, Amery A, Fagard R (1990) Isolated systolic hypertension in the elderly. *J Hypertens* **8**: 393–405.

27. Cruickshank JM (1992) The J curve lives *Lancet* **339**: 187.

28. D'Agostino RB, Belanger AJ, Kannel WB, Cruickshank JM (1991) Relation of low diastolic blood pressure to coronary heart disease in presence of myocardial infarction: the Framingham Study. *Br Med J* **303**: 385–389.

29. Staessen J, Bulpitt C, Clement D *et al.* (1989) Relation between mortality and treated blood pressure in elderly patients with hypertension: report of the European Working Party on High Blood Pressure in the Elderly. *Br. Med J* **298**: 1552–1556.

30. Weinberger MH (1992) Do no harm: antihypertensive therapy and the 'J' curve. *Arch Intern Med* **152**: 473–476.

31. Fletcher AE, Bulpitt CJ (1992) How far should blood pressure be lowered? *N Engl J Med* **326**: 251–254.

32. Morley JE (1991) Is low blood pressure dangerous? *J Am Geriatr Soc* **39**: 1239–1240.

33. Aronow WS (1992) Left ventricular hypertrophy. *J Am Geriatr Soc* **40**: 71–80.

34. Prior IAM, Evans JG, Harvey HPB *et al.* (1968) Sodium intake and blood pressure in two Polynesian populations. *N Engl J Med* **279**: 515–520.

35. Salmond CE, Joseph JG, Prior IAM *et al.* (1985) Longitudinal analysis of the relationship between blood pressure and migration: the Tokelau Island Migrant Study. *Am J Epidemiol* **122**: 291–301.

36. Marmot MG (1984) Geography of blood pressure and hypertension. *Br Med Bull* **40**: 380–386.

37. Anderson KM, Odell PM, Wilson PW, Kannel WB (1991) Cardiovascular disease risk profiles. *Am Heart J* **121** (Pt 2): 293–298.

38. Tosteson AN, Weinstein MC, Williams LW, Goldman L (1990) Long-term impact of smoking cessation on the incidence of coronary heart disease. *Am J Pub Health* **80**: 1481–1486.

39. Psaty BM, Koepsell TD, Manolio TA *et al.* (1990) Risk ratios and risk differences in estimating the effect of risk factors for cardiovascular disease in the elderly. *J Clin Epidemiol* **43**: 961–970.

40. LaCroix AZ, Lang J, Scherr P *et al.* (1991) Smoking and mortality among older men and women in three communities. *N Engl J Med* **324**: 1619–1625

41. Mariotti S, Capocaccia R, Farchi G *et al.* (1986) Age, period, cohort and geographical area effects on the relationship between risk factors and coronary heart disease mortality. *J Chronic Dis* **39**: 229–242.

42. LaCroix AZ, Omenn GS (1992) Older adults and smoking. *Clin Geriatr Med* **8**: 69–87.

43. Morris JN, Everitt MG, Pollard R, Chave SPW (1980) Vigorous exercise in leisure time: protection against coronary heart disease. *Lancet* **ii**: 1207–1210.

44. Paffenberger RS Jr, Hyde RT, Wing AL, Hsieh C-C (1986) Physical activity, all cause-mortality and longevity of college alumni. *N Engl J Med* **314**: 605–613; **315**: 399–401.

45. Leon AS, Connett J, Jacobs DR Jr, Rauramaa R (1987) Leisure-time physical activity levels and risk of coronary heart disease and death. The Multiple Risk Factor Intervention Trial. *JAMA* **258**: 2388–2395.

46. Ekelund L-G, Haskell WL, Johnson JL *et al.* (1988) Physical fitness as a predictor of

cardiovascular mortality in asymptomatic North American men. *N Engl J Med* **319**: 1379–1384.

47. Slattery ML, Jacobs DR Jr (1988) Physical fitness and cardiovascular disease mortality. The U.S. Railroad Study. *Am J Epidemiol* **127**: 571–580.
48. Forman DE, Manning WJ, Hauser R *et al.* (1992) Enhanced left ventricular diastolic filling associated with long-term endurance training. *J Gerontol* **47**: M56–58.
49. Siconlfi SF, Lasater TM, McKinlay S *et al.* (1985) Physical fitness and blood pressure: the role of age. *Am J Epidemiol* **122**: 452–457.
50. Morey MC, Cowper PA, Feussner JR *et al.* (1991) Two-year trends in physical performance following supervised exercise among community-dwelling older veterans. *J Am Geriatr Soc* **39**: 549–554.
51. Schwartz RS, Shuman WP, Larson V *et al.* (1991) The effect of intensive endurance exercise training on body fat distribution in young and older men. *Metabolism* **40**: 545–551.
52. Larsson B, Svardsudd K, Welin L *et al.* (1984) Abdominal adipose tissue distribution, obesity and risk of cardiovascular disease and death: 13 year follow up of participants in the study of men born in 1913. *Br Med J* **288**: 1401–1404.
53. Posner JD, Gorman KM, Gitlin LN *et al.* (1990) Effects of training in the elderly on the occurrence and time to onset of cardiovascular diagnoses. *J Am Geriatr Soc* **38**: 205–210.
54. Hagberg JM, Graves JE, Limacher M *et al.* (1989) Cardiovascular responses of 70- to 79-yr-old men and women to exercise training. *J Appl Physiol* **66**: 2589–2594.
55. Coats AJS, Adamopoulos S, Meyer TE *et al.* (1990) Effects of physical training in chronic heart failure. *Lancet* **335**: 63–66.
56. Sullivan MJ, Higginbotham MB, Cobb FR (1988) Exercise training in patients with severe left ventricular dysfunction: hemodynamic and metabolic effects. *Circulation* **78**: 506–515.
57. Shabetai R (1988) Beneficial effects of exercise training in compensated heart failure. *Circulation* **78**: 775–776.
58. Editorial (1991) Fair of face and sick at heart. *Lancet* **338**: 1366–1367.
59. Evans JG (1984) Epidemiology. In *Heart Disease in the Elderly*, Martin A Cramm AJ (eds). Wiley, Chichester, pp. 19–20.
60. Aronson MK, Ooi WL, Morgenstern H *et al.* (1990) Women, myocardial infarction and dementia in the very old. *Neurology* **40**: 1102–1106.
61. Krauss RM (1989) Lipoproteins and coronary heart disease. *Postgrad Med* Special Report, April: 54–57.
62. Walsh BW, Schiff I, Rosner B *et al.* (1991) Effects of postmenopausal estrogen replacement on the concentrations and metabolism of plasma lipoproteins. *N Engl J Med* **325**: 1196–1204.
63. Matthews KA, Meilahn E, Kuller LH *et al.* (1989) Menopause and risk factors for coronary heart disease. *N Engl J Med* **321**: 641–646.
64. Farish E, Rolton HA, Barnes JF, Hart DM (1991) Lipoprotein (a) concentrations in postmenopausal women taking norethisterone. *Br Med J* **303**; 694.
65. Wing RR, Matthews KA, Kuller LH *et al.* (1991) Weight gain at the time of menopause. *Arch Int Med* **151**: 97–102.
66. Gordon T, Kannel WB, Hjortland MC, McNamara PM (1978) Menopause and coronary heart disease: The Framingham Study. *Ann Intern Med* **89**: 157–161.
67. Sarrell PM (1990) Ovarian hormones and the circulation. *Maturitas* **12**: 287–298.
68. Barrett-Connor E, Khaw K-T (1988) Endogenous sex hormones and cardiovascular disease in men. *Circulation* **78**: 539–545.
69. Duell PB, Bierman EL (1990) The relationship between sex hormones and high-density lipoprotein cholesterol levels in healthy adult men. *Arch Intern Med*

150: 2317–2320.

70. Witteman JCM, Grobbee DE, Kok FJ *et al.* (1989) Increased risk of atherosclerosis in women after the menopause. *Br Med J* **298**: 642–644.
71. Gruchow HW, Anderson AJ, Barboriak JJ, Sobocinski KA (1988) Postmenopausal use of estrogen and occlusion of coronary arteries. *Am Heart J* **115**: 954–963.
72. McFarland KF, Boniface ME, Hornung CA *et al.* (1989) Risk factors and noncontraceptive estrogen use in women with and without coronary disease. *Am Heart J* **117**: 1209–1214.
73. Sullivan JM, Zwaag RV, Hughes JP *et al.* (1990) Estrogen replacement and coronary artery disease. *Arch Intern Med* **150**: 2557–2562.
74. Barrett-Connor E, Bush TL (1989) Estrogen replacement and coronary heart disease. *Cardiovasc Clin* **19**(3): 159–172.
75. Wilson PWF, Garrison RJ, Castelli WP (1985) Postmenopausal estrogen use, cigarette smoking and cardiovascular morbidity in women over 50. *N Engl J Med* **313**; 1038–1043.
76. Stampfer MJ, Willett WC, Colditz G *et al.* (1986) Postmenopausal estrogen and heart disease: letter in reply. *N Engl J Med* **315**:135–6.
77. Wilson PWF (1989) Prospective studies: The Framingham Study. *Postgrad Med* Special Report, April: 51–52.
78. Stampfer MJ, Colditz GA, Willett WC *et al.* (1991) Postmenopausal estrogen therapy and cardiovascular disease. *N Engl J Med* **325**: 756–762.
79. Goldman L, Tosteson ANA (1991) Uncertainty about postmenopausal estrogen: time for action not debate. *N Engl J Med* **325**: 800–802.
80. Editorial (1991) More than hot flushes. *Lancet* **338**: 917–918.
81. Ross RK, Pike MC, Henderson BE *et al.* (1989) Stroke prevention and oestrogen replacement therapy. *Lancet* **i**: 505.
82. Henderson BE, Paganini-Hill A, Ross RK (1991) Decreased mortality in users of estrogen replacement therapy. *Arch Intern Med* **151**: 75–78.
83. Moon TE (1991) Estrogens and disease prevention. *Arch Intern Med* **151**: 17–18.
84. Evans JG (1986) Medicine in society. *Ageing Soc* **6**: 87–89.
85. Criqui MH, Suarez L, Barrett-Connor E *et al.* (1988) Postmenopausal estrogen use and mortality: results from a prospective study in a defined, homogeneous community. *Am J Epidemiol* **128**: 606–614.
86. Mitchell JRA (1988) Diet and coronary disease: is there any connection? In *Advanced Medicine: 24*, Sheppard MC (ed.). Royal College of Physicians London, Baillière Tindall, London, pp. 351–360.
87. Anderson KM, Castelli WP, Levy DL (1987) Cholesterol and mortality: 30 years of follow-up from the Framingham Study. *JAMA* **257**: 2176.
88. Wilson PWF, Kannel WB, Anderson KM, Castelli WP (1990) Cholesterol and CHD in the elderly: the Framingham cohort. *Circulation* **82**: SIII, 576.
89. Shipley MJ, Pocock SJ, Marmot MG (1991) Does plasma cholesterol concentration predict mortality from coronary heart disease in elderly people? 18 year follow up in Whitehall study. *Br Med J* **303**: 89–92.
90. Benfante R, Reed D (1990) Is elevated serum cholesterol level a risk factor for coronary heart disease in the elderly? *JAMA* **263**: 393–396.
91. Rossouw JE, Bangdiwala S, Gordon DJ *et al.* (1990) Plasma lipids as predictors of CHD in older men and women: the LRC follow-up study. *Circulation* **82**: SIII, 346.
92. Rubin SM, Sidney S, Black DM *et al.* (1990) High blood cholesterol in elderly men and the excess risk for coronary heart disease. *Ann Intern Med* **113**: 916–920.
93. Shaw, K-T (1990) Serum lipids in later life. *Age Ageing* **19**: 277–279.
94. Forette B, Tortrat D, Wolmark Y (1989) Cholesterol as risk factor for mortality in elderly women. *Lancet* **i**: 868–870.

95. Cohen DL, Mindell JS (1992) Cardiovascular disease and high cholesterol in old age. *Rev Clin Gerontol* **2**: 1–2.
96. Garber AM, Littenberg B, Sox HC *et al.* (1991) Costs and health consequences of cholesterol screening for asymptomatic older Americans. *Arch Intern Med* **151**: 1089–1095.
97. Harris T, Cook EF, Kannel WB, Goldman L (1988) Proportional hazards analysis of risk factors for coronary heart disease in individuals aged 65 or older. *J Am Geriatr Soc* **36**: 1023–1028.
98. Anderson KA, Odell PM, Wilson PWF, Kannel WB (1990) Cardiovascular disease risk profiles. *Am Heart J* **121**: 293–298.
99. Pryor DB, Shaw L, Harrell FE *et al.* (1991) Estimating the likelihood of severe coronary artery disease. *Am J Med* **90**: 553–562.
100. Anderson KA, Odell PM, Wilson PWF, Kannel WB (1990) An updated coronary risk profile. *Circulation* **82**: SIII; 393.
101. Rose G, Shipley M (1990) Effects of coronary risk reduction on the pattern of mortality. *Lancet* **335**: 275–277.
102. Hallgrimsson J, Tulinus H (1979) Chronic non-rheumatic aortic valvular disease: a population study based on autopsies. *J Chronic Dis.* **32**: 355–363.
103. Campbell M (1970) Natural history of atrial septal defect. *Br Heart J* **32**: 820–826.
104. Landi F, Cipriani L, Cocchi A *et al.* (1991) Ostium secundum atrial septal defect in the elderly. *J Am Geriatr Soc* **39**: 60–63.
105. Bisno AL (1991) Medical progress: group A streptococcal infections and acute rheumatic fever. *N Engl J Med* **325**: 783–793.
106. Strasser T (ed.) (1987) Valvular heart disease. In *Cardiovascular Care of the Elderly*. World Health Organization, Geneva, p. 96.
107. Kennedy RD, Andrews GR, Caird FI (1977) Ischaemic heart disease in the elderly. *Br Heart J* **39**: 1121–1127.
108. Sherrid M, Goyal A, Delia E *et al.* (1991) Unsuspected mitral stenosis. *Am J Med* **90**: 189–192.
109. Strasser T (ed.) (1987) Infective endocarditis. In *Cardiovascular Care of the Elderly*. World Health Organization, Geneva, pp. 101–104.
110. King JW, Nguyen VQ, Conrad SA (1988) Results of a prospective statewide reporting system for infective endocarditis. *Am J Med Sci* **295**: 517–527.
111. Young SEJ (1987) Aetiology and epidemiology of infective endocarditis in England and Wales. *J Antimicrob Chemother* **20**: (SA): 7–14.
112. Wells AU, Fowler CC, Ellis-Pegler RB *et al.* (1990) Endocarditis in the '80s in a general hospital in Auckland, New Zealand. *Q J Med* **76**: (279): 753–762.
113. Steckelberg JM, Melton J, Ilstrup DM *et al.* (1990) Influence of referral bias on the apparent clinical spectrum of infective endocarditis. *Am J Med.* **88**: 582–588.
114. Hickey AJ, Wolfers J, Wilcken DEL (1981) Mitral valve prolapse: prevalence in an Australian population. *Med J Austr* **1**: 31–33.
115. Knight PV, Ballantyne D (1984) Idiopathic mitral valve prolapse in the elderly. *J Clin Exp Gerontol* **6**: 75–82.
116. Taylor J, Rodger JC (1991) Floppy mitral valves in elderly patients: clinical features and associated echocardiographic findings. *Age Ageing* **20**: 80–84.
117. Sainsbury R, White T, Wray R (1981) Echocardiography in elderly patients with systolic murmurs. *Age Ageing* **10**: 225–230.
118. Mills P, Rose J, Hollingsworth J *et al.* (1977) Long-term prognosis of mitral valve prolapse. *N Engl J Med* **297**: 13–18.
119. Scott RB, Mitchell MC (1988) Aging, alcohol and the liver. *J Am Geriatr Soc* **36**: 255–265.
120. Moushmoush B, Abi-Mansour P (1991) Alcohol and the heart: the long-term effects

of alcohol on the cardiovascular system. *Arch Intern Med.* **151**: 36–42.
121. Manolio TA, Levy D, Garrison RO *et al.* (1991) Relation of alcohol intake to left ventricular mass: the Framingham Study. *J Am Coll Cardiol* **17**: 717–721.
122. Anderson P (1988) Excess mortality associated with alcohol consumption. *Br Med J* **297**: 824–826.
123. Klatsky AL, Friedman GD, Siegelaub AB (1981) Alcohol and mortality. *Ann Intern Med* **95**: 139–145.
124. Shaper AG, Wannamethee G, Walker M (1988) Alcohol and mortality in British men: explaining the U-shaped curve. *Lancet* **ii**: 1267–1273.
125. Annotation (1988) Alcohol and mortality the myth of the U-shaped curve. *Lancet* **ii**: 1292–1293.
126. Shaper AG (1991) Alcohol and ill health: the continuing debate. *Br J Addict* **86**: 381.
127. Cullen K (1991) Alcohol and mortality. *Lancet* **337**: 363–364.
128. Marmot M, Brunner E (1991) Alcohol and cardiovascular disease: the status of the U shaped curve. *Br Med J* **303**: 565–568.
129. Rimm ER, Giovannucci EL, Willett WC *et al.* (1991) Prospective study of alcohol consumption and risk of coronary disease in men. *Lancet* **338**: 464–468.
130. Razay G, Heaton KW, Bolton CH, Hughes AO (1992) Alcohol consumption and its relation to cardiovascular risk factors in British women. *Br Med J* **304**: 80–83.
131. McKenna W, Deanfield J, Farqui A *et al.* (1981) Prognosis in hypertrophic cardiomyopathy: role of age and clinical, electrocardiographic and hemodynamic features. *Am J Cardiol* **47**: 532–538.
132. Koch J-P, Maron BJ, Epstein SE, Morrow AG (1980) Results of operation for obstructive hypertrophic cardiomyopathy in the elderly. *Am J Cardiol* **46**: 963–966.
133. Krasnow N, Stein RA (1978) Hypertrophic cardiomyopathy in the aged. *Am Heart J* **96**: 326–336.
134. Aronow WS, Kronzon I (1988) Prevalence of hypertrophic cardiomyopathy and its association with mitral annular calcium in elderly patients. *Chest* **94**: 1295–1296.
135. Matsushita S, Kuroo M, Takagi T *et al.* (1988) Cardiovascular disease in the aged: overview of an autopsy series. *Japan Circ J* **52**: 442–448.
136. Coughlin SS, Szklo M, Baughman K, Pearson TA (1990) The epidemiology of idiopathic dilated cardiomyopathy in a biracial community. *Am J Epidemiol* **131**: 48–56.
137. Michels VV, Moll PP, Miller FA *et al.* (1992) The frequency of familial dilated cardiomyopathy in a series of patients with idiopathic dilated cardiomyopathy. *N Engl J Med* **326**: 77–82.
138. Tunstall-Pedoe H (1991) Coronary heart disease. *Br Med J* **303**: 1546–1547.
139. Webb S, Impallomeni MG (1987) Cardiac failure in the elderly. *Q J Med* **64**: 641–650.
140. McMurray J, Dargie HJ (1991) Coronary heart disease. *Br Med J* **303**: 1546.
141. Smith WM (1985) Epidemiology of congestive heart failure. *Am J Cardiol* **55**: 3A–8A.
142. Taffet GE, Teasdale TA, Bleyer AJ *et al.* (1992) Survival of elderly men with congestive heart failure. *Age Ageing* **21**: 49–55.

3 Economics and Health Policy

NICK BOSANQUET[a] **AND ANNA ZAJDLER**[b]

[a] *St Mary's Hospital Medical School and* [b] *Imperial College, University of London, UK*

The aim of this chapter is to appraise how the new international culture of health economics and health management will affect treatment of clinical heart disease in old age.

The central priority of health economics is the idea of improving choice in a world where resources are scarce and there are many competing uses for them. This improvement in choice can be achieved by attention to four general themes with associated concepts (1).

DEMAND FOR HEALTH

Economists distinguish between the demand for health and the demand for health services. Individuals seek to improve their stock of health by various kinds of investment. They make decisions about lifestyle and they may allocate varying amounts of time and energy to improving health. Health is affected by individual decisions about smoking, alcohol, exercise and road safety. Social programmes and incentives can also affect these decisions. Thus the UK has low speed limits on the road and a lower level of deaths and injuries from accidents than Germany. The productivity of health services has to be assessed against other alternative ways of bringing about improvements in health outcomes.

EFFECTIVENESS AND HEALTH BENEFITS

Economists have a range of different possible measures. Some of them are economic, involving measurement of lost output from early mortality. This kind of calculation was used to support nineteenth-century public health programmes for clean water and sanitation and is still used to support the case for public health programmes in developing countries. The most common measure now is in terms of reduced mortality but there is increasing emphasis on utility-based measures in terms of improved quality of life. These define quality of life in terms of a range of day-to-day activities and allows responses to be weighted together into an overall score. The quality-adjusted life year, or QALY, is an index which health economists have developed which weights survival and freedom from pain

Geriatric Cardiology. Principles and Practice. Edited by A. Martin and A. J. Camm
© 1994 John Wiley & Sons Ltd

together into one composite measure. Economists are unusual in their interest in 'psychometrics' which has been a way of dealing with the difficulty of measuring output and the return to investment.

ASSESSMENT OF 'EFFICIENCY' OR RELATIVE COST

An effective treatment is one which increases health benefit. An efficient programme is one which delivers effective treatment at the lowest cost. This could be a matter of early detection of disease, or of changing location of treatment. Treatment in a day hospital might be more efficient than treatment as an inpatient.

DEVELOPMENT OF INCENTIVES TO HEALTH CARE PROVIDERS

Economists have been critical of health care agencies on the grounds that they have concentrated on administrative routines and 'blank cheque' financing rather than seeking to promote more effective and efficient treatment. Economists were most active to start with in designing incentives to greater efficiency in terms of cost containment. They are now also urging adoption of incentives to greater effectiveness such as the setting of health targets and the measurement of health needs.

These general concepts have been translated into decision-making techniques using different measures of cost and benefit.

Cost analysis

This can cover direct budgetary costs to health agencies. It would also be possible to measure money costs and psychic costs to patients. No attempt is made to collect evidence on benefits.

Cost–benefit analysis

This measures costs and benefits in money terms. The earliest forms of the analysis concentrated on benefits in reduced costs of medical treatment and production gains from an earlier return to work. This is the ideal form of economic evaluation but one which is very difficult to use.

Cost-effectiveness analysis

This method measures output in terms of health gain with measures such as 'cases successfully treated', reductions in mortality and years of life gained. This is the most common form used by medical scientists and researchers and is being used increasingly by health policy makers.

Cost utility analysis

This is the newest form of evaluation and can be applied to a wider range of programmes through measuring changes in quality of life. It can be used to assess benefits from programmes that are in part palliative, such as chemotherapy for advanced cancer or for treatment of chronic illness, which causes loss of quality of life but which does not reduce mortality. It can also allow the patient's own views and preferences to be taken into account so that patients can define what is quality of life for them.

These concepts have also been translated into decision-making techniques, incentives and guidelines to managers. Again there is a common culture, not least because of individual carriers such as Professor Alain Enthoven of Stanford University, who had a fundamental impact on thinking in the UK, Sweden and the Netherlands and the work of the OECD in a series of reports (2). Among the most influential of these concepts are the following.

The DRG or diagnosis-related group

This divides all hospital treatment into 467 different diagnoses and standard costs are attached to each. Hospitals are then reimbursed according to these standard costs. The aim is to increase efficiency and to lower cost.

The cash limit

This sets an annual budget which the health provider cannot exceed. The aim is to ensure budgetary control. This has been a key element in UK policies and has also been used in the French hospital system.

Increased co-payment

This shifts more of the burden of payment directly on to the consumer. Controlled experiments carried out by the Rand Corporation in the USA suggested that almost any element of payment would lead to a fall in demand of about 20% (3). This system has been used to reduce costs of Medicare by increasing amounts paid by elderly Americans for hospital treatment. It has also been applied to prescribing in Denmark, Germany and the UK, where patients have been asked to pay more in direct charges.

General management

The UK has pioneered the use of business management approaches in health services, stressing the setting of aims, the achievement of targets together with rewards for performance. This implies a stronger role for managers relative to professionals. The old role of the manager or administrator in many health systems was similar to that of a caddy on a golf course.

Provider competition

This is designed to increase both effectiveness and efficiency. Providers are expected to offer more attractive programmes with higher health benefits. They are also expected to offer lower costs. Provider competition was a strong theme in the US health system from 1980 onwards and the concept is now being used in the UK and in the Netherlands. The UK internal market system is trying to harness provider competition to local health needs. Purchasers will have freedom to buy services to meet local health needs from a range of providers, public and private.

Health systems are moving from short-term cost containment to longer-term measures designed to increase effectiveness. The first-generation of systems involving the use of DRGs and cash-limited budgets have generally succeeded in containing costs in Germany and in the UK and for hospitals, although not ambulatory care in France. The most rapid movement in second-generation systems involving provider competition has come in the UK, Sweden and the Netherlands. In the past countries may have been content to contain spending; now they may even be prepared to reduce it unless it can be related clearly to health aims, as is particularly clear in Sweden.

The new culture has already begun to have a major impact on the use of resources in the treatment of cardiac disease among younger patients. Among the major areas of change are the following.

Impact on cardiology

There is a shift towards health promotion and the reduction of risk factors through primary care. There is consensus on the importance of changes in lifestyle in contributing to these aims through reductions in smoking and moves to a low-fat diet. There is less agreement on the possible role of prescribing to lower cholesterol. Clinical judgement is, however, leading to a substantial increase in prescribing even in the absence of agreed results from formal trials. This leads to additional pressure on budgets. Forecasts for additional spending on drugs affecting hypertension point to a rise from $5.9 billion in 1989 to $8.9 billion in 1995 within the developed world (4). Much of this is likely to be the result of greater activism in trying to reduce premature mortality among younger patients.

Within active treatment there is an international consensus on the benefits of early resuscitation after acute attacks. Three out of five deaths from acute myocardial infarction occur outside the hospital. There are a variety of interventions which could substantially reduce mortality. These include community education in resuscitation, but most benefits have been established for paramedic or mobile coronary care unit programmes which produce rapid access to advanced life support systems such as defibrillation. Reductions in mortality have been reported from such programmes both in the USA and in the UK. In the UK ambulance personnel have been retrained in advanced resuscitation and ambulances re-equipped (5). In the USA there have been programmes to quicken response time by special coronary care units.

Cardiac surgery has been an expanding area of treatment throughout the developed world. Concern about low treatment rates in the UK was partly based on comparisons with the USA, and since 1986 an official target has been set of 300 coronary artery bypass graft (CABG) operations per million. Economists have carried out cost utility analyses on cardiac surgery showing that it represents good value per QALY. Such studies have helped to support expansion both of CABG surgery and of the heart transplant programme in the UK (6,7).

Coronary care units began as a controversial programme in the 1950s, with some evidence from trials showing that survival was as good or better at home, but there has been much less controversy recently. Yet such units are still expensive to equip and are heavy users of highly qualified manpower.

Cardiac care has attracted attention because of its high unit costs. Information generated by fund-holding GPs within the UK internal market points to cardiac surgery as the most expensive of all specialties, with prices in 1990 such as £3256 for pacemaker implant and £6040 for valve replacement. It is also among the three most expensive specialties for outpatient consultations. Heart transplants may cost as much as £15 000 (7).

As well as its high unit cost, cardiac care has a potential for large total expenditure with large numbers potentially eligible and with likely increases over time both as demography and as expectations change. Some high-cost procedures involve treatment of small groups or of rare conditions. Procedures which are both high cost and potentially in demand from large numbers present severe problems for resource allocation. There are a number of such procedures in cardiac treatment. It is hardly surprising that the field has attracted much attention from managers and economists, with effort devoted to appraisal and evaluation of programmes.

The results of such studies have generally supported expansion of activity. Although covering disparate types of care they have used a common methodology in relating costs to benefits, often measured in terms of QALYs (6). Yet such studies will give much clearer and more positive signals for the treatment of younger people. The high costs of the procedures can be justified in terms of the substantial number of life years gained. The effect may be in fact to create some deterrent to treatment of older patients where life expectancy is inevitably much shorter.

The pattern of treatment of older patients (over 75) is in fact very different, with much more care being given to patients with multiple pathology and chronic illness. One study for the UK looked at how patterns of treatment differed by diagnosis and age group in 1985. For people over 75 the DRG codes were concentrated in medical specialties and seemed related to serious long-term illness. Of the 26 most common DRG codes only one—fracture of the hip and pelvis—was found in a surgical specialty. Ten per cent of admissions were in the broad groups of 'spec. cerebrovascular disorder Exc. TIA' and 'heart failure and shock'. High treatment rates for very elderly people are the result of emergency admissions for degenerative illness rather than of an increasing availability of elective treatment (8).

Within primary care treatment for elderly patients seems to be mainly maintenance therapy for people with chronic illness. The central drive towards reducing risk factors is not currently seen as relevant to the needs of elderly patients. The main resource use is in prescribing. People over 75 received on average 24 prescription items per person in 1988 as compared to 12 for people aged 65–74 and five per person for younger age groups covering all types of therapy (9). Data on morbidity would suggest that much of this additional prescribing was for cardiovascular problems; however, there is little assessment or monitoring of either the costs or the benefits of these long-term and recurrent therapies. There has also been little attention to the long-term treatment problems of elderly people in nursing homes, where the effects of inactivity in lifestyle may compound those arising from multiple pathology and ill health.

The care of elderly patients has not, therefore, been affected by the same forces which have challenged and reshaped programmes for younger patients. They are not prime candidates for major surgery, not only from lack of benefits in terms of expected QALYs but because of concern about postoperative complications. They may not seem likely candidates for primary care programmes designed to lower risk factors and there may even be arguments about the ethics of intensive resuscitation. In the absence of evidence or stimulus towards active treatment, the main emphasis is on long-term maintenance therapy.

There is likely to be increasing concern, however, both about the costs and the benefits of current programmes. Expectations of active treatment from elderly patients themselves will increase as will demands from relatives. There may well be greater concern about the effects of repeat prescribing and over-medication; and views about lifestyle may change as the morbidity curve changes towards the pattern predicted by Fries (10) with improved health in later life.

IMPLICATIONS FOR CARDIOVASCULAR SERVICES

The concepts and the systems of health economics are likely to reshape decision making in each of the main areas of treatment of clinical heart disease for elderly patients.

Peripheral vascular disease

This is an area of care which has been relatively neglected under the old systems of treatment. Many of those suffering from peripheral vascular disease had little ability to articulate or demand new programmes.

Research has established the extensive prevalence of venous disease in developed countries (11). At least 25% of the population in the UK suffer from varicose veins. A study in Tubingen showed similar results for Germany.

Twenty-three per cent of men and 49% of women over the age of 18 were assessed as suffering from varicose veins. The prevalence of venous ulcers is 1.5 per 1000 in the UK and as much as 10 per 1000 for people over 75.

There has been little attention given to the effects of peripheral vascular disease on quality of life. One study of people with vascular disease who had been referred for treatment to an outpatient clinic suggested that effects on quality of life were likely to be considerable. The results of this investigation (using the Nottingham Health Profile) show that patients with peripheral vascular disease have many problems with functioning—low levels of energy, pain, sleep disturbance and limitations on physical mobility being the most serious (12). Women tended to score higher, particularly on sleep and energy problems, and those aged 50–59 tended to score higher than any other age group on all sections of the profile. The study concluded that the quality of life of patients with peripheral vascular disease is 'much impaired'. Well over half had to curtail their hobbies and interests, more than a third had problems carrying out household tasks and almost a third reported effects on social life, sex life and holidays.

Currently patients with peripheral vascular disease in the UK get maintenance therapy which may well not be very effective and which has a long-term recurrent cost. A recent study in London has shown that it costs £5000 over 5 years to treat patients with chronic venous ulcers (13).

The economics of peripheral vascular disease

The pattern of care is set by the perceptions of providers about cost and benefit and the level of demand of patients.

The care programme has a high long-term cost but one that is invisible to providers in the short term. There is very little incentive to save costs in the short term, especially as these can be divided between different agencies for prescribing, bandages and home nursing. There is little incentive to do more treatment given perceptions of the low benefits of current treatment.

The field is a static one in terms of incentives towards change. Short-term costs are not large enough to trigger any strong local efforts towards cost containment. Patients' expectations are low. Benefit measures in terms of reduced mortality or QALYs are not really relevant in this area and their use would not supply any clear incentive towards change. Improvement in this area will require new and compelling evidence on costs and benefits. Costs would have to be measured and presented in terms of treatment over a period of several years. The case for innovation will have to be developed through using measures of quality of life and of social functioning which would be suitable for chronic illness. Above all, the field needs more innovation and more definition of effective local programmes. Providers have to be convinced that there would be returns to increased effort and they would require assurance that they can get returns through simple treatment programmes which would not have opportunity costs for other groups of patients.

New programmes could be linked to new measures to increase the demand for health by encouraging patient activity and patient involvement in treatment. The element of patient motivation is important and even in peripheral circulation greater activity would be helpful. Any programme of 'innovation' has to show how improvement could be maintained permanently and relapse prevented. Thus health economics concepts give an opportunity for a new start in this field, with new incentives to providers.

Peripheral arterial disease

This is an important source of morbidity which is even more neglected than peripheral venous disease. Evidence from autopsies in the UK, the USA and Sweden shows that severe atherosclerosis is common (14). For the UK 15% of men and 5% of women had severe disease resulting in stenosis of more than half the diameter of at least one artery. Intermittent claudication was more variable but with a prevalence of at least 2% in many places. It was more common in men than in women. For these people the prevalence of ischaemic heart disease varied between 20% and 52% and was between two and four times higher than in normal subjects. These people were also much more likely to have strokes. In one study in Basle, 12% of male survivors with peripheral arterial disease developed a stroke during 11 years of follow-up compared to 4% of controls. Overall, the risk of death was about two to three times that of age- and sex-matched populations. Among males with intermittent claudication followed up in population studies, 5-year cumulative mortality rates ranged from 4.8% to 17%.

There is little evidence in Europe about costs of treatment for people suffering from this disease. However, there has been a recent very detailed survey in the USA which concluded that peripheral arterial occlusive disease of the extremities (PAODE) 'is an important cause of morbidity and health care expenditures among the elderly' (15). The survey used very detailed data from the National Vital Statistics System to assess impact. Between 1984 and 1987 about 229 000 men and 184 000 women per year were discharged with a diagnosis of chronic PAODE. Numbers of admissions to hospital and surgical procedures have increased substantially since 1979. The review suggests that as a result of population ageing and advances in surgical techniques there will be further increases. There is likely to be an increase in hospital treatment in Europe, but in general this has received even less attention than peripheral venous disease. With peripheral venous disease, the visible symptoms compel some attempt at treatment. Within primary care there was more interest in the topic in the 1970s when Rose and others developed a simple self-administered questionnaire on chest pain and intermittent claudication (16). This questionnaire proved to be a highly accurate predictor of later mortality from coronary heart disease (CHD) but it seems to be little used.

How does the current approach relate to perceptions of costs and benefits? Current treatment costs are underestimated and unrecorded. In many cases they are probably concealed in emergency admissions of elderly patients with multiple pathology. There is little definition of possible benefits in terms of reduced mortality from early detection and treatment. The programme not only lacks innovation; it lacks any settled consistent or organized pattern of activity at all. There are therefore many opportunities to direct the attention of policy makers to this area of care and to translate priorities into economic terms. Health agencies could seek to invest in early detection and treatment in order to reduce the need for often costly and ineffective hospital treatment of elderly patients. They could seek to target high-risk groups such as those with intermittent claudication for treatment by physicians; and they could collect more evidence on health benefits and on quality of life. Health economics could give a new focus and a new sense of urgency to future programme development in this area of care.

Coronary heart disease (CHD)

Disease here is seen as presenting a huge burden in terms of premature mortality. For men, 41% of life years under age 65 arise from CHD and diseases of the circulatory system. For women the proportion is 27% (17). Official UK reports showed CHD to be the single most important cause of premature death (18). However, a new consensus is emerging which sees a strictly limited role for active treatment, even though the UK reduction of CHD through local actions is seen as the single greatest priority for NHS managers and professionals.

This consensus draws on a large amount of research done over the past two decades in Britain and the USA. The Framingham Study in the USA is now entering its fifth decade. The British Regional Heart Study began in 1978 as a prospective study of heart disease and stroke in middle-aged men drawn at random from general practice registers in 24 towns. The study was designed in order to assess reasons for the marked differences in mortality from CHD between towns (29). In practice the study has produced much material on risk factors and on reasons for differences in prevalence. The three key risk factors are seen as cigarette smoking, cholesterol level and blood pressure, with smoking and cholesterol as the most important.

These results have not been translated into any strongly defined treatment programme. The researchers have in fact made a promising development of a weighted scoring system which allows identification of people at high risk. Under this system it is possible to detect the top quintile of patients who have a one in ten chance of an acute attack within 5 years. The Framingham Study has had rather similar results to the British studies in identifying risk factors, but American professionals have drawn very different conclusions about treatment pro-grammes. The American study has led to an active programme to lower cholesterol levels and to reduce blood pressure through drug treatment as well as programmes to change lifestyles through diet, exercise and reduction in smoking. The UK approach stresses change in lifestyle, with little role for drug treatment (20). There is also little consensus in the UK on the benefits of screening for elevated blood cholesterol (20). Professional inertia had provided a further braking effect along with scientific doubt on any action at the local level.

There are already some signs, however, of change in decision making and some shift towards more active treatment of elderly patients. Some trials of treatment of hypertension for patients between 65 and 74 have supported use of diuretics (21). This area of care is likely to see the development of shared care and treatment protocols between hospital consultants and family doctors. There will also be more investigation and treatment in an ambulatory or primary care setting stimulating the development of new equipment and technology.

In secondary care, more elderly patients will be considered for cardiac surgery and other active treatment programmes. Developments of non-invasive techniques in treatment and less traumatic methods in surgery will also help in increasing treatment rates. Treatment of chronic heart failure and 'multiple pathology' in very elderly people will remain an important and, in fact, a growing area of care. Treatment programmes for the younger elderly will become less distinctive. The same range of treatments will become available to them, both in terms of active treatment in the community to reduce risk factors and in access to investigation and surgery in secondary care. Resource constraints have limited access by elderly patients. For the 1990s new programmes for reducing risk factors should reduce demand for extensive treatment among younger patients. Some success has already been shown in reducing the incidence of strokes. These changes should release resources which will allow active treatment of many more elderly patients.

Stroke

This is an important cause of mortality which has been receiving some more recent attention from policy makers. Strokes were responsible for 12% of all deaths in the late 1980s. The background, however, supplies greater cause for optimism than with other major causes of death such as CHD and cancer. In the UK there have been major falls in the number of deaths in younger people from stroke. For the UK the reduction in mortality in people under 65 was 32% between 1980 and 1989. The change in the UK has been comparable to that in the USA. The improvement could be due to reduced smoking and to better treatment of high blood pressure. Possible targets for the further reduction in stroke mortality suggest a further 30% reduction in mortality by the year 2000 and a 25% reduction in the death rate for the 65–74 age group (18).

Stroke is also responsible for extensive disability. Stroke-related illness takes up nearly 10% of NHS beds and accounts for 7.7 million lost working days each year (18); but there is little focus either at the national level or locally on how gains might be achieved in terms of increased quality of life. The main emphasis is on specialized rehabilitation services rather than on any drug treatments.

A health economics perspective can supply a more positive view of current programmes. Benefits are being achieved even if the reasons for progress are not very clear. Costs of possible new programmes can be estimated by reference to specifics in age groups and risk factors. The opportunities for positive definition of new programmes in this field are considerable, especially in terms of accelerating recovery and reducing long-term disability.

IMPLICATIONS FOR CHANGE IN CLINICAL TREATMENT OF HEART DISEASE

In the 1980s, treatment programmes were affected by decision systems such as cost utility analysis; the 1990s are likely to be a period of developing impact for new types of management systems and incentives. Health care providers are faced with much tougher constraints on spending, with increased expectations of health benefit. Health agencies are essentially seeking to achieve higher health benefits.

Local doctors are working within greater funding constraints, often with less staff and facing greater scrutiny of their professional decisions. The demands are to improve quality while reducing cost. They may also feel more concerned about liability and thus more ready to follow peer group guidelines. In every country in Europe the freedom of action of the professional is under review and constraint from health managers and health agencies. The development of information technology is making it much easier to review and assess decisions.

Health agencies are under greater pressure from national ministries of finance. There is already a common European culture and contact between ministries of health. The old distinctions between insurance-based and government-funded NHS systems are becoming less clear.

Yet the phase of static expenditure may well be temporary. Long-term population shifts involving rising numbers of elderly people and increases in expectations of active treatment are likely to increase expenditure (22). There are major opportunities for specifying new programmes in most of the areas set out above.

One important part of programme definition will be in relating pharmaceutical treatment to lifestyle changes. The shift to greater demand for health is likely to be a permanent one, with much greater concern for lifestyle factors. Integration with Eastern Europe is likely to sharpen this emphasis even further given the need for low cost programmes. Companies could seek to relate future development much more explicitly to these factors, which would allow much clearer and more ambitious targets in terms of benefit.

There are particular opportunities in programme development in chronic illness, especially peripheral vascular disease and PAODE. These are currently invisible programmes where greater use of quality of life measures could sharpen perceptions of costs and benefits.

At the local level, family doctors and health agencies will be seeking to improve patient care. They will seek guidance in effective practice management for the reduction of risk. This would relate drug treatment to instruments and protocols for ensuring that practices can select and manage high-risk groups effectively. There would be particular opportunities for doing this in high-risk communities in older industrial areas in the UK, in Germany and in France.

Physicians in primary care will also be seeking to develop new joint programmes with secondary care. Without secondary care, purchasers are likely to seek a more integrated approach to treatment. The likely patterns of change in secondary care can be summarized as follows for the UK (23):

1. There will be an increased demand for hospital treatment from the very elderly. District health authorities are likely to insist on an integrated approach to treatment covering support after discharge as well as treatment in hospital.
2. There will be more information available to purchasers on quality as well as on cost, and more sensitivity to differences in quality. There are likely to be more accurate adjustments to outcome or mortality indicators.
3. There is likely to be more interest in prevention and in programmes for positive health reflecting the new obligations placed on GPs in the new contract. The climate will be one in which the benefits of 'high-tech' medicine will come increasingly under question. The demand will be for quality and preventive care. This may raise opportunities for new kinds of programmes in pathology and diagnostic services, but may well mean patient resistance to increasing inpatient care.
4. A new funding system will switch resources to areas of growing population and away from large cities. Areas with highest costs will also face the greatest funding constraints.
5. There will be intense competition for marginal patients. Purchasing agencies in areas of expanding population will have the funds and the flexibility to contract for new services.

The scenario includes relative increases in manpower and capital costs, changes in patterns of health care towards new links between secondary and primary care and a shift in culture towards preventions. The 'Health Enterprise' of the 1990s will have greater integration between hospital and community services, earlier discharge and more day treatment, and with greater emphasis on health promotion. It will also be a world of decentralized public enterprise with clearer quality standards policed by an independent agency.

Thus physicians and managers in care of clinical heart disease will face new challenges in innovation.

Outlook for the 1990s: a summary

The 1990s will see new challenges to health care providers in both the public and the private sectors, as sweeping changes in incentives begin to take effect. The new arm's-length relationship between purchasers and providers will be critical to the new system. Purchasers will be seeking to buy more clearly specified services to higher-quality standards. The new contracting systems will affect services for all groups, but for elderly patients the effect will be greater because of the enlarged role of local government in preparing plans for social care. The role of the family doctor will be increased through new assessments for people over 75.

The new climate will stimulate innovation for new kinds of consumer-orientated service to improve health, mobility and quality of life. For the private sector this is likely to mean increasing scope for joint ventures with public sector agencies in Britain. It will also mean growing international markets as health care systems in different European countries move in the same broad direction and as a shift takes place in expectations among elderly people. The 1990s are likely to see a worldwide revolution in health services for elderly people.

Acknowledgement

The author would like to thank Frances Daniels for assistance.

REFERENCES

1. McGuire A, Henderson J, Mooney M (1988) *The Economics of Health Care: An Introductory Text*. Routledge, London.
2. Enthoven A (1985) *Some Reflections on Management in the NHS*. Nuffield Provincial Hospital Trust.
3. Newhouse J *et al.* (1981) Some interim results from a controlled trial of cost sharing in health insurance. *N Engl J Med* **305**: 1501–1507.
4. Market Letter (1990). *Hypertension Market Forecasts to 1995*. July 30th, IMS London, p. 27.
5. Wright K (1985) *Extended Training of Ambulance Staff*. Discussion Paper No. 2, University of York.
6. Williams A (1985) Economics of coronary artery bypass grafting. *Br Med J* **291**: 326–9.
7. DHSS (1985) *Costs and Benefits of the Heart Transplant Programmes at Harefield and Papworth Hospital*. HMSO, Research Report No. 12.
8. Bosanquet N, Gray A (1989) *Will You Still Love Me? New Opportunities for Health Services for Elderly People in the 1990s and Beyond*. National Association of Health Authorities, Birmingham.
9. ABPI (1990) *Trends in Usage of Prescription Medicines by the Elderly and Very Elderly Between 1977 and 1988*. ABPI, London.
10. Fries JF (1980) Ageing, natural death and the compression of morbidity. *N Engl J Med* **303**: 130.
11. Franks PJ, Wright DDI, McCollum CN (1989) Epidemiology of venous disease: a review. *Phlebology* **4**: 143–51.
12. Hunt SJ *et al.* (1982) Subjective health of patients with peripheral vascular disease. *Practitioner* **226**: 133–136.
13. Moffatt CJ, Franks PF, Bosanquet N *et al.* (1991) *The Provision of Innovation in Venous Ulcer Management to the Elderly Population in the Community*. Report to the King Edward's Hospital Fund for London.

14. Fowkes FGR (1988) Epidemiology of atherosclerotic arterial disease in the lower limbs. *Eur J Vascular Surg* **2**: 283–291.
15. Gillum RF (1990) Peripheral arterial occlusive disease of the extremities in the United States: hospitalization and mortality. *Am Heart J* **120**: 1414–1418.
16. Rose G, McCartney P, Reid DD (1977) Self-administration of a questionnaire on chest pain and intermittent claudiction, *Br J Prev Soc Med* **31**: 42–48.
17. Godfrey C, Hardman G, Maynard M (1989) *Priorities for Health Promotion: An Economic Approach.* Discussion Paper 59, CHE, University of York.
18. Department of Health (1991) *The Health of the Nation.* HMSO, London, Cm 1523.
19. Shaper AG (1989) The British Regional Heart Study. *MRC News.* No. 45: 16–17.
20. O'Brien B (1991) *Cholesterol and Coronary Heart Disease: Consensus or Controversy?* Office of Health Economics, London.
21. MRC (1992) Medical Research Council trial of treatment of hypertension in older adults: principal results. *Br Med J* **304**: 405–411.
22. OECD (1988) *Reforming Public Pensions.* OECD, Paris.
23. Bosanquet N (1990) *Investing in Health Care for the 1990s: A Case Study in Planning for an NHS Trust.* Health Policy Unit Discussion Paper 2, Carden Publications Limited, Chichester.

Part II

EXAMINATION

4 Communicating with Elderly People

IAN R. HASTIE
St George's Hospital Medical School, London, UK

Good communication with elderly people is essential in providing them with the best health care possible. Elderly people are not a different race from the rest of the population but, of course, are individuals who happen to have been alive longer. Most of our attitudes are formed in childhood and adolescence, and elderly people grew up in times that were very different from the present day. Their ideas of, and attitudes towards, doctors, nurses, social services, therapists and hospitals were different from those held by the present younger generation. Health and social care had to be paid for unless charity was relied upon and this usually implied an inferior service. The doctor has always been looked up to, if not put on a pedestal, and everything the doctor said was accepted, usually without question. Hospitals tended to be places where people only went if they were severely ill, and whereas most people entering hospital in today's world quite rightly expect to be made better, if not cured, this was not the case in the past. Consequently, elderly people today may still be in awe, if not fear, of hospitals and anything to do with medical services, and this may hinder effective communication and make the provision of health care more difficult.

They tended therefore to consult a doctor only if they had a major complaint, any minor illness being treated at home by themselves or members of their family. This tendency is still carried through to today. Unfortunately, this in combination with a lot of elderly people themselves ascribing complaints just to 'getting older' may lead to an elderly person not seeking advice early enough in the course of an illness.

The attitude of not talking about bodily functions still pervades to this day, resulting in elderly people having some reluctance to talk about personal functions such as defaecation and micturition. It may therefore be necessary to approach questions on these functions from different angles in order to get an accurate reply. Asking a patient 'if they are suffering from urinary incontinence' may be met with a negative reply, whereas, they may reply positively to asking them 'if they sometimes find that they cannot get to the toilet in time and have damp underclothes'. Personal language and the use of words is continually evolving but this mainly occurs in the first half of life. There are therefore words that may be used when people are young that during their lifetime change their

Geriatric Cardiology. Principles and Practice. Edited by A. Martin and A. J. Camm
© 1994 John Wiley & Sons Ltd

meaning completely, leading to difficulties in comprehension during a person's later years. An example is that it may be important and relevant to a patient's diagnosis to know whether or not the patient is homosexual; however, using the modern euphemism of asking if the patient is 'gay' may have a totally different meaning if asked to an 80-year-old as opposed to a 30-year-old. It is important that we speak to elderly people in their language and not our own, but at the same time we should not be condescending.

The attitude of the interviewer towards elderly people may have a great bearing on the interviewer's ability to communicate with them. There may be a very negative attitude towards old age, which may be brought on by fear of ageing and death, in younger members of our society who tend to be youth-orientated. These negative attitudes to old age are then extrapolated to the elderly as a group and as individuals and gives the prejudice of ageism. It is important to conquer these thoughts if good communication with older people is sought.

Derogative terms in the doctor/patient relationship such as 'Pop', 'Gramps' or 'Love', should not be used. Elderly people should be addressed by their title—Mr, Mrs, Miss, etc.—and their surname. A lot of elderly women lost boyfriends or fiancées in the First or Second World War and subsequently never married. Remaining a spinster may have been out of respect of their lost loved one, or because they never met anyone else that they wished to marry, or of course that there were just too few men of the same age due to the terrible slaughter of men, especially in the First World War, within their late teens and early 20s. It is therefore important to these people that they should be addressed by the correct title of Miss rather than be called Mrs. Sometimes a close relationship develops between a doctor or health care provider and the patient and in this case the patient may ask that they are called by their first name. However, first names should not be used unless requested by the patient as it may be seen as a sign of familiarity or condescension when the patient is looking for a more professional relationship.

Part of a good relationship, and therefore good communication between a doctor and the patient, is achieved by the general appearance of the doctor. Uniforms, such as a white coat, although institutional, will often enhance this relationship in the eyes of older people, who expect their doctor to be smartly dressed and to look the part. All of this helps to build up the confidence of the elderly patient with the doctor and thereby enable the optimum health care to be provided.

Ageing is not a sudden phenomenon that occurs at 65 or 70, but is a relative concept that is occurring throughout a person's life. Illness is not special to the older age groups, although the pattern of illness does tend to change as people reach later life. First, the elderly person may suffer from multiple pathological processes occurring at the same time. There may be a combination of medical and social pathology and they must be seen as interconnecting in the same person, rather than looked upon as separate diagnoses. This is important when considering treatment for the various aspects of multiple pathology as there may be unwanted interactions between them. Second, the same disease that is seen in a younger person may give a different presentation in an older patient. Illnesses in this group may not appear with classical symptoms but may occur with one of the patterns of presentation often seen in elderly people such as falling, incontinence of urine, confusion or failure to cope at home.

It may be difficult to know whether a problem occurring in an older patient is due to the ageing process which is accepted as normal, or a pathological process which is accepted as abnormal. To unravel the differences there are four concepts that must be present in order to put a problem down to ageing rather than to pathology (1). These concepts are:

1. *Universality*: the phenomenon must occur in all old people rather than in individual groups, although the degree of effect may vary between individuals.
2. *Intrinsicality*: the phenomenon must be due to causes occurring from within the body rather than to extrinsic, external or environmental causes.
3. *Deleteriousness*: the process of ageing is one of decline and therefore there must be an element of the phenomenon being deleterious to people.
4. *Progressiveness*: the onset must be gradual as the person becomes older and should not occur suddenly.

PROCESS OF COMMUNICATION AND NORMAL AGEING

Normal pathways of communication are complex and some parts are better understood than others. Disorders of the communication pathways in elderly people include deficits in language, hearing, comprehension, speech and voice. These deficits may occur singly but, as multiple pathology increases with increasing age, then two or more of these deficits may occur in the same individual, thereby producing a handicap which may be greater than the sum of each of the individual deficits would produce alone.

Language production

Changes may occur due to both normal ageing and pathological neurological conditions. Once speech is learnt in childhood then people speak automatically until the presence of a disorder causes a breakdown in these automatic pathways, producing a deficit which may or may not be able to be overcome by hard work and concentration. Language production may be classified into four areas:

1. *Phonology*: the selection and production of various sounds that are put together to make words. In addition to simple mono-tonous sounds, different intonation can be added so that normal speech patterns are achieved. Phonology remains unchanged with normal ageing.
2. *Syntax*: words are put together to produce a sentence, the grammatical and

structural make-up of which is the syntax. There is some evidence that with increasing age there may be a decrease in the length of grammatical utterances (2). However, syntax is probably mainly unchanged as people age.

3. *Semantics*: words and sentences have a meaning, and semantics is the use of a vocabulary to produce this meaning, and with normal ageing there is a decline. In normal elderly people the changes in semantic usage are identified by an increasing use of pronouns and a decrease in the use of proper nouns associated with increasing numbers of references with ambiguous meanings (3).

4. *Pragmatics*: in a social situation language is used as an interaction between different individuals. There has been little investigation of the effects of increasing age on pragmatics although it has been shown that in a conversation elderly people tend to share less information (3).

Perception

Information is obtained from the environment, and perception is the ability of acquiring this information and its interpretation. With increasing age there is an associated decline in performing cerebral functions and of registering external stimuli, in addition to a reduction in sensory function. All of these combine to increase the time it takes for an elderly person to respond to a given stimulus and provides a decrease in the quality of the information. Therefore as age increases, in order to produce an equivalent reaction to younger age groups there is a need for larger changes in the stimuli.

Hearing

The ability to hear declines with increasing age due both to physiological and superimposed pathological causes. Deafness causing a demonstrable problem is common in elderly people and has been estimated as occurring in a third of people over the age of 65, rising to a half of those over 80 years of age.

Hearing loss of the high frequencies starts in early adulthood. With increasing age there is a greater impairment in the high frequencies but also a gradual spreading of this impairment to lower frequencies (4). Males have an average of up to five times greater hearing loss than females.

This may be related to increased environmental or occupational noise damage. Vowels tend to be of longer duration and of lower frequency range, whereas consonants are generally of shorter duration with a higher frequency range. For understanding, speech consonants are more important than vowels. Consequently, there is a close relationship between the decrease in higher frequencies with age and the decreased ability to hear speech properly but this is not totally consistent. The noises of speech may be heard but distinguishing the noises may be difficult. This, however, does not correlate well with either pure tone audiograms or speech articulation tests. This may be due to an increase in the time that is needed by the higher listening centres in order to identify the messages from the noises received (5). It was found that in elderly people, as opposed to younger subjects, if the speed of speech was increased then there was a decreased ability to understand that speech (6). With increasing age there is also a decrease in nerve velocity, all producing a delay in transmission of the information.

Sound waves entering the external auditory meatus are transmitted mechanically through the middle ear and are registered by the basilar membrane and receptor cells in the cochlea. Here the mechanical energy is changed into nerve impulses which are transmitted along the auditory nerve to the auditory cortex of the temporal lobes. Sound waves use three characteristics in order to convey information: frequency, intensity and timing. Other factors may then affect the reception of the speech and its discrimination.

Frequency sensitivity

Although high frequencies deteriorate first with increasing age, the ability to discriminate between different frequencies deteriorates to a greater extent for the lower frequencies. The absolute threshold for hearing declines with increasing age, and again this is greater in men. There is also cross-sectionally a decline from 250 Hz to 80 kHz as age increases from 18 to 65 years (7).

Intensity discrimination

Young adults have a mean speech reception threshold of 18.5 dB, whereas elderly people up to 74 years of age have a speech reception threshold of 42 dB (8). However, as changes occur throughout the auditory system with increasing age and at different rates, the intensity discrimination may vary considerably between different elderly individuals.

Sound localization

It is important to be able to focus on the sound source as, in addition to pinpointing the origin of the sound it also helps to distinguish that sound from surrounding noise. This is useful when hearing speech against background interference.

Two factors help achieve this. First, although minute there is often a time delay in sound reaching each ear unless the sound source is being faced. Second, the intensity of sound from a single source can be compared in both ears. Sound localization can be affected if both ears have a different ability to hear, either by an increased deafness in one ear as opposed to the other, or an unequal deterioration in central auditory pathways on each side.

Loudness recruitment

Loudness recruitment occurs in sensineural deafness due to damage in the sensory cells of the inner ear (9). Loudness recruitment occurs when sounds are amplified and discrimination becomes more difficult. It has been estimated that approximately half of all elderly people who have difficulty in hearing suffer from loudness recruitment (10).

Hypersensitivity

In elderly people with hearing problems an increase in the intensity of sound may produce discomfort or even pain in the sufferer. This may occur at a sound level which is normal and causes no problems to younger people. Hypersensitivity commonly occurs when people are using a hearing aid and either the volume is turned up or the speaker speaks too loudly.

Environmental effects of speech discrimination

From 20 to 60 years of age the ability to understand speech remains relatively constant, but by the time 80 years is reached there is an approximately 25% reduction in discrimination (11). Also, as the speech intensity is increased elderly people tend to show a lower rate of improvement in discrimination. Even when the degree of pure tone hearing loss is held constant, a progressive decline in the correct perception of phonetically well-balanced words with increasing age has been demonstrated (12). This is in a quiet environment; however, under adverse environmental conditions elderly people, due to, for example, reverberation and echoes, are even less able to discriminate speech.

Pathological changes

Outer ear

With increasing age the pinna increases both in length and breadth. Atrophic changes may be found in the supporting walls of the external auditory meatus, although both these have not been shown to have any functional significance. Wax is produced normally in the external auditory canal but with increasing age this tends to become harder and therefore less likely to clear naturally. In one study it was found that out of 283 elderly people with impaired hearing, 49 had both ears blocked by wax and a further 61 had only one ear blocked (13). Wax in the external auditory canal tends to attenuate low-frequency sound in the first instance.

Middle ear

There is a thickening and decreased elasticity in the tympanic membrane and a decrease in the movement of the joints between the auditory ossicles (14). Otosclerosis is commonly found, with new bone formation tending to immobilize the footplate of the stapes within the oval window. This is more often found in women than men and may require a stapedectomy if severe. Atrophy of the tensor tympany muscle is also seen.

Inner ear

Specific age-related changes in the inner ear have been identified (15) and a complex number of other changes have been shown by other workers:

1. *Sensory*: within the cochlea atrophy and degeneration of hair cells and their supporting cells and the organ of Corti in the basal coil of the cochlea have been identified. This degeneration seems to be slowly progressive from middle age onwards and the audiogram shows an abrupt high tone loss.
2. *Neural*: there is a loss of neurones throughout the cochlea but this is worse in the basal coil. This can start at any age and leads to poor speech discrimination rather than a threshold loss on a pure tone audiogram.
3. *Vascular*: starting between 20 and 50 years of age there is a slowly progressive loss of hearing due to vascular changes. This produces a flat audiogram pattern but with good speech discrimination. Atrophy of the stria vasculares with corresponding deficiencies in the properties of the endolymphatic fluid is also seen.
4. *Mechanical*: there is atrophy of the vibrating structures of the cochlea partition.

Brain pathways

Some of the hearing loss associated with increasing age has a central cause with no involvement of the inner ear (16). Also reported are simple atrophy of the VIIIth cranial nerve, a diminished number of neuronal cells in the auditory pathways and a bilateral loss of ganglion cells in the cortex of the temporal lobes, although normal stratification was retained.

Hearing deficits

Conductive hearing loss

Problems occurring in the outer/middle ear produce hearing loss of a conductive pattern. The sufferer can comfortably hear other people if they talk loudly enough and often hears better in a noisy environment rather than a quiet one. Common causes producing a conductive hearing loss are: wax in the external auditory meatus; a rigid oscilla chain; and diminished function of the Eustachian tube.

Sensorineural loss

This occurs when there is a problem with either the inner ear or the VIIIth cranial nerve. Higher frequencies are lost in comparison to lower ones. The sufferer may also experience loudness recruitment. The listener thinks people are shouting at him or her and will often say so, even though the speaker may be speaking normally. Often the low frequencies are heard but the listener misses higher frequencies, therefore believing that the speaker has poor enunciation.

Presbyacusis

There is a decrease in hearing with advancing age usually starting in the fourth decade. Although it may be classed as an ageing phenomenon it is uncertain why some elderly people get progressively severe loss of hearing whilst others find that the changes are minimal. Sufferers experience a decrease in hearing high-pitched sounds and also have trouble differentiating between sounds, especially in noisy environments. It has been considered that the following criteria need to be satisfied before the syndrome of presbyacusis can be diagnosed (10):

1. There is no history of previous ear disease, and examination of the ear and nose is normal.
2. There is no past medical history of a severe generalized disease.
3. The sufferer is over 60 years of age.
4. The audiogram shows a sensorineural hearing deficit.
5. There is a gradual increase in loss of high frequencies on the pure tone audiogram.
6. At the point of testing there should be a history of progressive hearing loss of no longer than 10 years.
7. Bone conduction is almost equal to air conduction of sound.
8. Air conduction of sound should not differ by more than 15 dB at any frequency when one ear is compared to another.
9. On average there should be a 10–60 dB hearing loss for pure tones in the range 50–200 Hz.

It has been estimated that advanced signs of presbyacusis are seen in 13% of people over the age of 65 (17).

Conclusion

Elderly people who suffer from a combination of ageing problems have a greater chance of social withdrawal and isolation than younger people. Conversation between elderly people may be difficult as both may be suffering from problems of hearing in addition to deficits in localization, attention and comprehension in a situation of background noise (18). In addition impaired vision may lead to difficulty in lip-reading or partial lip-reading, and physical impairment may produce decreased mobility. Thus isolation can occur with consequent pathological depression. Problems have been highlighted with acoustics in rooms that are occupied by elderly people, and more attention should be paid to acoustics in these circumstances. This is of particular importance in institutions where, as well as poor acoustics, there is an increased prevalence of deafness in the residents and this may lead to one of the unrecognized factors for institutionalization.

ADAPTATIONS TO AID COMMUNICATIONS WITH ELDERLY PEOPLE

Good communication is possible with some people even in adverse conditions. However, the doctor can aid good communication by taking account of the environment, the positioning of the communicator and non-verbal language. The environment in which the communication is occurring should be quiet, excluding most external distractions such as televisions and radios. General noise can also be distracting and, therefore, it can be appreciated that an open general ward is not the best environment. The elderly person should preferably be sitting comfortably without the glare of bright lights, which will produce constant constriction of the pupils with diminished vision, which will decrease the input from non-verbal communication and any attempt to lip-read.

The doctor should also be comfortable, preferably at the same eye level as the elderly person and about 2–3 feet away. Talking from a higher position and too far away such as from the end of the bed will only hinder good communication. Sitting on a patient's bed used to be frowned upon but when communicating with older people the benefits will be appreciated. Any light that is available should be on the doctor's face rather than shining directly onto the elderly person, nor should it be coming from behind the doctor's head to produce only a silhouette. Good light on the doctor's face will enable the elderly person to have the best opportunity to see any facial expressions and non-verbal communication. Many people will enhance their understanding by partial lip-reading and it is therefore important that the lips are not obscured whilst talking, either by the habit of putting a hand to the mouth, or placing pencils, fingers or anything else around that area. Chewing can also be distracting to the lip movements, especially chewing gum. As well as making lip-reading difficult, turning the head away whilst talking to an elderly person, especially if there are other people around or if the doctor is distracted himself, not only leads to difficulties in lip-reading but also produces a muffled voice. The doctor should speak distinctly, with a voice that is only slightly raised to the level that he would normally use speaking to someone at a distance of 5–6 feet. He should not shout as this will not help comprehension and may produce discomfort or pain to the patient, due to loudness recruitment and hypersensitivity.

Non-verbal communication often occurs at a subconscious level yet is extremely important. The shaking of hands when the doctor and patient first meet helps to break down barriers and start to forge a rapport between the two. Touch is probably the most emotional and direct form of non-verbal communication and quite often the hand on the patient's shoulder, or the holding of the patient's hand will lead to a much closer understanding and better communication between the doctor and his patient. Of course, too much touching can have an adverse affect and this may be enhanced by cultural differences. The doctor who smiles and has a pleasant manner will often communicate better with his patients than those who are gruff and fierce. The experienced interviewer will always appear to be paying attention and showing an interest in what the patient is saying, even if he is only in fact half paying attention and thinking about the next question, or possible differential diagnosis. Eye contact will be maintained, often with a slight lean towards the patient and an occasional nod of the head in agreement. This will give a message to the patient that the doctor is interested and has a personal concern. This can be enhanced if the doctor appears to spend time with the patient and does not always appear in a rush, producing a caring attitude in the eye of the patient. Quite often the doctor can undo the good intentions if he has a negative attitude towards elderly people—ageism. There may be many causes for this but there has to be a recognition on behalf of the doctor of his own fears about growing older, as this is of the utmost importance in establishing good effective communication with older people. Body language can be seen in both patient and doctor. The fearful patient will sit in a retracted position with arms folded and legs crossed, and it is a challenge to the doctor to overcome these boundaries in order to communicate effectively. The doctor needs to be alert to these non-verbal forms of communication in the patient but also in himself. The hunched shoulders or pointed finger may enhance a perfectly valid point that the doctor is making, but the patient may unwittingly perceive a hidden message in the gesture. The ultimate aim is to produce a close rapport between the doctor and patient, as with this good communication ensues.

It is important that patients are given information about their illness, treatment and medication. Unfortunately, sometimes too much information can be given at any one time and this can lead to poor understanding. As elderly people suffer from multiple pathology they are often taking several different medications at any one time and have difficulties in maintaining compliance unless the information is kept simple. If a quantity of information needs to be given to the patient then this can often be reinforced if written down. The patient's response to too much information, without proper reinforcement, may well be to decide to ignore all or part of it, leading to a breakdown in communications.

PATHOLOGICAL PROBLEMS

Specific pathological problems affecting reception and expression lead to some of the most difficult areas in communication.

Dysphasia/aphasia

Almost every right-handed and many left-handed people have all or most of their functions of language situated in the left hemisphere (20). There are a few truly left-handed people whose language function is found in the right hemisphere. However, in the vast majority of people damage occurring to the left hemisphere gives disruption to the many complex pathways producing aphasia or, to a lesser degree, dysphasia. The processes of reception of stimuli, their decoding, the formulation of a response and production of that response are very complex and over the years problems occurring with these processes have been given a mainly functional terminology.

Receptive aphasia/dysphasia

This is also known as sensory or Wernicke's aphasia. There are varying degrees of difficulty in understanding the spoken or written word. The pathological lesion produces damage to Wernicke's area, which is in the posterior part of the superior temporal gyrus. The patient may be able to understand the meaning of a sentence or paragraph but not any word taken in isolation, and words that are not used frequently by the patient are often most affected. There is an association with paraphrasia, with the production of fluent speech which is not understandable and often including inappropriate jargon.

Expressive aphasia/dysphasia

This is also called motor or Broca's aphasia. Problems occur with expression, often with a difficulty in finding words or using wrong words and in producing normal fluent speech. Sensory input appears to be dissociated from expressive output, although automatic responses and speech often remain, e.g. counting and saying that they are well if asked the question 'How are you?' Damage is seen in Broca's area, which is situated in the third frontal convolution of the left hemisphere.

Although in elderly people each may occur separately it is usual to find both expressive and receptive deficits present, although one type may be dominant (21). As well as difficulty in speech, there may also be problems in various degrees with reading and writing. People suffering from receptive aphasia may not be able to understand a simple command such as 'stand up', but may be able to imitate and understand a simple visual command such as the interviewer gesturing to the patient and demonstrating standing.

Anomia

Often in association with aphasia there may be an inability to find specific words. Anomia is when this is out of proportion to other symptoms.

Agraphia and alexia

Both agraphia and alexia may occur separately, or coexist, or be part of the total aphasia syndrome. In a previously normal person alexia is the inability to read and agraphia the inability to write. Three groups of alexia are defined (20):

1. *Parietal/temporal alexia*: occurs with coexisting agraphia, creating difficulties in both reading and writing.

2. *Occipital alexia*: occurs when only reading difficulties are present and there is no agraphia, although the patient may be unable to remember what they have written as they cannot read their writing.
3. *Frontal alexia*: often occurs in conjunction with expressive dysphasia.

Dysarthria

Neuromuscular dysfunction produces an inability to produce the coordinated movements of respiration, articulation, phonation, resonance and rhythm that are needed in order to produce the intelligent speech that the patient knows and wishes to say. The different types of dysarthria are classified according to the type of lesion and the type of deficit produced (22).

Spastic dysarthria

This occurs with bilateral upper motor neurone lesions and is part of the syndrome of pseudo-bulbar palsy. Speech is slow and slurred, with indistinct articulation and a weak voice.

Ataxia adysarthria

Pathology such as a stroke, tumour, trauma, or degeneration to the cerebellum produces ataxia dysarthria, with a voice described as being slow and slurred with jerky monotonous, staccato speech.

Hyperkinetic dysarthria

This is due to an extra-pyramidal lesion and if often seen in chorea, or with degeneration of the extrapyramidal system. Speech becomes hesitant and jerky, especially with variations in loudness, rate and accuracy of articulation. The speech pattern is produced by involuntary movements affecting normal speech.

Hypokinetic dysarthria

This is seen in extrapyramidal lesions such as Parkinsonism. Phrases tend to be short, with a weak voice, indistinct articulation, monotonous and with an increasing rate of speech. Treatment, as with the other symptoms of Parkinsonism, is with dopaminergic drugs, although there is a danger that too much medication may produce similar speech problems to those that are being treated.

Flaccid dysarthria

This occurs with lower motor neurone lesions, and the presentation of the dysarthria depends to a greater extent on which lower motor neurone is affected of the cranial nerves V, VII, X and XII. Speech tends to have indistinct articulation which is excessively nasal.

Mixed dysarthrias

With increasing age and increasing pathology there is often a combination of different lesions producing a mixture of dysarthrias.

Dysphonia

With dysphonia there is a problem with the structures of voice production. This commonly occurs in younger subjects due to infections of the throat but this is less common in elderly people except for *Candida*, which may be seen in association with other illnesses or due to medications, such as oral antibiotics. With increasing age there is an increasing risk of carcinomas of the tongue, lips and larynx, producing dysphonia. Treatment for the different types of dysphonia is the same for any age group but depends on the underlying pathology.

Drugs

Drugs usually affect speech in one of three ways. Many drugs, especially those with anticholinergic action, can produce a dry mouth with subsequent dysphonia. Sedative drugs of one sort or another are too frequently used in older people, with the subsequent slowing and slurring of speech as well as the other sedative symptoms. The major tranquillizers and dopaminergic drugs may often produce involuntary movements which lead to difficulty in speech production.

SPECIAL CIRCUMSTANCES

Dementia

Dementia is a syndrome that needs further elucidation. Specific diagnosis is not often easy; however, it is necessary for prognosis and management (23). People suffering from dementia syndrome by definition have a poor memory. When they speak it tends to be in short phrases or even single words, and occasionally they use words that are closely associated but in fact wrong. In the later stages of dementia the patient will often become mute. Perseveration—the inappropriate and repetitive use of words or phrases—and echolalia—the echoing of other people's speech—is common. In the early stages of dementia in people who do not have English as their first language it is often found that they revert to their original language even if English has been spoken for many years. People speaking to sufferers of dementia should use simple words in short sentences and be careful with sarcasm or humour or introducing proverbs as these may be taken literally.

Institutionalization

Institutions have changed dramatically in recent years and there is now much more concern for residents having autonomy. However, even the best homes still have some rules and regulations and therefore there is no room for complacency. Residents who are housebound often lose contact with the outside world and normal variation in weekly events is lost, so that one day may seem very similar to another. This can cause problems of communication, especially when formal testing of the person's mental state uses knowledge that is assumed, but may not in fact be present. If every day seems the same then asking which day of the week it is may have little significance. This is equivalent to when younger people are on holiday and they have difficulty remembering which day it is. In institutions the commonest verbal contact with the residents are commands. Men tend to be spoken to less than females except with the ethnic minorities, where females are spoken to less than males. There are also many questions by residents that are not answered. This may be because the care staff are too busy, just do not bother, or have poor communication skills. Therefore all institutions should critically examine their communication patterns (24).

Terminally Ill

Improved communication between medical and nursing staff will improve the general understanding of the needs of individual dying patients and enable more appropriate treatment to be given (25). Elderly people are often aware that they are dying sometimes even before the doctor has come to that conclusion. Unfortunately, patients' questions at this time may be wrongly interpreted as being morbid and this will often deny them the help and understanding that they require. Elderly people are often more realistic about death than those younger people who are caring for them. The doctor should ask himself, 'at what point does the patient wish to know that he or she is dying and what does the patient wish to know about the illness?' This would then enable the patient to decide how much he or she wishes to know and at what pace that information is given. The relatives and carers also need to be told but this should not be in lieu of telling the patient, but in association with them. Sometimes carers insist that the patient is not told and, although this is not binding on the doctor, time needs to be spent explaining to them why it is best that the patient knows and is not kept in the dark. This will help to prevent barriers being erected between the carers and the patient and the doctor. Support and understanding can then be given to both the patient and carers together. All patients will go through the stages of awareness—understanding and realization—but at different time-scales. Communication with dying people requires sympathy, reassurance and time, preferably given by staff that they know, and form a relationship with. Four phases have been described that a dying patient goes through: disbelief, denial, anger and resentment (26). Staff and carers should be aware of these phases and communicate accordingly, leading finally to acceptance. Different ethnic groups may have different attitudes towards death and bereavement and therefore communication techniques may need to be amended for these individuals (27).

Bereavement

The chances of bereavement increase with increasing age and, although this is obvious and elderly people accept mortality more readily, bereavement can nevertheless be just as much of a shock in older people as in the young. Death preceded by a period of illness is common in the older age groups and if handled correctly can greatly help the bereaved person. Problems that may be important to the non-bereaved may fade into insignificance with the bereaved, and vice versa, and this may lead to communication difficulties. These, however, can be worked through with sensitivity, patience and understanding on behalf of the doctor. Grieving is natural but working with a bereavement counsellor may still be beneficial even in the early stages.

Non-English speakers

Communication is just as important with this group of elderly people, whose numbers are increasing. Many are moving from one country to another and are not speaking the recipient country's language. Although elderly people are quite able to learn a new language, given the commitment and training, there may be many reasons why this does not occur. Quite often it is due to younger members of the family organizing their lives for them and therefore there is no necessity to learn the new language. This leads to isolation, which can be very frightening when the elderly person becomes ill. Even a simple 'Good morning' by the doctor in their own language can help to break down this isolation, which will also be helped by the many non-verbal forms of communication. Families will often be able to translate as younger members may have learnt English; however, hospitals and other institutions should have a list of people who can communicate in a foreign language.

TREATMENTS AND IMPROVEMENTS

Hearing aids

Amplification of normal sound can produce a harsh or painful noise due to loudness recruitment and hypersensitivity. Loss of the consonants, which are of higher frequency, improves very little with amplification, therefore speech may remain poorly understood. Hearing aids of different types, however, can be of help. These are of two basic designs.

Acoustic amplification

In the past these have been the mainstay of helping deaf people with such instruments as the ear trumpet. However, recent advances have meant that these are now little used. It must be remembered that stethoscopes are a form of acoustic amplifier and these are often of use to the doctor with a moderately deaf person, as the earpieces can be put into the patient's ear and the doctor can then speak through the bell. This gives little speech distortion and is a useful technique in the one-to-one situation.

Electronic amplification

These are basically of two types: those worn on the body, and those worn behind the ear. Both of these may use either bone or air conduction as their route for the sound. Although air conduction is most often used, bone conduction can be beneficial if there is an external ear problem. Hearing aids are very useful in the face-to-face situation when the sufferer may also use other non-verbal forms of communication as an adjunct to understanding. However, with long distances other extraneous noises are also amplified and these can lead to distortion in communication. The controls on electronic amplifiers tend to be fairly small and these can cause problems if there are any other disabilities, such as arthritic hands or Parkinsonian tremors. Good maintenance and back-up are imperative both for care of the hearing aid and also in order to provide good advice to the patient. Both the microphone and earpiece become dirty and clogged very easily, requiring regular cleaning. Although the life of batteries is increasing these will need regular replacement, and the sufferer should be encouraged to keep the hearing aid switched on, rather than switched off in an attempt to conserve the batteries and therefore leading to poor communication. Hearing aid whistle is a common problem and is due to acoustic feedback between the microphone and the earpiece. This is caused by either the volume being too high or the earpiece ill-fitting, both of which can be easily remedied.

Modern electronics enable more than simple amplification to be provided in the newer hearing aids. Amplification of different frequencies and selective controls have enabled hearing aids to be produced that suit the individual, but this requires the setting up of audiology centres. Some sufferers themselves, by being experimental, can be very adaptive with this modern equipment (28). In presbyacusis there is a loss of high frequency with difficulty in hearing consonants, and therefore there is a need for selective amplification. Without this selection low-frequency speech and loud speech would be amplified to too great a level and sudden loud noises, such as an overhead aeroplane, would also be amplified to an uncomfortable level. Some hearing aids are binaural, amplifying sounds to both ears from the same source; however, a better effect, especially enabling better localization of sound, is the use of a separate hearing aid for each ear. It must be remembered that to some people hearing aids are socially unacceptable as they denote a disability, and this often has to be overcome to provide good communication with the sufferer.

Non-wearable hearing aids, which are basically a microphone, amplifier and earphone, should be available in every ward, outpatient department or setting where deaf people may be encountered.

When talking to a person wearing a hearing aid make sure that the hearing aid is turned on and set to the 'M' for microphone setting. Make sure that if the hearing aid is of the body type the amplifier and microphone are not behind layers of clothing, but clipped on the outside with the microphone pointing forwards. Don't be tempted to pick it up and use it as an audio microphone as this will cause distortion. Don't shout, but slightly raise the voice to a level that you would use if you were 4–5 feet away. Enunciate clearly and don't rush your speech. This will often give the wearer the optimum conditions for hearing in order to aid communication.

Other Aids to Communications

Other aids to communication are available and these may take the form of pictures or cards with words printed clearly on them. Also available now are mechanical or electronic communication devices, that use a written printout, artificial voice or simple visual display. Most modern hearing aids also have a 'T' setting, which is for a telephone loop, and this is now available in most public telephones, some domestic telephones and a number of cinemas and theatres. Understanding television even with hearing aids used to be a problem, but the introduction of subtitles has gone a long way to help this.

Reality orientation

Reality orientation is something that we all do every day of our lives. Nevertheless, it specifically helps elderly people to keep a realistic idea of their environment and to be more aware of everyday matters. This is done frequently by reinforcing the truth and can occur every day on a one-to-one basis, or through group meetings. These groups should preferably be small and are found to be especially useful for the confused elderly and may often reawaken an interest in past memories. Evaluation of group reality orientation sessions has been tried and, although this is difficult, small improvements are seen, especially with the mildly confused, in some measures of cognitive function (29), and in staff morale and their improved attitudes to elderly people (30). Benefits of day-to-day reality orientation are in the main to inform and orientate the elderly person to his or her environment and to form closer communication links between the elderly person and the carers.

Speech therapy

Speech therapy plays an important role in communication disorders of elderly people. Speech therapists are not only able to assess, diagnose and treat the various problems of communication, but they can also advise carers and other members of staff on how they can help the patient with the treatment and enable them to communicate better. Age is no bar and some speech therapists specialize in elderly patients.

REFERENCES

1. Strehler BL (1962) *Time Cells and Ageing.* Academic Press, New York.
2. Walker VG, Hardiman CJ, Hendrick DL, Holbrook A (1981) Speech and Language characteristics of an ageing population. In *Speech and Language: Advances in Basic Research and Practice*, Vol. 6, Lars NJ (ed.). Academic Press, New York, pp. 143–202.
3. Ulatowska HK, Cannito MP, Hayashi MM, Fleming SG (1985) Language abilities in the elderly. In *The Aging Brain: Comunication in the Elderly*, Ulatowska HK (ed.). College-Hill Press, San Diego, pp. 125–139.
4. Hinchcliffe R (1959) Correction of pure-tone audiograms for advancing age. **73**: 830–832.
5. Fournier JE (1953) Sur le mécanisme de la conduction osseuse. *Ann Otolar Par.* **70** (8–9): 527–543.
6. Calearo C, Lazzaroni A (1957) Speech intelligibility in relation to the speed of the message. *Laryngology* **67**: 410–419.
7. Corso JF (1963) Age and sex differences in pure-tone thresholds. *Arch Otolaryngol* **77**: 385–405.
8. Corso JF (1967) Confirmation of the normal threshold for speech on C.I.D. Auditory Test W–Z. *J Acoust Soc Am* **29**: 368–370.
9. Williams BT (1970) Medical Assessment. In *Helping the Aged*, Goldberg EM (ed.). Allen & Unwin, London.
10. Pestalozza G, Shore I (1955) Clinical evaluation of presbycusis on the basis of different tests of auditory function. *Laryngology* **65**: 1136–1163.
11. Feldman RM, Reger SN (1987) Relations among hearing, reaction time and age. *J Speech Hearing Research* **10**: 479–495.
12. Jerger J (1973) Audiological findings in aging. *Otorhinolaryngology* **20**: 115–124.
13. Williams BT (1970) Medical Assessment. In *Helping the Aged*, Goldberg EM (ed.). Allen & Unwin, London.
14. Plomp R, Duquesnoy AJ (1980) Room acoustics for the aged. *J Acoust Soc Am* **68**: 1616–1621.
15. Gacek RR, Schuknecht HF (1969) Pathology of presbycusis. *Int Audiol* **8**: 199–209.
16. Hallpike CS (1962) Vertigo of central origin. *Proc R Soc Med* **55**: 364–370.
17. Corso JF (1977) Auditory perception and communication. In *Handbook of the Psychology of Aging*, Birren JE, Schare KW (eds). Van Nostrand Reinholt, New York, pp. 535–536.
18. Maurer JF, Rupp RR (1979) *Hearing and Aging: For Intervention.* Grune & Stratton, New York.
19. Plomp R, Duquesnoy AJ (1980) Room acoustics for the aged. *J Acoust Soc Am* **29**: 368–370.
20. Benson DF (1979) *Aphasia, Alexia and Agraphia.* Clinical Neurology and Neurosurgery Monographs, Churchill Livingstone, Edinburgh.
21. Shewan CM (1982) To hear is not to understand: auditory processing deficits and

factors in influencing performance in aphasic individuals. In *Speech and Language: Advances in Basic Research and Practice*, Vol. 7, Lass NJ (ed.). Academic Press, New York, pp. 1–70.

22. Darley FL, Aronson AE, Brown JR (1975) *Motor Speech Disorders*. Saunders, Philadelphia.
23. Homer AC, Honavar M, Lantos PL *et al.* (1988) Diagnosing dementia: do we get it right? *Br Med J* **297**: 894–896.
24. Jones DC, Jones G Van A (1985) Communication between nursing staff and institutional elderly. *Perspectives* Fall: 12–14.
25. Graham H, Livesley B (1983) Dying as a diagnosis: difficulties of communication and management in elderly patients. *Lancet* **ii** (September), 670–672.
26. Kubler-Ross E (1977) *On Death and Dying*. Tavistock Publications, London.
27. Speck PW (1978) Cultural factors and grief. In *Loss and Grief in Medicine*, Baillière Tindall, London, pp. 113–148.
28. Hodge PH (1991) Inventive amplification. *Sound Barrier* **46**: 9.
29. Schwenk MA (1979) Reality orientation for the institutionalised aged: does it help? *Gerontologist* **19**: 373–377.
30. Smith BJ, Barker HR (1972) Influence of a reality orientation training program on the attitude of trainees. *Gerontologist* **12**: 262–264.

5 Clinical Examination

AUBREY LEATHAM
Wimpole Street, London, UK

An accurate history is still the most important part of diagnosis and management of cardiovascular disease in the elderly, and must precede clinical examination and investigation. Questioning may be more difficult in the elderly, and extra time may have to be spent in finding out what the patient himself, or herself, has noticed to be wrong. Why was a doctor consulted in the first place? The findings at a routine examination are usually much less important, particularly for treatment. It is often necessary to question a relative. After unguided history taking, direct questions may have to be asked about the following symptoms.

Pain in the chest

Ischaemic cardiac pain is usually related to increased cardiac work (as indicated by heart rate and systolic blood pressure) caused by exertion or emotion and is brief, being confined to that period of time of increased physical or emotional work. Whilst typically a tightness across the chest, ischaemic pain may be limited to one area, e.g. sternum, left scapula, one or both arms. Pain limited to one side of the chest and not immediately related to increased cardiac work is seldom due to cardiac ischaemia. It may be respiratory in origin or much more often is skeletal in origin and tends to last for hours at a time. A common cause is cervical spondylosis with root stimulation, and presumably the actual cause of the discomfort is secondary intercostal muscle spasm. Central sternal discomfort is much more difficult to evaluate. Apart from cardiac ischaemia, it may be due to oesophageal irritation from acid reflux and is usually then dominant at night in the reclining position and radiates vertically rather than across the chest.

Brief attacks (e.g. 0.5–5 minutes) of ischaemic pain without infarction may occur at rest and particularly at night, when they are relieved by sitting up. There are three principal causes:

1. Impending myocardial infarction (occurring in the next few days, thought to be due to transient obstruction of a narrow vessel relieved temporarily by natural lysis).
2. During a period of unstable angina and accompanied by severe angina of effort and may or may not culminate in infarction. Nocturnal attacks may be

Geriatric Cardiology. Principles and Practice.   Edited by A. Martin and A. J. Camm
© 1994 John Wiley & Sons Ltd

caused by increased cardiac work from restlessness, tachycardia, dreaming or possibly by suboxygenation from inefficient respiration.

3. Coronary spasm: this is relatively rare and is much more common in women than in men. It is usually benign but is associated with severe coronary disease in about half the patients with Prinzmetal's syndrome, in which ischaemic pain is associated with elevation of the S–T segment of the electrocardiogram (ECG) without infarction.

Dyspnoea on exertion

There are many causes:

1. Cardiac: raised left atrial and pulmonary venous pressure due to mitral stenosis or poor left ventricular function.
2. Respiratory: airways disease, bronchospasm or parenchymatous disease.
3. Obesity.
4. Anaemia.

Dyspnoea at rest

If the left atrial pressure is mildly or moderately elevated from mitral stenosis or impaired left ventricular function, a further increase may exceed the oncotic pressure exerted by the plasma proteins and will cause pulmonary oedema, relieved by reducing the right atrial pressure by sitting, standing, or moving from a bed to a chair. There are two main precipitating factors.

The first factor is tachycardia, causing shortening of the available ventricular filling time (e.g. paroxysmal atrial tachycardia or atrial fibrillation), particularly with old age when the left ventricle becomes more stiff. Tachycardia by itself, however, does not cause dyspnoea at rest even in old age if there is no disparity between the two ventricles.

The second factor is increased venous return resulting from maintaining the reclining position for several hours (e.g. middle of the night), in association with a relatively intact right ventricle increasing the flow of blood to the lungs. The patient is awakened by shortness of breath which makes him sit or stand, and lasts for minutes or an hour or two. With high pressures there is an irritating cough which may be accompanied by frothy white sputum, and this may be tinged with blood. The title of cardiac asthma is appropriate since the bronchial irritation may cause bronchospasm, and indeed at first sight and without a knowledge of the previous history bronchial asthma may be misdiagnosed, particularly as this may occur for the first time in old age. More often the problem is to differentiate anxious subjects who wake for other reasons and *later* notice difficult breathing. Patients with elevated pulmonary venous pressure learn to increase the number of pillows. If slipping down from elevated pillows does not produce awakening by dyspnoea, then the history of the requirement of increased pillows is probably spurious and the patient may be sleeping high because of nasal obstruction or bad advice. With anxiety, close questioning usually reveals that the problem is difficulty in getting a satisfactory deep breath and this may produce irregular sighing respiration or overbreathing, with all its secondary side-effects.

Palpitations: awareness of the heart beat from irregularity or increased rate

At least half the normal population have ectopic beats at times. These may be atrial or ventricular in origin and are usually premature, causing omission of the next sinus beat; the sequence is more easily diagnosed by auscultation than by palpation of the pulse. The irregularity of atrial fibrillation is often not noticed unless fast or associated with left ventricular disease causing increased resistance to filling, with short diastoles, or with mitral stenosis, when it will cause shortness of breath.

Paroxysmal tachycardia usually occurs spontaneously, though occasionally it is related to exertion or to a sudden movement. There may be symptoms from hypotension but no dyspnoea at rest or ischaemic pain in the absence of coronary disease. Thus these attacks are usually easily differentiated from emotional tachycardia.

Faints, dimming, or loss of consciousness

Simple 'benign' faints are usually life-long and often the tendency is inherited. They are gradual in onset and injury is rare. With sinoatrial disease (brady/tachy syndrome) the attacks of sinus slowing seldom cause loss of consciousness, usually occur at rest, and tend to be benign unless they occur during an activity such as driving; they may be interspersed with long periods of normality and therefore difficult to diagnose. Sudden attacks of complete loss of consciousness when cardiac in origin are usually due to atrioventricular conduction defects with constant evidence in the ECG of atrioventricular conduction delay or bundle branch block, but they may be secondary to high-rate tachycardias, usually ventricular. These matters are discussed in greater detail in Chapter 20.

Other causes of a sudden fall in blood pressure causing loss or dimming of consciousness are painless myocardial infarction, pulmonary embolism or an acute gastrointestinal bleed. The exclusion of epilepsy, where there is no fall of blood pressure or pallor, may be a problem and it should be remembered that fits may be secondary to sudden cerebral anoxia (e.g. Stokes–Adams attack).

The sudden onset of rotation from a primary disturbance of vestibular function is another cause of a 'dizzy turn', which should not be confused with dimming of consciousness. Occasionally, however, a fall in the blood pressure may produce rotation, perhaps because the vestibular apparatus is susceptible.

PHYSICAL EXAMINATION

Examination is best performed with the patient relaxed and reclining comfortably at an angle of 30–40° from the horizontal.

General appearance

Peripheral cyanosis due to lowered peripheral blood flow increasing oxygen extraction is extremely common in older people as a response to cold and diminished physical activity. It is only of significance when the patient is ill with a low cardiac output. The detection of *central cyanosis* requires daylight and examination of the tongue and interior of the mouth. It may be useful to have a 'control patient' who is known not to have central cyanosis. Exercise will increase central but not peripheral cyanosis. The presence or absence of anaemia, the type of respiration and shape of the chest, and the presence or absence of finger clubbing should be noted.

Arterial pulse (Figure 1)

Palpation of the radial pulse is used to analyse rate and rhythm, though much greater accuracy in detecting changes of rhythm is achieved by auscultation. It is convenient to palpate both right and left radial pulses simultaneously to check that they are approximately equal. Palpation of the *carotid pulse* is far superior for analysing the form of the pulse wave. The neck must be completely relaxed and angled slightly backwards, with the nape of the neck comfortably supported on a small pillow. Aortic systolic murmurs are common in the elderly, caused by unimportant stiffening of aortic cusps, and a normal sharp upstroke to the carotid pulse excludes significant aortic stenosis. Conversely, a *slow rising* carotid pulse is diagnostic of aortic stenosis, in the absence of a low cardiac output state. Analysis of the upstroke of the brachial pulse, best done with elbow flexed, is useful when the carotid pulse is difficult to feel. The brachial pulse is also the optimum pulse for detecting a *bisferiens pulse*, which is diagnostic of aortic stenosis combined with aortic regurgitation.

An *abnormally sharp* arterial pulse is best detected at the periphery and suggests increased stroke volume of the left ventricle and aortic 'run-off' from aortic regurgitation or other arteriovenous communication (including patent ductus arteriosus), but may be hard to diffferentiate from the big pulse pressure caused by rigid great vessels in old age. *Inspiratory diminution* of the arterial pulse is found in asthma owing to the large swings in intrathoracic pressure, and with cardiac tamponade where the diastolic volume of the heart is limited and inspiratory filling of the right heart diminishes left ventricular filling (Figure 2). Finally, *pulsus alternans* is regular in rhythm but the beat-to-beat amplitude varies from large to small (Figure 3).

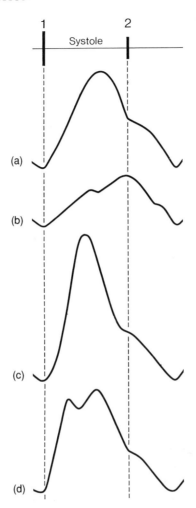

Figure 1. The arterial pulse waves. (a) Normal. (b) Slow rising. (c) Sharp ('water-hammer'). (d) Bisferiens. 1 and 2—first and second heart sounds. Reproduced with permission from Blackwell Scientific Publications

The arterial pressure

The use of an inflatable cuff, 12.5 cm wide for the average arm, and a mercury manometer, are still the standard recommendations for indirect measurement. The importance of multiple readings, including some with complete relaxation, cannot be over-emphasized. While a diastolic pressure of 95 mmHg or more is regarded as abnormal, the upper limit for a normal systolic pressure in subjects over 65 with diminished elasticity of the great vessels is debatable. A figure above

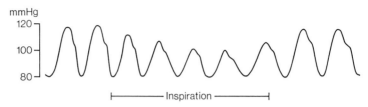

Figure 2. Pulses paradoxus: marked diminution of pulse amplitude during inspiration. Reproduced with permission from Blackwell Scientific Publications

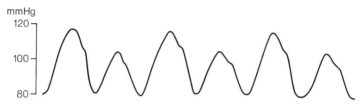

Figure 3. Pulsus alternans: alternate large- and small-amplitude pulses. Reproduced with permission from Blackwell Scientific Publications

160 mmHg systolic under relaxed conditions may prove to be undesirable. In elderly patients with episodes of dimming of consciousness, it is essential to take a standing pressure.

Examination of the fundi

Ophthalmoscopes with a narrow beam make it possible to examine the retina in a shaded room without dilatation of the pupil in most subjects. While papilloedema and retinopathy are now rare findings owing to the success of hypotensive therapy, the state of the retinal arterioles gives useful information, being fairly well correlated with mean diastolic pressure and degree of left ventricular hypertrophy. The retinal arterioles are normal with transient emotional hypertension. While mild arteriovenous crossing changes may be seen normally in old age, irregularity of lumen of arterioles (Figure 4) is diagnostic of diastolic hypertension.

Venous pressure and pulse waveform

The free transmission of the right atrial pressure pulse to the deep veins of the neck gives immediate visual information on the state of the right heart. With normal right atrial pressures the venous pressure is visible just above the clavicles (Figure 5) when the patient is reclining comfortably at 30–40° with the neck muscles completely relaxed. With right heart failure the height of the venous pulse above the sternal angle may be estimated fairly accurately, provided that the top of the wave can be clearly seen and differentiated from the underlying

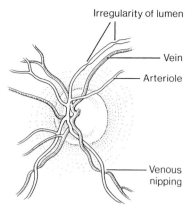

Figure 4. Irregularity of lumen of a retinal arteriole and nipping of veins at arteriovenous crossings indicate sustained diastolic hypertension. Reproduced with permission from Blackwell Scientific Publications

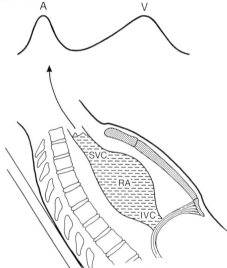

Figure 5. Jugular venous pulse rising unimpeded from RA to great veins just above level of the clavicle at 30–40°. SVC = superior vena cava; IVC = inferior vena cava. Reproduced with permission from Blackwell Scientific Publications

carotid pulse. A useful point is that the dominant movement of the venous pulse is inwards (the 'y' descent following the opening of the tricuspid valve), whereas carotid movement is outwards. Gentle pressure over the base of the neck with fingers or stethoscope tubing stops venous pulsation but not arterial. Pressure on the abdomen raises venous pressure but not the arterial. Full superficial veins are no indication of the deep venous pressure, and a high pressure seen in the left jugular vein only may be simply due to partial obstruction of the innominate vein by the arch of the aorta (Figure 6), disappearing as the mediastinum moves down with a deep inspiration.

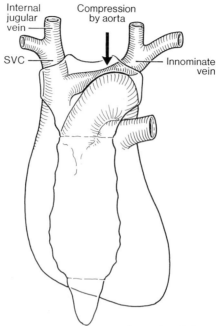

Figure 6. Jugular venous pressure may appear elevated and damped on the left owing to compression of the innominate vein by the aortic arch. SVC = superior vena cava. Reproduced with permission from Blackwell Scientific Publications

Thus an estimate of the height of the venous pressure is probably the most rewarding physical sign in the examination of the cardiovascular system. With the common problem of oedema of the ankles, a normal pressure excludes right heart failure, and an elevated pressure indicates right heart failure, or pericardial constriction, or hypervolaemia (superior mediastinal obstruction if there is no pulsation).

The waveform of the venous pulse is also of value in clinical diagnosis (Figure 7). The 'a' wave from right atrial contraction precedes the carotid upstroke (timed by palpation on the other side of the neck). The 'v' wave is due to the gradual rise of pressure in the right atrium when the tricuspid valve is shut in ventricular systole and is followed by the abrupt 'y' descent when the valve opens and is the most obvious wave in the normal venous pulse. With tricuspid stenosis or right ventricular hypertrophy (Figure 7b) the 'a' wave is prominent (even giant) and the 'y' descent slow. With tricuspid regurgitation (Figure 7c) transmission of the right ventricular pressure pulse to the right atrium causes a large pansystolic wave in the neck.

With ventricular ectopics stimulation of the atria is retrograde and delayed so that atrial contraction coincides with ventricular contraction and a closed tricuspid valve. This causes a large and sharp 'a' wave, aptly described as a cannon wave (Figure 7f). In a patient with an irregular pulse the presence of cannon waves excludes atrial fibrillation. Sporadic cannon waves occur when-

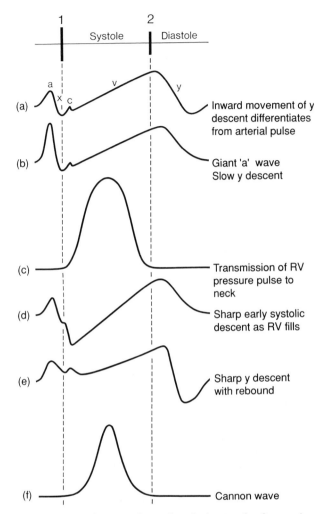

Figure 7. Jugular venous pulse waveforms in relation to the first and second sounds. (a) Normal. (b) Tricuspid stenosis; RV hypertrophy. (c) Tricuspid regurgitation. (d) Tamponade; constrictive pericarditis without calcification. (e) Constrictive pericarditis with calcification. (f) Atrial contraction during RV systole. Reproduced with permission from Blackwell Scientific Publications

ever there is a dissociation between atrial and ventricular contraction as in complete atrioventricular block or ventricular tachycardia. They occur regularly and rapidly with nodal tachycardia.

Palpation of the precordial impulse

While the position of the outward movement of the left ventricle forming the apex depends on several factors, and particularly the presence or absence of

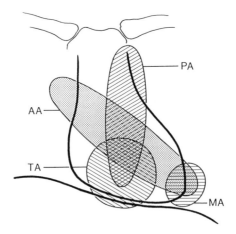

Figure 8. Sites for auscultation. MA = mitral area; TA = tricuspid area; AA = aortic area; PA = pulmonary area. Reproduced with permission from Blackwell Scientific Publications

scoliosis, the 'feel' of the left ventricle, particularly when the patient lies on the left side, gives very useful information. A sharp lift indicates hyperkinetic contraction from overloading (mitral regurgitation or aortic regurgitation) or anxiety, and a sustained lift indicates hypertrophy. The same applies to palpation of the right ventricle at the lower left sternal edge, tricuspid regurgitation and atrial septal defect with left to right shunt producing hyperkinetic impulses, and right ventricular hypertrophy a sustained impulse. With biventricular hyper-trophy these outward movements are separated by a small area of inward movement over the septum.

Auscultation

The stethoscope chestpiece should have a rigid diaphragm for detecting high-frequency sounds and murmurs, and a bell which, when applied lightly to the chest wall, transmits low-frequency sounds, e.g. ventricular filling sounds, and low-frequency diastolic murmurs such as a mitral diastolic murmur. The earpieces must fit comfortably and well; transmission of sound is more efficient through double tubing, and the patient should be in a comfortable reclining position, tipped partly to the left for auscultation at the apex.

The auscultatory areas are shown in Figure 8. The site of maximum intensity of a sound or murmur is useful but does not always decide its origin, e.g. the murmur of aortic stenosis is frequently loudest at the apex. The direction of selective spread (e.g. axilla in mitral regurgitation) and the effect of respiration are also useful factors to take into account.

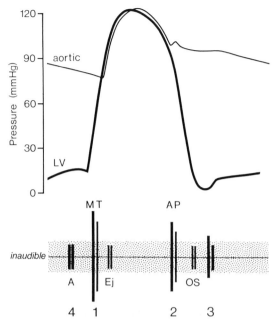

Figure 9. The heart sounds and their relation to the LV and aortic pressure pulses (RV pulse occurs 10–20 ms later). Left-sided events precede right except for RA contraction (sinus node in RA) and RV ejection (low pressure in PA). 4 and A = atrial sounds (right and left); 1 = first sound, mitral (M) and tricuspid (T) components: Ej = ejection sounds (pulmonary and aortic); 2 = second sound, aortic (A) and pulmonary (P) components; OS = opening snaps of mitral and tricuspid valves; 3 = third sounds (left and right). Only those sounds spreading beyond the shaded area are audible in a normal subject. Reproduced with permission from Blackwell Scientific Publications

HEART SOUNDS (Figure 9)

There are two groups of sounds, each with a different mechanism of production and different acoustic characteristics, making identification easy.

Valve sounds are of high frequency and best heard with the rigid diaphragm of the stethoscope. They coincide with the final halt of opening and closing valves as shown by echocardiograms taken simultaneously with phonocardiograms. The following valve sounds will be discussed separately: first heart sounds and ejection sounds, and second heart sounds and opening snaps.

Ventricular filling sounds are of low frequency and therefore more difficult to hear because of the poor sensitivity of the hearing mechanism to low-frequency sound. They are best heard with a large bell and comprise the rapid filling third heart sounds and the atrial or fourth heart sounds.

Thus there are six heart sounds (four from the valve, two from ventricular filling) and since left and right ventricular contraction are slightly asynchronous, 12 sounds must be considered.

Valve sounds

First heart sounds

Close splitting of the first sound into a louder mitral and softer tricuspid component can be heard at the lower left sternal edge (tricuspid area) in most normal subjects (Figure 10a). Contraction of the left ventricle first causes closure of the mitral valve, and the intensity of the sound caused by the final halt of the closing valve depends on its relation to the left ventricular pressure pulse, which starts slowly and later becomes rapid (Figure 11). Thus mitral closure is soft

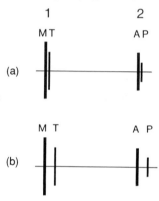

Figure 10. First heart sounds. (a) Physiological splitting of first sound. (b) Wide splitting of first (and second) sounds. (Right bundle branch block, pacing from LV, LV ectopic.) M and T = mitral and tricuspid components of first sound. A and P = aortic and pulmonary components of second sound. Reproduced with permission from Blackwell Scientific Publications

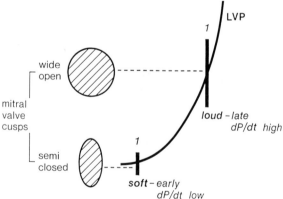

Figure 11. Variations in intensity of first sound depend on the position of the cusps of the AV valves (mainly mitral) at the start of contraction. A wide open valve takes longer to reach its final closure point (causing the sound), which therefore occurs on a later and steeper part of the LVP (LV (pressure) pulse) with greater velocity. A semi-closed valve reaches its final closure point early when pressure change is slower. Reproduced with permission from Blackwell Scientific Publications

when early, and this occurs when the leaflets are already semi-closed at the onset of left ventricular systole (e.g. low flow, long diastole). Conversely, mitral closure is loud when delayed until the steeper part of the left ventricular pressure pulse and this occurs when the leaflets are wide open at the end of diastole (high flow or high left atrial pressure from mitral stenosis). The intensity of the first sound also varies with the P–R interval. Atrial contraction reopens the leaflets, and if the P–R interval is long enough (0.2 s or more) the eddies from ventricular filling semi-close the valve (Figure 12) before ventricular contraction, resulting in a soft first sound. With a short P–R interval the valve is wide open at the start of ventricular contraction and closure is therefore delayed until the later, steeper part of the left ventricular pressure pulse, and the sound is loud. In practice the commonest cause of a loud first sound is a short P–R interval and if this is absent it is important to look for other evidence of mitral stenosis.

Varying intensity of the first sound occurs with an irregular rhythm (e.g. atrial fibrillation), being loud following a short diastole (cusps open—mitral closure late) and soft with long diastoles (cusps semi-closed—mitral closure early). With regular rhythm, varying intensity of the first sound indicates varying relationship between atrial and ventricular contraction (e.g. complete atrioventricular dissociation).

The second or tricuspid component of a split first heart sound (Figure 10) is much softer and often confined to the tricuspid area, though louder with sternal

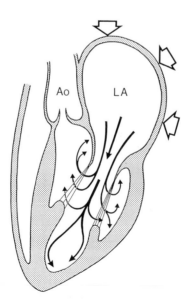

Figure 12. Reopening and closing of mitral valve following left atrial (LA) contraction (broad arrows). Ao = aorta. Reproduced with permission from Blackwell Scientific Publications

depression when the heart is closer to the stethoscope. The influence of P–R interval on intensity is less than on the left side of the heart since right atrial contraction is less efficient than left atrial because of greater 'run-off'. Tricuspid closure is loud, however, with high rates of flow such as with a left-to-right shunting atrial septal defect. Splitting of the first sound is abnormally wide if tricuspid closure is delayed from right bundle branch block, left ventricular pacing, or when a ventricular ectopic is left-sided (Figure 10b).

Ejection sounds in early systole (Figure 13) are heard when the aortic or pulmonary valves have restrictive cusp tissue which cannot fold into the vessel wall during ejection; they coincide with the halt of the upgoing valve on the echo and disappear when the valve becomes rigid and calcified. Aortic ejection sounds are best recognized at the apex and occur soon (60 ms) after the mitral component of the first sound and when isolated are due to a congenitally bicuspid aortic valve. When heard in association with aortic regurgitation the sound indicates that the cause of the regurgitation is almost certainly a bicuspid valve.

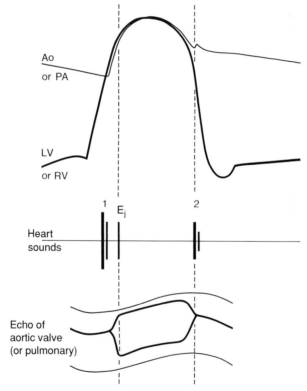

Figure 13. Ejection sounds (Ej) occur on the upstroke of the aortic or pulmonary pressure pulse and coincide with the final half of the opening aortic (or pulmonary) valve on the echo. Reproduced with permission from Blackwell Scientific Publications

When splitting of the first heart sound is wide from right bundle branch block, the later tricuspid component may simulate an aortic ejection sound but is maximal in the tricuspid area rather than at the apex. Pulmonary ejection sounds occur with pulmonary valve stenosis and are earlier in systole because of the short isovolumic time of the right ventricle.They also occur with pulmonary hypertension (mechanism unknown) and are much later then because of the prolonged isovolumic time of the right ventricle.

Mid- or late systolic sounds, either isolated or preceding a late systolic murmur, are heard with stretched, floppy, prolapsing mitral valves.

Second heart sounds (Figure 14)

The normal inspiratory splitting of the second sound heard in the pulmonary area is due to delay in closure of the pulmonary valve from the inspiratory increase in stroke volume of the right ventricle, but is less easily detected in older subjects because the intensity of the sounds tends to be reduced (probably because of hyperinflation), and a relatively soft pulmonary component may not be audible. P2 is loud and delayed in atrial septal defect and the splitting is 'fixed' (Figure 14d, equal inspiratory delay of A2 and P2). P2 is late in right bundle branch block (Figure 14b), right heart failure and pulmonary stenosis (Figure 14c). The splitting is also wide in mitral regurgitation when A2 is early because of diminished resistance to left ventricular outflow (Figure 14e). Reversed splitting of the second sound due to delay of A2 is easily picked up in the pulmonary area and tricuspid areas since the split is maximal in expiration and diminishes on inspiration as P2 delays (Figure 14f). It is usually obvious in left bundle block but also occurs with prolongation of left ventricular systole from relatively unimportant systolic hypertension. An abnormally loud P2 from pulmonary hypertension exceeds A2 in intensity in the pulmonary area and is transmitted to the mitral area (Figure 14g).

Opening snaps (Figure 15)

The final halt of the opening of the mitral and tricuspid valves produces minor vibrations which become increased in intensity and audible when movement of the cusps valve is abnormally rapid, or the resistance to inflow (cusp fusion) is increased. In practice an audible opening snap is the best physical sign of mitral stenosis (Figure 18) but unfortunately is less obvious or absent in the older age groups when the valve is rigid and calcified. Soft mitral snaps may be audible with rapidly moving cusps in mitral regurgitation, and tricuspid snaps are heard with tricuspid stenosis, atrial septal defect, and Ebstein's anomaly. Snaps are high frequency and similar in quality to P2 but later (0.1 s after A2) and are heard over a wider area, usually including the apex. In difficult cases a search should be made for three high-frequency sounds in rapid succession during inspiration (A2, P2, opening snap) and two in expiration (fused A2 and P2 and opening snap).

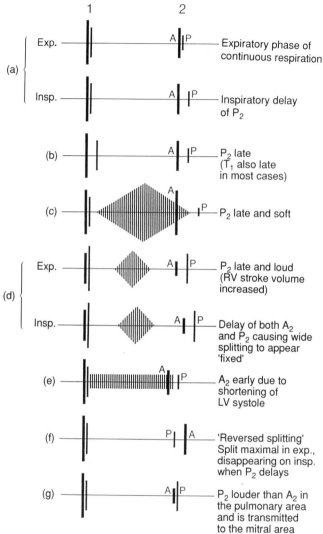

Figure 14. Second heart sound in pulmonary area. (a) Normal. (b) Right bundle branch block. (c) Pulmonary stenosis. (d) Atrial septal defect. (e) Mitral regurgitation. (f) Left bundle branch block; aortic stenosis; systolic hypertension. (g) Pulmonary hypertension. Reproduced with permission from Blackwell Scientific Publications

Ventricular filling sounds (Figure 16)

These low-frequency sounds, best heard with a stethoscope bell, are caused by the halting of the ventricular wall following ventricular filling. There are two varieties.

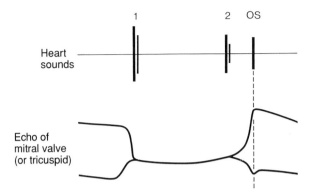

Figure 15. Opening snaps of the mitral (or tricuspid) valve coinciding with the final halt of the opening valve on the echo. Reproduced with permission from Blackwell Scientific Publications

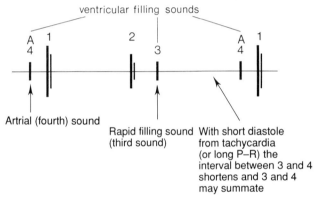

Figure 16. Ventricular filling sounds. Reproduced with permission from Blackwell Scientific Publications

Rapid filling third heart sound

A third heart sound is normally heard over the apex of the left ventricle in children and young adults under good auscultatory conditions with the patient inclined to the left. The sound is about 150 ms after A2 and becomes inaudible (though recordable) in middle age as the ventricle stiffens and filling becomes less rapid. It becomes audible again with increased rate of filling from high left atrial pressure from left ventricular failure or mitral regurgitation (without stenosis). Third sounds are heard over the right ventricle at the lower left sternal edge with right ventricular failure and tricuspid regurgitation.

Atrial or fourth sound

This sound coincides with the halt of the extra ventricular filling which follows atrial contraction and is never audible with a normal heart (though it can be recorded), unless the P–R interval is long (causing summation with rapid filling). When heard it is a useful indication of ventricular hypertrophy (e.g. cardiomyopathy or hypertension) or fibrosis (e.g. myocardial infarction). An atrial sound may be difficult to differentiate from the first component of a split first sound when this is of low frequency (e.g. P–R interval of 200 ms or more) and a phonocardiogram is then required to show the relation of the sound to the QRS complex.

Summation of atrial and third vibrations causing an audible sound occurs with shortening of diastole from tachycardia (rates of 90 or more) or a long P–R interval (more than 220 ms), and then has no significance.

HEART MURMURS (Figure 17)

Murmurs are caused by turbulence of blood flowing through valves or ventricular outflow tracts. They are classified by their relation to the heart sounds and phases of the cardiac cycle.

1. Systolic
     Midsystolic (ejection)
     Pansystolic (regurgitant)
2. Diastolic
     Early diastolic (regurgitant)
     Mid- or delayed diastolic (ventricular filling)
     Atrial systolic (presystolic–ventricular filling)
3. Continuous
4. Pericardial friction rub

The site of maximum intensity is useful (see Figure 8) but may be misleading (e.g. aortic ejection murmurs are often maximal at the apex). Large pressure gradients generate high-velocity and high-frequency murmurs and small pressure gradients low-velocity and low-frequency murmurs. The intensity is conveniently graded into four grades: 1 = soft; 2 = moderate; 3 = loud; 4 = very loud and palpated as a thrill.

Systolic murmurs

Midsystolic (ejection) murmurs

From the left or right ventricular outflow tract or valves, these are recognized by the cessation before the relevant component of the second heart sound as outflow diminishes before valve closure (Figure 17a). Left ventricular ejection murmurs

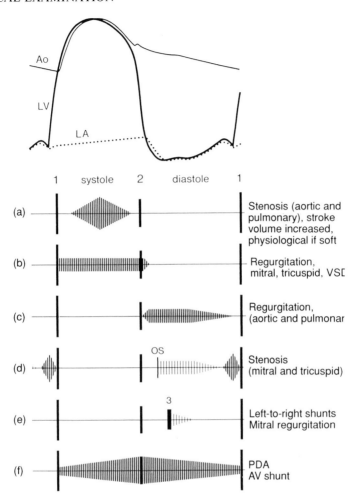

Figure 17. Murmurs and their relation to the pressure pulses. (a) Midsystolic ejection (high frequency). (b) Pansystolic (high frequency). (c) Regurgitant early diastolic (high frequency). (d) Ventricular filling across obstruction (low frequency). (e) Ventricular filling from increased flow or turbulence (low frequency). (f) Continuous. Reproduced with permission from Blackwell Scientific Publications

are common in the elderly and often maximal at the apex and only distinguishable from mitral regurgitant murmurs by their relation to the second heart sound. Soft ejection murmurs (grade 1 or 2) are caused by stiffening of aortic cusps without obstruction (aortic sclerosis). Loud murmurs (grade 3 or 4) usually indicate aortic stenosis and are accompanied by a slow rising carotid pulse and left ventricular hypertrophy. Assessment may be difficult if all heart sounds and murmurs are reduced in intensity by hyperinflation or a thick chest wall. Ejection murmurs vary in intensity with varying stroke volume (e.g. atrial fibrillation).

Even with stenosis the murmur is soft when the preceding diastole is short (e.g. premature beat) or with low cardiac output from left ventricular failure even in regular rhythm. Indeed aortic stenosis should always be thought of as a possibility with unexplained left ventricular failure and no obvious murmur during a period of very low cardiac output. The diagnosis of aortic stenosis may also be difficult if A2 (the sole component of the second sound at the apex) is reduced in intensity by calcification. Differentiation from mitral regurgitation is then achieved by palpation of the carotid pulse. The presence or absence of left ventricular hypertrophy is very useful unless there is associated systolic hypertension, which could equally be the cause and is so common in the elderly. Left ventricular ejection murmurs may also be caused by increased stroke volume from aortic regurgitation without obstruction. Subaortic obstruction may produce similar ejection systolic murmurs. Congenital causes are rare in the older age groups but hypertrophic cardiomyopathy is an occasional cause and is differentiated from aortic valve stenosis by its sharp arterial pulse, and the ejection murmur is later.

Right ventricular ejection murmurs are uncommon in the older age groups except in a left-to-right shunting atrial septal defect, where the increased stroke volume produces a moderately loud midsystolic murmur audible in the pulmonary area and over most of the precordium because of the dilated right ventricle. Further evidence of atrial septal defect lies in the palpable hyperkinetic right ventricle, and the wide fixed splitting of the second sound, and this diagnosis should be considered with unexplained heart failure and atrial fibrillation even in the elderly.

Pansystolic (regurgitant) murmurs

From mitral or tricuspid regurgitation or from a left-to-right shunting ventricular septal defect, these murmurs continue right up to and beyond the relevant valve closure sound (Figure 17b) in keeping with the pressure gradient from the left ventricle to left atrium. Thus A2 is inaudible at the apex when a mitral systolic murmur is loud. Here the intensity of the murmur bears no relation to the severity of the mitral regurgitation and the murmur is fairly constant with varying stroke volume. An apical murmur confined to late systole, however, is nearly always an indication of only mild mitral regurgitation.

Diastolic murmurs

Early diastolic (regurgitant) murmurs (Figure 17c)

These murmurs start immediately after aortic or pulmonary valve closure when the valve is regurgitant and continue throughout diastole, unless the regurgitation is trivial, because of the pressure gradient between great artery and ventricle.

The murmur of aortic regurgitation is high pitched because of the large pressure gradient between aorta and left ventricle and is therefore best heard with a rigid diaphragm chestpiece. It is usually maximal near the fourth left interspace over the aortic valve, but is maximal superiorly and to the right of the sternum if the aorta is dilated. The murmur is best heard with the patient sitting forward in held expiration (the noise of respiration has the same frequency). The presence of an aortic ejection sound indicates that there is a biscupid aortic valve which is probably the cause of the regurgitation. The presence of an additional apical diastolic murmur does not necessarily indicate that the mitral valve is also affected and therefore that the aetiology is rheumatic, since the apical murmur may be due to the Austin Flint phenomenon (aortic regurgitant jet forcing the anterior cusp of the mitral valve into the ventricular filling stream).

Pulmonary regurgitation is usually secondary to a dilated valve ring from pulmonary hypertension when it is high pitched because of the high-velocity regurgitant jet and is then indistinguishable from the murmur of aortic regurgitation, except that it is usually maximal about the third left space rather than the fourth. It is differentiated from aortic regurgitation by looking for evidence of pulmonary hypertension (right ventricular hypertrophy and an enlarged main pulmonary artery on X-ray) with no sharp arterial pulse or left ventricular hypertrophy.

Mid-(delayed) diastolic (ventricular filling) murmurs (Figure 17d,e)

These murmurs are low-frequency rumbles due to low-velocity forward flow, and are best heard with the bell chestpiece gently applied. They start appreciably after the second sound, occurring during the rapid filling phase after isovolumic relaxation. Respiration should not be halted as this diminishes flow. They may be due to obstruction, and with mitral stenosis the murmur is maximal at the apex with the patient inclined to the left (Figure 18). The murmur begins after the opening snap and is long if the stenosis is severe, but short if mild because there is then no gradient in late diastole. Duration is much more important than intensity for assessing severity. With tricuspid stenosis the murmur is maximal at the lower left sternal edge and increased by inspiration.

Short ventricular filling murmurs (Figure 17e) may also be caused by high rates of flow without obstruction as with severe mitral regurgitation or with left-to-right shunts (patent ductus arteriosus and ventricular septal defect). Tricuspid flow murmurs are maximal at the left sternal edge and during inspiration and may be secondary to tricuspid regurgitation or left-to-right shunting atrial septal defect. Flow murmurs are always short since there is no prolongation of ventricular filling.

Ventricular filling murmurs may also be caused by turbulence as with vegetations from acute rheumatic valvulitis and also with severe aortic regurgitation due to the regurgitant jet from the aortic valve striking the anterior cusp of the mitral valve (Austin Flint murmur).

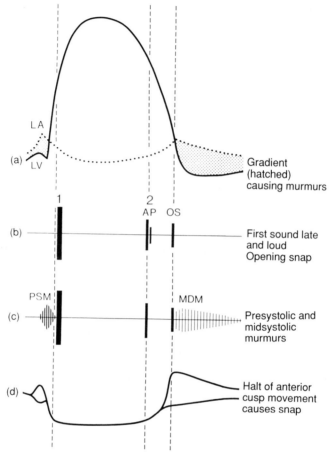

Figure 18. Mitral stenosis: auscultatory findings. A = aortic; P = pulmonary; OS = opening snap; MDM = mid-diastolic murmur; PSM = presystolic murmur. (a) Pressure pulses. (b) Lower left sternal edge. (c) Apex. (d) Echo of mitral valve. Reproduced with permission from Blackwell Scientific Publications

Atrial systolic (presystolic) murmurs

These are caused by increased flow from atrial contraction immediately preceding the first sound. The best example is mitral stenosis (Figure 17d).

Continuous murmurs (Figure 17f)

These murmurs are due to a communication in the circulation with a continuous pressure gradient throughout the cardiac cycle. They may be caused by a patent ductus arteriosus or by any arteriovenous fistula.

Pericardial friction rub

Pericarditis without appreciable effusion causes a 'murmur', usually of a quality different from an intracardiac murmur, and sounding closer to the stethoscope. It coincides with heart movement in midsystole and during ventricular filling (rapid filling phase in mid-diastole and in atrial asystole). All three components are louder during inspiration, when increased flow of blood into the heart increases the friction. They may also be louder with increased pressure on the stethoscope.

THE PRACTICAL VALUE OF ANALYSIS OF THE HEART SOUNDS AND MURMURS IN GERIATRIC MEDICINE

Heart sounds

A loud first heart sound, particularly in association with atrial fibrillation, may be due to mitral stenosis (acute rheumatic fever was common up to the 1940s) and a close search should be made for an opening snap and a mitral diastolic murmur since unsuspected mitral stenosis in the elderly is a not uncommon cause of thromboembolism. Wide splitting of the first (and second) sounds may be due to right bundle branch block, which is occasionally evidence of important disease of the conducting tissue causing syncope. Varying intensity of the first sound with regular rhythm is diagnostic of atrioventricular dissociation. An isolated aortic ejection sound indicates that the aortic valve is biscuspid and may become stenotic from calcium deposition, or become infected. Wide 'fixed' splitting of the second heart sound raises the possibility of an atrial septal defect, which is not uncommon as a cause of atrial fibrillation and heart failure in the elderly, but may be difficult to distinguish from a late P2 from heart failure or right bundle branch block. The finding of reversed splitting of the second sound is an indication of prolongation of left ventricular systole, and the commonest cause is left bundle branch block which is nearly always an indication of myocardial disease or an important defect in conduction.

A third sound after middle age is useful evidence for potential or actual left ventricular failure in the absence of mitral regurgitation. An atrial sound raises the possibility of hyptertrophic cardiomyopathy or in hypertensives is a useful indication that the average pressure has been high enough to cause hypertrophy and to warrant therapy.

Heart murmurs

An aortic ejection murmur is common in elderly subjects due to increasing rigidity and calcification in aortic cusps. Biscuspid valves deteriorate in this way 10–20 years before the normal tricuspid valve. In the vast majority the stiffening is not sufficient to cause significant stenosis and the carotid pulse and left ventricle remain normal. With a moderate or loud ejection murmur (which may be maximal at the apex) significant stenosis will invariably produce slowing of the carotid upstroke and almost invariably left ventricular hypertrophy clinically and on the electrocardiogram. Palpation of the carotid pulse is the best sign since in old people with rigid great vessels this pulse is normally sharp. Furthermore, left ventricular hypertrophy is not specific to aortic stenosis. An echocardiogram is extremely useful in doubtful cases showing calcification of the valve (except with rheumatic aortic stenosis when calcium may be absent), and Doppler gradients assessed by an expert are very useful.

Apical pansystolic or late systolic murmurs are also common in the elderly because floppy valves tend to become regurgitant with the passage of years. The murmur by itself is no indication of severity except that a late systolic murmur indicates that the regurgitation is mild. Doppler assessment, even when aided by colour, is extremely difficult and the electrocardiogram is insensitive. Thus in the presence of a loud apical pansystolic murmur, attention should be concentrated on the presence or absence of a hyperkinetic left ventricle on palpation, of a third heart sound as a measure of the rate of ventricular filling, and above all the end systolic dimension and force of contraction of the left ventricle on the echocardiogram.

ACKNOWLEDGEMENTS

I am grateful to Blackwell Scientific Publications for permission to reproduce the figures from *Lecture Notes on Cardiology* by Aubrey Leatham, Catherine Bull and Mark V. Braimbridge, 3rd edition, 1991. The auscultatory diagrams are adapted from phonocardiograms published in *Auscultation of the Heart and Phonocardiography*, 2nd edition, Churchill Livingstone, 1975, and Figure 4 from The retinal vessels in hypertension, *Quarterly Journal of Medicine*, 1949; 18: 203, by Aubrey Leatham.

6 Echocardiography

STEPHEN J. D. BRECKER AND PAUL J. OLDERSHAW
Royal Brompton National Heart and Lung Hospital, UK

Since its introduction into clinical medicine over 20 years ago, the use of ultrasound has expanded dramatically to become a major diagnostic tool in cardiology. Echocardiography is able to provide detailed information about cardiac anatomy and physiology, and is a cheap, safe, non-invasive procedure, particularly suitable for elderly patients. Its non-invasive nature makes it convenient as a means of investigating patients during follow-up, and repeated measurements may be made over the course of many years.

TECHNICAL ASPECTS

Ultrasound, by definition, has a frequency above that perceived by the human ear (20 kHz), and most cardiac applications utilize frequencies between 2 and 7.5 MHz. Ultrasonic compression waves are generated by piezoelectric crystals, which vibrate at a predetermined frequency when a short-pulse electric voltage is applied to them. Such waves are transmitted as longitudinal vibrations through tissue. When the wave encounters a boundary between two tissues of differing physical properties, such as blood and valvular tissue, a percentage of the energy is reflected. Returning compression waves impinging upon the crystals will generate small electric signals, so enabling the transducer to act as a microphone. The electrical information thus obtained is then classically displayed in one of two formats, known as M-mode and two-dimensional echocardiography.

MODALITIES OF ECHOCARDIOGRAPHY

M-mode echocardiography

M- or motion-mode echocardiography produces a recording of motion along a thin slice through the heart, and is derived from a single beam of ultrasound of high frequency. Using such a beam, the maximum sampling rate (i.e. rate of emission and receipt of sound from the crystals) will be limited by the time taken for an impulse to travel to the deepest cardiac structure, and back again. This imposes a *maximum* repetition rate of approximately 3000 per second, and the usual sampling rate of M-mode is 1000 pulses per second. This represents one of

Geriatric Cardiology. Principles and Practice. Edited by A. Martin and A. J. Camm
© 1994 John Wiley & Sons Ltd

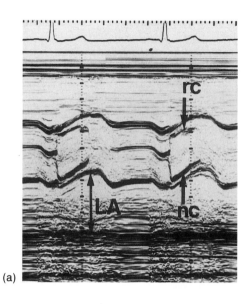

(a)

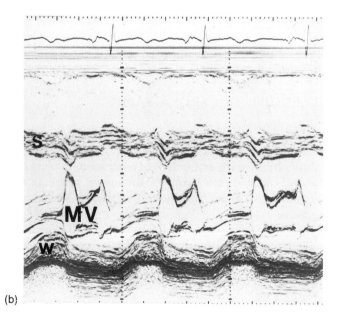

(b)

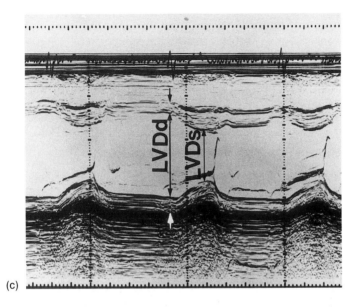

(c)

Figure 1. (a) (opposite) M-mode echocardiogram of the aorta, aortic valve and left atrium from a normal subject. The aortic valve is seen between the anterior and posterior aortic roots with the right coronary cusp (rc), and the non-coronary cusp (nc) open widely in systole, almost in apposition with the aortic walls. The left atrium (LA) is posterior to the aorta and its dimension is measured at end ejection (double arrows). (b) (opposite) M-mode echocardiogram from a normal subject obtained through the basal region of the left ventricle, showing the septum (s) and the left ventricular cavity, with the anterior and posterior leaflets of the mitral valve (MV) and the posterior LV wall (w). (c) M-mode echocardiogram of the normal left ventricle at the tips of the mitral leaflets, showing end-diastolic dimension (LVDd), end-diastolic septal and posterior wall thicknesses, and left ventricular end-systolic dimension (LVDs). Note the similar excursion of the septum and posterior wall. Parts (a)–(c) reproduced by permission of Blackwell Scientific Publications, Inc., from St John Sutton and Oldershaw (eds) (1989), *Textbook of Adult and Pediatric Echocardiography and Doppler*

the highest degrees of temporal resolution available for clinical measurement, and provides a large amount of information from a localized segment of the heart. Echoes are printed onto moving photosensitive paper, which can be kept as a permanent record.

Three standard M-mode cuts are commonly used in routine examination, obtained by altering the transducer angulation on the chest wall. These are: (i) at the level of the aortic root with left atrium behind (Figure 1a); (ii) at the mitral leaflets (Figure 1b); and (iii) through the left ventricular cavity, just below the level of the tips of the mitral leaflets (Figure 1c). M-mode echocardiography enables cavity dimension and wall thickness to be accurately determined, and with simultaneous phono- and electrocardiography physiological measurements of wall motion and time intervals may be obtained. The M-mode echocardiogram, far from becoming obsolete, contributes significant information unobtainable in any other way. Computer analysis of M-mode traces provides further information such as peak rate of cavity dimension increase, and rate of posterior wall thinning, which are physiologically useful measures of left ventricular diastolic function.

Two-dimensional or cross-sectional echocardiography

Two-dimensional or cross-sectional echocardiography produces a 'realtime' image of the heart, and is the modality of choice for displaying anatomy. It does so by acquiring echoes from a sector made up of approximately 100 lines, each with a frame rate of approximately 30 per second. With *phased array* transducers, the beam of ultrasound is steered electrically by firing sequential beams of ultrasound from an array of crystals. *Mechanical* scanners utilize rotating crystals which fire up to 30 times per second, so producing an image.

Echocardiographic access to the heart is limited to only four sites utilizing the transthoracic approach. These comprise the parasternal position, the apex, the subcostal approach (beneath the ribs) and the suprasternal notch. Not all views will be obtainable from every patient, and versatility of approach will enable the maximum information to be obtained. A series of standardized views from each approach has evolved to form the complete transthoracic two-dimensional study. The parasternal views examine the left ventricle, aorta and left atrium, either in long (Figure 2) or short axis. Transducer angulation will demonstrate three levels of short-axis image: the aortic valve (Figure 3a), mitral orifice (Figure 3b) and left ventricular cavity (Figure 3c). The apical approach will provide a four-chamber view (Figure 4), and by angulating the transducer upwards will allow a four-chamber with left ventricular outflow/aortic root view (the so-called 'five-chamber view') to be obtained (Figure 5). The subcostal view may prove invaluable in elderly patients, in whom obesity, lung disease, chest wall deformities or kyphoscoliosis may prevent images being obtained from the above approaches. The suprasternal view may provide information about the great arteries, including aneurysms and aortic dissections, but in a significant number of patients it will prove impossible to obtain diagnostic images from this approach.

Doppler echocardiography

Doppler echocardiography is an application of cardiac ultrasound which enables the position, direction and velocity of blood flow within the heart to be accurately assessed. Ultrasound waves, when reflected by a moving object (i.e. red blood cells), will return with a frequency different from that of the emitted ultrasound.

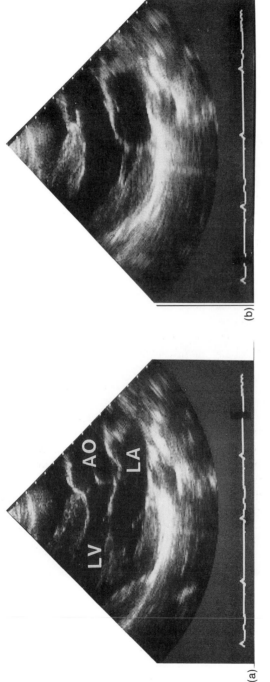

Figure 2. (a) Two-dimensional echocardiogram of the long axis of the left ventricle in a normal subject in diastole, showing the aortic valve, the mitral leaflets and subvalve tensor apparatus, the septum and the posterior LV wall. The thoracic aorta is visible posterior to the atrioventricular groove at the left ventricular–left atrial junction. (b) Two-dimensional echocardiogram of the long axis of the left ventricle in a normal subject in systole. The aortic valve leaflets open and are retracted into their respective sinuses of Valsalva. The mitral valve is in the closed position with the left atrium posterior to the aorta. Parts (a) and (b) reproduced by permission of Blackwell Scientific Publications, Inc., from St John Sutton and Oldershaw (eds) (1989), *Textbook of Adult and Pediatric Echocardiography and Doppler*

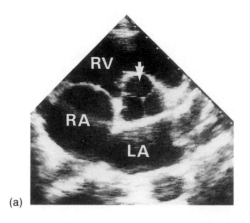

(a)

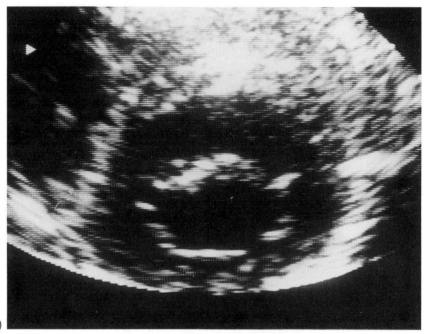

(b)

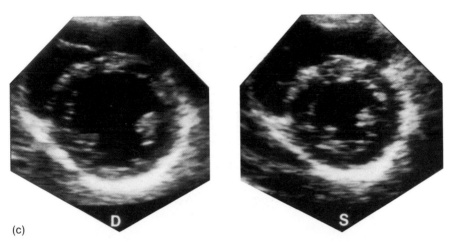

(c)

Figure 3. (a) (opposite) Two-dimensional echocardiogram of the short-axis view of the aorta at aortic valve level in diastole, showing the three aortic valve leaflets. The right coronary cusp is superior (arrow), the non-coronary cusp is on the left, and the left coronary cusp is on the right. The left atrium is posterior, the tricupsid valve is on the left, and the right ventricular outflow tract wraps around the aorta superiorly. (b) (opposite) Two-dimensional echocardiogram of the short-axis view of the left ventricle through the basal segment, showing the mitral valve open in diastole. (c) Two-dimensional echocardiogram of the short-axis view from a patient with a normal left ventricle. The view is at the level of the papillary muscles. D = diastole, S = systole. Parts (a) and (c) reproduced by permission of Blackwell Scientific Publications, Inc., from St John Sutton and Oldershaw (eds) (1989), *Textbook of Adult and Pediatric Echocardiography and Doppler*

The difference between the transmitted and reflected frequencies represents the Doppler frequency shift, and is proportional to the velocity of the moving object.

Three applications of Doppler echocardiography are commonly used.

Continuous wave

Ultrasonic energy is continuously transmitted and received by separate crystals in the same transducer. All the information along the line of the ultrasound beam is displayed, permitting the calculation of the peak velocity of blood. Experience and a smooth, complete spectral envelope will confirm that the angulation of the transducer along the line of maximal velocity is correct.

Pulsed wave

A pulse of waves is emitted, and information from a specific point or 'sample volume' is received. The peak recordable velocity is limited by the *pulse repetition frequency*. Any flow with velocities above this will be misinterpreted as being in the opposite direction. This technical problem is known as *aliasing*. For analysis of normal transmitral or transtricuspid flow, pulsed wave Doppler is the mode of choice, allowing flow at a specified depth to be examined.

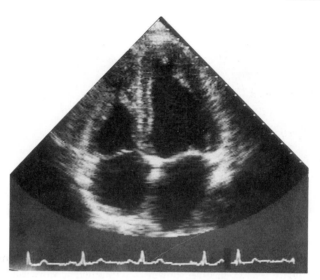

Figure 4. Two-dimensional echocardiogram of the apical four-chamber view in systole, showing the closed tricupsid and mitral valves. Reproduced by permission of Blackwell Scientific Publications, Inc., from St John Sutton and Oldershaw (eds) (1989), *Textbook of Adult and Pediatric Echocardiography and Doppler*

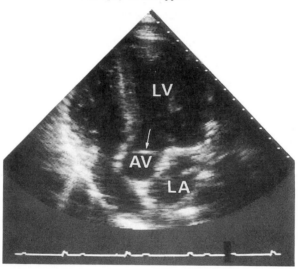

Figure 5. Two-dimensional echocardiogram obtained from the apex, showing the five-chamber view. The fifth chamber is the left ventricular outflow tract. The other four chambers include the right and left ventricles and right and left atria. The aortic valve (arrow) can be seen in the closed position. Reproduced by permission of Blackwell Scientific Publications, Inc., from St John Sutton and Oldershaw (eds) (1989), *Textbook of Adult and Pediatric Echocardiography and Doppler*

Colour flow mapping

Pulsed Doppler information about many different points can be superimposed upon a cross-sectional or M-mode echocardiogram. The direction of flow is assigned a colour, and a 'flow map' can be displayed in real time on the two-dimensional image (Figure 6).

ADJUNCTIVE TECHNIQUES

Transoesophageal echocardiography

A recent development has been to place a small phased array transducer (5 MHz) to the tip of a standard gastroscope, to enable imaging from a transoesophageal approach. This technique demonstrates anatomy with a high degree of spatial resolution, and provides excellent image quality in almost every patient. Pulsed wave Doppler and colour flow mapping allow useful physiological information to be obtained, and the latest developments are the addition of continuous wave Doppler and biplane capability. The technique of transducer placement is similar to that of upper gastrointestinal endoscopy, but is performed blind. Operators must therefore be familiar with endoscopic techniques. Patients must be free of oesophageal pathology, and be nil by mouth for at least 4 hours before the procedure. Explanation of the technique and the sensations that the patient will experience by a confident operator may permit the procedure to be performed on an outpatient basis without sedation. Elderly patients tolerate the technique at least as well as the young, and in some instances better. Whilst avoidance of benzodiazepine is desirable in the elderly, some patients will require sedation.

Contrast echocardiography

The rapid intravenous injection of 5–10 ml of saline, agitated with a small amount of the patient's blood, will show up as a stream of moving echoes produced by the microbubbles within the fluid. If a right-to-left shunt is present, the contrast echoes may be demonstrated in the left heart, either on the two-dimensional image or on M-mode. This represents a sensitive, cheap, non-invasive method of investigation of a possible intracardiac shunt. Methods such as this represent a significant advantage in the elderly, who might otherwise require cardiac catheterization.

ADVANTAGES AND LIMITATIONS OF ECHOCARDIOGRAPHY

In order to maximize comfort to patient and operator, and to enhance the capabilities of the investigation, a dedicated area should be assigned to echocardiography. The room should be large enough to contain the equipment, patient and operator comfortably. It should be maintained at a comfortable temperature, and be capable of being darkened sufficiently to make the display

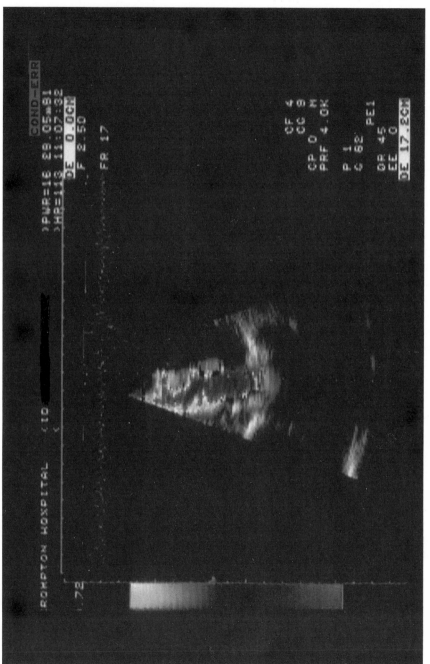

Figure 6. Two-dimensional echocardiogram with Doppler colour flow mapping. The image is obtained from the apex, and shows a xenograft in the mitral position. Turbulent flow through the xenograft is demonstrated by aliasing within the colour flow jet

visible. Under these circumstances elderly patients find the investigation atraumatic. In many situations, high-quality echocardiography removes the need for cardiac catheterization in the routine assessment of patients with valvular heart disease; under certain circumstances, catheterization may not even be required prior to surgery (1). However, performance and interpretation of the recordings require a degree of technical expertise and experience, particularly so in the Doppler assessment of valvar stenosis, where the importance of recognizing when the signal is 'off-axis' (and thus underestimating the peak velocity) is paramount. By combining M-mode and cross-sectional information with that obtained from the Doppler examination, it should be possible to grade the severity of valvular lesions with a high degree of accuracy. Diagnostic images may not be obtainable in a small number of patients, and the transoesophageal approach should be considered if important clinical decisions rest on the findings.

Apart from the need for an experienced operator, and the minority of patients in whom an echocardiographic window will not be possible, limitations of the technique are few. It is clearly important to place the information obtained into the clinical context. Trivial degrees of valvular incompetence may be over-interpreted, and it possible to miss significant Doppler gradients by under-estimation. It is important to be aware that echocardiography cannot rule out the presence of thrombus, vegetation or a diagnosis of infective endocarditis.

THE NORMAL AGEING PROCESS

When performing echocardiography on elderly patients, it is important to recognize features associated with the normal ageing process. In both the aortic and mitral valve, calcification is a recognized age-related finding. Calcification of the mitral ring and dilatation and calcification of the aortic arch may also occur. The incidence of mitral leaflet prolapse is between 5% and 10% in some series (2), and autopsy series suggest that the incidence increases with age (3). On Doppler studies, trivial mitral, tricuspid and aortic regurgitation of no clinical significance may be detected in all age groups, but are particularly common in the elderly. An increase in left ventricular mass also occurs, which may be associated with loss of compliance. The Doppler A/E ratio of transmitral filling may become reversed because of changing diastolic properties of the myocardium with increased age (4,5).

DISEASE PROCESSES IN THE ELDERLY

Valvular disease

Aortic valve disease

Aortic sclerosis and stenosis
The normal aortic valve has a characteristic appearance on M-mode and two-dimensional echocardiography (Figures 1a, 2 and 3a). The leaflets are thin

102

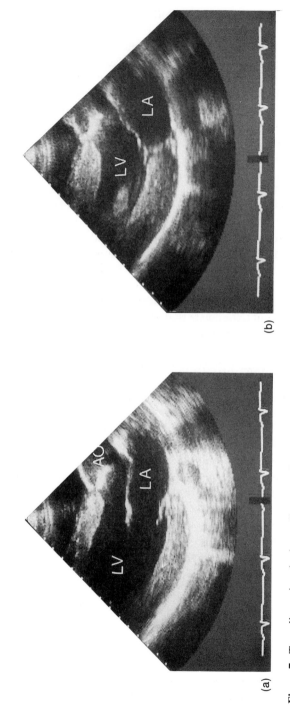

Figure 7. Two-dimensional echocardiogram of the long axis of the LV of a patient with severe aortic stenosis, in diastole (a) and in systole (b), showing the calcified immobile aortic valve, normal cavity size and severe concentric hypertrophy. Reproduced by permission of Blackwell Scientific Publications, Inc., from St John Sutton and Oldershaw (eds) (1989), *Textbook of Adult and Pediatric Echocardiography and Doppler*

and mobile, open fully, and give rise to a thin line of echoes in diastole as the edges of the right and non-coronary cusp coapt. Over the age of 65, thickening, fibrosis and mild calcification of the aortic valve are common. All three cusps may be affected, and mobility so reduced. So-called 'aortic sclerosis' refers to such age-related changes, and does not give rise to haemodynamic disturbance. In this condition a characteristic murmur may be audible, but no valvular gradient detected on Doppler. In some cases, although cusp fusion classically does not occur, calcification may progress further reducing cusp mobility, and so give rise to a significant pressure gradient and outflow tract obstruction. Such changes are then known as senile tricuspid aortic stenosis. When advanced, the appearances are striking and identical to those occurring with degeneration of a bicuspid aortic valve, namely the aortic leaflets are characteristically thickened, heavily calcified and have reduced mobility (Figure 7). Aortic stenosis is thus diagnosed when, in addition to calcification of the aortic valve, there is restriction of cusp mobility. On cross-sectional echocardiography, the aortic valve orifice of a calcified valve may be visualized and the severity estimated (6). However, lesser degrees of stenosis may be difficult to assess without Doppler. Secondary effects of the valvular obstruction include post-stenotic dilatation of the aorta and left ventricular hypertrophy (Figure 8) which, although usually concentric, may be asymmetric. Echocardiography provides the most convenient assessment of accompanying ventricular disease, and may remove the need for left ventricular angiography.

Doppler echocardiography has now become a standard by which to quantify the severity of aortic stenosis, and excellent correlation exists between gradients obtained from invasive and non-invasive techniques (7,8). Using the modified Bernoulli equation, the pressure gradient across the valve may be calculated from the measured peak velocity (Figure 9). A high-velocity jet over 3.5 m/s indicates severe aortic stenosis (equivalent to a gradient of 50 mmHg), and some would consider invasive studies to be both unnecessary and risky in such patients. If a good-quality Doppler signal demonstrates a normal or only slightly elevated velocity, then severe stenosis may be excluded. Invasive confirmation may be required for some patients between these two extremes (8). An estimate of the aortic valve area may be made by using the continuity equation. This is based on the principle that if the volume of blood per unit time flowing across the stenosed valve remains constant, then the volume flow per unit time in the left ventricular outflow tract, and in the proximal aortic root, will be equal. The flow velocity integral in the outflow tract and distal to the valve can be recorded, and if the cross-sectional area of the outflow tract is determined valve area can be calculated, as outlined in the equation below:

$$A_a \times FVI_a = A_{lvot} \times FVI_{lvot}$$

where A_a is the aortic valve area, FVI_a is the flow velocity integral of flow distal to the aortic valve, A_{lvot} is the area of the left ventricular outflow tract, and FVI_{lvot} is the flow velocity integral of flow recorded from the outflow tract. The aortic valve

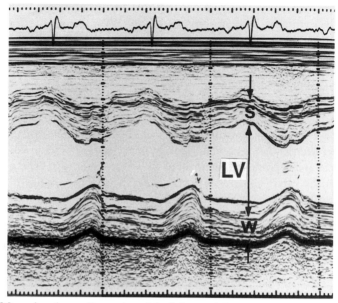

Figure 8. M-mode echocardiography of the left ventricle, at the tips of the mitral valve leaflets, from a patient with moderately severe aortic valve stenosis. The LV cavity is of normal size, and endocardial motion of the septum and posterior left LV wall are normal and equal. The septum (S) and left ventricular posterior wall thicknesses (W) are equivalently increased, indicating moderate concentric LV hypertrophy. Reproduced by permission of Blackwell Scientific Publications, Inc., from St John Sutton and Oldershaw (eds) (1989), *Textbook of Adult and Pediatric Echocardiography and Doppler*

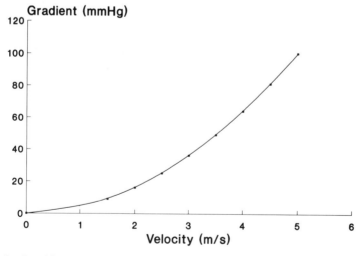

Figure 9. Graphical representation of the relationship between the peak velocity and pressure gradient, derived from the modified Bernoulli equation (gradient = $4 \times \text{velocity}^2$)

area is thus calculated:

$$A_a = \frac{A_{lvot} \times FVI_{lvot}}{FVI_a}$$

The diameter of the left ventricular outflow tract is measured below the aortic valve, and the area calculated assuming the outflow tract to be circular.

Although senile calcific aortic stenosis on a tricuspid valve will account for the vast majority of cases seen in the elderly population, some cases will be due to calcification of a congenitally bicuspid valve, and the remainder will be due to previous rheumatic fever. A bicuspid valve has certain characteristics when non-calcified such as an eccentric diastolic closure line on M-mode, and an ejection click on phonocardiography, but when heavily calcified it may not be possible to distinguish a bicuspid from a tricuspid valve.

Aortic regurgitation

Echocardiography is extremely sensitive in detecting aortic regurgitation, and may provide clues to the aetiology (Table 1). Qualitative assessment of the severity is possible, and although definitive indices are lacking, serial measurement of left ventricular internal cavity dimensions may aid follow-up and decisions regarding timing of aortic valve replacement.

The pathognomonic M-mode sign of aortic regurgitation is high-frequency fluttering on the anterior leaflet of the mitral valve (Figure 10). This is caused by the regurgitant jet impinging upon the leaflet during diastole. It does not relate to the severity of the condition but merely identifies its presence. The left ventricular cavity dimensions can be measured and will increase progressively in significant aortic regurgitation. Increased septal and posterior wall motion reflect a volume-overloaded left ventricle. Left ventricular hypertrophy may be evident, although an increase in wall thickness may not be obvious if the increased muscle mass has been 'dispersed' by a dilating ventricle. In cases of infective endocarditis, vegetations may be visible and seen to prolapse into the left ventricular outflow tract in diastole. In addition, root abscesses and cusp perforation may be

Table 1. Causes of aortic regurgitation

Valve cusp disease
  Rheumatic fever
  Infective endocarditis
  Rheumatoid arthritis
  Trauma

Aortic root disease
  Idiopathic root dilatation
  Aortic dissection/dissecting aneurysm
  Marfan's syndrome
  Ankylosing spondylitis
  Other HLA B27-associated arthropathies (Reiter's, psoriasis, ulcerative colitis)
  Syphilis

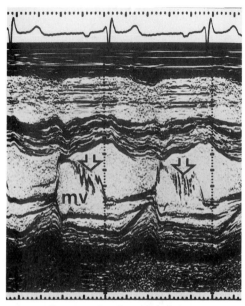

Figure 10. M-mode echocardiogram showing high-frequency diastolic flutter of the anterior mitral valve leaflet due to aortic regurgitation (arrows). This patient had moderately severe aortic stenosis with mild aortic regurgitation. Diastolic flutter of the mitral valve (mv) does not correlate with the severity of aortic regurgitation. Reproduced by permission of Blackwell Scientific Publications, Inc., from St John Sutton and Oldershaw (eds) (1989), *Textbook of Adult and Pediatric Echocardiography and Doppler*

seen. Transoesophageal echocardiography is proving to be more sensitive in the detection of vegetations, particularly when evaluating infected prosthetic valves (9). A particularly useful sign in *acute* severe aortic regurgitation is premature mitral valve closure (10), caused by free regurgitation into a non-compliant ventricle. The pressure rises in mid-diastole, so leading to closure of the valve. A further useful M-mode sign of severe regurgitation is premature aortic valve opening (11). This is caused by the left ventricular diastolic pressure rapidly exceeding aortic diastolic pressure.

Cross-sectional echocardiography will demonstrate aortic root pathology, and biplane transoesophageal echocardiography is particularly useful in the diagnosis of aortic dissection. Doppler provides the most sensitive tool for detection of aortic regurgitation, and clinically insignificant lesions may be found in a sizeable minority of elderly patients. Flow mapping using pulsed Doppler, and colour flow may provide semi-quantitative indices of the severity, as may the shape of the envelope on spectral display of continuous wave doppler. In cases of severe regurgitation, the pressures in the aorta and left ventricle may approach one another rapidly at end-diastole. The pressure gradient and thus peak velocity of the regurgitant signal will fall, so giving rise to a sloped rather than a flat-topped signal (Figure 11).

107

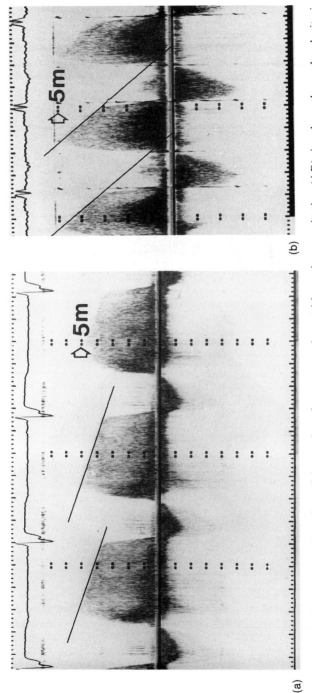

(a)

(b)

Figure 11. Continuous wave Doppler velicity tracings from two patients with aortic regurgitation (AR), in whom the peak velocity is approximately 5 m/s. The deceleration rate (indicated by the slope) is markedly slower in (a)—the pressure half-time ($t_{1/2}$) of 520 ms indicates mild AR. In (b) the deceleration rate is rapid, with a $t_{1/2}$ of 200 ms, indicating that the aortic regurgitation is severe. Reproduced by permission of Blackwell Scientific Publications, Inc., from St John Sutton and Oldershaw (eds) (1989), *Textbook of Adult and Pediatric Echocardiography and Doppler*

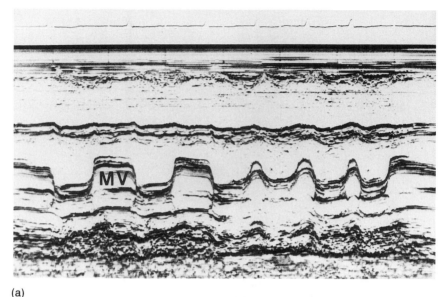

(a)

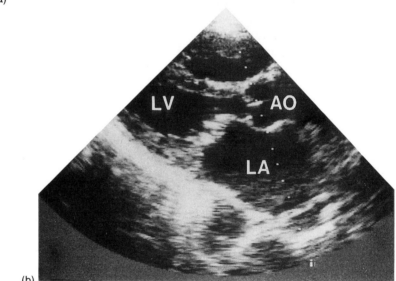

(b)

Figure 12. (a) M-mode echocardiogram from a patient with severe calcific rheumatic mitral stenosis with atrial fibrillation, showing variation in the EF slope with cycle length. There is also calcification of the mitral subvalve apparatus. (b) Two-dimensional echocardiogram of the LV long axis in diastole showing heavily calcified mitral valve leaflets with severely restricted motion. Aortic valve leaflets are also thickened. The left atrium is markedly enlarged. Parts (a) and (b) reproduced by permission of Blackwell Scientific Publications, Inc., from St John Sutton and Oldershaw (eds) (1989), *Textbook of Adult and Pediatric Echocardiography and Doppler*

Mitral valve disease

Mitral stenosis

Although new cases of rheumatic heart disease are rare in the UK, there remain a large number of elderly patients with long-standing rheumatic mitral stenosis, some of whom will have undergone previous mitral valvotomy in the past 30 years. Routine examination and follow-up assessment are best done with echocardiography. Classical rheumatic mitral stenosis has a characteristic appearance on M-mode and two-dimensional studies (Figure 12a,b). The valve leaflets are thickened and the commissures are fused. The posterior leaflet is tethered and pulled anteriorly in diastole, and bowing of the leaflets occurs. Cusp mobility is reduced and may be assessed from both M-mode and two-dimensional appearances. There is a reduced diastolic closure rate of the valve, manifest as a reduced 'E–F' slope. The left atrium will be enlarged and thrombus may be present. The pattern of left ventricular filling is abnormal and a reduced rate of dimension increase may be demonstrated from computer analysis of digitized M-mode traces (12).

Valve area may be calculated from the two-dimensional image using planimetry, although this technique has the limitations of subjective interpretation of the valve orifice boundaries, which may be ill defined. Doppler provides an excellent quantitative assessment of the severity of mitral stenosis (Figure 13), and the peak, mean and end-diastolic pressure gradient across the valve can be accurately measured. Characteristic features are an increased peak velocity, reduced rate of velocity decline and prolonged pressure half-time. The mitral pressure half-time is the time interval over which the velocity falls from its peak value to the peak value divided by the square root of two. This has been related to the mitral valve area by the following equation:

$$\text{mitral valve area (cm}^2) = 220/\text{pressure half-time (ms)}$$

The normal value for this is less than 100 ms (Figure 14).

Mitral regurgitation

Mitral regurgitation is most easily detected using Doppler echo techniques, although its presence may be suggested if there is a dilated and active left ventricle, particularly if the left atrium is dilated. Echocardiography is also useful in determining the aetiology (Table 2). Many cases of mitral regurgitation are still rheumatic in origin and characteristic appearances of a rheumatic mitral valve have already been discussed. Vegetations may be obvious in cases of infective endocarditis. A 'floppy' mitral valve is a common finding in otherwise normal individuals, with an incidence of approximately 5%. Echocardiographic criteria for the diagnosis of mitral valve prolapse (13) should include M-mode evidence of posterior displacement or 'hammocking' of one or both leaflets, in systole (Figure 15a). Excessive diastolic motion of the redundant leaflet may be evident. On two-dimensional studies displacement of the cusp coaption point is

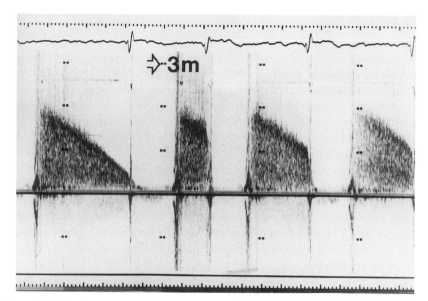

Figure 13. Continuous wave Doppler signal from a patient with rheumatic mitral stenosis in atrial fibrillation. The peak velocity varies little (1.8–2.0 m/s), consistent with a gradient of approximately 13–16 mmHg in early diastole. The velocity decays to zero by end-diastole with long cycle lengths, so that there is equilibration of the pressures across the mitral valve at end-diastole. Consecutive velocity signals in atrial fibrillation show zero gradient after long cardiac cycles, but 4–5 mmHg gradients with short cycle lengths. Reproduced by permission of Blackwell Scientific Publications, Inc., from St John Sutton and Oldershaw (eds) (1989), *Textbook of Adult and Pediatric Echocardiography and Doppler*

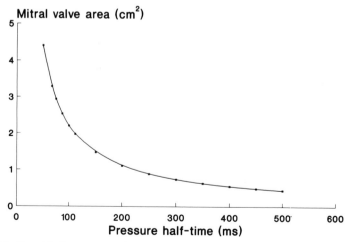

Figure 14. Graphical representation of the relationship between the Doppler pressure half-time (PHT) and calculated mitral valve area (MVA) (derived from the relationship MVA = 220/PHT)

Table 2. Causes of mitral regurgitation

Cusps	Congenital abnormality
	Rheumatic fever
	Infective endocarditis
	Floppy valve—redundant leaflet
	Post-valvotomy/valvuloplasty
	Trauma
Chordae	Redundant—floppy valve
	Ruptured
Papillary muscle	Dysfunction
	Rupture
Valve ring	Dilatation
	Annulus calcification

best made from the parasternal long-axis view (Figure 15b). Prolapse may be judged to occur if either leaflet or the coaption point is displaced more than 2 mm behind the mitral annulus. Only a minority will have mitral regurgitation, which may be detected on Doppler and colour flow mapping. Chordal rupture may occur in association with mitral valve prolapse, and multiple flickering echoes from the unsupported cusp or free chordae may be seen. Chordal perforation or rupture may of course be evident in the absence of any abnormality of the mitral valve itself. Papillary muscle dysfunction may be caused by ischaemia or ventricular dilatation, and scarring or cavity enlargement may be evident on cross-sectional echocardiography. If papillary muscle rupture has occurred, then on transoesophageal echocardiography the disrupted papillary muscle may be visualized, for example following myocardial infarction. Functional mitral regurgitation is frequently present in dilated cardiomyopathy and although valve ring dilatation undoubtedly plays an important role, the precise mechanisms underlying this are by no means clear. Mitral annulus calcification, an important cause of mitral regurgitation in the elderly, is discussed below.

Whatever the cause, the severity of the mitral regurgitation may be difficult to determine. The left ventricular dimensions and wall motion are useful clues. In cases of severe regurgitation, the left ventricle will be dilated and show vigorous contraction, characteristic of volume overload (Figure 16). An increase in septal and posterior wall motion are indicators of the increased ejection fraction. Pulsed Doppler and colour flow mapping are semi-quantitative, although the indices of regurgitant jet length, area and width may not prove as useful as initially thought. A useful sign of severity is the length of time that the mitral regurgitant signal (on continuous wave Doppler) persists beyond the aortic component of the second heart sound (recorded on phonocardiography). An interval of less than 55 ms between A2 and the cessation of retrograde flow predicts severe regurgitation (14).

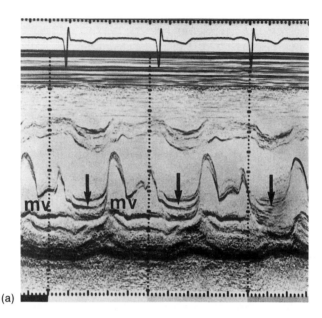

(a)

Figure 15. (a) M-mode echocardiogram showing holosystolic bowing or hammocking of the mitral valve leaflets (arrows). Two-dimensional echocardiography demonstrated hyolosystolic mitral valve prolapse. (b) (opposite) Two-dimensional echocardiogram of the left ventricular long axis from a different patient, showing the plane of the mitral valve annulus, designated by a line joined by arrows. The leaflets of the mitral valve prolapse onto the left atrial side of that plane in systole, indicating the presence of mitral valve prolapse. Parts (a) and (b) reproduced by permission of Blackwell Scientific Publications, Inc., from St John Sutton and Oldershaw (eds) (1989), *Textbook of Adult and Pediatric Echocardiography and Doppler*

Mitral annulus calcification

This is a common degenerative condition in the elderly, more often found in females (15). On M-mode echocardiography, a dense band of echoes is present behind the mitral valve, anterior to the posterior left ventricular wall. The calcification may encircle the valve and progress to involve the posterior leaflet, so causing mitral regurgitation. Calcification may interfere with normal mitral ring motion and cause functional mitral stenosis (16). It may also extend into the base of the heart, involving the aortic root or conducting system, causing heart block. The severity of the calcification may be assessed from M-mode and cross-sectional echocardiography (Figure 17), and may range from a small dense mass adjacent to the posterior mitral leaflet, to a large encircling collection of calcium capable of producing both stenosis and incompetence. Massive annular calcification may protude into the atrium or ventricle, and mimic a tumour.

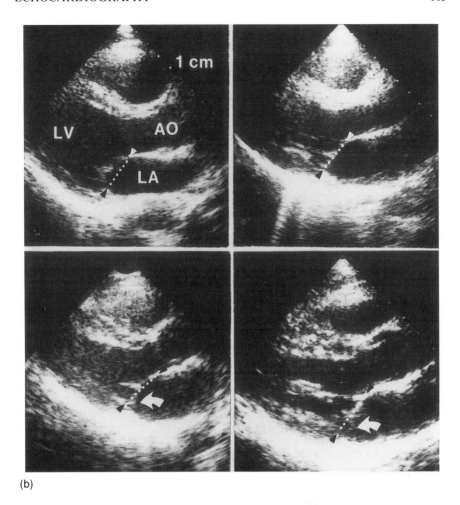

(b)

Infective endocarditis

Endocarditis in the elderly may present in an atypical way with little in the way of a classical history or physical signs; as a result the diagnosis is often missed or not considered. Echocardiography has proven to be a valuable method for detection and assessment of patients with this condition. Detection of vegetations, assessment of valvular incompetence and investigation of complications are all potential uses. Vegetations appear as echogenic masses attached to valve leaflets (Figure 18), or occasionally other intracardiac structures, but only vegetations greater than 2 mm will be visible. The distinction between a mitral valve vegetation and mitral leaflet redundancy may, however, be difficult, because both may produce thickening of the leaflet on M-mode, and both flail leaflet and vegetation may prolapse. On two-dimensional echocardiography, a vegetation

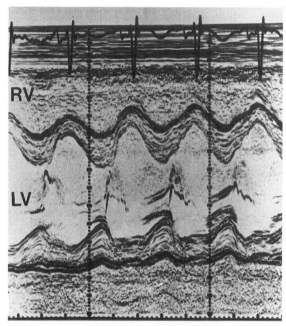

Figure 16. M-mode left ventricular echocardiogram from a patient with chronic severe mitral regurgitation, showing a dilated left ventricular cavity, a vigorous contraction pattern due to volume overload, and increased excursion of the septum and posterior left ventricular wall. The anterior mitral valve leaflet is thickened in this patient because of mitral valve vegetative endocarditis. Reproduced by permission of Blackell Scientific Publications, Inc., from St John Sutton and Oldershaw (eds) (1989), *Textbook of Adult and Pediatric Echocardiography and Doppler*

may appear to arise from a stalk, and flop around independently of the cusp itself, although clearly its motion will be related to it.

The diagnosis of endocarditis is ultimately a clinical one, and echocardiography can add support to that diagnosis in a positive way, by demonstrating likely vegetations in a patient with other evidence of the disease. Conversely, the diagnosis should not depend upon the echo findings alone, as some patients with endocarditis will have no detectable vegetations. Flail mitral leaflets, torn aortic cusps, ruptured chordae, and small mobile intracardiac tumours and thrombi may all be mistaken for vegetations, and experience, together with the clinical index of suspicion, are important factors in the interpretation of echocardiographic images of suspected vegetation. The finding of possible vegetations in an otherwise completely well patient may represent healed endocarditis. In established endocarditis, serial echocardiography may demonstrate slow growth or resolution of a vegetation, the development of paravalvular abscesses, or valve leaflet aneurysm formation. Regurgitant jets should be looked for with continuous wave and colour Doppler, although jets may be eccentric if damage to the valve is focal, or if cusp perforation has occurred. In addition, the

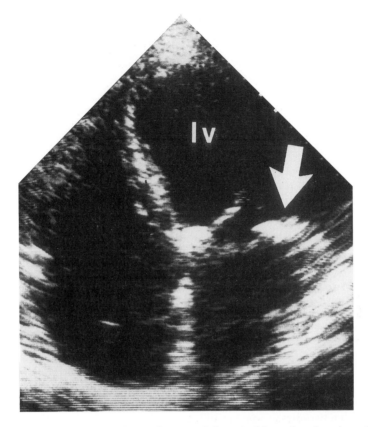

Figure 17. Two-dimensional echocardiogram of the apical four chamber view, showing mitral annular calcification (arrow). Reproduced by permission of Blackwell Scientific Publications, Inc., from St John Sutton and Oldershaw (eds) (1989), *Textbook of Adult and Pediatric Echocardiography and Doppler*

assessment of the severity of the regurgitant lesion is possible, both from the condition of the left ventricle, and the features discussed above in relation to aortic and mitral regurgitation. Ring abscesses are common in patients with aortic vegetations and indicate severe involvement of the cusps and paravalvular tissues (17). As has been stated already, the sensitivity of detection of vegetations and abscesses is increased markedly if the transoesophageal approach is used. Prosthetic valve endocarditis is discussed below.

Prosthetic valves

An increasingly large number of elderly patients are now undergoing valve replacement, and many are now in their second decade post replacement. Echocardiography is the investigation of choice for routine follow-up of such

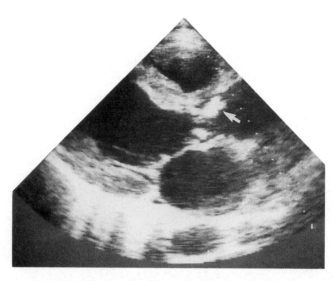

Figure 18. Two-dimensional echocardiogram of the parasternal long axis from a patient with aortic valve endocarditis. Vegetations are visualized involving both the aortic valve leaflets. Reproduced by permission of Blackwell Scientific Publications, Inc., from St John Sutton and Oldershaw (eds) (1989), *Textbook of Adult and Pediatric Echocardiography and Doppler*

patients, and is an integral part of the assessment of suspected prosthetic valve malfunction. Many bioprostheses show signs of malfunction after approximately 10 years, and such patients should be kept under regular review. Assessment begins with a two-dimensional examination of the prosthesis itself, the paravalvular tissues and pattern of motion. In cases of endocarditis where the valve sewing ring is damaged, the whole prosthesis may 'rock', leaving a gap through which a large paravalvular leak may occur. The operator should be familiar with the typical appearances of the common types of prosthesis in use. Most bioprostheses are mounted on a stent which has a characteristic appearance (Figure 19). Mechanical valves are of many designs, the major ones being ball and cage (Starr–Edwards), monocuspid tilting disc (Bjork–Shiley) or bileaflet tilting disc (St Jude). M-mode recordings through each prosthesis give rise to characteristic appearances. The left ventricular cavity should be measured, and signs of volume overload (implying valve regurgitation) looked for. A particularly useful M-mode sign of prosthetic mitral regurgitation is normalization of septal motion. In the postoperative state this will be reversed with a non-leaking valve, but the movement normalizes as the left ventricle becomes volume overloaded (Figure 20). Doppler and colour flow are used to detect valve regurgitation, and this is one area where transoesophageal studies are of particular value. Prosthetic valve regurgitation may be notoriously difficult to detect with Doppler from the transthoracic approach owing to the marked eccentricity of the jet. In patients with clinical and M-mode evidence of prosthetic

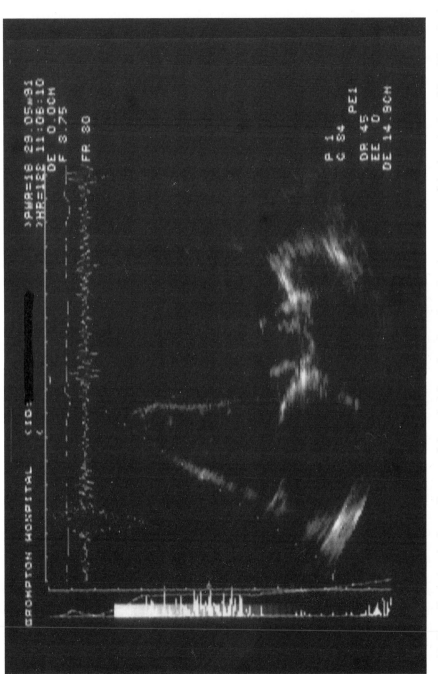

Figure 19. Two-dimensional echocardiogram of the apical four-chamber view, showing a xenograft in the mitral position. The valve is mounted on a stent, which can be seen to protrude into the left ventricle

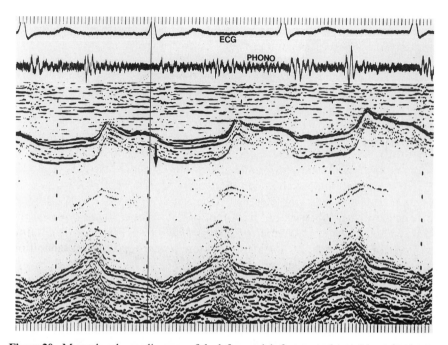

Figure 20. M-mode echocardiogram of the left ventricle from a patient with a mitral valve replacement and severe prosthetic mitral regurgitation. Septal motion, which should be reversed following mitral valve replacement, has 'normalized' due to the left ventricular volume overload. The septal motion is posterior during systole (arrow)

valve regurgitation, but no detectable Doppler signal, the transoesophageal technique should be considered. Conventional Doppler of forward transprosthesis flow enables detection of stenosis, and this is of particular importance in bioprostheses in the aortic position, which are prone to calcify.

Hypertensive heart disease

Blood pressure is known to rise with age, and its prevalence in an elderly population is high. Echocardiography is a sensitive way of assessing its sequelae in the heart, namely left ventricular hypertrophy. On two-dimensional echo this appears as concentric hypertrophy of the septum and posterior wall, and the thickness may be accurately measured from M-mode. Abnormalities of left ventricular filling on Doppler may be present, reflected as an increase in the atrial contribution to filling (18). An interesting group of elderly patients with hypertension has recently been described as having 'hypertensive hypertrophic cardiomyopathy of the elderly' (19). Predominantly black females, these patients were demonstrated to have severe concentric cardiac hypertrophy, a small left ventricular cavity, and supernormal indices of systolic function. The majority of these patients presented with chest pain or dyspnoea. This syndrome is important to recognize as patients treated with vasodilators tend to deteriorate, while those receiving β-blockers or calcium antagonists obtain symptomatic relief.

Cardiomyopathies

Dilated cardiomyopathy

The principal features of dilated cardiomyopathy are an enlarged left ventricular cavity with reduced amplitude of septal and posterior wall motion (20). All four chambers are usually enlarged, and there is global hypokinaesia (Figure 21). These features are similar in both idiopathic and ischaemic cardiomyopathy. On M-mode there is in addition increased separation between the E point of the anterior mitral leaflet and the left side of the septum. The cavity dimensions may be measured, and repeated serially during follow-up. The low cardiac output may be manifest as reduced aortic root motion, reduced mitral cusp separation, and slow drifting together of the aortic leaflets. Segmental wall motion abnormalities are suggestive of an ischaemic aetiology. On cross-sectional echocardiography, thrombus may be visualized within the cardiac chambers in some patients.

Both mitral and tricuspid regurgitation may be commonly detected on Doppler in dilated cardiomyopathy.

Hypertrophic cardiomyopathy

The two characteristic M-mode echocardiographic features of hypertrophic cardiomyopathy (HCM) are systolic anterior motion of the mitral valve (SAM) (21) and asymmetric septal hypertrophy (ASH) (22,23). SAM has been correlated with obstruction to outflow (24), but it has also been found in other conditions. In the obstructive variety of HCM, hypertrophy is usually asymmetric, whilst the non-obstructive variety is more often characterized by concentric hypertrophy. Two-dimensional echocardiography is useful in demonstrating the profile and site of the hypertrophied septum, and the narrowing of the outflow tract (Figure 22). If the hypertrophy is concentric, the cavity may become obliterated in systole. The echo intensity of the abnormal muscle may be increased, or speckled. A third echo feature of HCM is midsystolic closure of the aortic valve (25), although this finding, together with fluttering of the leaflets, is also found in discrete subaortic stenosis. In any event, this characteristic is indicative of a significant outflow tract gradient.

Systolic function is usually normal; however, indices of diastolic function are characteristically abnormal (26). Doppler ultrasound is of considerable value in demonstrating the presence of an outflow tract gradient, and of mitral regurgitation, which is often found.

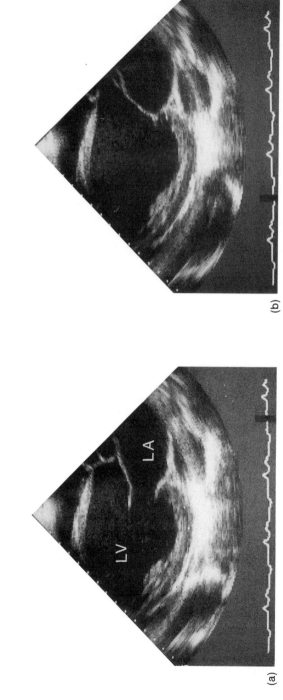

Figure 21. Two-dimensional echocardiogram of the LV long axis in dilated cardiomyopathy showing a greatly enlarged chamber in diastole (a) and little change in size in systole (b). The mitral valve opens, but with a much increased distance between the anterior leaflet tip and the left side of the septum (increased E point—septal separation). Reproduced by permission of Blackwell Scientific Publications, Inc., from St John Sutton and Oldershaw (eds) (1989), *Textbook of Adult and Pediatric Echocardiography and Doppler*

Restrictive cardiomyopathy and senile amyloid

Restrictive cardiomyopathy is an uncommon entity characterized by thickening of the left ventricular wall, enlarged atria, and a normal left ventricular cavity size. The primary physiological disturbance is that of restricted left ventricular filling, associated with abnormal wall thinning and reduced compliance. The commonest specific form of restrictive cardiomyopathy in an elderly population is amyloid heart disease. There is infiltration of the myocardium with deposits of amyloid which appear as speckling within the thickened septum and free wall of the left ventricle. Systolic function is characteristically normal, but there are marked disturbances in diastolic function with a reduction in peak left ventricular filling rate (27). Infiltration causes both thickening and thinning of the posterior wall of the left ventricle to be reduced, and there is increased epicardial excursion in parallel to the endocardium (Figure 23). These features, without evidence of left ventricular hypertrophy on the ECG, are strongly suggestive of amyloid.

'Senile amyloid' refers to the common degenerative condition of amyloid deposition in an ageing heart. It should be considered in any elderly patient with cardiac failure refractory to diuretics, or in those with a normal cardiothoracic ratio on chest X-ray.

Diseases of the aorta

In young children it is often possible to examine the entire aorta with echocardiography; however, in the elderly it may be difficult to display more than a small length. Multiple views may be necessary from the transthoracic approach. Transoesophageal echocardiography represents a significant advance in studying the aorta, and is increasingly used in the diagnosis of dissection—a condition which is not uncommon in the elderly hypertensive patient.

Aneurysm and dilatation

The proximal ascending aorta is usually well visualized from the parasternal long-axis view, and its dimensions may be measured from M-mode traces. The suprasternal approach enables the arch to be visualized, and occasionally the origin of the head and neck vessels can be defined. The normal ascending aortic root dimension is 2.1–3.4 cm (28), and dilatation is easy to recognize.

Dissection

Two-dimensional echocardiography may be useful in the diagnosis of aortic dissection (29) and may permit visualization of the intimal flap as an additional set of echoes from the aortic wall (Figure 24). Doppler echocardiography may detect aortic regurgitation, which is often present in such cases, and colour flow

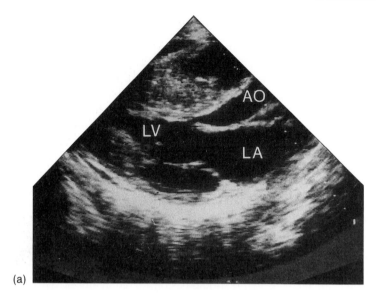

(a)

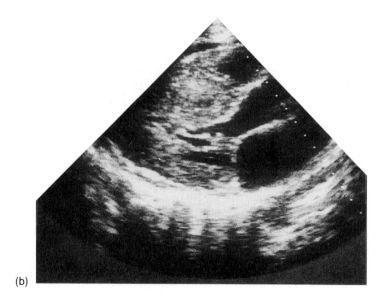

(b)

Figure 22. Two-dimensional echocardiogram from two patients with hypertrophic cardiomyopathy. There is extreme asymmetric septal hypertrophy compared to the inferior wall in diastole (a and c), which is still apparent in systole (b and d). There are bright spots within the septum, which are specular reflections representing either fibrosis

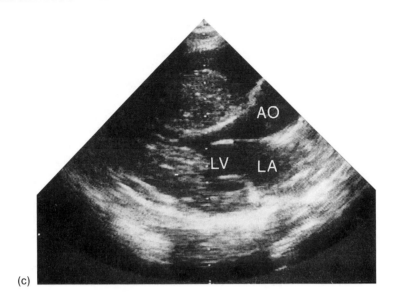

(c)

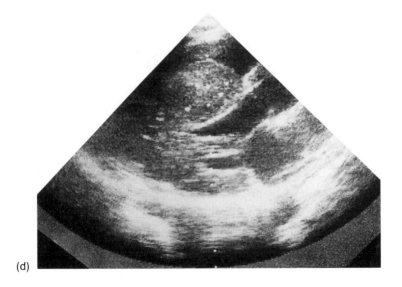

(d)

or myocardial fibre disarray. Reproduced by permission of Blackwell Scientific Publications, Inc., from St John Sutton and Oldershaw (eds) (1989), *Textbook of Adult and Pediatric Echocardiography and Doppler*

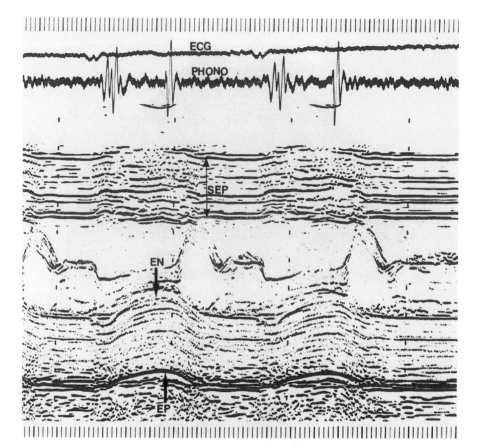

Figure 23. M-mode echocardiogram of the left ventricle at the level of the tips of the mitral leaflets, from a patient with cardiac amyloid. Note the marked hypertrophy of the septum (SEP) and posterior wall, but low-voltage complexes on the ECG. The endocardium (EN) and epicardium (EP) are indicated. Note the lack of systolic thickening and diastolic thinning of the posterior wall, typical of cardiac amyloid

mapping may display flow in a false lumen (30). In addition, pericardial fluid is often present, and well demonstrated echocardiographically.

Pericardial disease

Pericardial effusion

Echocardiography is the investigation of choice for demonstrating pericardial fluid. An echo-free space is present on both M-mode and two-dimensional echocardiography (Figure 25a,b), and may be demonstrated both anteriorly and posteriorly, with relation to the left ventricle. The width of the echo-free space

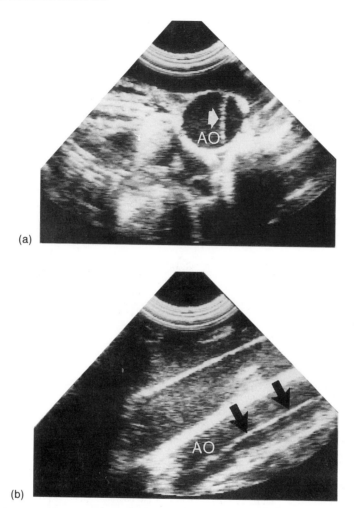

(a)

(b)

Figure 24. Two-dimensional echocardiogram, obtained intraoperatively, of an aortic dissection showing the descending thoracic aortic lumen with an intimal flap in cross-section (a, arrow), and in long axis (b, arrows). Reproduced by permission of Blackwell Scientific Publications, Inc., St John Suttom and Oldershaw (eds) (1989), *Textbook of Adult and Pediatric Echocardiography and Doppler*

relates approximately to the amount of fluid present, and the two-dimensional image provides information about location and consistency of the fluid. Strands of fibrin may be seen in loculated effusions. Some clinicians use the two-dimensional image to guide aspiration.

When the amount of fluid present within the pericardium reaches a certain point, the intrapericardial pressure will rise and interfere with ventricular filling. Reliable and sensitive echocardiographic features of tamponade are collapse or indentation of the right ventricular (31) or right atrial (32) free wall in early

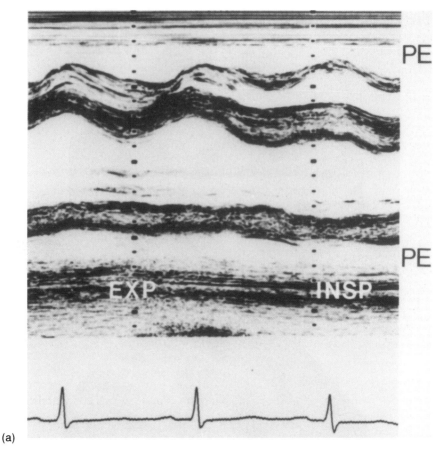

(a)

Figure 25. (a) M-mode echocardiogram of a patient with a large pericardial effusion (PE) seen both anteriorly and posteriorly. There is reciprocal variation in RV and LV sizes, with decreased RV size and increased LV size during expiration (EXP), with the reverse occurring during inspiration (INSP). (b) (opposite) Two-dimensional echocardiogram of a patient with a pericardial effusion (PERI EFF). Parts (a) and (b) reproduced by permission of Blackwell Scientific Publications, Inc., from St John Sutton and Oldershaw (eds) (1989), *Textbook of Adult and Pediatric Echocardiography and Doppler*

diastole. A further useful sign is the fall in aortic Doppler flow velocity with inspiration—the echocardiographic demonstration of pulsus paradoxus.

Pericardial constriction

The most useful echocardiographic finding in pericardial constriction is thickening of the pericardium (33). Other features, such as reduced diastolic outward motion of the posterior left ventricular wall, are not specific. The recognition of pericardial constriction may thus be difficult, and may depend upon the

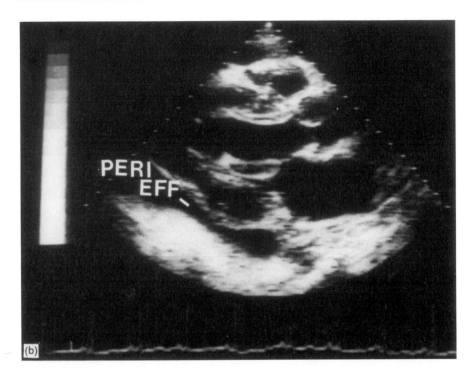

recognition of a number of suggestive features. However, a particularly useful technique is the recording of the jugular venous pulse, which characteristically shows a deep and dominant 'x' descent in pericardial constriction. This is unusual in cases of restrictive cardiomyopathy, with which constriction is often confused.

On the two-dimensional image, the sudden and abrupt outward motion of the ventricular wall during diastole reflects the abnormal physiology, with premature termination of rapid filling. A combination of effusion with the characteristics of constriction may occur in so-called effusive-constrictive pericarditis, which may have a variety of aetiologies.

CONCLUSIONS

Echocardiographic techniques have advanced enormously in the last 20 years, such that it now represents an indispensable part of cardiological investigation. It is particularly suited to the study of elderly patients because of its non-invasive nature. The information obtained often provides the clinician with sufficient details to formulate a management plan, and serial studies may be conveniently performed to monitor progression of disease processes, increasingly common in an ageing population.

Acknowledgements

We are indebted to Dr Martin St John Sutton and Dr Derek G. Gibson for their advice and for allowing us to reproduce illustrations.

REFERENCES

1. St John Sutton MG, St John Sutton M, Oldershaw P *et al.* (1981) Valve replacement without preoperative cardiac catheterisation. *N Engl J Med* **305**: 1233–1238.
2. Savage DD, Garrison RJ, Devereux RB *et al.* (1983) Mitral valve prolapse in the general population. I. Epidemiologic features: the Framingham Study. *Am Heart J* **106**: 571–576.
3. Davies MJ, Moore BP, Braimbridge MV (1978) The floppy mitral valve: study of incidence, pathology, and complications in surgical, necropsy, and forensic material. *Br Heart J* **40**: 468–481.
4. Bryg RJ, Williams GA, Labovitz AJ (1987) Effect of aging on left ventricular diastolic filling in normal subjects. *Am J Cardiol* **59**: 971–974.
5. Kuo LC, Quinones MA, Rokey R *et al.* (1987) Quantification of atrial contribution to left ventricular filling by pulsed Doppler echocardiography and the effect of age in normal and diseased hearts. *Am J Cardiol* **59**: 1174–1178.
6. Weyman AE, Feigenbaum H, Dillon JC, Chang S (1975) Cross-sectional echocardiography in assessing the severity of valvular aortic stenosis. *Circulation* **52**: 828–834.
7. Currie PJ, Seward JB, Reeder GS *et al.* (1985) Continuous-wave Doppler echocardiographic assessment of severity of calcific aortic stenosis: a simultaneous Doppler–catheter correlative study in 100 adult patients. *Circulation* **71**: 1162–1169.
8. Yeager M, Yock PG, Popp RL (1986) Comparison of Doppler-derived pressure gradient to that determined at cardiac catheterization in adults with aortic valve stenosis: implications for management. *Am J Cardiol* **57**: 644–648.
9. Mugge A, Daniel WG, Frank G, Lichtlen PR (1989) Echocardiography in infective endocarditis: reassessment of prognostic implications of vegetation size determined by the transthoracic and the transesophageal approach. *J Am Coll Cardiol* **14**: 631–638.
10. Ambrose JA, Meller J, Teicholz LE, Herman MV (1978) Premature closure of the mitral valve: echocardiographic clue for the diagnosis of aortic dissection. *Chest* **73**: 121–123.
11. Weaver WF, Wilson CS, Rourke T, Caudill CC (1977) Mid-diastolic aortic valve opening in severe acute aortic regurgitation. *Circulation* **55**: 145–148.
12. Gibson DG, Brown D (1973) Measurement of instantaneous left ventricular dimension and filling rate in man, using echocardiography. *Br Heart J* **35**: 1141–1149.
13. Devereux RB, Kramer-Fox R, Shear MK *et al.* (1987) Diagnosis and classification of severity of mitral valve prolapse: methodologic, biologic, and forensic considerations. *Am Heart J* **113**: 1265–1280.
14. Bradley JA, Gibson DG (1988) Assessment of the severity of mitral regurgitation from the dynamics of retrograde flow. *Br Heart J* **60**: 134–140.
15. Nair CK, Aronow WS, Sketch MH *et al.* (1983) Clinical and echocardiographic characteristics of patients with mitral annular calcification. *Am J Cardiol* **51**: 992–995.
16. Osterberger LE, Goldstein S, Khaja F, Lakier JB (1981) Functional mitral stenosis in patients with massive mitral annular calcification. **64**: 472–476.
17. Buchbinder NA, Roberts WC (1972) Left sided valvular active infective endocarditis: a study of 45 necropsy patients. *Am J Med* **53**: 20–35.

18. Ruddy TD, Zusman RM, Dighero RH *et al.* (1986) Increased contribution of atrial systole to left ventricular diastolic filling in hypertensive patients. *Clin Res* **34**: 485A.
19. Topol EJ, Traill TA, Fortuin NJ (1984) Hypertensive hypertrophic cardiomyopathy of the elderly. *N Engl J Med* **312**: 277–283.
20. Corya BC, Feigenbaum H, Rasmussen S, Black MJ (1974) Echocardiographic features of congestive cardiomyopathy compared with normal subjects and patients with coronary artery disease. *Circulation* **49**: 1153–1159.
21. Shah PM, Taylor RD, Wong M (1981) Abnormal mitral valve coaption in hypertrophic obstructive cardiomyopathy: proposed role in systolic anterior motion of mitral valve. *Am J Cardiol* **48**: 258–262.
22. Henry WL, Clark CE, Epstein SE (1973) Asymmetric septal hypertrophy: echocardiographic identification of the pathognomonic anatomic abnormality of IHSS. *Circulation* **47**: 225–233.
23. Henry WL, Clark CE, Roberts WC *et al.* (1974) Differences in distribution of myocardial abnormalities in patients with obstructive and nonobstructive asymmetric septal hypertrophy (ASH): echocardiographic and gross anatomic findings. *Circulation* **50**: 447–455.
24. Henry WL, Clark CE, Glancy DL, Epstein SE (1973) Echocardiographic measurement of the left ventricular outflow gradient in idiopathic hypertrophic subaortic stenosis. *N Engl J Med* **288**: 989–993.
25. Krajcer Z, Orzan F, Pechacek LW *et al.* (1978) Early systolic closure of the aortic valve in patients with hypertrophic subaortic stenosis and discrete subaortic stenosis: correlation with preoperative and postoperative hemodynamics. *Am J Cardiol* **41**: 823–829.
26. St John Sutton MG, Tajik AJ, Gibson DG *et al.* (1977) Echocardiographic assessment of left ventricular filling and septal and posterior wall dynamics in idiopathic hypertrophic subaortic stenosis. *Circulation* **57**: 512–520.
27. St John Sutton MG, Reichek N, Kastor JA, Giuliani ER (1982) Computerized M-mode echocardiographic analysis of left ventricular dysfunction in cardiac amyloid. *Circulation* **66**: 790–799.
28. Triulzi M, Gillam LD, Gentile F *et al.* (1984) Normal adult cross-sectional echocardiographic values: linear dimensions and chamber areas. *Echocardiography* **1**: 403–426.
29. Victor MF, Mintz, GS, Kotler MN *et al.* (1981) Two dimensional echocardiographic diagnosis of aortic dissection. *Am J Cardiol* **48**: 1155–1159.
30. Dagli SV, Nanda NC, Roitman D *et al.* (1985) Evaluation of aortic dissection by Doppler color flow mapping. *Am J Cardiol* **56**: 497–498.
31. Armstrong WF, Schilt BF, Helper DJ *et al.* (1982) Diastolic collapse of the right ventricle with cardiac tamponade: an echocardiographic study. *Circulation* **65**: 1491–1496.
32. Gillam LD, Guyer DE, Gibson TC *et al.* (1983) Hydrodynamic compression of the right atrium: a new echocardiographic sign of cardiac tamponade. *Circulation* **68**: 294–301.
33. Schnittger I, Bowden RE, Abrams J, Popp RL (1978) Echocardiography: pericardial thickening and constrictive pericarditis. *Am J Cardiol* **42**: 388–395.

7 Clinical Electrocardiography and Electrophysiology in the Elderly

A. JOHN CAMM[a], DEMOSTHENES KATRITSIS[a] AND DAVID E. WARD[b]

[a]St George's Hospital Medical School, London, UK
[b]St George's Hospital, London, UK

The progressive loss of organic function which reflects ageing cannot be predicted by chronological age or any other physiological index. Consequently, no standard or good definition of 'elderly' exists and in contemporary society the elderly population conventionally comprises those who are in their seventh decade of life or beyond. The term 'senescence' is used to denote the normal process of growing old (60–75 years), in contrast to 'senility' which is pathologic old age, whereas 'old age' usually refers to persons who have exceeded the 75th year (1) and the 'very old' denotes subjects older than 80 years. Another problem encountered in clinical studies of the elderly is the difficulty in defining 'normal' in this population. The concept of normality, particularly as it relates to the electrocardiogram (ECG) of the elderly, has been analysed in detail by Simonson (2,3). The distinction between the natural involutionary ageing process and a deviation which results in disease is not always possible and most of the time remains a matter of conjecture. Rarity of occurrence has often been used to connote disease, but could equally well represent an extreme of the shifting spectrum of normality. An analysis of the electrocardiographic findings in apparently normal elderly people is therefore essential for the appreciation of deviations which might be potentially associated with disease.

CONVENTIONAL ELECTROCARDIOGRAPHY

Electrocardiographic surveys in the elderly

In 1931, Willius published results of an electrocardiographic survey of 700 patients, between 75 and 96 years of age. No information was provided about electrocardiographic findings in patients with apparently normal hearts, but in 385 with evident heart disease there were T wave changes in 25%, atrioventricular (AV) conduction abnormalities in 11%, and atrial fibrillation in 18%.

Asymptomatic old people with apparently normal hearts were subsequently

Geriatric Cardiology. Principles and Practice. Edited by A. Martin and A. J. Camm
© 1994 John Wiley & Sons Ltd

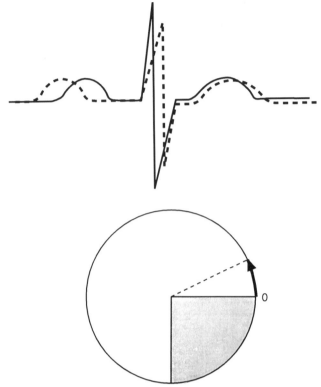

Figure 1. Typical ECG changes in the elderly. Please note left axis deviation, PR prolongation and T-wave flattening

investigated by Gelman and Brown (4), who compared ECGs from 60 old subjects with those from normal schoolchildren, and discovered long P–R intervals, wide and split QRS complexes, depressed ST segments and flat or inverted T waves. Levitt (5) also detected ST or T wave abnormalities in 26 out of 100 patients over 79 years old with no evidence of cardiorespiratory, renal or systemic disease on clinical, historical and biochemical findings. Eliaser and Kondo (6), studying active, asymptomatic persons between the ages of 70 and 92 years, found left axis deviation, low QRS voltage, sinus bradycardia and T wave flattening so common that they regarded them as normal, in contrast to AV and bundle branch block, infarction patterns and right axis deviation which were sufficiently rare to be regarded as abnormal. Following studies showed that heart rate decreases with age and that female heart rates were faster than males (7), and that ectopic activity could be detected in up to 25–28% in elderly people with no cardiac symptoms (8,9). However, electrocardiographic abnormalities occurred more frequently in those with hypertension or radiographically enlarged hearts (10). A follow-up study (11) of elderly patients with normal ECG showed that although mortality was clearly related more to cardiac enlargement than to electrocardiographic abnormalities, there was a higher mortality rate in those with abnormal ECGs but otherwise normal hearts. As a result Fox (11) proposed that the criteria of normality should be the same for elderly as for non-elderly adult groups. However, by 1950 it was obvious that in most series of usually ambulant and apparently healthy individuals electrocardiographic abnormalities were present in one-half to two-thirds of cases. Gavey (8) therefore accepted that minor changes such as prolonged P–R interval or T wave flattening were entirely consistent with healthy old age (Figures 1 and 2).

In general, investigations of electrocardiographic tracings from the elderly have reported a prevalence of abnormal ECGs ranging from nil (12) to 98% (13). The overall average prevalence of abnormal tracings among subjects over 70 years of age in the reported series is approximately 52% but several methodological differences make the interpretation of all these trials difficult. Different diagnostic and electrocardiographic criteria have been employed by various investigators. For example, Fisch *et al.* (14) used the criteria of the New York Heart Association whereas Kennedy and Caird (15) applied the Minnesota code (16). Some, such as Michie (17), have regarded isolated ventricular premature beats as normal but others have not. Furthermore, even after the introduction of the unipolar precordial leads, not all investigators have used 12-lead ECGs (18); it has been shown, however, that a six-limb tracing in the elderly can miss up to 22% of major diagnostic information compared with conventional 12-lead ECGs (19). Finally, the surveyed population in several studies was rather small, thus creating certain problems for statistical verification of the apparent results (20,21).

Specific findings

First-degree atrioventricular block

The prevalence of a P–R interval prolonged beyond 0.22 s increases with age (21,22). In a broad range of geriatric patients the prevalence is approximately 5% (14) to 10% (23) but in nonagenarians the prevalence rises to 35% (24). First-degree AV block is not usually associated with clinical heart disease (14) and when first-degree AV block is an isolated finding it is not associated with an adverse prognosis (25).

Left axis deviation

Several studies have demonstrated an age-related trend towards left axis deviation (26,27) (Figure 1). Progressive leftward shift in the middle-aged (28) and the elderly (29) has been confirmed by longitudinal studies (Figure 3). A leftward axis is found more commonly in men than in women and does not necessarily imply underlying cardiac pathology. Mihalick and Fisch (23) noted a definite increase in left axis deviation with advancing years but no correlation with cardiovascular disease could be documented. Kulbertus *et al.* (22) showed a

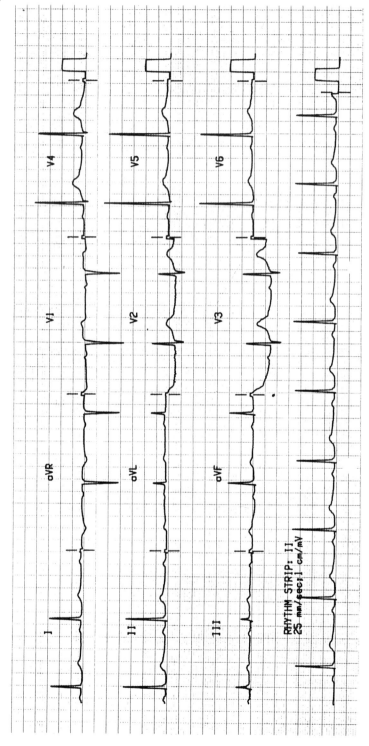

Figure 2. ECG from an 80-year-old man with apparently normal heart. Note the borderline PR and QT intervals

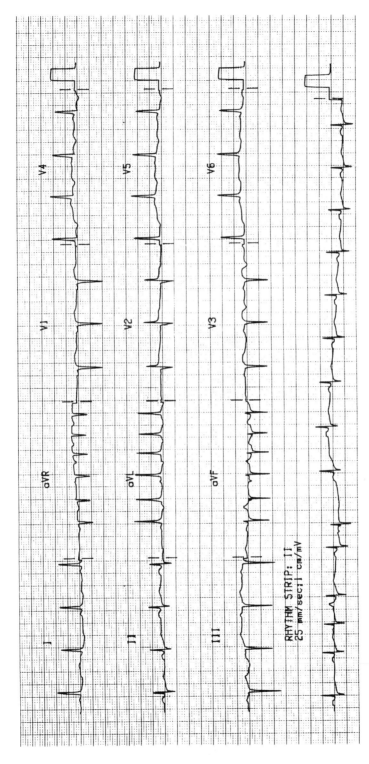

Figure 3. ECG from a 76-year-old woman. Left axis deviation and frequent atrial ectopics

clear linear increase in left axis deviation with age but they could only correlate this with aortic knuckle calcification and dilatation. In the younger age group left axis deviation is not often preceded by myocardial infarction (30) and in the old, brown atrophy of the heart may be the only pathology (31). A sclero-degenerative process of the subjunctional conduction system is frequently associated with the development of hemiblocks in the elderly population (32), which may occur in both normal and patient groups (33).

In other studies this finding has been documented in patients with cardiovascular disease but not in apparently normal elderly subjects (34–36). It seems that left axis deviation in the elderly is probably related to underlying coronary disease and hypertension (17,35,37,38) rather than to skeletal deformation (e.g. kyphoscoliosis) and pulmonary disease as has been suggested (23,39,40). In a postmortem correlation study of 353 cases with left axis deviation, Bahl *et al.* (38) found coronary disease in 85%. Irrespective of the possible association of left axis deviation with cardiovascular disease, isolated left axis shift carries no adverse prognosis. Campbell *et al.* (41) studied the ECGs of 2254 ambulant old people and noted no excess mortality in the 36 cases with left axis deviation alone over a 3-year follow-up period. No increased mortality from left axis deviation even in association with right bundle branch block (RBBB) was noted by Kulbertus *et al.* (22). The risk of development RBBB (30) or other forms of conduction disturbances is also slight.

Bundle branch block

The prevalence of bundle branch block in the fit elderly population varies between 3% and 5% (41,42) compared with 1% in young military populations (43). In hospitalized and institutionalized populations bundle branch block is found in 10–15% (14,23,33). In almost all series RBBB occurs slightly more often than left bundle branch block (LBBB). In the elderly bundle branch block is usually due to fibrosis and sclerosis of the conduction system (44,45) rather than to ischaemic heart disease. RBBB has little or no adverse effect on prognosis (46,47) whereas the survival of elderly patients with LBBB is generally worse than that of age-matched controls (22). Interestingly, in the large series of relatively well subjects reported by Campbell *et al.* (41) LBBB was associated with only a slightly worse prognosis than was RBBB (48).

Ventricular hypertrophy

Although the ECGs of the elderly often show low voltage, increased voltages have also been noted in a high proportion. Indeed, in the studies by Taran and Szilagyi (49) and Kulbertus *et al.* (22) left ventricular hypertrophy (LVH) was the most common abnormality (10–40%). In the latter study its prevalence was higher in women, increased almost exponentially with age and paralleled the distribution of systemic hypertension. The relationship of LVH with age and hypertension had also been noted in the Framingham study (50). The reported prevalence obviously depended on the diagnostic criteria used and ranged usually around 20% (17,51), and a prevalence as low as 1% has been also reported (23). Campbell *et al.* (41) have shown that LVH associated with ST segment changes as well as voltage changes is associated with a mortality almost four times larger than expected.

Right ventricular hypertrophy seems to have a smaller prevalence in old age compared with middle age (22,41).

Myocardial infarction

The prevalence of electrocardiographic patterns consistent with old myocardial infarction varies from less than 3% (14) to 11% in the very old (24). However, there is no strong evidence that myocardial infarction patterns occur more frequently as age advances beyond 70 years. At least 50% of subjects with myocardial infarction electrocardiographic patterns have no previous history of myocardial infarction (52) and less than 20% of elderly patients with acute myocardial infarction present with classical symptoms (53). In the elderly, Q waves denote a worse prognosis, and a twofold risk has been documented by Campbell *et al.* (41).

Arrhythmias

Many studies have recorded a high prevalence of cardiac arrhythmias in the elderly. Harris (54) has introduced the phrase 'cardiac paradox of the senior citizen' to describe the increasing frequency of cardiac disease in elderly patients associated with a decreasing clinical significance. As many as one-third of persons over 70 years may have a cardiac arrhythmia (55,56). The most common disturbances appear to be ventricular premature beats followed by atrial fibrillation and atrial premature beats (Figure 3). Pooled data from nearly 2500 ECGs in patients over 70 disclosed ventricular ectopic beats in approximately 8% of them (57). Within apparently healthy members of the Baltimore Longitudinal Study of Aging (BLSA), isolated ventricular ectopy occurred at rest in 17% of subjects over 80, compared with only 2.5% in those aged 20–30 (58).

The prevalence of atrial fibrillation ranges from 2–3% in relatively fit elderly subjects living at home (15,22) to 5–15% in hospitalized or institutionalized subjects (23). The prevalence of atrial fibrillation is higher in the very old, i.e. nonagenarians (approximately 30% (24)) and the sick elderly (22% (59)). About one-half of subjects with atrial fibrillation have demonstrated heart disease during life (14) and 40% of cases show cardiomegaly (22). At autopsy, up to 76% of those with atrial fibrillation during life have been found to have pathological features of ischaemic, hypertensive or valvular heart disease (60). Atrial fibrillation certainly reduces life expectancy in nonagenarians (24) and may have a generally poor prognosis (61). Although prognosis is more likely to depend on the aetiology of the atrial fibrillation, the additional risk of thromboembolic events associated with atrial fibrillation represents an independent risk factor.

AMBULATORY (24-HOUR) ELECTROCARDIOGRAPHY

Cardiac rhythm in the normal elderly population

The technique for ambulatory electrocardiographic monitoring utilizing a small, portable tape recorder was introduced by Holter in 1961, and systematic studies in the elderly have been conducted since the early 1980s. Ambulatory electrocardiography of adult populations has revealed that the prevalence of arrhythmias increases with age, and this was confirmed in the apparently healthy elderly population by several studies as discussed below. Although it is difficult to compare the findings of these reports because of methodological differences in arrhythmia definitions and in definition of the 'normal' population, their findings were remarkably similar in several important respects. Ventricular arrhythmias were frequent, sinus bradycardia was uncommon, and second- and third-degree atrioventricular block was very uncommon (Table 1).

Abnormalities of sinus function

The dynamics and range of sinus rhythm have been considered in detail by Fleg and Kennedy (62) and to a lesser extent by ourselves (63) and Clee et al. (64). All of these studies agree that the mean heart rate of the elderly subject is approximately 72 beats/min and, as in younger age groups (65–67) that the sinus rate in women is approximately 6–7 beats/min faster than in men. After total autonomic blockade (68) there is no difference between the heart rates of men and women, which suggests that the faster heart rate of men is due to autonomic influences.

   Although sinus bradycardia (<60 beats/min) occurred in a substantial proportion of patients (30–90%), marked sinus bradycardia (<40 beats/min) was documented in only 2–4% of the subjects studied, whereas marked sinus pauses (>2 seconds) were virtually absent (62,63) (Table 2). It is generally assumed that the sinus rate falls with increasing age but, although this tendency has been documented by some investigators (69,70), most agree that the decline

Table 1. Summary of prevalence of arrhythmias found in the apparently normal elderly population

Common	Intermediate	Uncommon
Atrial ectopic beats	Atrial fibrillation	Sinus pauses
Slow atrial tachycardia	Ventricular tachycardia	Sinus bradycardia
Ventricular ectopic beats		Complete heart block

Table 2. Prevalence of sinus pauses and sinus bradycardia in the largest reported studies

Author	No.	Age	Definition of study group	Sinus bradycardia (%)	Sinus pauses (%)
					(<40 beats/min) (>2 s)
Camm et al. (63)	106	75–95	Ambulatory, elderly subjects living at home No acute illness	4	0
Fleg and Kennedy (2)	98	60–85	Normal physical, ECG, chest X-ray, exercise test No cardiovascular medications	2	0
Manyari et al. (81)	86	60–96	Normal physical, ECG, chest X-ray, biochemistry, M-mode echo, spirometry No cardiovascular medication	0	0

in heart rate with increasing adult age is hardly significant (71). Simonson and Keys (26) failed to demonstrate any difference in the sinus rates of younger and older men (approximately 30 years' difference in age). Although occasional sinus bradycardia unassociated with overt underlying heart disease (72) may occur in the elderly, it is certainly not usual in apparently healthy old people, and is mostly confined to the elderly sick (73). Interestingly, sinus bradycardia has been also noted in the very young age groups, such as medical students and neonates (74). Whether the dysfunction of the sinus node is a result of gradual degeneration of the dominant pacemaker or is related to the increased incidence of coronary artery disease is unknown. Kostis et al. (75) documented that the reduction in the maximum heart rate was associated with lower exercise tolerance in the aged. The heart rate at rest was not reduced and the heart rate response to sudden maximal exercise was exaggerated rather than attenuated. Thus in this age group this finding might represent a specific group with chronotropic incompetence (76).

In the study by Camm et al. (63), but not in that of Fleg and Kennedy (62), there was a marked reduction in the dynamic range of heart rate. This difference possibly occurred because we studied significantly older subjects who were likely to have been more immobile. However, in our subjects there was also a very low incidence of sinus arrhythmia which has been shown to decrease with age (77), and the absence of sinus arrhythmia may be due to latent myocardial disease, age-related partial autonomic paresis or degenerative sinus node disease, indicating a variety of sick or 'lazy' sinus node disease (Figure 4). The age-related decline in sinus rate variability has been demonstrated by others as well (70,78).

140

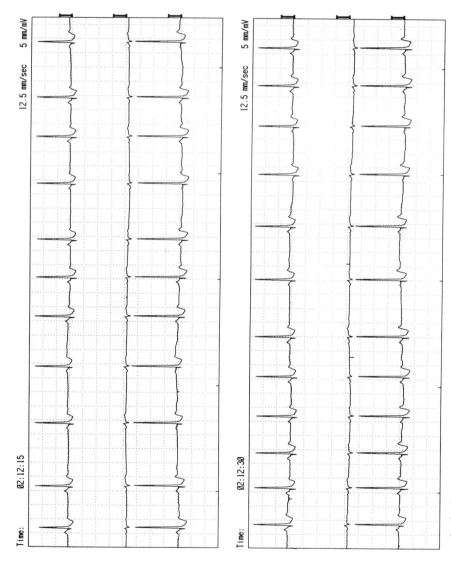

Figure 4. Sinus arrhythmia

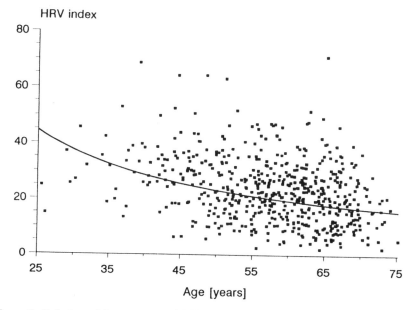

Figure 5. Relation of heart rate variability with age (Malik and Camm, unpublished observations)

Hrushesky *et al.* (79) suggested that respiratory sinus arrhythmia can be utilized as a measure of cardiac age. His studies indicated that the amplitude of the respiratory sinus arrhythmias fell approximately 10% per decade. According to our unpublished observations, heart rate variability also decreases with advanced age (Figure 5).

Atrioventricular block

High degrees of AV block are rarely found in apparently healthy old people (62,63,80). Intermittent complete heart block has been reported in these studies with a frequency ranging from 1% to 4%. Sinus arrest has also been extremely rare in these studies, thus making ventricular pauses a very rare finding in normal elderly subjects.

Supraventricular arrhythmias

Most studies have excluded subjects with atrial fibrillation. Atrial fibrillation (Figure 6) was detected in approximately 11% of our population (63), which consisted of subjects aged more than 70 years, whereas Manyari *et al.* (81) detected paroxysmal atrial fibrillation in only 3% of their patients, who had a broader age spectrum (60–96). Atrial ectopic activity was detected from

142

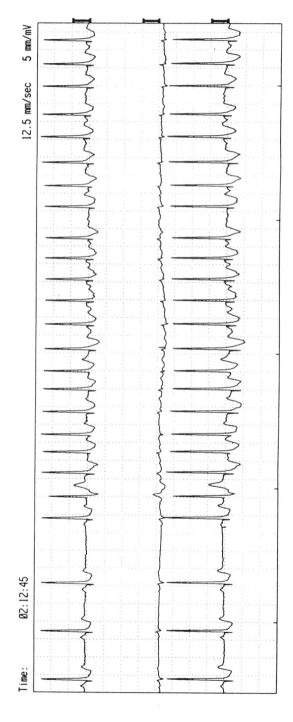

Figure 6. Episode of paroxysmal AF

143

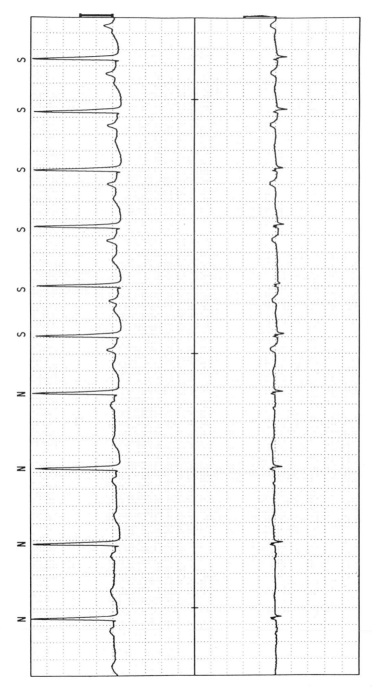

Figure 7. Slow atrial tachycardia, typical of the old age

approximately 25% (63,81) to 100% (82) of patients in various series. Fleg and Kennedy (62) and Manyari *et al.* (81) also recorded a relatively slow atrial tachycardia (Figure 7) in 30% of their patients and considered this arrhythmia as a benign variant. Atrial flutter was also seen in the series of Abdon (83) and Fleg and Kennedy (62). Left atrial dilatation, a normal development in healthy elderly subjects, seems to play a significant role in the pathophysiology of the increased incidence of atrial arrhythmias seen in this age (81).

Prognostic implications

The prognostic significance of atrial fibrillation in the elderly has been the subject of much dispute. The follow-up study of Martin *et al.* (84) showed evidence for increased mortality for those who had atrial fibrillation, although only one of the eight, out of 106, subjects died from an identifiable cardiovascular cause. This study also confirmed that the incidence of atrial fibrillation increases with age since 17% of our survivors, all over the age of 80 years, had proven atrial fibrillation. Kulbertus *et al.* (61), using conventional electrocardiography, discovered a threefold increase in mortality in subjects with lone atrial fibrillation compared with age-matched controls in sinus rhythm. It is not clear whether this can be attributed to the increased risk of thromboembolism associated with the arrhythmia.

Supraventricular ectopic beats (up to 100 per hour) or paroxysmal atrial tachycardia do not appear to have any long-term prognostic significance in subjects between 60 and 85 years old without apparent cardiac disease (85).

Ventricular arrhythmias

Ventricular arrhythmias may be a common finding at any age (74,86–88), but as age advances there is an almost exponential increase in the frequency of ventricular extrasystoles (89). Although most investigators have quantified and graded ventricular arrhythmias using a modification of the method suggested by Lown and Wolf (90), the exact grading system has been different for each study. Table 3 details the prevalence of frequent ventricular ectopic beats and ventricular tachycardia (Figure 8) in the largest reported series so far. Ventricular ectopic activity in general can be found from 35% (91) to 100% (80) of apparently normal elderly people. Complex ventricular arrhythmias are less frequent, whereas ventricular tachycardia can be seen in up to 4% of asymptomatic patients (Table 3). Thus ventricular ectopy, simple and complex, is frequent in elderly ambulant patients. Although the mechanism for the increase in ventricular premature beats (VPBs) with advancing age is uncertain, theoretical possibilities include latent coronary artery disease, left ventricular hypertrophy or dilatation, elevated plasma catecholamines and a relative prolongation of the Q–T interval (58). However, in practice, myocardial ischaemia secondary to coronary disease is an improbable cause for the majority

Table 3. Prevalance of ventricular arrhythmias in the largest reported studies

Author	No.	Age	Definition of study group	Frequent VPBs Definition	(%)	VT (%)
Clee *et al.* (64)	50	>60	Active asymptomatic No CV medication	1 VPB/100 SB	26	NA
Camm *et al.* (63)	106	75–95	Ambulatory, elderly subjects living at home	100 VPB/h	12	4
			No acute illness	10 VPB/h	26	
Abdon *et al.* (91)	77	47–92	Asymptomatic	1 VPB/10 SB	8	0
Fleg and Kennedy (62)	98	60–85	Normal physical, ECG, chest X-ray, exercise test No CV medications	60 VPB/h 30 VPB/h	7 12	4
Kantelip *et al.* (82)	50	>80	Normal physical, ECG, biochemistry Bo CV medication	50–100 >100	10 4	2
Manyari *et al.* (81)	86	60–96	Normal physical, ECG, chest X-ray, biochemistry, M-mode echo, spirometry No CV medication	>50/24 h	35	2

CV = cardiovascular, VPB = ventricular premature beat, VT = ventricular tachycardia, SB = sinus beats, NA = not available.

of ventricular ectopics in the elderly (58,63), whereas the effect of hypertension and left ventricular hypertrophy is controversial (63,64,81,92,93). Recently, Manyari *et al.* (81) in a study of 86 normal elderly subjects detected ventricular arrhythmias in 55 (64%) subjects but the frequency and complexity of ventricular arrhythmias did not correlate with the ventricular mass index. Tea and coffee consumption appear to be irrelevant to the incidence of VPBs in the elderly, whereas the effect of tobacco is disputed (63,64).

Prognostic implications

Prognostic inferences from the results of ambulatory ECG recordings in elderly subjects are weak and rather contradictory. Several studies (94,95) have failed to demonstrate any significant relationship between symptoms, sudden death and ventricular ectopics. Martin *et al.* (84) have followed up the cohort of elderly, apparently healthy subjects originally reported by Camm *et al.* (63). Over a follow-up period of approximately 2.5 years, 67% of the 28 patients with frequent ventricular ectopics had died, whereas only 36% of those without such ectopics had died. However, these are crude survival statistics and the relevance

146

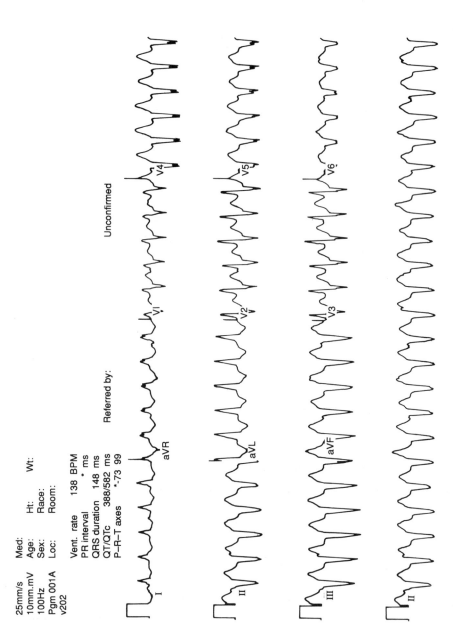

Figure 8. Ventricular tachycardia in a 75-year-old man, probably due to ischaemic heart disease

of other factors was not assessed; the excess mortality may be due to associated heart disease rather than the ectopic activity itself. Fleg and Kennedy (85) also failed to detect any long-term prognostic significance of ventricular ectopic beats (up to 30 VPB/h) in subjects between 60 and 85 years old without apparent cardiac disease. Generally, ventricular ectopic activity noted on 24-hour ECG monitoring is not clearly associated with an adverse prognosis in this age group or in any other (96), unless coupled with overt coronary artery disease (58), and routine therapeutic intervention is not justified.

Ambulatory electrocardiographic monitoring in symptomatic patients

In the aged patient it has proved difficult to establish a direct correlation between symptoms, such as dizziness, lightheadedness, vertigo, fits, faints and falls and transient cardiac arrhythmias. There are several reasons for this. First, forgetfulness, physical infirmity and mental disability often result in inability to complete the diary or log of daily events and symptoms. Second, even when diaries or event markers have been meticulously completed there is often no exact relationship between a cardiac arrhythmia and the symptoms which may be caused by such rhythms. For example, although a sustained tachycardia or asystolic episode may result in a syncopal spell in an ambulant subject the same arrhythmia may cause no symptoms when the patient is recumbent. As a result, most investigators have searched recordings for arrhythmias which may be responsible for such symptoms and, therefore, are referred to as 'pertinent' or 'predisposing' arrhythmias. Third, in the elderly, symptoms are often multifactorial in aetiology. In the same patient, dizziness may result from a tachycardia, from a bradycardia, or from vertebrobasilar insufficiency. However, in practical terms, treatment of the predominant arrhythmia may well solve many of the patients' symptomatic problems.

Cardiac arrhythmias and central nervous system symptoms

Both tachycardias and bradycardias (97–100) significantly reduce cerebral blood flow and may thus give rise to cerebral symptoms (101), especially in the elderly where associated cerebrovascular disease is common. Such symptoms may be due to reduction in cerebral blood flow or to cerebral infarction (100).

In a retrospective survey of 290 symptomatic patients who received a cardiac pacemaker for disturbances of cardiac rhythm, Reed et al. (102) established that 239 (82%) had suffered generalized (81%) or focal (1.4%) cerebral symptoms prior to pacemaker implantation. Conversely, of 39 patients presenting with cerebral ischaemia Walter et al. (103), using 10-hour ambulatory ECG monitoring, found cardiac arrhythmias which possibly provoked the ischaemic episodes in 10 patients (25%). In subsequent studies on patients with cerebral symptoms evaluated by ambulatory electrocardiographic monitoring, predisposing arrhythmias were noticed from 23% (104) to almost half (105) of the cases.

McHenry *et al.* (106) investigated 10 patients with cerebrovascular insufficiency and identified six of the patients to have cardiac arrhythmias which were thought to be relevant to their neurological presentation. However, eight patients had also had cardiovascular disease—usually carotid artery stenosis. The interplay between limitations of local flow (stenosis) and reduced cardiac output (arrhythmia) is probably responsible for focal rather than generalized ischaemic attacks.

Although arrhythmias do occur in a substantial proportion of patients presenting with transient ischaemic attacks, a causal relationship is difficult to establish since significant arrhythmias also occur in many normal elderly subjects. McCarthy and Wollner (107) attempted to compare symptomatic patients with age-matched control subjects and found arrhythmias to be more common in the symptomatic group. However, the control group was small and no firm conclusions should be drawn from such a study. Rai (94) compared 20 asymptomatic control subjects with 20 patients complaining of 'funny turns', 'collapse' and 'falls'. Both groups had a wide range of arrhythmias on the 24-hour ECG recordings but the symptomatic group had rather more serious arrhythmias. A much larger investigation conducted by De Bono *et al.* (108) compared 89 patients with transient non-focal central nervous system symptoms with 109 control (but not necessarily 'normal') subjects. In the elderly (>60 years) cohort, which comprised 18 patients and 31 controls, there was a high prevalence of arrhythmias but there was no excess of arrhythmias in the patient group. Clark *et al.* (109) analysed ambulatory ECGs in 98 consecutive patients complaining of dizziness or syncope. Although 41 subjects suffered symptoms during the recording, there was a poor correlation with arrhythmias. So far, the largest series of ambulatory monitoring findings in the elderly is the one reported by Nelson *et al.* (110). This group analysed the records of 1238 patients with a mean age of 78 years, from their computerized Holter recording database. The majority of these patients had known or suspected heart disease and less than 5% had 'normal' electrocardiographic monitor recordings. Bradyarrhythmias were detected in 12.5% of the patients, supraventricular arrhythmias in 55%, complex ventricular ectopics (Lown class 3 or greater) in 88%, and ventricular tachycardia in 8% of the patients. When a symptom occurred in this population during the ECG monitoring, approximately half of the patients had an associated arrhythmia recorded at the time of the symptom. Bradyarrhythmias accounted for 4% of patients with dizziness and 29% of patients with syncope. Tachyarrhythmias were recorded in 13% of patients with dizziness, in 21% of patients with syncope, in 17% with palpitation and in 5% with chest pain. However, arrhythmias that are potentially capable of causing symptoms occurred concurrently with a symptom at a frequency of 2–5% (5% of bradyarrhythmias, 3% of supraventricular arrhythmias and 2% of ventricular arrhythmias). This poor symptom–arrhythmia correlation underlines the difficulties encountered in interpreting Holter monitoring in symptomatic elderly, as previously discussed.

The relevance of arrhythmias to the genesis of symptoms of central nervous system insufficiency may also be partially assessed from the response of treatment directed at these arrhythmias. In most studies (111,112) the prescription of antiarrhythmic treatment guided by the results of ambulatory electrocardiographic monitoring has been generally successful.

In conclusion, the discovery of sustained arrhythmias on ambulatory recordings of elderly patients with central nervous system symptoms suggests, although does not prove, that the symptoms may be related to the arrhythmia and specific therapy should be considered. Conventional ECGs are unlikely to disclose such rhythm disturbances and 24-hour ECG monitoring is necessary for this purpose (104). Longer recordings are generally not warranted (91). Although the cost-effectiveness of ambulatory electrocardiographic recording has been questioned (109,113,114), this investigation gives a definitive yield of therapeutically important information and should be performed in all cases of recurrent fits, faints or falls (115). In occasional cases, trans-telephonic ECG monitoring, tilt testing and invasive electrophysiology testing may also be required.

Cardiac arrhythmias and psychiatric symptoms

A so-called chronic encephalopathy due to heart block was described by D'Allesio et al. (116), and Lassers et al. (117) noted that depressant mental function associated with heart block due to myocardial infarction could be improved by artificial pacing. A case of acute psychosis related to complete AV block which was effectively suppressed by cardiac pacing has also been reported (118). Duncan and Stevenson (119) and Clark (120) have described the association between mental symptoms and paroxysmal ectopic tachycardias, whereas in a systematic evaluation of electroencephalogram and ambulatory ECG correlates in patients with sick sinus syndrome or AV block, significant bradycardia was generally associated with excessive slow wave activity (100). Cases of dementia and even Parkinsonism have been attributed to AV block and ventricular bradycardia (100,121). The causative relation between arrhythmias and dementia, however, has not been substantiated in other studies (83,122). Since potentially harmful bradyarrhythmias were only seen in association with atherosclerotic cerebral disease it is probable that atherosclerosis was responsible for the arrhythmias.

Cardiac arrhythmias and accidents

Comparisons between X-ray department records of patients with arrhythmias and a history consistent with Stokes–Adams attacks and of age-matched control patients have shown higher accidents and a slight preponderance of fractures in the former group (123). Increased risk of femoral neck fractures has also been noticed in elderly patients suffering cardiac arrhythmias, although the evidence for this association has been disputed (95,124).

INVASIVE ELECTROPHYSIOLOGY IN THE ELDERLY

Studies in the apparently normal population

Sinus node recovery time

Kulbertus *et al.* (125) have studied the sinus node function of 30 patients with atherosclerosis, aged between 52 and 72, without any clinical suggestion of sinus node disease or AV node disease. Atrial pacing rates up to 120 beats/min produced the maximum sinus nodal suppression, in contrast to younger adults in whom the degree of suppression increased up to pacing rates of 150 beats/min (126). Maximum post-pacing pauses ranged from 680 to 1600 ms and, when corrected for heart rate, from 110 to 680 ms. The upper normal 'cut-off' proposed by this group for the elderly was 1500 ms, i.e. more or less similar to ordinary adult populations. Higher recovery times (up to 1660 ms) for patients without evidence of sinus nodal dysfunction have been reported by other (127,128). Vallin (128) reported the results of sinus node recovery times in 18 volunteer elderly subjects, aged 52–76 years of age, who were clinically normal and had normal biochemical and cardiovascular evaluation including an ECG and bicycle ergometer stress test. Sinus node recovery times ranged from 870 to 1675 ms whereas corrected values ranged from 235 to 510 ms. Thus in the elderly an upper limit of normal for the uncorrected sinus node recovery time should be longer than the 1400 ms suggested by Rosen *et al.* (129) for a younger adult group. The value of 1680 ms, originally recommended for adult populations by Dhingra *et al.* (130), would seem to be particularly applicable to the elderly. Because most of the increased sinus node recovery time is due to prolongation of the basic cycle length, a maximum normal corrected recovery time of 525 ms (131) would suffice for both elderly and younger adult subjects. Vallin (128) suggested that the upper limit of normal for the corrected maximum value should be increased to 545 ms and also that a more precise evaluation of sinus node function could be achieved by autonomic blockade with atropine (0.02 mg/kg) and propranolol (0.01 mg/kg), the upper normal limit of corrected sinus node recovery time under these circumstances being 505 ms.

In a systematic evaluation of the effect of age on the sinus node recovery time, Pop and Fleishman (132) studied 110 patients without overt sinus node dysfunction and without AV conduction disturbances. They observed a small but progressive increase in the recovery time up to the age of 70 years and a small but significant reduction after 70 years.

Sinoatrial conduction time

Sinoatrial conduction time is known to increase in youth (133), but is not further influenced by old age. Usual reported values range from 195 ms (134) to 167 ms (135).

Intracardiac conduction intervals and refractory periods

With the exception of the intra-atrial conduction time (P–A interval) which may be prolonged up to 65 ms in the elderly, as opposed to the upper normal limit of 55 ms in adults, there is little difference between populations (136). Similarly, atrial and AV nodal effective refractory periods in the aged match those in the adult population in general (136), whereas a significant prolongation of right atrial functional refractory period has been reported by Padaletti *et al.* (135). Kulbertus *et al.* (125) estimated the Wenckebach periodicity point in their cohort of 30 relatively normal elderly patients. In seven patients AV conduction persisted up to the maximum rate of 180 beats/min, and in six Wenckebach periodicity was encountered at pacing rates as low as 120 beats/min, whereas in the adult population in general this does not occur at rates less than 130 beats/min (129).

Invasive electrophysiological tests in abnormal or symptomatic elderly patients

Sick sinus syndrome

Several studies of elderly patients with sick sinus syndrome have reported a prolongation of the maximum sinus node recovery time (127) and, although inconsistently, of the sinoatrial conduction times (134,137) compared with patients without sick sinus syndrome.

Bifascicular block

Bifascicular block in the elderly may not represent a serious threat to life and rarely indicates imminent progression to advanced AV block, even in the presence of a prolonged H–V interval (138). The rather better prognosis in the elderly may indicate that intraventricular block in this patient group is more likely to be due to degenerative fibrosis than to coronary artery disease (139).

Wolff–Parkinson–White syndrome

Results in the elderly with Wolff–Parkinson–White syndrome are similar to adult patients in general, although Ueda *et al.* (140) have reported somewhat longer refractory periods of the accessory pathway and delayed conduction times in 10 elderly (50–82 years) patients with the syndrome. Thus the P to delta interval in four of these elderly patients exceeded 120 ms.

CONCLUSIONS

Electrocardiographic abnormalities typical of old age include slight prolongation of the P–R interval (up to 0.22 s), leftwards QRS axis (up to −30), and T wave flattening. However, abnormalities of the adult ECG are also abnormal in old age and have similar prognostic implications. The prevalence of atrial fibrillation increases with age and probably reflects fibrosis or amyloid infiltration of the atrial myocardium. Its significance is not certain but recent evidence suggests that it is associated with a slightly adverse prognosis.

Ambulatory electrocardiography has shown that the prevalence of both supraventricular and ventricular ectopic beats increases almost exponentially with age. Both supraventricular and ventricular ectopic beats appear to be asymptomatic and their prognostic importance is unknown. Bradycardias (sinus bradycardia, sinus arrest, sinoatrial exit block and second- or third-degree AV block) are rare in normal elderly subjects. Thus slow heart rate in symptomatic patients usually indicates the need for corrective therapy.

In normal elderly patients intracardiac electrophysiological testing reveals results similar to the adult population as a whole.

In conclusion, conventional ECGs and electrophysiological findings may be interpreted similarly in the young and elderly patients. Ambulatory electrocardiographic data from the aged, however, must be interpreted with caution because marked bradycardia is less common and ventricular ectopic activity is much more common than in younger subjects.

REFERENCES

1. Harris R (1986) Aging and the cardiovascular system. In: *Clinical Geriatric Cardiology: Management of the Elderly Patient*. Lippincot, Philadelphia, pp. 1–31.
2. Simonson E (1958) The normal variability of the electrocardiogram as a basis for differentiation between 'normal' and 'abnormal' clinical electrocardiography. *Am Heart J* **55**: 80–103.
3. Simonson E (1966) The concept and definition of normality. *Ann NY Acad Sci* **134**: 541–558.
4. Gelman I, Brown S (1937) Electrocardiographical characterisation of the heart in old age and in childhood. *Acta Med Scand* **91**: 378–396.
5. Levitt G (1939) The electrocardiogram in the aged. *Am Heart J* **18**: 692–696.
6. Eliaser M, Kondo BO (1941) The electrocardiogram in later life. *Arch. Intern. Med.* **67**: 637–646.
7. Taran LM, Kaye M (1944) Electrocardiographic studies in old age. *Ann Intern Med* **20**: 954–960.
8. Gavey CG (1949) The cardiology of old age. *Lancet* **ii**: 725–735.
9. McNamara RJ (1949) A study of the electrocardiogram in persons over 70. *Geriatrics* **4**: 150–160.
10. Fox TT, Klements SJ, Mandel EE (1942) Electrocardiographic changes in old age. *Ann Intern Med* **17**: 236–244.
11. Fox TT (1949) On the significance of the normal electrocardiogram in old age. *Ann Intern Med* **31**: 120–124.
12. Jensen J, Smith M, Cartwright ED (1932) The electrocardiogram in late middle life. *Am Heart J* **7**: 718–724.
13. Duthoit A, Warembourg H (1938) L'electrocardiogramme du vieillard. *Arch Mal Coeur* **31**: 34–45.
14. Fisch C, Genovese PK, Dyke RW *et al.* (1957) The electrocardiogram in persons over 70. *Geriatrics* **12**: 616–620.

15. Kennedy RD, Caird FI (1972) The application of the Minnesota code to population studies of the electrocardiogram in the elderly. *Gerontol Clin* **14**: 5–16.
16. Blackburn H, Keys A, Simonson E *et al.* (1960) The electrocardiogram in population studies: a classification system. *Circulation* **21**: 1160–1175.
17. Michie I (1970) Electrocardiographic changes in the elderly. *Genontol Clin* **12**: 193–202.
18. Sidney KH, Shephard RJ (1977) Training and electrocardiographic abnormalities in the elderly. *Br Heart J* **39**: 1114–1120.
19. Evans JG, Tunbridge WMG (1976) Information loss in limb lead electrocardiograms compared with twelve-lead tracings in a population survey among the elderly. *Age Ageing* **5**: 56–61.
20. Pipberger HC, Schneiderman MA, Klingeman JD (1968) The love at first sight effect in research. *Circulation* **38**: 822–825.
21. Simonson E (1972) The effect of age on the electrocardiogram. *Am J Cardiol* **29**: 64–73.
22. Kulbertus HE, De Leval-Rutten F, Albert A *et al.* (1981) Electrocardiographic changes occurring with advancing age. In *What's New in Electrocardiography*, Wellens HJJ, Kulbertus HE (eds). Martinus Nijhoff, The Hague, pp. 300–314.
23. Mihalick MJ, Fiusch C (1974) Electrocardiographic findings in the aged. *Am Heart J* **87**: 117–128.
24. Bowers D (1969) Electrogram of nonagenarians. *Geriatrics* **24**: 89–92.
25. Rodstein M, Brown M, Wolloch L (1968) First degree atrioventricular heart block in the aged. *Geriatrics* **23**: 159–165.
26. Simonson E, Keys A (1952) The effect of age and body weight on the electrocardiogram of healthy men. *Circulation* **6**: 749–761.
27. Hiss CG, Lamb LE, Allen MF (1960) Electrocardiographic findings in 67,375 asymptomatic subjects. X. Normal values. *Am J Cardiol* **6**: 200–231.
28. Harlan WR, Graybiel A, Mitchell RE *et al.* (1967) Serial electrocardiograms: their reliability and prognostic validity during a 24 year period. *J. Chronic Dis.* **20**: 853–867.
29. Bachman S, Sparrow D, Smith LK (1981) Effect of ageing on the electrocardiogram. *Am J Cardiol* **48**: 513–516.
30. Rabkin SW, Mathewson FAL, Tale RB (1979) Natural history of marked left axis deviation. *Am J Cardiol* **43**: 605–611.
31. Katz LN, Saphir O, Strauss H (1935) The electrocardiogram in brown atrophy of the heart. *Am Heart J* **10**: 542–545.
32. Rosenbaum MB, Eliziari MV, Lazzari JO (1970) The hemiblocks: new concepts of intraventricular conduction block on human anatomical physiological and clinical studies. Tampa Tracings, Florida.
33. Saurez RM, Saurez RM (1961) The electrocardiogram in aged Puerto Ricans. *J Am Geriat Soc* **9**: 645–650.
34. Gormon PA, Catalayud JB, Abrahams S, Caveres CA (1964) Effects of age and heart disease on the QRS axis during the seventh through the tenth decades. *Am Heart J* **67**: 39–43.
35. Eliot RS, Millhon WA, Millhon J (1963) The clinical significance of uncomplicated marked left axis deviation in men without known disease. *Am J Cardiol* **12**: 767–771.
36. Curd GW, Hicks WM, Gyorkey F (1961) Marked left axis deviation: indication of cardiac abnormality. *Am Heart J* **62**: 462–469.
37. Grant RP (1956) Left axis deviation: an electrocardiographic–pathologic correlation study. *Circulation* **14**: 233–249.
38. Bahl OP, Walsh TJ, Massie E (1969) Left axis deviation: an electrocardiographic study with post-mortem correlation. *Br Heart J* **31**: 451–456.

39. Olbrich O, Woodford-Williams E (1953a) The normal precordial electrocardiogram in the aged. *J Gerontol* **8**: 40–55.
40. Olbrich O, Woodford-Williams E (1953b). The effect of change of body position on the precordial electrocardiogram in young and aged subjects. *J Gerontol* **8**: 56–62.
41. Campbell A, Caird FI, Jackson TFM (1974) Prevalence of abnormalities of the electrocardiogram in old people. *Br Heart J* **36**: 1005–1011.
42. Edmands RE (1966) An epidemiological assessment of bundle branch block. *Circulation* **34**: 1081–1087.
43. Johnson RI, Averill KH, Lamb LE (1960) Electrocardiographic findings in 67,375 asymptomatic individuals. *Am J Cardiol* **6**: 143–167.
44. Lenegre J (1964) Etiology and pathology of bilateral bundle branch block in relation to complete heart block. *Progressive Cardiovasc Discoveries* **6**: 409–444.
45. Lev M (1964) Anatomic basis for atrioventricular block. *Am J Med* **37**: 742–748.
46. Rodstein M, Gubner R, Mills JP *et al.* (1951) A mortality study in bundle branch block. *Arch Intern Med* **87**: 663–668.
47. Fleg JL, Das DN, Lakatta EG (1983) Right bundle branch block: long-term prognosis in apparently healthy men. *J Am Coll Cardiol* **1**: 887–982.
48. Caird FI, Campbell A, Jackson TFM (1974) Significance of abnormalities of electrocardiogram in old people. *Br Heart J* **36**: 1012–1018.
49. Taran LM, Szilagyi N (1958) Electrocardiographic changes with advancing age. *Geriatrics* **13**: 352–358.
50. Kannel WB, Gordon T, Offutt D (1969) Left ventricular hypertrophy by electrocardiogram: prevalence, incidence and mortality in the Framingham study. *Ann Intern Med* **71**: 89–105.
51. Gelfand M (1957) The octogenarian electrocardiogram. *Geriatrics* **12**: 136–161.
52. Foulds Ak (1966) *Medicine in Old Age*. Pitman, London.
53. Pathy MS (1977) Clinical presentation of myocardial infarction in the elderly. *Br Heart J* **29**: 190–199.
54. Harris R (1964) Cardiac parodox of the senior citizen. A phenomenon of age. *N.Y. State J. Med.* **1964**: 2461–2464.
55. Lamy PP, Kitler ME (1971) The geriatric patient: age-dependent physiologic and pathologic changes. *J Am Geriat Soc* **19**: 871–879.
56. Storch S, Tang ZT (1954) Cardiac arrhythmias in the aged. *Am Pract* **5**: 367–373.
57. Fisch C (1981) Electrocardiogram in the aged: an independent marker of heart disease? *Am J Med* **70**: 4–6.
58. Fleg JL (1988) Ventricular arrhythmias in the elderly: prevalence, mechanisms, and therapeutic implications. *Geriatrics* **43**: 23–29.
59. Patel K (1977) Electrocardiographic abnormalities in the sick elderly. *Age Ageing* **6**: 163–167.
60. Inoue H, Ohkawa S, Ueyama C *et al.* (1982) Clinicopathologic study on determinants of the amplitude of atrial fibrillation waves in the geriatric population. *Am Heart J* **103**: 1382–1384.
61. Kulbertus H, De Leval-Rutten F, Barsch P, Petit JM (1983) Is lone atrial fibrillation benign in the elderly? *J Am Coll Cardiol* **1**: 583 (abstract).
62. Fleg JL, Kennedy HL (1982) Cardiac arrhythmias in a healthy elderly population: detection by 24-hour ambulatory electrocardiography. *Chest* **81**: 302–307.
63. Camm AJ, Evans KE, Ward DE, Martin A (1980) The rhythm of the heart in acute elderly subjects. *Am Heart J* **99**: 589–603.
64. Clee MD, Smith N, McNeill GP, Wright DS (1979) Dysrhythmias in apparently healthy elderly subjects. *Age Ageing* **8**: 173–176.
65. Clarke JM, Hamer J, Shelton JR *et al.* (1976) The rhythm of the normal human heart. *Lancet* **ii**: 508–512.

66. Sobotka PA, Mayer JH, Bauernfeind RA *et al.* (1981) Arrhythmias documented by 24-hour continuous ambulatory electrocardiographic monitoring in young women without apparent heart disease. *Am Heart J* **101**: 753–759.

67. Bjerregaard P (1983) Mean 24 hour heart rate, minimal heart rate and pauses in healthy subjects 40–79 years of age. *Eur Heart J* **4**: 44–51.

68. Jose AD, Collison D (1970) The normal range and determinants of the intrinsic heart rate in man. *Cardiovascular Res* **4**: 160–167.

69. Brandfonbrener M, Landowne M, Shock NW (1955) Changes in cardiac output with age. *Circulation* **12**: 557–566.

70. Cinelli P, de Scalzi M, Fabiano F *et al.* (1983) Risk factors in chronoelectrocardiology. *IRCS Med Sci* **11**: 316–362.

71. Landowne M, Brandfonbrener M, Shock NW (1955) The relation of age to certain measures of performance of the heart and the circulation. *Circulation* **11**: 567.

72. Agruss ND, Rosin EY, Adolph RJ, Rowler NO (1972) Significance of chronic sinus bradycardia in elderly people. *Circulation* **46**: 924–930.

73. Kirk JE, Kvorning SA (1952) Sinus bradycardia: a clinical study of 515 consecutive cases. *Acta Med Scand* (Suppl) **266**: 625–652.

74. Southall DP, Orrell MJ, Talbot FJ *et al.* (1977) Study of cardiac arrhythmias and other forms of conduction abnormality in newborn infants. *Br Med J* **ii**: 579–599.

75. Kostis JB, Moreyra AE, Amendo MT *et al.* (1982) The effect of age on heart rate in subjects free of heart disese. *Circulation* **65**: 141–145.

76. Katritsis D, Camm AJ (1993) Chromotropic incompetance. A proposal for definition and diagnosis. *Br Heart J* **70**: 400–402.

77. Faulkner JM (1980) The significance of sinus arrhythmias in old people. *Am J Med Sci* **180**: 42–47.

78. Schering *et al.* 1974

79. Hrushesky WJM, Fader D, Schmitt O *et al.* (1984) The respiratory sinus arrhythmia: a measure of cardiac age. *Science* **224**: 1001–1004.

80. Glasser SP, Clark PI, Applebaum HJ (1979) Occurrence of frequent complex arrhythmias detected by ambulatory monitoring: findings in an apparently healthy asymptomatic elderly population. *Chest* **75**: 565–568.

81. Manyari DE, Peterson C, Johnson D *et al.* (1990) Atrial and ventricular arrhythmias in asymptomatic active elderly subjects: correlation with left atrial size and left ventricular mass. *Am Heart J* **119**: 1069–1076.

82. Kantelip JP, Sage E, Duchene-Marullaz P (1986) Findings on ambulatory electrocardiographic monitoring in subjects older than 89 years. *Am J Cardiol* **57**: 398–401.

83. Abdon NJ (1981) Frequency and distribution of long-term ECG-recorded cardiac arrhythmias in an elderly population, with special reference to neurological symptoms. *Acta Med Scand* **209**: 175–183.

84. Martin A, Benbow LJ, Butrous G *et al.* (1984) Five year follow-up of 106 elderly subjects by means of long-term ambulatory monitoring. **5**: 592–595.

85. Fleg JL, Kennedy HL (1992) Long-term prognostic significance of ambulatory electrocardiographic findings in apparently healthy subjects greater than or equal to 60 years of age. *Am J Cardiol* **70**: 748–751.

86. Brodsky M, Wu D, Denes P *et al.* (1977) Arrhythmias documented by 24 hour continuous electrocardiographic monitoring in 50 male medical students without apparent heart disease. *Am J Cardiol* **39**: 390–395.

87. Kostis JB, McCrone K, Moreyra AE *et al.* (1981) Premature ventricular complexes in the absence of identifiable heart disease. *Circulation* **62**: 1541–1356.

88. Bjerregaard P (1982) Premature beats in healthy subjects 40–79 years of age. *Eur Heart J* **3**: 493–503.

89. Sherman H, Sandberg S, Fineberg HV (1982) Exponential increase in age-specific prevalence of ventricular dysrhythmia among males. *J Chronic Dis* **35**: 743–750.

90. Lown B, Wolf M (1971) Approaches to sudden death from coronary heart disease. *Circulation* **44**: 130.

91. Abdon NJ, Johansson BW, Lessem J (1981) Predictive use of routine 24-hour electrocardiography in suspected Adams–Stokes syndrome. Comparison with cardiac rhythm during symptoms. *Br Heart J* **47**: 533–558.

92. Celentano A, Galderisi M, Mureddu GF *et al.* (1988) Arrhythmias, hypertension and the elderly: Holter evaluation. *J Hypertens* **6** (Suppl 1): S29–S32.

93. Kawecka-Jaszck K, Dubiel JP, Skoczen M *et al.* (1990) Ventricular arrhythmias and electrocardiographic patterns of the left ventricular morphology in elderly patients with arterial hypertension. *Eur J Clin Pharmacol* **39** (Suppl. I): S47–S48.

94. Rai GS (1982) Cardiac arrhythmias in the elderly. *Age Ageing* **11**: 113–115.

95. Kirkland JL, Faragher EB, Dos Santos AGR, Lye M (1983) A longitudinal study of the prognostic significance of ventricular ectopic beats in the elderly. *Gerontology* **29**: 199–201.

96. Crow R, Prineas R, Blackburn H (1981) The prognostic significance of ventricular ectopic beats among the apparently healthy. *Am Heart J* **101**: 241–248.

97. Corday E, Irving DW (1960) Effect of cardiac arrhythmias on the cerebral circulation. *Am J Cardiol* **6**: 803–808.

98. Sulg A, Cronqvist S, Schuller H, Ingvar DH (1969) The effect of intracardiac pacemaker therapy on cerebral blood flow and electroencephalogram in patients with complete atrioventricular block. *Circulation* **39**: 487–497.

99. Samet P (1973) Haemodynamic sequelae of cardiac arrhythmias. *Circulation* **47**: 399–407.

100. Otsuka K, Yanaga T, Ichimaru Y, Seto K (1972) Observations of the effect of arrhythmias on the cerebral function by recordings of 24 hour continuous electrocardiograms: comparison between the sick sinus syndrome and atrioventricular block. *Jpn Heart J* **23**: 469–478.

101. Barnes AR (1926) Cerebral manifestations of paroxysmal tachycardia. *Am J Med Sci* **171**: 489–495.

102. Reed RL, Sickert RG, Meredith J (1973) Rarity of transient focal cerebral ischaemia in cardiac dysrhythmia. *JAMA* **223**: 893–895.

103. Walter PF, Reid SK, Wegner NK (1970) Transient cerebral ischaemia due to arrhythmia. *Ann Intern Med* **72**: 471–474.

104. Jonas S, Klein I, Dimant J (1977) Importance of Holter monitoring in patients with periodic cerebral symptoms. *Ann Neurol* **1**: 470–474.

105. Van Durme JP (1975) Tachyarrhythmias and transient cerebral ischaemic attacks. *Am Heart J* **89**: 538–540.

106. McHenry LC, Toole JF, Miller HS (1976) Long term ECG monitoring in patients with cerebrovascular insufficiency. *Stroke* **7**: 264–269.

107. McCarthy ST, Wollner L (1977) Cardiac dysrhythmias: treatable cause of transient cerebral dysfunction. Lancet **ii**: 202–203.

108. De Bono DP, Warrlow CP, Hayman NM (1982) Cardiac rhythm abnormalities in patients presenting with transient non-focal neurological symptoms: a diagnostic grey area? *Br Med J* **284**: 1437–1439.

109. Clark PI, Glasser SP, Spoto E (1980) Arrhythmias detected by ambulatory monitoring: lack of correlation with symptoms of dizziness and syncope. *Chest* **77**: 722–725.

110. Nelson RD, Ezri M, Denes P (1984) Disturbances of cardiac rhythm and conduction. In *Cardiovascular Disease in the Elderly*, Messerli FH (ed.). Martinus Nijhoff, The Hague, pp. 83–107.

111. Tzivoni D, Stern S (1975) Pacemaker implantation based on ambulatory ECG monitoring in patients with cerebral symptoms. *Chest* **67**: 274–278.
112. Levin EB (1976) Use of Holter electrocardiographic monitor in the diagnosis of transient ischaemic attacks. *J Am Geriatr Soc* **24**: 516–521.
113. Gibson TC, Levy AM (1982) Ambulatory EKC monitoring as a screening test in patients with syncope. *Circulation* **66** (Suppl. II): 73 (abstract).
114. Kapoor WN, Karpf M, Maher Y *et al.* (1982) Syncope of unknown origin. *JAMA* **247**: 2687–2691.
115. Camm AJ, Levy AM (1983) Evaluation of syncope. *Br Med J* **286**: 895.
116. D'Allesio DJ, Benchimol A, Dimond EG (1965) Chronic encephalopathy related to heart block: its correction by permanent cardiac pacemaker. *Neurology* **15**: 499.
117. Lassers BW, Anderson JL, George M *et al.* (1968) Haemodynamic effects of artificial pacing in complete heart block, complicating acute myocardial infarction. *Circulation* **38**: 308.
118. Lavy S, Stern S (1969) Transient neurological manifestations in cardiac arrhythmias. *J Neurol Sci* **9**: 97–102.
119. Duncan DH, Stevenson IP (1950) Paroxysmal arrhythmias: a psychosomatic study. *Geriatrics* **5**: 259–267.
120. Clark ANG (1970) Ectopic tachycardia in the elderly. *Gerontol Clin* **12**: 203–212.
121. Abdon N-J (1977) Unrecognised intermittent bradycardias in patients treated for senile dementia. In *Cardiac Pacing: Proceedings of the Vth International Symposium (Y. Watanabe, ed.)*. Excerpta Medica, Amsterdam, pp. 93–97.
122. Emerson TR, Milne JR, Gardner AJ (1981) Cardiogenic dementia—a myth? *Lancet* **ii**: 743–744.
123. Nilsson BE, Abdon NJ (1980) Episodic cardiac arrhythmia and accident rate. *Acta Med Scand* **208**: 69–71.
124. Abdon NJ, Nilsson BE (1980) Episodic cardiac arrhythmia and femoral neck fracture. *Acta Med Scand* **208**: 73–76.
125. Kulbertus HE, De Leval-Rutten F, Mary L, Casters P (1975) Sinus node recovery time in the elderly. *Br Heart J* **37**: 420–425.
126. Mandel W, Hayakawa H, Danzig R, Marcus HS (1971) Evaluation of sinoatrial node function in man by overdrive suppression. *Circulation* **44**: 59–66.
127. Okimoto T, Veda K, Kamata C *et al.* (1976) Sinus node recovery time and abnormal post-pacing phase in the aged patients with sick sinus syndrome. *Jpn Heart J* **17**: 290–301.
128. Vallin HO (1980) Autonomous influence on sinus node and AV node function in the elderly without significant heart disease: assessment with electrophysiological and automonic tests. *Cardiovasc Res* **14**: 206–210.
129. Rosen KM, Loeb HS, Sinno MZ *et al.* (1971) Cardiac conduction in patients with symptomatic sinus node disease. *Circulation* **43**: 836–844.
130. Dhingra RC, Rosen KM, Rahimtoola SH (1973) Normal conduction intervals and responses in sixty-one patients using His bundle recording and atrial pacing. *Chest* **64**: 55–59.
131. Narula OS, Samet P, Javier RP (1972) Significance of sinus-node recovery time. *Circulation* **45**: 140–158.
132. Pop T, Fleischmann D (1978) Sinus node recovery time after atrial pacing. In *The Sinus Node*, FIM (ed.). Martinus Nijhoff, The Hague, pp. 23–35.
133. Kugler JD, Gilette PC, Mullins CE, McNamara DG (1979) Sinoatrial conduction in children: an index of sinoatrial node function. *Circulation* **59**: 1266–1267.
134. Ueda K, Kamato C, Matsuo H *et al.* (1977) A study on sinoatrial conduction in the aged. *Jpn Heart J* **18**: 143–153.
135. Padaletti L, Michelucci A, Franchi F, Fradelli GA (1982) Sinoatrial function in old

age. *Acta Cardiol* **37**: 11–21.

136. Ward DT and Camm AJ (1987) *Clinical Electrophysiology of the Heart.* Arnold, London.
137. Ueda K, Takayanagi K, Matsuo H *et al.* (1978) Sinoatrial response to premature atrial stimulation during atrial pacing in aged patients with and without sinus node dysfunction. *Jpn Heart J* **19**: 677–686.
138. Inoue H, Ueda K, Ohkawa S *et al.* (1979) Electrophysiologic study and prognosis of chronic bifascicular block. *Jpn Heart* **20**: 141–151.
139. Ginks W, Leatham A, Siddons H (1979) Prognosis of patients paced for chronic atrioventricular block. *Br Heart J* **41**: 633–636.
140. Ueda K, Kitano K, Mifune J *et al.* (1977) Clinical and electrophysiologic studies on the Wolff–Parkinson–White syndrome in aged cases. *Jpn Heart J* **18**: 798–811.

8 Ambulatory Electrocardiography in the Elderly Patient

JOHN M. MORGAN[a] AND PAUL J. OLDERSHAW[b]
[a] *Southampton General Hospital, Southampton, UK*
[b] *Royal Brompton National Heart and Lung Hospital, London, UK*

INTRODUCTION AND BACKGROUND

The purpose of this chapter is to consider the use of ambulatory electrocardiography in the assessment of palpitation, syncope or dizziness in the elderly patient.

Prolonged periods of electrocardiographic recording, longer than that afforded by the standard 12-lead electrocardiogram (ECG), may be necessary to document paroxysms of abnormal cardiac rhythm that give rise to symptoms of palpitation or impaired consciousness. The practical use of ambulatory electrocardiography in this context was first reported by Holter (1). The early systems devised by him consisted of portable magnetic tape 'electrocardiorecorders' which weighed less than 2 kg and were able to record continuously for periods of up to 10 hours.

Modern equipment

Since the introduction of those early devices, advances in technology have resulted in the development of many types of sophisticated equipment (2,3). The common modern devices are battery-powered cassette tape recorders which are able to continuously record two ECG leads for a period of 24–48 hours. The signals recorded may be AM or FM analogue though more recent devices can also convert the signal to a digital format for storage. The recorder device itself is usually equipped with an internal clock together with calibration and event marker facilities.

Intermittent ambulatory ECG recorders are either patient- or time-activated and record only short segments of the ECG for later reproduction. Other devices allow a 'memory loop' to be recorded by the patient when symptoms are experienced, and the recorded ECG can then be transmitted telephonically to a central recording station. These latter devices allow ECG monitoring over prolonged periods and may document infrequently occurring arrhythmias.

Geriatric Cardiology. Principles and Practice. Edited by A. Martin and A. J. Camm
© 1994 John Wiley & Sons Ltd

However, their use has not been validated in the same way as standard ambulatory electrocardiography.

Analysis

There are a considerable variety of analyser and printout formats available. The principle of analysis is that all recorded QRST intervals are compared with a normal template, the analysing computer using standard criteria to identify abnormality of QRS timing and morphology. The smaller amplitude of the atrial signal makes its detection more difficult, so that analysis of atrial activity alone can be unreliable unless an oesophageal electrode is used. Confirmation by a technician or physician that events flagged by the computer are abnormal is necessary for thorough analysis and exclusion of artefacts. Though some softwear packages also have the ability to analyse pacemaker activity, the complexity and subtlety of modern pacemaker programming are such that rigorous analysis of paced rhythms by using the computerized techniques now available is unreliable.

Hard copy from ambulatory ECGs varies greatly but may include standard-size ECGs, compressed-size and -speed ECGs, graphic displays, or tables of heart rate and detected arrhythmias.

Monitoring period

Most centres limit recording periods to 24 hours, at least at the time of first presentation of the patient. However, there is evidence that 48-hour monitoring may be more appropriate. Bass and colleagues (4) reported that an immediate second period of 24-hour ambulatory monitoring identified arrhythmia in significantly more patients but that the incremental yield from a further third 24-hour period of monitoring was small. Age over 65 years was the only other patient variable noted by these authors to increase the likelihood of diagnosis of significant arrhythmia by ambulatory electrocardiography.

Investigation cost

The cost of 24-hour monitoring is not small. In the USA each 24-hour period of monitoring has been estimated to cost approximately $350. At the time of writing there are no similar costings available in the UK but the cost is not likely to be less given the capital expenditure and maintenance costs which are necessary, in addition to the cost of technician time.

CLINICAL APPLICATIONS OF AMBULATORY ELECTROCARDIOGRAPHY

Since the introduction of the technique, ambulatory electrocardiography has found several applications in clinical practice. These include detection of cardiac arrhythmias, correlation of arrhythmia with patients' symptoms, guidance of antiarrhythmic therapy, assessment of prognosis, and detection and management of myocardial ischaemia. Not surprisingly, these applications have generated a very large literature which debates the value of the technique and its role relative to other investigational tools such as electrophysiology study.

Use of ambulatory monitoring in patients with symptoms of unknown aetiology

Early reports of the usefulness of ambulatory electrocardiography in diagnosing arrhythmia suggested that the investigation held great promise because apparently diagnostic information was obtained in the majority of reported patients (5–7). However, many of the documented arrhythmias had been asymptomatic during the period of ambulatory monitoring. Asymptomatic arrhythmias commonly occur in normal individuals (8,9). Their relevance in patients who have symptoms suggestive of arrhythmia but electrocardiographically documented arrhythmia that is unaccompanied by symptoms is uncertain. This may lead to confusion in clinical practice and it is not uncommon for physicians to refer patients for further assessment of benign arrhythmia, such as asymptomatic short periods of sinus arrest occurring during sleep. For the ambulatory ECG to be diagnostic then the patient's symptoms must coincide with the recorded arrhythmia. A recent review of published studies suggested that the ambulatory ECG is diagnostic by this criterion in about a quarter of patients studied (10). These authors noted that episodes of palpitation correlating with patient symptoms were more frequently diagnosed than episodes of syncope. Arrhythmias, unaccompanied by symptoms but recorded during monitoring, may reveal a correct diagnosis, but should be interpreted in the light of the patient's underlying structural heart disease, the prognostic implications of the identified arrhythmia and the prevalence of similar arrhythmias in patients without symptoms.

Use of the ambulatory electrocardiogram in assessing patient prognosis

There is evidence from several studies that ambulatory electrocardiography is useful in the assessment of risk stratification after acute myocardial infarction, though left ventricular ejection fraction and the signal-averaged ECG are likely to be more useful predictors according to recent evidence (11–14). There is no evidence that ambulatory electrocardiography is useful in determining prognosis in patients with coronary disease without myocardial infarction (15,16), and the occurrence of ventricular arrhythmia in patients with dilated cardiomyopathy is not an independent predictor of patient prognosis (17,18). However, there is some evidence to suggest that patients with hypertrophic cardiomyopathy may be identified as being at high risk of sudden death by recording ventricular arrhythmia during ambulatory electrocardiography (19,20).

Use of the ambulatory electrocardiogram in assessing efficacy of antiarrhythmic therapy

There is inherent variability in ambulatory electrocardiography recordings within patients. In the best hands, variability between and within observers interpreting recordings can demonstrate discrepancies of as much as 25% for the assessment of arrhythmia episodes within a given set of recordings (2). Thus quality-control practices need to be carefully observed if ambulatory electrocardiography is to be used to assess the efficacy of a therapeutic intervention. Even in these circumstances the reduction in frequency of arrhythmia necessary to demonstrate a beneficial effect of therapy varies in prospective studies from as low as 63% (21) to as high as 93% (220). Thus considerable caution must be used in interpreting the information derived from a single patient. If paired recordings are to be used to assess the therapeutic efficacy the reproducibility of arrhythmia in an individual at baseline must be assessed, and a major reduction in arrhythmia frequency is necessary to demonstrate an effect of treatment.

Several studies have assessed the effect of antiarrhythmic therapy in asymptomatic patients with documented ventricular ectopy but have not demonstrated any prognostic benefit from therapy in such patients (10). The role of ambulatory electrocardiography has not been defined in the assessment of patients with previously identified sustained ventricular tachycardia or ventricular fibrillation because no therapeutic approach has been identified as superior. Thus the relative value of ambulatory electrocardiography compared with invasive electrophysiology study has yet to be decided. Recent reports suggest that electrophysiology study may be superior at identifying a reduction in morbidity but not mortality after a therapeutic intervention. The Electrophysiology Study Versus Electrocardiographic Monitoring Study (ESVEM) recently reported that ambulatory electrocardiography is superior for the assessment of antiarrhythmic drug therapy, but its findings are contentious and potentially flawed. For the moment, the investigational and management approaches must be tailored to individual patients. Management options will be limited as much by pragmatic considerations (such as the cost-effectiveness of ablative procedures or implantable defibrillator devices) as by interpretation of the investigational data.

Use of the ambulatory electrocardiogram in assessing myocardial ischaemia

Electrocardiography has only recently been employed in the assessment of myocardial ischaemia. The technical challenges of ST segment analysis are inherently great than those posed by QRS morphology recognition because of variability in ST segments with posture and activity, and distortion due to signal-to-noise ratio, phase shift and frequency response (23,24). Nevertheless ambulatory electrocardiography has been applied to the study of asymptomatic ('silent') ischaemia and has identified patient populations who suffer ischaemic events despite the absence of cardiac symptoms. The importance of these events in determining patient prognosis and the value of therapeutic interventions in such patients are debated. Clearly, in asymptomatic patients these arguments revolve around prognostic considerations which may be of lesser importance in the elderly when, in the absence of a symptomatic indication for therapeutic intervention, the benefit/risk ratio of treatment may be disadvantageous.

ARRHYTHMIA IN THE ELDERLY POPULATION

There are many cardiac and non-cardiac causes of dizziness, presyncope, syncope and palpitation (25). Most elderly patients susceptible to cardiac arrhythmia will have underlying structural heart disease and their management may consist principally of the investigation and treatment of that condition rather than the complicating arrhythmia.

Supraventricular arrhythmias

The commoner supraventricular arrhythmias are sinus bradycardia (usually as a feature of sinus node disease (Figure 1) and atrial fibrillation (Figure 2).

Sinus node disease and sick sinus syndrome are more prevalent in elderly patients and may present as a cause of syncope or alternating bradycardia and tachycardia. Pacemaker therapy is reserved in this disorder for symptomatic patients (with dizziness, presyncope or syncope). A fall in heart rate is reported to be a normal feature of the ageing process (26) and, if an isolated finding, is usually

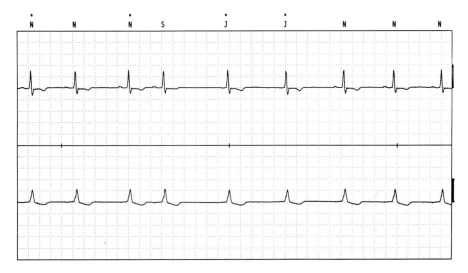

Figure 1. Sinus bradycardia with atrial ectopic activity. This was the peak heart rate achieved during 24-hour ambulatory monitoring

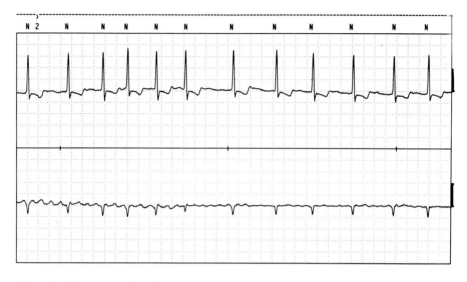

Figure 2. Flutter recording from a patient with paroxysmal atrial fibrillation. Palpitations were recorded in the patient's diary at the time of recordings

considered to be benign. However, other causes of sinus bradycardia (such as hypothyroidism, jaundice and drug therapy) should always be considered. Carotid sinus hypersensitivity is reported to be more prevalent in older patients (27) and this is also true of the malignant vasovagal syndrome.

Atrial fibrillation deserves particular attention as adequate management can be problematic. Atrial fibrillation occurs in around 30% of patients in chronic care institutions (28), the majority of whom have evidence of structural heart disease. As a complication of thyrotoxicosis, atrial fibrillation is almost exclusively present in older patients (29) and may sometimes be the only clinical manifestation of the disorder. Digoxin remains the mainstay of therapy in the elderly although recently attention has again been directed to the role of sotalol as a prophylaxis and as a means of limiting the ventricular response rate to atrial fibrillation (30). The use of aspirin or formal anticoagulation as prophylaxis against embolic events in paroxysmal or established lone atrial fibrillation remains a topic of debate. Recently a multicentre study from the USA has shown prognostic benefit from treatment with either aspirin or low-dose warfarin for prevention of thromboembolic events (31) and suggests that warfarin therapy may be superior, although these data are not necessarily applicable to elderly patients in the UK. Atrial flutter (Figure 3) similarly complicates structural heart disease, but is less prevalent and requires similar management approaches. Other types of atrial tachycardia are uncommon. Presentation of re-entrant supraventricular tachycardia due either to an accessory bypass tract or atrioventricular nodal re-entry is infrequent in the elderly.

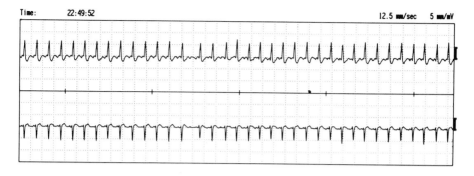

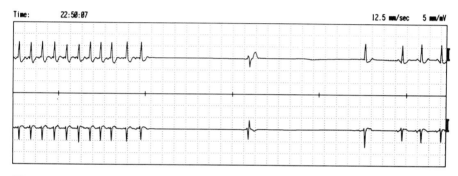

Figure 3. Paroxysmal atrial flutter recorded during ambulatory monitoring. Note spontaneous cessation followed by long sinus node recovery time suggesting sinoatrial disease

Ventricular arrhythmias

The prevalence of ventricular ectopy increases with age (32) but does not require therapy unless particularly symptomatic. Sustained ventricular arrhythmias (Figure 4) may require drug or other therapy, but principally on symptomatic rather than prognostic grounds in elderly patients, and management of the underlying cardiac condition is the first requirement.

Atrioventricular conduction disease

First-degree heart block increases in prevalence with age but there is no strong evidence that it is a marker of heart disease or prognosis (33) in the elderly population. Second- or third-degree block (Figure 5) is less frequent and, while permanent cardiac pacing may be required on symptomatic grounds, prognosis is usually determined by any underlying cardiac disease (34).

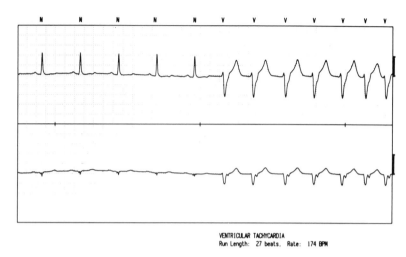

VENTRICULAR TACHYCARDIA
Run Length: 27 beats. Rate: 174 BPM

Figure 4. Sustained ventricular tachycardia associated with symptomatic palpitations on patient diary card

Application of ambulatory electrocardiography in the elderly and correlation of arrhythmia with symptoms

It is well recognized that paroxysmal cardiac arrhythmia can cause a variety of symptoms in the elderly, such as syncope, dizziness, falls, palpitation and paroxysmal breathlessness (35,36). Distinction of cardiac arrhythmia from other causes of impaired consciousness in the elderly may be problematic. The ECG will be diagnostic in less than 10% of such patients. However, paroxysmal arrhythmia may often be asymptomatic and not a cause of symptoms in the elderly patient (28,37), so that detection of an arrhythmia does not necessarily

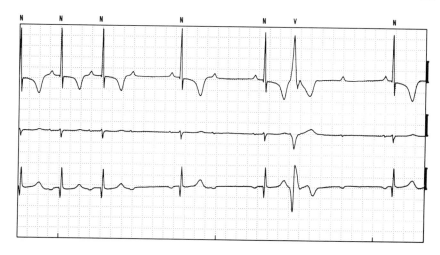

Figure 5. Second-degree heat block captured on 24-hour ambulatory monitoring in a patient with a history of syncope

determine the aetiology of infrequent episodes of syncope, presyncope or dizziness unless the arrhythmia is recorded during a symptomatic episode. Therefore identification of an arrhythmia which is not associated with symptoms during ambulatory electrocardiography may present a clinical dilemma. Rana and colleagues (38) recently reported their experience of the use of ambulatory electrocardiography in the investigation of symptoms which appeared to be cardiac in nature in a population of patients over the age of 60 years. Almost all had episodes of syncope, dizziness or palpitation though a small number had also experienced chest pain. The ambulatory ECG was useful in identifying a diagnosis in only 12% of their series. Only 9% of patients had symptoms accompanying the recorded arrhythmia but the ambulatory ECG was considered to have influenced patient management in 16% of patients. These authors noted that symptoms were more likely to occur at the time of tachycardia rather than bradycardia. Furthermore, in more than a quarter of patients with abnormal ambulatory ECGs, the same abnormality was apparent on the resting ECG (though in the majority of such instances this was a bradycardia rather than tachycardia). However, despite the low yield of the investigation in this population of patients, these authors concluded that ambulatory electrocardiography was a useful tool in the investigation of such patients. In particular they considered the main advantages of the technique to be that it is inexpensive and minimally disturbing to patients.

CONCLUSIONS

The ambulatory ECG is useful in the assessment of impaired consciousness and palpitation in the elderly patient. However, it is important that the limitations of the technique are appreciated. When arrhythmia and symptoms occur together, the ECG is diagnostic. This will occur in the minority (less than 25%) of patients. In all other circumstances, the results of ambulatory monitoring must be interpreted in the wider clinical context. A 48-hour period of monitoring will increase the diagnostic yield of the investigation.

REFERENCES

1. Holter NJ (1961) New method for heart studies. *Science* **134**: 1214.
2. Pratt CM, Eaton T, Francis M, Pacificio A (1988) Ambulatory electrocardiographic recordings: the Holter monitor. *Curr Probl Cardiol* **13**: 521.
3. Fisch C, DeSanctis RW, Dodge HT *et al.* (1989) Guidelines for ambulatory electrocardiography: a report of the American College of Cardiology/American Heart Association Task Force on Assessment of Diagnostic and Therapeutic Cardiovascular Procedures (Subcommittee on Ambulatory Electrocardiography). *J Am Coll Cardiol* **13**: 249.
4. Bass *et al.* (1986)
5. Goldberg AD, Raftery EB, Cashman PM (1975) Ambulatory electrocardiographic records in patients with transient cerebral attacks or palpitation. *Br Med J* **4**: 569.
6. Lipski J, Cohen L, Espinoza J *et al.* (1976) Value of Holter monitoring in assessing cardiac arrhythmias in symptomatic patients. *Am J Cardiol* **37**: 102.
7. Gordon M, Huang M, Gryfe CI (1982) An evaluation of falls, syncope, and dizziness by prolonged ambulatory cardiographic monitoring in a geriatric institutional setting. *J Am Geriatr Soc* **30**: 6.
8. Barrett PA, Peter CT, Swan HJ *et al.* (1981) The frequency and prognostic significance of electrocardiographic abnormalities in clinically normal individuals. *Prog Cardiovasc Dis* **23**: 299.
9. Glasser S, Clark PI, Applebaum H (1979) Occurrence of frequent complex arrhythmias detected by ambulatory monitoring: findings in an apparently health asymptomatic elderly population. *Chest* **75**: 565.
10. DiMarco JP, Philbrick JT (1990) Use of ambulatory electrocardiographic (Holter) monitoring. *Ann Interm Med* **113**: 53–68.
11. Kostis JB, Byington R, Friedman LM *et al.* (1987) Prognostic significance of ventricular ectopic activity in survivors of acute myocardial infarction. *J Am Coll Cardiol* **10**: 231.
12. Kostis JB, Wilson AC, Sanders MR, Byington RP (1988) Prognostic significance of ventricular ectopic activity in survivors of acute myocardial infarction who receive propanolol. *Am J Cardiol* **48**: 815.
13. Bigger JT, Weld FM, Rolnitzky LM (1981) Prevalence, characteristics and significance of ventricular tachycardia (three or more complexes) detected with ambulatory electrocardiographic recording in the late hospital phase of acute myocardial infarction. *Am J Cardiol* **48**: 815.
14. Kleiger RE, Miller JP, Bigger JT Jr, Moss AJ (1987) Decreased heart rate variability and its association with increased mortality after acute myocardial infarction. *Am J Cardiol* **57**: 256.
15. Ruberman W, Weinblatt E, Goldberg JD *et al.* (1980) Ventricular premature complexes in prognosis of angina. *Circulation* **61**: 1172.
16. Califf RM, McKinnis RA, Burks J *et al.* (1982) Prognostic implications of ventricular arrhythmias during 24 hour ambulatory monitoring in patients undergoing cardiac catheterisation for coronary artery disease. *Am J Cardiol* **50**: 23.
17. Huang SK, Messer JV, Denes P (1983) Significance of ventricular tachycardia in

idiopathic dilated cardiomyopathy: observations in 35 patients. *Am J Cardiol* **51**: 507.

18. Kron J, Hart M, Schual-Berke S *et al.* (1988) Idiopathic dilated cardiomyopathy: role of programmed electrical stimulation and Holter monitoring in predicting those at risk of sudden death. *Chest* **93**: 85.

19. Maron BJ, Savage DD, Wolfson JK, Epstein SE (1981) Prognostic significance of 24 hour ambulatory electrocardiography monitoring in patients with hypertrophic cardiomyopathy: a prospective study. *Am J Cardiol* **48**: 252.

20. McKenna WJ, England D, Doi YL *et al.* (1981) Arrhythmia in hypertrophic cardiomyopathy. I: Influence on prognosis. *Br Heart J* **46**: 168.

21. Raeder EA, Hohnloser SH, Graboys TB *et al.* (1988) Spontaneous variability and circadian distribution of ectopic activity in patients with malignant ventricular arrhythmia. *J Am Coll Cardiol* **12**: 656.

22. Pratt CM, Theroux P, Slymen D *et al.* (1987) Spontaneous variability of ventricular arrhythmias in patients at increased risk for sudden death after acute myocardial infarction: consecutive ambulatory electrocardiographic recordings of 88 patients. *Am J Cardiol* **59**: 278.

23. Bragg-Remschel DA, Anderson CM, Winkle RA (1982) Frequency response characteristics of ambulatory ECG monitoring systems and their implications for ST segment analysis. *Am Heart J* **103**: 20.

24. Shook TL, Balke CW, Kotilainen PW *et al.* (1987) Comparison of amplitude-modulated (direct) and frequency-modulated ambulatory techniques for recording ischaemic electrocardiographic changes. *Am J Cardiol* **60**: 895.

25. Critchley EMR, Wright JS (1983) Evluation of syncope. *Br Med J* **286**: 500.

26. Brandfonbrener RA, Amat-y-Leon F, Dhingra RC *et al.* (1955) Chronic nonparoxysmal sinus tachycardia in otherwise healthy persons. *Ann Intern Med* **91**: 702.

27. Nathanson MH (1946) Hyperactive cardioinhibiting carotid sinus reflex. *Ann Intern Med* **77**: 491.

28. Camm AJ, Evans KE, Ward DE *et al.* (1980) The rhythm of the heart in active elderly subjects. *Am Heart J* **12**: 21.

29. Staffurth JS, Gibberd MB, Hitton PS (1965) Atrial fibrillation in thyrotoxicosis treated with radioiodine. *Postgrad Med J* **41**: 663.

30. Bavernfiend RA, Welch WJ (1990) New hope in atrial fibrillation. *J Am Coll Cardiol* **15**: 708.

31. Stroke Prevention in Atrial Fibrillation Investigators (1991) Stroke prevention in atrial fibrillation study: final result. *Circulation* **84**: 527.

32. Svanborg A (1977) Seventy year old people in Gothenburg: a population study in an industrialised Swedish city, II. General presentation of social and medical conditions. *Acta Med Scand* (Suppl): 611.

33. Rodstein, M, Brown M, Wollock L (1968) First degree atrioventricular block in the aged. *Geriatrics* **23**: 159.

34. Ginks W, Leatham A, Siddons H (1979) Prognosis of patients paced for chronic atrioventricular block. *Br Heart J* **41**: 633.

35. McCarthy ST, Wollner L (1977) Cardiac dysrhythmias: treatable cause of transient cerebral dysfunction in the elderly. *Lancet* **ii**: 202.

36. Gordon M (1978) Occult cardiac dysrhythmias associated with falls and dizziness in the elderly: detection by Holter monitoring. *J Am Geriatr Soc* **26**: 418.

37. Taylor IC, Stout RW (1983) Is ambulatory cardiography a useful investigation in elderly people with 'funny turns'? *Age Ageing* **12**: 211.

38. Rana MZK, Dunstan EJ, Allen SC (1989) Ambulatory electrocardiography in the elderly: an audit. *Br J Clin Pract* **43**: 341.

9 The Chest Radiograph

ALAN G. WILSON
St George's Hospital, London, UK

This chapter considers the signs produced on a chest radiograph by heart disease. Many of the findings are common to heart disease in patients of all ages but those peculiar to or common in old age are given emphasis.

TECHNICAL CONSIDERATIONS

A number of technical factors influence the appearance of the chest radiograph and need to be understood to avoid misinterpretation.

Projection

Frontal views are best taken posteroanteriorly with the X-ray source behind the patient. The posteroanterior (PA) view is ideal because the heart is close to the film and essentially unmagnified, whereas in the anteroposterior (AP) projection it is magnified to an indeterminate degree. By convention, radiographers make a record on radiographs if they are not PA. Other ways of identifying a PA film are: (i) the position of the name label (in some departments only); (ii) medial scapular margins generally overlap the lungs on AP views, but clear or just about clear the lung margins on PA views.

Erect versus supine

Cardiac disease is much more reliably assessed with an erect rather than with a supine radiograph. The main differences between these two views are: (i) the gravitationally induced gradient in vessel size is present on erect films but cannot be appreciated on supine radiographs (see section 'Pulmonary venous hypertension'); (ii) pleural pathology (both effusion and pneumothorax) are easier to detect on erect radiographs; (iii) in the supine position the upward movement of abdominal contents compresses and distorts the mediastinum, including the heart; (iv) air–fluid levels are not appreciated on supine radiographs. By convention radiographers make a record on radiographs that are not erect. In cases of doubt the position of the gastric air bubble is of help, being

Geriatric Cardiology. Principles and Practice. Edited by A. Martin and A.J. Camm
© 1994 John Wiley & Sons Ltd

subdiaphragmatic on erect views and remote from the diaphragm (antral) on supine views.

Supine and many AP radiographs are taken with portable apparatus and for technical reasons they are often unable to achieve the ideal 2 m tube–film distance and this is another factor that magnifies the cardiac image.

Rotation

Rotation around the long axis of the body alters apparent cardiac size and affects the prominence of various mediastinal structures, particularly the hila and aorta. The degree of rotation can be assessed from the relative position of the clavicular heads and the intervening dorsal vertebra. Rotation on a transverse axis through the body often results in lordotic projections that bring the main pulmonary artery into prominence and make the heart look globular.

Lung volume

Chest radiographs are taken at total lung capacity but for a variety of reasons this may not be achieved. Under these circumstances the diaphragm is high and the heart, lying more horizontally than usual, appears spuriously large. Vascular crowding may be misinterpreted as pulmonary pathology (especially consolidation) and the gravitational gradient in size of vessels disappears. It is usual to assess lung volume by relating anterior rib ends to the diaphragmatic border. In the mid-clavicular line this border should lie between the anterior ends of the fifth to seventh ribs.

Film density

Optical density of radiographs, particularly AP and portable ones, can vary considerably. Account must be taken of under- and over-exposure particularly when assessing pulmonary vascularity and oedema to avoid misinterpretation.

ANATOMICAL COMPONENTS OF THE MEDIASTINAL SILHOUETTE

In order to detect enlargement of various cardiac chambers and great vessels it is essential to know the components of the mediastinal silhouette.

Border-forming structures on the right from above downwards are superior vena cava, ascending aorta (beyond 40 years of age) and right atrium. Age-related lengthening (unfolding) of the aorta becomes especially pronounced in the elderly. High on the right the border is variably formed by the innominate artery or the right brachiocephalic vein.

On the left the border-forming structures, from above down, are the left subclavian artery, the aortic arch and the main pulmonary artery. Just below the level of the left main stem bronchus the left atrium is border-forming for a short segment before the left ventricle takes over, continuing down to the diaphragm.

The cardiac outline is poorly marginated on the lateral chest radiograph because few of the cardiac borders are tangential to a lateral X-ray beam. The principal border-forming structures are the right ventricle low down behind the sternum giving way to the right ventricular outflow tract and the main pulmonary artery, which passes obliquely backwards to the hilar region in the mid chest. The right ventricular outflow tract and the main pulmonary artery often have a well-defined upper border, interrupted after a variable distance by the ascending aorta. The posterior aspect of the heart on the lateral chest radiograph, particularly superiorly, lacks clarity due to overlapping pulmonary veins. As a general rule in the upper two-thirds the left atrium is border-forming and in the lower third the left ventricle.

HEART SIZE

Heart size is an important clue to the presence of heart disease. Detecting small hearts is rarely helpful clinically but identifying large ones is extremely useful and usually indicates cardiac abnormality. There are a number of important exceptions to this rule (Table 1).

Heart size may be assessed subjectively or objectively by measuring transverse cardiac diameter or cardiac volume (1). Cardiac area/volume has little advantage over simple diameter measurement (2) and is rarely used. Various authors give ranges for the transverse cardiac diameter. In one series of 200 young to middle-aged adults 93% ranged between 9.5 and 13.9 cm, and these authors concluded rather arbitrarily that for adult males the upper limit should be 13.4 cm and for females 12.4 cm. These data highlight a significant problem in using absolute diameters. For example, a subject may start with a transverse diameter of 10 cm and with the development of cardiac disease the transverse diameter increases to 13 cm, but this is a figure that still falls in the normal range.

Table 1. 'Spurious' causes of cardiac enlargement in adults

Technical	Radiograph: AP, supine, rotated
Cardiac fat pads	
High diaphragm	Shallow inspiration
	Intra-abdominal disease
Skeletal	Depressed sternum, straight back, scoliosis
Racial	In Afro-Caribbeans
Athletes	
Bradycardia	
Pericardial effusion	

There are two ways around this problem: one is to assess change on serial radiographs, and this is discussed later; the other is to narrow the range of normality by relating cardiac size to height and body weight (3) since, in general, small people have small hearts and large people large ones. This would work well except that height and weight data are often not available at the time of reading a radiograph and there is a general reluctance to consult complicated nomograms. To overcome this it has become common practice to use the transverse diameter of the chest as a normalizing function and to express heart size as a ratio of transverse cardiac diameter to tranverse chest diameter. There is some inconsistency in the way that the chest diameter is measured (3–5) but the best option is probably to measure the maximum width above the costophrenic angles using the inner rib margin as endpoint. However, measuring the cardiothoracic ratio (CTR) is by no means ideal as the chest and cardiac diameter have a non-linear relationship (6) and furthermore the data establishing normal ranges are poor.

Faced with this generally rather unsatisfactory situation most film readers adopt a pragmatic approach and take CTRs of 50% or less as normal with borderline/mild enlargement of 50–55%, moderate 55–60% and marked more than 60%. This works quite well except at the extremes of life. In old age, particularly beyond 75 years of age and in females, the CTR increases. There are two elements to this increase: a small one, measured in millimetres, due to a real increase in transverse cardiac diameter (5,7–10); and a larger one due to reduction in the transverse diameter of the chest (4,5,10). In the elderly, particularly in females, it is quite common to have a CTR of more than 50% or even 60% with a normal heart. Thus in the elderly it makes more sense to use absolute cardiac diameters, and to make this a reasonably sensitive method as already discussed height/weight nomograms should be used (3). As a rule it is unusual to have a transverse cardiac diameter of more than 15 cm in an adult and such a measurement should be treated with suspicion unless the patient is 6 feet (183 cm) or more and 180 pounds (82 kg) or more (3). Some authors take 15.5 cm as their threshold measurement (11).

If previous radiographs are available it is possible to assess change in cardiac transverse diameter, eliminating reliance on absolute measurements or CTR. A difference in transverse cardiac diameter of 1.5 cm is taken as significant given unrotated films of comparable magnification and level of inspiration (12). Much of this 1.5 cm is accounted for by systolic–diastolic size variation (13).

CHAMBER ENLARGEMENT

Identifying specific chamber enlargement is a key step in assessing the chest radiograph for cardiac disease. The chest radiograph is very good for assessing the left atrium (LA), less good for the left ventricle and poor for the right ventricle and right atrium.

Left atrium

The radiographic signs of LA enlargement are:

1. A double density seen through the right heart with a convex border laterally and inferiorly (Figure 1). If the LA is greatly enlarged there is often concordance between the right lateral wall of both atria and the double border is lost. One clue to LA enlargement in this circumstance is the increased density of the right heart compared with the left. Occasionally the right upper venous trunk generates a short convex border within the right atrial shadow. This is usually a rather modest affair but if there is doubt about its significance the distance between this border and the left main stem bronchus can be

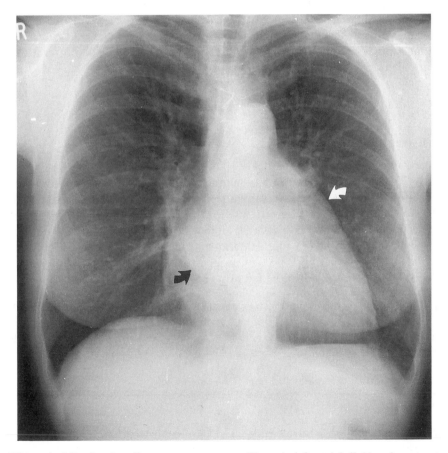

Figure 1. Mitral valve disease, post surgery. There is left atrial (LA) enlargement, indicated by prominence of the LA appendage (white arrow) and a convex border (black arrow) within the right atrial shadow. The right hilum has a 'squared off' appearance (large upper venous trunk) and upper zone vessels are enlarged

measured (endpoints are from halfway along the convexity to the nearest part of the inferior margin of the left main stem bronchus). This should measure less than 7.0 cm (14).

2. A general increase in density in the region of the LA on the frontal radiograph.
3. A carinal angle of 80° or more.
4. An upward lifting of the distal left main stem bronchus so that it becomes horizontal.
5. A prominence of the LA appendage (Figure 1). This borders the cardiac silhouette for a short segment immediately below the left main stem bronchus. Mild appendage enlargement straightens this segment of the silhouette and with increasing enlargement the segment becomes locally convex. Appendage enlargement is essentially confined to rheumatic heart disease (15) and its degree does not correlate with overall LA enlargement (15).
6. On lateral view the upper two-thirds of the cardiac silhouette moves backwards and the left main stem bronchus is elevated and displaced backwards (normally it continues in the same straight line as the trachea).

The main causes of LA enlargement are given in Table 2. In all except rheumatic mitral valve disease, enlargement is mild or at most moderate and proportionate to that of other chambers.

Left ventricle

The left ventricle forms the left cardiac border from the LA appendage to the diaphragm. When the left ventricle enlarges the heart volume increases and the left border becomes longer, the cardiac apex moving downwards and outwards (Figure 2) (16). On lateral view the inferior third of the posterior cardiac border projects backwards and downwards. Similar changes are produced by hypertrophy but tend to be less marked, and sometimes all that is seen is a rather rounded left ventricular contour. Causes of left ventricular enlargement are essentially the same as those of left atrial enlargement (Table 2).

Right ventricle and right atrium

Assessment of the size of these chambers from the plain radiograph is very unreliable and essentially plays no part in assessing adult heart disease.

Table 2. Principal causes of left atrium (LA) enlargement

Mitral valve disease
Aortic valve disease
Stiff left ventricle (systemic hypertension, restrictive and hypertrophic cardiomyopathy)
Congestive cardiomyopathy
Ischaemic heart disease
Intracardiac shunt (Not ASD)
LA mass

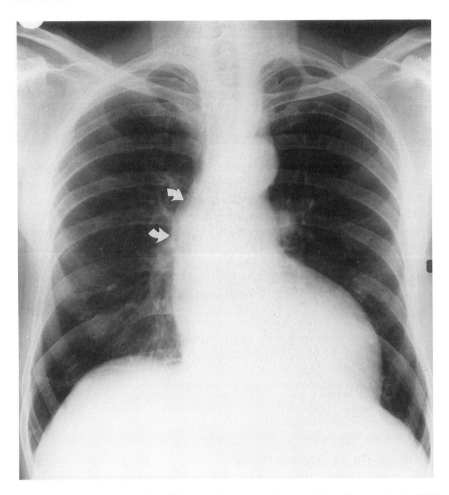

Figure 2. Aortic regurgitation. The heart is large, with a contour characteristic of left ventricular enlargement. The ascending aorta is prominent (arrows)

PULMONARY VENOUS HYPERTENSION

Pulmonary venous hypertension (PVHT) is a common finding in acquired adult heart disease. Its main causes are listed in anatomical sequence (Table 3). The main manifestations of PVHT are dilatation of upper zone vessels, interstitial and alveolar oedema and pleural effusion.

Dilatation of upper zone vessels

In the normal erect chest radiograph upper zone vessels, both arteries and veins, are smaller than lower zone ones of a similar generation. Diameters of 1 and

Table 3. Principal causes of pulmonary venous hypertension (PVHT)

Pulmonary veins	Veno-occlusive disease, constrictive pericarditis
Left atrium/mitral valve	LA mass
	Mitral stenosis/regurgitation
Left ventricle	Ischaemic heart disease
	Cardiomyopathy
	Stiff left ventricle (e.g. systemic hypertension)
Aortic valve disease	Aortic stenosis/regurgitation

4 mm or 2 and 5 mm in upper and lower zones would be typical. As pulmonary venous pressure rises upper zone vessels dilate and eventually become bigger than lower zone ones—so-called flow diversion or redistribution, the hallmark of PVHT (Figure 1). During this process upper and lower zone vessels may pass through a phase when they are of equal size, and confusion with the plethoric lungs of a shunt is then possible. At the same time that upper zone veins dilate, distension of the more proximal upper venous trunk flattens off the V-shaped lateral border of the right hilum (Figure 1).

Interstitial oedema

The interstitium of the lung is an interconnecting connective tissue framework that has peripheral (subpleural, interlobular) and central (peribronchial and perivascular) components. When pulmonary venous pressure rises sufficiently tissue fluid accumulates in the interstitium, making various components visible on the radiograph as opacities.

Laminar 'effusions'

Waterlogging of the visceral subpleural space gives a band of soft tissue density several millimetres wide parallel to the chest wall in and above the costophrenic angle. It is a common finding in PVH and assessing its size is a useful way to follow therapeutic response in heart failure.

Septal B lines (Kerley B lines)

These well-known opacities occur particularly in the costophrenic angles and are straight, horizontal lines 1–2 cm long and 1–5 mm thick (Figure 3). They differ from small vessels in that they, (i) touch the pleural, (ii) do not branch and (iii) appear unduly dense for their width. Septal B lines are not specific for raised pulmonary venous pressure (see Table 4).

Septal A lines

These are much less common than B lines and are due to oedema of deeper lung septa. They occur mainly in the mid/upper zone and are thin, long (2–5 cm) unbranching lines that point towards the hilum.

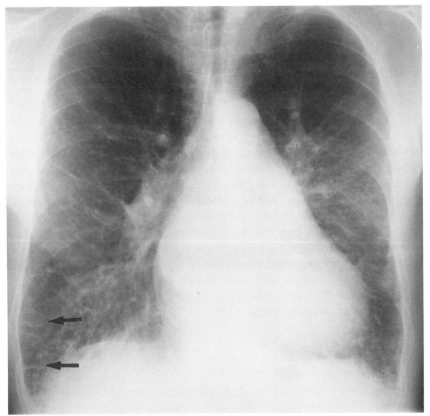

Figure 3. Raised pulmonary venous pressure. A patient with long-standing mitral valve disease and pulmonary arterial hypertension also has evidence of interstitial oedema, with profuse interstitial opacities particularly in the lower zones, blurring vessels together with classical septal B lines (arrows)

Table 4. Principal causes of septal lines

PVHT
Lymphangitis carcinomatosa
Central lymphatic obstruction (e.g. hilar mass)
Diffuse fibrosis (e.g. pneumoconiosis)
Pneumonia
Pulmonary haemosiderosis

Septal D lines (17)

A variety of other line opacities are seen when the lung interstitium is waterlogged. These thin, linear or slightly wedge-shaped opacities may be long or short and orientated in various directions. They are seen in the lower zones particularly projected over the heart in lateral view.

At the same time that septal lines appear pulmonary vessels become hazy and ill defined (Figure 3) due to oedema of the perivascular space, and bronchi appear cuffed—a feature that is best appreciated as wall thickening in end-on airways (18).

Alveolar oedema

When tissue fluid collects in alveoli it produces airspace or alveolar oedema. Radiologically this is like other airspace filling processes (e.g. pneumonia, pulmonary haemorrhage) giving the radiological signs of consolidation. This is characterized by an opacity with (i) ill-defined margins, (ii) nondescript shape, (iii) tendency to confluence, and (iv) the presence of an air bronchogram (or air alveologram). Pulmonary oedema due to PVH differs from non-oedema consolidation in that it tends to be extensive, bilaterally symmetrical and may have a perihilar (bat-wing) distribution. It can change rapidly in extent and distribution from hour to hour or with diuretic therapy. However, it is difficult to establish 'rules' for cardiogenic pulmonary oedema. Some consider a purely central pattern is unusual and that bibasal predominance with a perihilar component is much more common (19), while focal forms with unilateral and lobar patterns are well recognized (1,20).

Pleural effusion

Pleural effusions are common in heart failure. They vary from small to large and are usually fairly symmetrical or slightly bigger on the right side. Occasionally pleural fluid is loculated in either the major or, more characteristically, the minor fissure. This gives a rounded or lenticular opacity that often looks rather mass-like and may come and go as heart failure fluctuates—so-called 'phantom tumour'.

There is debate about the pathogenetic mechanism underlying pleural effusion in heart failure. Most authors suggest that a mixture of right and left heart failure is necessary, while a recent study showed a much better correlation with elevated left-sided rather than right-sided pressures (21).

Other features of pulmonary venous hypertension

Two types of intrapulmonary nodule may occasionally be seen in chronic PVH, particularly that associated with mitral valve disease. In pulmonary haemosiderosis (22) numerous soft tissue nodules, about 1–2 mm in diameter, are distributed fairly evenly throughout the lungs. High-density nodules, on the other hand, are seen with pulmonary ossification in which nodules are mid- and lower zone predominant, about 10–100 in number and of variable size (range 1–10 mm).

In some patients the major signs of PVHT develop and regress in an orderly fashion, upper zone vessel distension appearing with LA pressures in the order of 16–22 mmHg, interstitial oedema at 22–30 mmHg and alveolar oedema above 30 mmHg. However, this idealized relationship does not always hold and is affected by (i) the duration, rate of onset and cause of the pulmonary venous hypertension, (ii) the lag between changes in pressure and radiological signs, and (iii) diuretic treatment. Patients on diuretics, for example, may have cardiac dyspnoea in the absence of oedema and with essentially normal pulmonary vessels (20).

ISCHAEMIC HEART DISEASE

Acute myocardial infarction

A radiograph in acute myocardial infarction (MI) is useful in excluding other causes for chest pain and in assessing complications and the degree of haemodynamic disturbance.

In acute MI heart size is commonly normal (even when there is gross pulmonary oedema) and the initial chest radiograph is completely normal in about 50% of patients. (23). A common early abnormality is redistribution of pulmonary vessel size, indicating mild pulmonary venous hypertension with a pulmonary artery diastolic pressure (equivalent to left atrial pressure) of at least 14 mmHg (24). Redistribution commonly disappears, leaving a normal chest radiograph, but in some patients signs of more marked pulmonary venous hypertension develop with signs of interstitial and/or alveolar oedema. In one group of 173 patients from a consecutive series of patients admitted with acute MI the chest radiographic finding during the first day of admission was 52% normal, 14% upper zone vascular redistribution, 22% interstitial oedema and 12% alveolar oedema (25). The radiographic signs of PVHT are a good gauge of the severity of acute MI (23) and they are good predictors of early and late mortality (25). Basal band opacities are not uncommon during the first few days following myocardial infarction and nearly always represent subsegmental areas of collapse rather than pulmonary embolism (26).

Complications of myocardial infarction

The most important are the following.

Mitral regurgitation

This is usually due to ischaemia or infarction of the posterior papillary muscle—a feature of posterior or inferior myocardial infarction. Radiographically there is usually some cardiomegaly and signs of pulmonary venous hypertension. Left atrial enlargement is often absent or mild. If the onset of mitral regurgitation is very acute, as with papillary muscle rupture, overall heart size and left atrial size can be normal despite gross alveolar oedema (27).

Ventricular septal defect

This occurs most commonly between 4 and 21 days after infarction (27). Plain chest radiography usually shows a large heart with interstitial and/or alveolar oedema (28). Upper zone vessels are dilated but often obscured by pulmonary shadowing. The expected finding of pulmonary plethora is rarely seen except in treated patients in whom pulmonary oedema has cleared.

True left ventricular aneurysm

This usually follows occlusion of the left anterior descending artery and typically affects the apical and anterolateral part of the left ventricle (Figure 4) (29). Probably at least 50% of true aneurysms show no characteristic radiological findings, and in these cases all that may be seen is a large heart with a configuration suggesting left ventricular enlargement. When there are character-

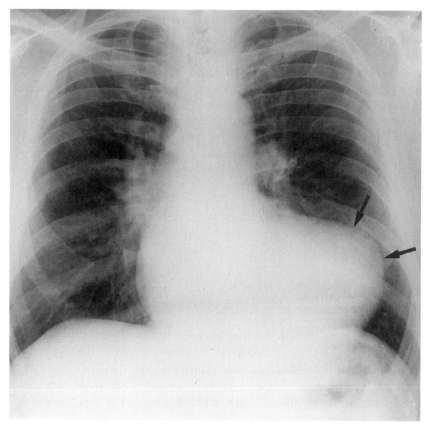

Figure 4. Left ventricular aneurysm. The left ventricular contour has an unusual shape, with an exaggerated local convexity (arrows)

istic findings they consist of a local bulge typically apical or low lateral in frontal view, expanding laterally or anteriorly on lateral view (30). Aneurysms sometimes calcify (see p. 199 (Figure 15)).

Left ventricular pseudo-aneurysm

These are much less common than true aneurysms and two-thirds occur with diaphragmatic or posterolateral infarcts. It is important that they are identified as they tend to rupture (31). The majority are associated with an abnormal cardiac contour, with a bulge typically affecting the lower posterior aspect of the heart on lateral view or the upper left cardiac border on frontal view (due to elevation of the heart). This contrasts with the findings in a true aneurysm.

Dressler's syndrome (postmyocardial infarction syndrome)

This occurs in a few per cent of patients after MI, typically at about 3 weeks (ranging from days to months (32)). Ninety per cent of patients have an abnormal chest radiograph with about 80% having pleural effusion (unilateral or bilateral), 50% basal consolidation and 50% pericardial effusion characterized by a large and rapidly changing cardiac silhouette.

MITRAL STENOSIS

In adults mitral stenosis (MS) is almost invariably rheumatic in origin. Non-rheumatic causes are rare and include left atrial myxoma and the carcinoid syndrome. The most important sign of MS is LA enlargement affecting both the LA itself and the appendage. Occasionally appendage enlargement occurs on its own and, very unusually, the LA can appear completely normal (33). The size of the LA correlates poorly with the degree of stenosis. Gross LA enlargement is not seen in pure mitral stenosis and it indicates additional mitral regurgitation. Heart size overall is normal or mildly increased in mitral stenosis but tends to be enlarged in old age and with pulmonary arterial hypertension or atrial fibrillation (1). Valve calcification usually indicates long-standing and gross valve disease (20). It is typically nodular or mottled and is best appreciated on screening (fluoroscopy). It is difficult to detect on plain radiographs, with the lateral view being the one of choice. In the lateral projection mitral valve calcification is usually projected below a line joining the hilum to the anterior diaphragmatic/sternal junction. The aorta is often rather small (23). With significant mitral stenosis there will be signs of pulmonary venous hypertension. Long-standing and severe mitral stenosis leads to pulmonary arterial hypertension (Figure 3) manifest by enlargement of the main and proximal left and right pulmonary arteries, with narrowing of lower zone muscular arteries. At this stage both right-sided chambers may become enlarged, with clinical evidence of tricuspid regurgitation.

MITRAL REGURGITATION

In contrast to mitral stenosis, mitral regurgitation (MR) has many causes (see Table 5). The onset of MR may be acute or chronic and these differ radiologically. In acute MR, seen typically with papillary muscle rupture (ischaemic heart disease) or chordal rupture (infective endocarditis, rheumatic heart disease, floppy valve), the heart and the LA are normal in size or only mildly enlarged despite the presence of gross pulmonary oedema (33). In chronic, significant MR the heart is enlarged with a contour suggesting left ventricular enlargement. LA enlargement is usually more obvious than with mitral stenosis (23) and may be massive, but its degree does not correlate with the severity of the MR. Severity correlates better with overall heart size if disease of the left ventricle can be excluded (1). Changes of pulmonary venous hypertension are less obvious with MR than with mitral stenosis, and the presence of obvious upper zone vessel dilatation indicates severe MR.

AORTIC STENOSIS

Critical aortic stenosis is an important diagnosis not to miss since it is life-threatening yet amenable to surgery. In the elderly, symptoms are often non-specific (34) and with falling cardiac output the characteristic signs may be difficult to elicit (35). In these circumstances plain radiographic findings are of importance.

The causes of aortic stenosis are listed in Table 6. A congenitally bicuspid aortic valve is the commonest cause of aortic stenosis (AS) in patients under 65 years of age if rheumatic heart disease is excluded (36). In adults stenosis in a bicuspid valve is strongly associated with valve calcification (Figure 5) and in subjects more than 40 years of age it is rare to have significant stenosis of a biscuspid aortic valve without radiologically detectable calcification (37) and by the time there is left heart failure calcification is a universal finding. The extent and density of the aortic valve calcification is a reliable predictor of the degree of stenosis (23), and radiological calcification usually indicates a gradient of at least 50 mmHg, though there are exceptions (20). On the frontal radiograph the aortic

Table 5. Principal causes of mitral regurgitation (MR)

Rheumatic heart disease	
Left venticular dilatation	
Papillary muscle dysfunction/rupture	Ischaemic heart disease
Floppy mitral valve (cusp prolapse)	Cryptogenic
	Familial
	Marfan's syndrome
Infective endocarditis	
Mitral annular calcification	
Left atrial myxoma	

Table 6. Causes of aortic stenosis (AS)

Rheumatic heart disease
Senile tricuspid aortic valve
Bicuspid aortic valve

Less important causes
Hypertrophic obstructive cardiomyopathy
Supravalvar AS
Subvalvar AS

---

valve is overlapped by dense mediastinal structures including the spine, and heavy aortic valve calcification can easily escape detection in this projection. The lateral radiograph must therefore be used for assessment, and in this view aortic valve calcification is projected on or above a line joining the hilum and the junction of diaphragm and sternum (Figure 5). Calcification may be irregularly nodular, lacking a distinct organization, but on occasions it is ring-like or partially ring-like with a crossing linear element either at the valve free margin or along the raphe that sometimes divides one of the cusps. Aortic valve calcification can spread to the anterior mitral valve leaflet, coronary ostia and the conducting tissue, causing dysfunction of these structures (37).

In patients over 65 years of age calcification in a tricuspid aortic valve becomes a commoner cause of AS. However, calcification in tricuspid valves does not necessarily cause AS, and an aortic murmur without a gradient is common (38). Senile calcification occurs fairly uniformly on the aortic side of the valve and is unaccompanied by commisural fusion (39). Mitral annular calcification is a frequent association—16/21 patients in one series (39)—and can be a source of error when aortic and mitral calcification is ascribed to annular calcification alone (35).

Aortic valve calcification in stenosis due to rheumatic heart disease tends to be relatively light.

Apart from valve calcification radiological changes in AS are best considered as those occurring in compensated disease and those occurring once left heart failure sets in. Without failure heart size is normal (Figure 5) or borderline large, often with a pronounced convexity to the left ventricular contour in its lower third (35). This latter finding indicates hypertrophy and on the lateral radiograph is accompanied by a convex bulge or the posterior heart border just above the diaphragm. The ascending aorta is prominent. However, this is a common finding in elderly patients due to age-related unfolding and hence it loses much of its usefulness as a sign. Even without unfolding the degree of ascending aortic prominence does not correlate with the aortic valve gradient and prominence may be seen with a gradient-free bicuspid aortic valve (37). With the onset of heart failure the heart and LA become enlarged and there are signs of pulmonary venous hypertension.

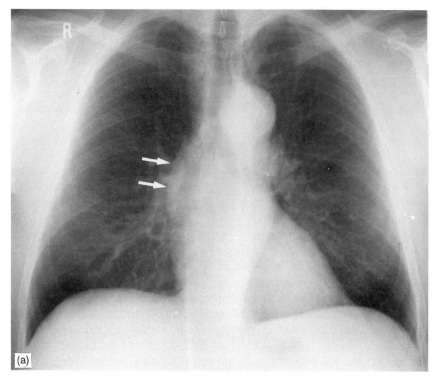

Figure 5. Aortic valve stenosis. (a) PA view shows a normal heart size with prominence of the ascending aorta (arrows). (b) (opposite) The lateral view shows heavy aortic valve calcification (arrow) typical of a bicuspid aortic valve and indicating significant stenosis. The calcification was not detectable on the PA radiograph. The calcification lies on a line joining the hilum to the anterior costophrenic angle and is a little more caudad than usual

AORTIC REGURGITATION

This may be due to lesions of the aortic wall or of the cusps. Principal causes are listed in Table 7. The main signs on the plain radiograph are a large heart with a left ventricular dilatation pattern (Figure 2). Sometimes the enlargement is predominatly downwards and the transverse diameter is not increased very much (1). There may be mild LA enlargement, present in 15% in one series (35). Ascending aortic dilatation is common and often more extensive than is seen in AS, involving the aortic arch as well. Dilatation is more pronounced when there is additional AS (rheumatic heart disease or biscuspid aortic valve) or when regurgitation is secondary to aortic wall disease (35). The regurgitant aortic valve may be calcified with disease of a rheumatic or bicuspid aetiology. In the latter instance, however, the degree of calcification is much less than with pure aortic stenosis (37). Pulmonary venous hypertension occurs late in the course of the

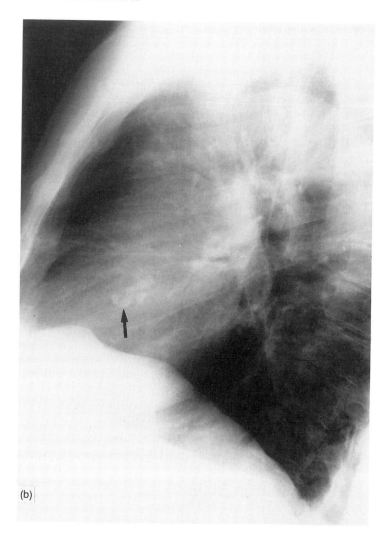

(b)

disease, and lung vacularity may be normal even with severe aortic regurgitation (23).

CARDIOMYOPATHY

Cardiomyopathy is conveniently divided into three types: (i) congestive or dilated; (ii) hypertrophic; and (iii) restrictive.

Congestive/dilated cardiomyopathy

The plain chest radiograph shows a heart that is large and which may be massive. All chambers are enlarged and there are no particular identifying radiological

Table 7. Causes of aortic regurgitation

Rheumatic heart disease
Infective endocarditis
Bicuspid aortic valve
Aortic dilatation
Connective tissue disorders including ankylosing spondylitis
Aortic trauma

Syphilis
Aortic dissection
Marfan's syndrome
Cystic medial necrosis
Idiopathic aortopathy

features. This latter point, curiously enough, has some diagnostic value, as other causes of moderate or markedly enlarged hearts tend to have characteristic features, e.g. a prominent ascending aorta in aortic regurgitation and a big LA with mitral regurgitation. At presentation there are usually signs of pulmonary venous hypertension but after treatment these often disappear and the heart may reduce considerably in size.

Hypertrophic cardiomyopathy

In this condition there is a reduction in left ventricular compliance, sometimes with systolic obstruction to left ventricular emptying, and the radiology varies depending on the particular mix of functional abnormality. A normal chest radiograph is probably the commonest finding and is seen in about half of the patients. The commonest abnormality is of a bulging or rounded left ventricular contour suggestive of left ventricular hypertrophy. Sometimes the left ventricular margin bulges locally high up just below the LA appendage and this is a rather characteristic finding. Later on in the course of the disease, particularly with the onset of atrial fibrillation, pulmonary venous pressure becomes raised and there is general cardiac enlargement with an element of selective LA enlargement (40). Other patients may show general cardiac enlargement without any specific features at all and these are indistinguishable from cases with congestive cardiomyopathy. A small subgroup with hypertrophic cardiomyopathy resemble mitral stenosis, having a normal heart size with selective LA enlargement and pulmonary venous hypertension (23).

Restrictive cardiomyopathy

Of the three varieties of cardiomyopathy this is the least common, and it shares some features with constrictive pericarditis. A variety of underlying causes have been identified (1). The heart size is commonly relatively normal though it can be enlarged in some forms. Selective LA enlargement reflecting the difficulty in filling the left ventricle in diastole is not uncommon and is accompanied by PVH. In some forms the disease is predominantly right-sided and in these circumstances PVH is absent, and the main features are of peripheral oedema, ascites and pleural effusion.

THE PULMONARY ARTERY AND PULMONARY ARTERIAL HYPERTENSION

The principal radiographic changes produced by pulmonary arterial hypertension (PAHT) are dilatation of the proximal elastic pulmonary arteries (particularly the main, and right and left) with or without narrowing of the more distal muscular pulmonary arteries.

Main pulmonary artery

On a frontal radiograph the contour of the segment where the main pulmonary artery is border-forming varies with body habitus and may be concave to lung, straight or *slightly* convex to lung. The main pulmonary artery (MPA) may become prominent on the basis of a real or apparent change in size. As with other great vessels (e.g. aorta) real increase in size may be due to (i) increased pressure, (ii) increased flow/stroke volume, (iii) increased wall compliance, and (iv) turbulence. The principal causes of a prominent MPA are listed in Table 8.

Pulmonary valve stenosis

This is one of the forms of congenial heart disease that may occasionally be seen in old age (41). The main finding on a chest radiograph (Figure 6) is prominence of the MPA (particularly its roof), with a large left and a normal right pulmonary artery. This odd combination of findings is due to selective propagation of turbulence to the roof of the MPA and down the left pulmonary artery. The heart size is typically normal.

Table 8. Causes of a prominent main pulmonary artery

'Spurious'	Displacement by large aortic root
	Lordotic or rotated (RAO or LPO) frontal radiograph
	Mediastinal mass
	Corrected transposition
Turbulence	Pulmonary valve stenosis
Compliance change	Aneurysm (rare, e.g. mycotic)
Increased pressure	PAHT
Increased flow/stroke volume	Shunts
	Pulmonary regurgitation

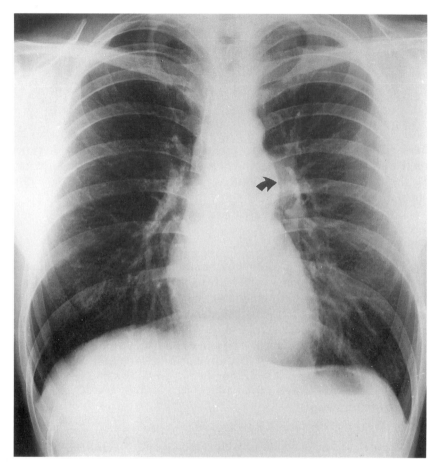

Figure 6. Pulmonary valve stenosis. The main pulmonary artery is prominent (arrow).
The left pulmonary artery is large but the right is normal (10 mm diameter, see p. 190). If
the main pulmonary artery prominence had indicated pulmonary artery hypertension
then both left and right pulmonary arteries would have been large

Pulmonary arterial hypertension

This is characterized by a prominent MPA (Figure 3) and big proximal right and
left pulmonary arteries. The interlobar part of the right pulmonary artery (just
proximal to its basal segment) can be measured, being well outlined by
air-containing lung laterally and air in the intermediate stem bronchus medially.
The measurement is taken across the vessel 1 cm distal to the apex of the V ('hilar
point') of the right hilum and has an upper range of 16 mm in males and 15 mm in
females. In some forms of PAHT the smaller muscular vessels beyond segmental
level constrict and become smaller than normal. The principal causes of PAHT
are listed in Table 9.

Table 9. Causes of pulmonary arterial hypertension (PAHT)

Hypoxia	Chronic airflow limitation
	Pickwickian syndrome
	Neuromuscular/skeletal disorders
	Altitude
Diffuse lung disease	Fibrosing alveolitis
	Sarcoidosis
	Pneumoconioses
	Others with obvious radiological lung changes
PVHT (p. 177)	
Shunts	Eisenmenger's shunt
Left-to-right shunt	
Pulmonary embolism	Thromboembolism
	Tumour/parasites
Arteritis	
Drugs/toxins	
Cryptogenic	

Shunts

Of the major left-to-right shunts—patent ductus arteriosus, ventricular septal defect (VSD) and secundum atrial septal defect (ASD)—the last is much the commonest one to be seen in adults (42) and survival into the ninth decade is recorded (41). Patients with secundum ASD may be asymptomatic even when they are old (43) and asymptomatic patients may present with an abnormal chest radiography (41). However, in general most patients are symptomatic after 40 years of age with complications such as tricuspid regurgitation, atrial fibrillation and incidental ischaemic heart disease (44).

The characteristic radiological signs of a secundum ASD (Figure 7) are: (i) large heart: in frontal view the heart is left-shifted and in lateral view the large right ventricle makes increased sternal contact; (ii) small aortic knuckle; (iii) the LA is typically of normal size in secundum ASD but as patients grow older there is a tendency for it to become enlarged, especially with concomitant atrial fibrillation and reducing left ventricular compliance (45); in fact with deteriorating left ventricular function signs of pulmonary venous hypertension may be seen, including septal lines (46); (iv) the main and proximal pulmonary arteries are enlarged, often markedly so, and vessels beyond decrease gradually in size to the periphery. The lungs are plethoric, with subsegmental and smaller lung vessels being increased in diameter equally in all lung zones.

Eisenmenger's syndrome

In Eisenmenger's syndrome there is PAHT with a reversed shunt. This implies pulmonary vascular resistance at systemic level and, while this is true with a VSD or patent ductus arteriosus, resistance is often less in ASD and the shunt is bidirectional (1).

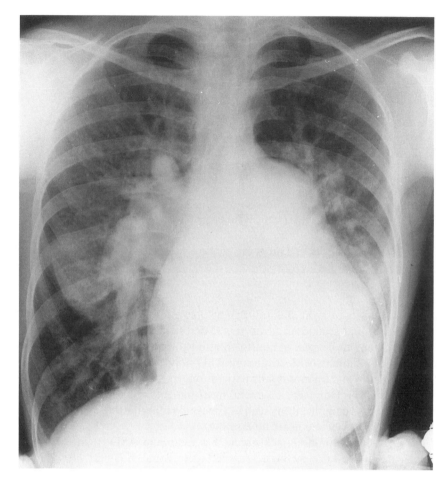

Figure 7. Atrial septal defect. The heart is enlarged, with greatly enlarged main and right and left pulmonary arteries. More distal vessels are also large and show no zonal size variation (plethora). The aortic arch is typically small and here cannot be identified

The findings in Eisenmenger's secundum ASD are greatly enlarged main, lobar and proximal segmental vessels. Distal segmental and peripheral arteries are reduced in size (47,48). The heart is usually greatly enlarged even though it may be smaller than before shunt reversal (48). There is a tendency for central arteries to enlarge with age alone in ASD and as patients get older it becomes more difficult to make haemodynamic predictions from their size (1).

Signs on the chest radiograph are useful in distinguishing among various types of Eisenmenger's syndrome (48).

THE AORTA

In middle-aged and elderly subjects parts of all three segments of the thoracic aorta are visible on the radiograph.

On a frontal radiograph of adults more than 40 years of age the ascending aorta often gives rise to a low-profile convexity midway along the right mediastinal silhouette between right atrium and superior vena cava. This is caused by the lengthening (and mild dilatation) of the aorta that occurs with age—so called aortic unfolding (Figure 8). Unfortunately an aneurysm of the ascending aorta can look identical and a lateral radiograph usually does not help resolve this dilemma. In general, mild prominence of the ascending aorta in a patient beyond 40 years of age with the rest of the aorta looking normal is assumed to be due to ageing alone. If the prominence is more than mild then it is to be expected that evidence of unfolding will be seen in the rest of the aorta and if this is not present then aneurysm of the ascending aorta should be suspected.

The arch of the aorta produces the aortic knuckle on the frontal radiograph. The distal arch is a frequent early site of calcification (Figure 9). This starts in a localized fashion at the pit related to the ligamentum arteriosum and later spreads around the wall in a circumferential fashion (49). It increases in prevalence with age (9) and is a local process that does not indicate generalized atheroma (1). The aortic diameter can be measured in the arch when the aorta forms a rounded opacity with a distinct lateral border against lung and a distinct medial one against the tracheal air column. There are no good measurement data for an elderly population. In a young to middle-aged group (upper limit 55 years of age) it was found that the diameter increased with age and in no case was the diameter more than 40 mm (50). In a group of men radiographed twice (mean interval of 17 years) the mean value for aortic diameter increased 4 mm between the ages of 48 and 65 years (34.6 mm to 38.6 mm). Unlike Felson, but in an older population, these authors found that 28% of subjects had an aortic diameter more than 40 mm at final examination (9).

The descending aorta has an interface with lung that in a young adult population is essentially straight, passing from the aortic knuckle downwards and medially to the midline at the level of the 12th thoracic vertebra. With age it unfolds and buckles out into the left lung simulating an aneurysm. Although on frontal view its medial wall is invisible, in lateral projection lung in front and behind the unfolded descending aorta clearly delineates its borders and allows assessment of its diameter (Figure 8). Occasionally the unfolded descending aorta buckles into the mediastinum and may even become border-forming low down on the right side of the mediastinal silhouette. Causes of a prominent ascending aorta are listed in Table 10.

Some of the entities appearing under the heading dilatation affect the arch and descending aorta as well as the ascending. These include atherosclerosis, which is characteristically more pronounced in the descending aorta, producing aneurysms with an uneven outline and irregular wall calcification. Athero-

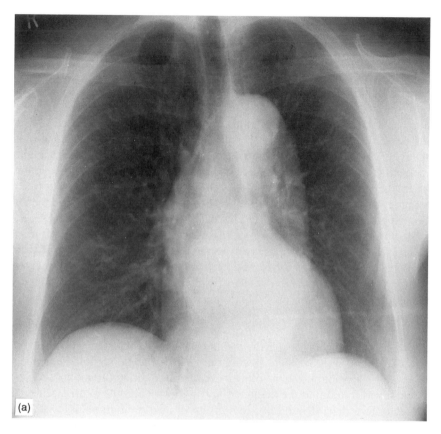

(a)

Figure 8. Unfolded aorta. (a) On the posteroanterior view the ascending and descending aorta are prominent. Since the medial border of the aorta is lost in the mediastinum it is not possible to say whether the aorta is unfolded, or aneurysmal, although the calibre of the arch (40 mm) adjacent to the trachea suggests unfolding. (b) (opposite) In lateral view lung in front and behind the aorta allows its calibre to be assessed and it is not significantly increased (36 mm)

sclerotic aneurysms contrast with syphilitic ones in which dilatation is more or less confined to the ascending aorta, and the marginal calcification is thin, even and curvilinear (Figure 10). Aortic regurgitation if marked often causes dilatation both of the ascending aorta and the aortic arch, while systemic hypertension tends to affect the whole aorta, particularly the arch (1). Traumatic aneurysms are rare and largely confined to the aortic isthmus (arch/descending aorta junction). Dissecting aneurysms (Figure 11) are subdivided into types A and B depending on whether the ascending aorta is or is not involved. In type B (corresponding closely to the former type III) the descending aorta from the left subclavian artery take-off downwards is dilated and in the acute situation there is often a left pleural effusion.

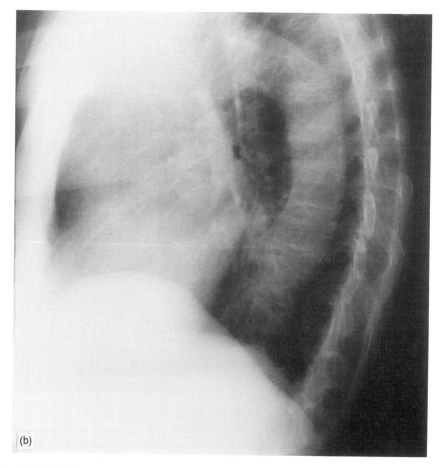

(b)

THE PERICARDIUM

Pericardial disease can be manifest by the development of pericardial effusion, thickening or calcification and may be complicated by cardiac tamponade or constrictive pericarditis.

Pericardial effusion

A list of the commoner causes is given in Table 11. A pericardial effusion may underlie any large cardiac silhouette, especially when there is no previous history of heart disease, and a search should be made for suggestive signs. Echocardiography is the definitive investigation in cases of doubt. The following chest radiographic findings are seen with subacute or chronic pericardial effusion:

1. Large cardiac silhouette, often grossly so, with a rather featureless envelope ('globular heart').

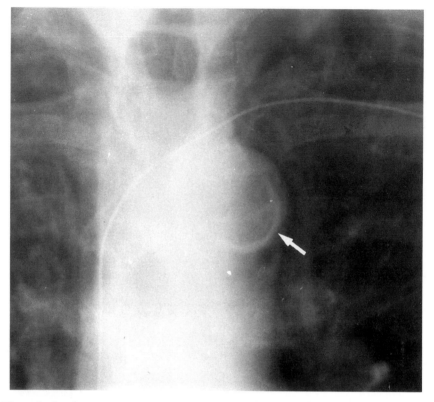

Figure 9. Aortic arch calicification. Local view of upper mediastinum in a patient with a pacemaker. Heavy C-shaped aortic arch calcification (arrow)

2. Surprisingly normal lungs and pulmonary vessels in the face of a large heart.
3. Rapid change in cardiac size over a few days.
4. A subtle band-like reduction of density along the inside of the cardiac border. This is occasionally seen and is due to the slightly lesser radiographic absorption of pericardial fluid compared with blood and myocardium (51).
5. Sometimes on a frontal radiograph the thin line of epicardial fat deep to the effusion can be seen as a thin dark band inside and roughly parallel to the cardiac envelope (52).
6. A sign with a similar basis is seen on the lateral radiograph. In about 20–30% of subjects there is enough mediastinal and epicardial fat to outline the anterior pericardium as a thin line of soft tissue density parallel to the sternum between it and the anterior aspect of the heart (Figure 12). This is normally up to 2 mm wide, and becomes wider with pericardial thickening or effusion (Figure 13) (53).
7. Widening of the subcarinal angle. This angle is rather variable—60° (10° SD)—making widening an insensitive sign. In pericardial effusion it may

Table 10. Prominent ascending aorta

Artefactual	Rotation into left anterior oblique position
Unfolding	
Dilatation	Systemic hypertension
	Aortic valve stenosis/bicuspid aortic valve
	Aortic regurgitation
	Atherosclerosis
	Inflammatory aneurysm (syphilitic, mycotic)
	Aortic dissection
	Cystic medial necrosis/idiopathic aortopathy
	Coarctation of aorta
	Congenital (patent ductus arteriosus, Fallot tetralogy, truncus arteriosus)

measure more than 80° or change significantly on a series of radiographs (54).
8. An isolated small left pleural effusion is common with a pericardial effusion (55).

When pericardial effusion causes tamponade, systemic veins dilate (superior vena cava and azygos). Tamponade often develops acutely without time for the pericardium to stretch, so that the heart may be normal in size or only mildly enlarged.

Constrictive pericarditis

Constrictive pericarditis is due to pericardial thickening, and the plain radiographic signs (Figure 14) are different from those of effusion:

1. The heart is normal in size or more commonly mildly enlarged.
2. About 50% of cases have a calcified pericardium (see 'Cardiovascular calcification').
3. The cardiac outline may be distorted in an unusual fashion with additional local irregularities due to pleuropericardial scars.
4. Evidence of raised systemic venous pressure due to right inflow obstruction is more common than signs of raised pulmonary venous pressure due to left-sided inflow obstruction.

CARDIOVASCULAR CALCIFICATION

A variety of cardiac and vascular lesions calcify and the prevalence of such calcifications increases markedly with age. The main causes of cardiovascular calcification are listed in Table 12 and the commoner and more important conditions are underlined. Moderate to marked calcification can be detected on the chest radiograph and, depending on the site, some are best or only appreciated in frontal view and others in lateral view. Minor calcifications are more likely to be detected by screening, which is more sensitive than the chest

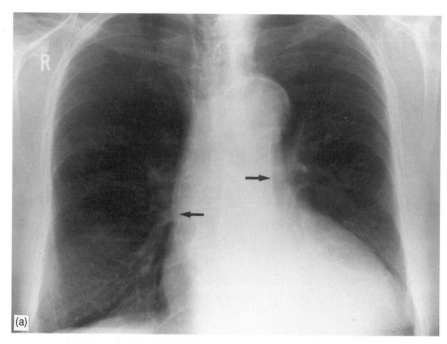

Figure 10. Syphilitic aortitis. (a) On the anteroposterior radiograph, both walls of the ascending aorta are outlined by their curvilinear calcification (arrows) which extends into the arch. The aorta is wide. The large heart with a contour suggesting left ventricular enlargement is secondary to aortic regurgitation. (b) (opposite) The aortic calcification is more clearly appreciated on the lateral view (arrows) and again the wide separation of the calcification indicates an aneurysm

radiograph. As patients become older extracardiovascular calcifications become commoner and these can be a source of confusion. This particularly applies to the nodular form of costal cartilage calcification seen typically in older females. It is usually possible to identify the nature of cardiovascular calcification by taking account of its morphology and position, which are commonly characteristic. Screening, which is now rarely used, usually clarifies the nature of dubious calcifications.

Pericardial calcification

This is usually the result of infective (or rarely non-infective) inflammation of the pericardium, particularly due to tuberculosis. It may also follow haemopericardium.

Calcification is commonly rather thick and coarse (Figure 14) but it can be fine and linear. It lies characteristically over the right-sided chambers and in the atrioventricular grooves covering the anterior and diaphragmatic surfaces of the heart (56). The surface of the left ventricle is only involved when there is extensive

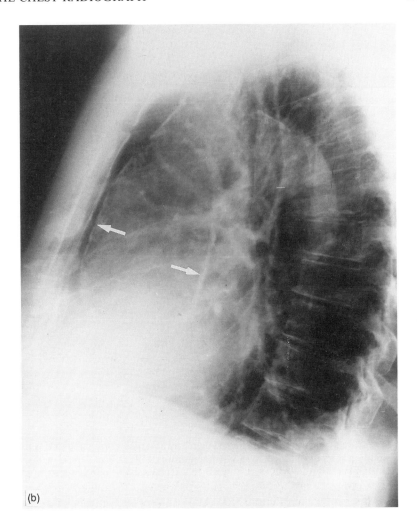

(b)

right-sided involvement, and the LA is usually spared. Fifty per cent of patients with constrictive pericarditis have radiologically detectable calcification (57). Not all patients with pericardial calcification have constriction and in one series only two-thirds had evidence of constriction (57).

Isolated pericardial plaques occasionally occur in patients with rheumatic heart disease and these are generally not a cause of constriction, but possible exceptions are recorded (58).

Myocardial and wall calcification

Calcification may occur in myocardial infarction and is usually near the cardiac apex (Figure 15) (56). It is thin and curvilinear and is often associated with an

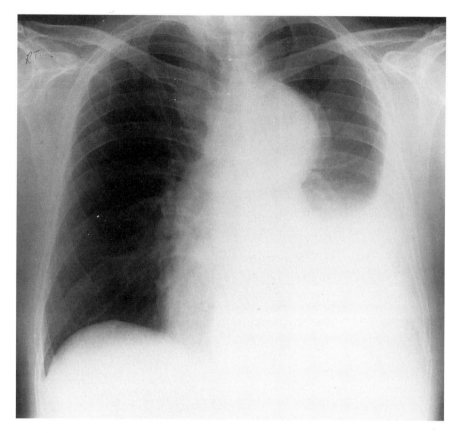

Figure 11. Acute aortic dissection. There is a greatly enlarged aortic arch in this patient. The descending aorta is hidden by a left haemothorax. This was a type A dissection starting in the ascending aorta, even though this segment does not appear prominent

abnormal left ventricular contour (59). About 5% of left ventricular aneurysms calcify (60,61). On the same ischaemic basis the apical parts of papillary muscles may calcify—particularly the posteromedial, which has only a single arterial supply (62).

Calcification occurs in the left atrial wall in rheumatic heart disease. It is generally thin and curvilinear.

Mitral annular calcification (MAC) is an important cause of cardiac calcification in old age (Figure 16). The overall prevalence in subjects over 50 years of age was 8.5% in one postmortem series, rising steeply with age to 17% in men and 43.5% in women over 90 years of age. It is two to three times more common and also more marked in females (63–65). It is generally considered to be a non-inflammatory 'degenerative' process though rheumatic heart disease, chronic renal failure and occasionally other diseases have been implicated in its pathogenesis (66).

MAC occurs in the region of the mitral annulus, initially as small calcified

Table 11. Causes of pericardial effusion

Infective pericarditis	Viral, tuberculous (other bacterial, fungal, protozoal)
Neoplasm	Metastasis (breast, lung)
Pericardial transudate	Heart failure
	Hypoproteinaemia
Rheumatic fever	
Postcardiac injury syndrome	Myocardial infarct
	Cardiac surgery
Postradiation	
Connective tissue disorders	Systemic lupus erythematosus (rheumatoid arthritis, systemic sclerosis, polyarteritis nodosa)
Myxoedema	
Uraemia	
Blood	Dissecting aneurysm of aorta
	Trauma

nodules or spicules which later coalesce to form a rigid curved bar up to 2 cm in diameter (64), sometimes with spread of calcification into the adjacent myocardium (65). The calcified deposits are generally confined to the C-shaped part of the mitral annulus that lies behind the posterior mitral valve orifice. Since the plane of the mitral annulus lies approximately midway between sagittal and coronal planes, established calcification is U-, J- or C-shaped both on the frontal and lateral chest radiograph, lying in the region of the mitral orifice (Figure 16). Rarely calcification is completely annular when it extends across the anterior mitral valve leaflet (67). Lesser degrees of calcification are seen with difficulty on the radiograph as small, discontinuous, linear or nodular calcifications in the region of the posterior mitral annulus (65). As might be expected, screening and echocardiography are more sensitive than the chest radiograph in the detection of MAC (65,66).

There are a number of recognized complications and associations of MAC. These are as follows.

Mitral regurgitation

Pansystolic murmurs are a common association, recorded in 73% of cases of MAC in one series (64). Significant mitral regurgitation is less common but occurs with heavy calcification, when the posterior mitral valve leaflet is invariably distorted and displaced towards the atrium. In the same postmortem series 89/258 cases (34%) showed changes of this degree (64). Significant mitral stenosis is recorded, but rarely (68).

Dysrrhythmias

Calcification may spread from the region of the annulus to that of the bundle of His and the atrioventricular node. Various dysrrhythmias may result (69) including complete heart block (70) and bundle branch block. Interestingly, in

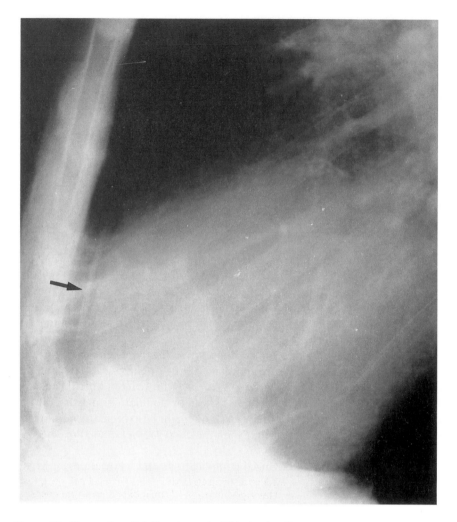

Figure 12. The pericardial line (arrow). This is the fibrous and serous pericardium outlined by the darker mediastinal and epicardial fat. When more than 2 mm thick it is abnormal, indicating pericardial fluid or thickening

one controlled series only the presence of right bundle branch block was shown to be a significant association (65). In the Framingham study a 12-fold increase in atrial fibrillation was recorded in patients with MAC (71).

Endocarditis

This can be infective (72) or thrombotic and sterile (64).

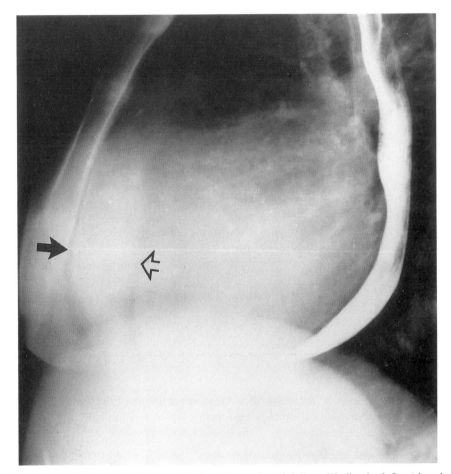

Figure 13. Pericardial effusion widening the pericardial line. Mediastinal fat (closed arrow) is separated from epicardial fat (open arrow) by 3 cm, indicating a large pericardial effusion

Systemic emboli

There is a recognized association between MAC and systemic embolization (69) and it seems likely that a number of different pathogenic mechanisms are involved.

Aortic valve calcification

Aortic valve calcification of the 'senile' variety occurs commonly with MAC. Thus on one echo-assessed series of patients with aortic valve calcification there was a 10-fold excess of patients with MAC (73), and looked at from the opposite

Table 12. Causes of cardiovascular calcification

Pericardium	'Constrictive' pericarditis[a]
	Rheumatic heart disease
	Asbestos exposure
Myocardium and wall	Myocardial infarct
	Rheumatic heart disease (LA)
	Surgical incision
	Mitral annulus
Endocardium	Jet lesion
Chamber cavity	Thrombus
	Myxoma
Valvular	Aortic (rheumatic heart disease, bicuspid, senile, homograft)
	Mitral (rheumatic heart disease)
	(Complicated pulmonary stenosis, homograft)
	Tricuspid (rheumatic heart disease)
Coronary artery	Atheroma
	Aneurysm, fistula
Pulmonary artery	Ductus arteriosus
	Pulmonary arterial hypertension
	Thrombus
Aorta	Atheroma
	Aortitis (syphilis, Takayasu)
	Knuckle

[a]Commoner conditions underlined.

standpoint 25–75% of patients with MAC have aortic valve calcification (74,75). The aortic valve calcification may be functionally significant (65).

Endocardial and chamber cavity calcification

Endocardial calcification, considered to be a 'jet' lesion, is seen rarely in mitral regurgitation as a localized linear plaque indistinguishable from rheumatic atrial wall calcification.

Valvular

Aortic and mitral valve calcification are discussed under aortic and mitral stenosis.

The stenotic pulmonary valve rarely calcifies in adults, usually when it is associated with septal defects (76).

Coronary artery calcification

Nearly all examples of coronary artery calcification (CAC) are due to calcification in atheromatous plaques. Calcification usually occurs proximally and is commoner on the left than the right (77). CAC is linear, plaque- or ring-like and may be detected on the chest radiograph but, not surprisingly, screening and cine radiography are several times more sensitive (78). Left CAC is best seen on the frontal chest radiograph in the 'CAC triangle' (78). This triangle overlies the left mid heart and has its apex at the left main stem bronchus, the medial side is the spine and the lateral the diagonal cardiac margin, while the base is a horizontal line at the 'shoulder of the left ventricle' (about one-third of the way from the left main stem bronchus to the diaphragm). About 40% of a series with CAC on screening had a positive CAC sign on the plain radiograph (78). Right CAC is probably best detected on the lateral chest radiograph.

CAC indicates atheroma but conclusions about the degree of underlying arterial stenosis is less certain. A number of studies show good correlation between CAC detected fluoroscopically and the severity and prognosis of underlying coronary artery disease (79,80), and it is generally accepted that widespread heavy calcification in younger patients (less than 50 years old) is associated with significant stenoses (1). In older patients, however, this relationship is much less certain and calcification can occur without significant stenosis (81).

Pulmonary artery

The ductus arteriosus may calcify in middle-aged or elderly patients outlining either the diverticulum at the aortic end of the ductus or the ductus itself as a linear, curved or circular calcified opacity (1).

Calcification in the pulmonary artery itself is rare but can be seen in two circumstances. Wall calcification occurs in atheroma associated with gross PAHT, especially that in Eisenmenger's syndrome. Calcification in the lumen of the central pulmonary arteries occurs uncommonly with long-standing thrombus.

VALVE PROSTHESES AND PACEMAKERS

Prosthetic valves

There is a great range of prosthetic valves available (Table 13). Uncomplicated homografts are invisible on chest radiographs. However, some go on to calcify, particularly in their walls, giving thin curvilinear calcifications visible on the plain radiograph. Valve function need not be impaired by this process. All other valves contain radio-opaque components. These allow the valve to be identified as a named type and usually indicate the direction of flow. Nearly all valves replaced in adults are either mitral (MVR) or aortic (AVR), and under most circumstances knowing the direction of flow in a prosthesis allows an unequivocal distinction on a chest radiograph. Other criteria that are helpful on a frontal radiograph are the largely *en face* view of a vertical prosthesis indicating an

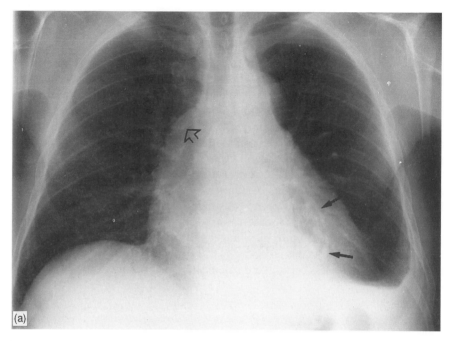

Figure 14. Constrictive pericarditis. (a) On the posteroarterior radiograph, the heart is, somewhat unusually, mildly enlarged with a large superior vena cava and azygos vein (open arrow) indicating raised systemic venous pressure. There is an apparently isolated left pleural effusion—a characteristic feature. Calcification (closed arrows) is not easy to detect. (b) (opposite) On the lateral view pericardial calcification is easy to see. It is peripheral, curvilinear and quite heavy and irregular. Again note the unilateral pleural effusion

MVR, and the profile view of an essentially horizontal prosthesis indicating an AVR. Valve position *per se* is not a reliable criterion (82).

Complications associated with prosthetic valves are of three types: (i) occluder dysfunction; (ii) cage and base ring dysfunction; (iii) systemic complications (83). Only a few of these are identifiable on the plain chest radiograph (strut fracture, calcification, disc wear and embolization, abnormalities of radio-opaque poppets) and most need fluoroscopy (screening), ultrasound or angiography for their detection.

Pacemakers

Cardiac pacemakers are commonly used in elderly patients, and chest radiography is a convenient way of assessing complications and some forms of malfunction.

Most pacemakers are of the transvenous, endocardial type, with a generator in the region of the axilla or chest wall, and a wire with a unipolar or bipolar tip

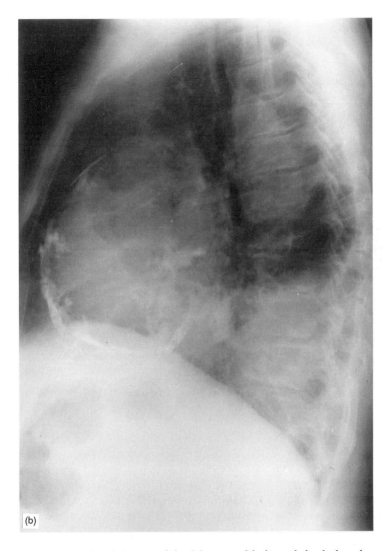

(b)

usually located in the right ventricle. More sophisticated dual-chamber pacing systems have two wires, with the tip of one in the right ventricle and the other in the right atrial appendage. Correctly positioned wires have a characteristic appearance on the PA and lateral chest radiograph (84,85). Chest radiography is used both at the time of the pacemaker insertion and during follow-up and is useful for detecting the following:

1. Immediate complications of insertion such as pneumothorax.
2. Electrode malposition with inadvertent placement in the coronary sinus, middle cardiac vein or right ventricular outflow tract (85,86).
3. Wire dislodgement: this usually occurs within hours or days of insertion.

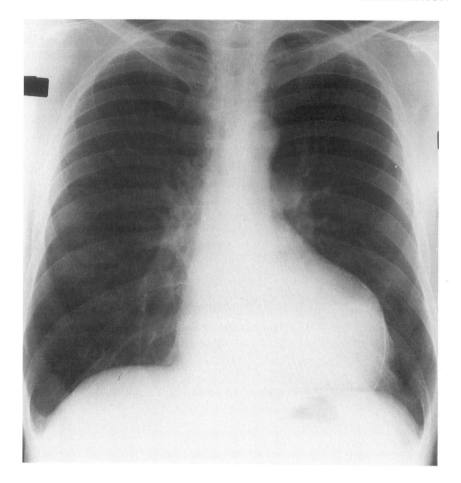

Figure 15. Calcified cardiac aneurysm. The left ventricular contour in its lower two-thirds is unduly convex and has a thin calcified rim. This is a typical position for a true left ventricular aneurysm

Displacement of the wire is sometimes a feature of the 'pacemaker twiddler's syndrome', which can also lead to wire fracture (84). This 'syndrome' is characterized by change in position of the generator, twisted or looped leads and sometimes wire withdrawal from the right ventricle.

4. Wire fracture: this is often surprisingly difficult to detect radiographically. It occurs typically at the generator connections, at sharp bends and at venous entry points (86).

5. Myocardial perforation: this is another early complication, often clinically obvious with failure to pace, somatic muscle stimulation and pericardial rub. Radiologically it may be suspected when the pacing wire tip is projected

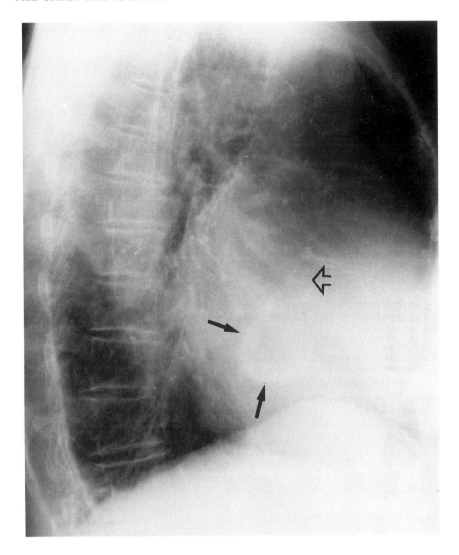

Figure 16. Mitral annular calcification. A lateral view shows the heavy C-shaped calcification of the mitral annulus in its characteristic position (closed arrows). There is also a little aortic valve calcification (open arrow)—a common association

outside or within 3 mm of the cardiac silhouette or epicardial fat (see 'Pericardial disease', p. 196) (87).
6. The chest radiograph also detects other possible complications such as infection in the generator bed and pulmonary emboli.
7. The radiographic appearance of the generator allows manufacturer, type and mode of action to be identified (86).

Table 13. Main types of valve replacement

Homograft	
Heterograft	
porcine	Hancock
	Carpentier–Edwards
bovine	
Caged ball valve	Starr–Edwards
Caged disc valve	
Tilting leaflet	Bjork–Shiley

REFERENCES

1. Jefferson K, Rees S (1980) *Clinical Cardiac Radiology*, 2nd edn. Butterworths, London.
2. Comeau WJ, White PDA (1942) Critical analysis of standard methods of estimating heart size from roentgen measurements. *AJR* **47**: 665–677.
3. Ungerleider HE, Gubner R (1942) Evaluation of heart size measurements. *Am Heart J* **24**: 494–510.
4. Cowan NR (1959) The heart lung coefficient in older people. *Br Heart J* **21**: 238–242.
5. Lauder IJ, Milne JS (1976) Study of heart size in older people. *Br Heart J* **38**: 1286–1290.
6. Ungerleider HE, Clark CP (1939) A study of the transverse diameter of the heart silhouette with prediction table based on the teleoroentgenogram. *Am Heart J* **17**: 92–102.
7. Cowan NR (1960) The transverse diameter of the heart in older people. *Br Heart J* **22**: 391–394.
8. Milne JS, Lauder IJ (1974) Heart size in older people. *Br Heart J* **36**: 352–356.
9. Ensor RE, Fleg JL, Kim YC *et al.* (1983) Longitudinal chest x-ray changes in normal men. *J Gerontol* **38**: 307–314.
10. Simon G (1965) The appearance of the chest radiograph in old persons. *Radiol Clin North Am* **3**: 293–297.
11. Rubens MB (1984) The chest X-ray in adult heart disease. *Cardiol Pract* November 6–18.
12. Simon G (1968) The limitations of the radiograph for detecting early heart enlargement. *Br J Radiol* **41**: 862–865.
13. Gammill SL, Krebs C, Meyers P *et al.* (1970) Cardiac measurements in systole and diastole. *Radiology* **94**: 115–119.
14. Higgins CB, Reinke RT, Jones NE, Broderick T (1978) Left atrial dimension on the frontal thoracic radiograph: a method for assessing left atrial enlargement. *AJR* **130**: 251–255.
15. Green CE, Kelley MJ, Higgins CB (1982) Etiologic significance of enlargement of the left atrial appendage in adults. *Radiology* **142**: 21–27.
16. Chikos PM, Figley MM, Fisher L (1977) Correlation between chest film and angiographic assessment of left ventricular size. *AJR* **128**: 367–373.
17. Kreel L, Slavin G, Herbert A, Sandin B (1975) Intralobar septal oedema: 'D'lines. *Clin Radiol* **26**: 209–221.
18. Don C, Johnson R (1977) The nature of significance of peribronchial cuffing in pulmonary edema. *Radiology* **125**: 577–582.
19. Milne ENC, Pistolesi M, Miniati M, Giuntini C (1985) The radiologic distinction of

cardiogenic and noncardiogenic edema. *AJR* **144**: 879–894.

20. Raphael MJ, Donaldson RM (1987) The plain chest X-ray in acquired heart disease in adults. *Br J Hosp Med* **37**: 211–219.

21. Wiener-Kronish JP, Matthay MA, Callen PW *et al.* (1985) Relationship of pleural effusions to pulmonary hemodynamics in patients with congestive heart failure. *Am Rev Respir Dis* **132**: 1253–1256.

22. Taylor HE, Strong GF (1955) Pulmonary hemosiderosis in mitral stenosis. *Ann Intern Med* **42**: 26–35.

23. Newell JD, Higgins CB, Kelley MJ (1980) Radiographic–echocardiographic approach to acquired heart disease: diagnosis and assessment of severity. *Radiol Clin North Am* **18**: 387–409.

24. Bennett ED, Rees S (1974) The significance of radiological changes in the lungs in acute myocardial infarction. *Br J Radiol* **47**: 879–881.

25. Battler A, Karliner JS, Higgins CB *et al.* (1980) The initial chest x-ray in acute myocardial infarction: prediction of early and late mortality and survival. *Circulation* **61**: 1004–1009.

26. Tudor J, Maurer BJ, Wray R, Steiner RE (1973) Lung shadows after acute myocardial infarction. *Clin Radiol* **24**: 365–369.

27. Higgins CB, Lipton MJ (1980) Radiography of acute myocardial infarction. *Radiol Clin North Am* **18**: 359–368.

28. Miller SW, Dinsmore RE, Greene RE, Doggett WM (1978) Coronary, ventricular, and pulmonary abnormalities associated with rupture of the interventricular septum complicating myocardial infarction. *AJR* **131**: 571–577.

29. Dubnow MH, Burchell HB, Titus JI (1965) Post-infarction ventricular aneurysm. *Am Heart J* **70**: 753–760.

30. Higgins CB, Lipton MR, Johnson AD *et al.* (1978) False aneurysms of the left ventricle. *Radiology* **127**: 21–27.

31. Van Tassel RA, Edwards JE (1972) Rupture of heart complicating myocardial infarction: analysis of 40 cases including nine examples of left ventricular false aneurysm. *Chest* **61**: 104–116.

32. Stelzner TJ, King TE, Antony VB, Sahn SA (1983) The pleuropulmonary manifestations of the post-cardiac injury syndrome. *Chest* **84**: 383–387.

33. Grainger RG (1970) Review article: an evaluation of conventional radiography in acquired heart disease. *Br J Radiol* **43**: 673–684.

34. Hancock EW (1977) Aortic stenosis, angina pectoris, and coronary artery disease. *Am Heart J* **93**: 382–393.

35. Klatte EC, Yune H, Burney B (1979) Radiographic manifestations of aortic stenosis and aortic valvular insufficiency. *Semin Roentgenol* **14**: 122–130.

36. Green CE, Kelley MJ (1980) A renewed role for fluoroscopy in the evaluation of cardiac disease. *Radiol Clin North Am* **18**, 345–357.

37. Roberts WC, Elliott LP (1968) Lesions complicating the congenitally bicuspid aortic valve. *Radiol Clin North Am* **6**: 409–421.

38. Edwards JE (1979) Pathology of acquired valvular disease of the heart. *Semin Roentgenol* **14**: 96–115.

39. Roberts WC, Perloff JK, Constantino T (1971) Severe valvular aortic stenosis in patients over 65 years of age. *Am J Cardiol* **27**: 497–506.

40. Chapman, AH, Raphael MJ, Steiner RE, Oakley CM (1978) Unusual chest X-ray appearances in hypertrophic cardiomyopathy. *Clin Radiol* **29**: 9–16.

41. Perloff JK, Lindgren KM (1974) Adult survival in congenital heart disease. Part 1. Common defects with expected adult survival. *Geriatrics* **29** (April): 94–104.

42. Nejat M, Greif E (1976) The aging heart: a clinical review. *Med Clin North Am* **60**: 1059–1078.

43. Markman P, Howitt G, Wade EG (1965) Atrial septal defect in the middle-aged and elderly. *Q J Med* **34**: 409–426.
44. Kaplan S (1985) The adult with congenital heart disease. *Semin Roentgenol* **20**: 151–159.
45. Green CE, Gottdiener JS, Goldstein HA (1985) Atrial septal defect. *Semin. Roentgenol.* **20**: 214–225.
46. O'Reilly G, Jefferson K (1976) Septal lines in pure right heart failure. *Br J Radiol* **49**: 123–125.
47. Rees RSO, Jefferson KE (1967) The Eisenmenger syndrome. *Clin Radiol* **18**: 366–371.
48. Rees S (1968) The chest radiograph in pulmonary hypertension with central shunt. *Br J Radiol* **41**: 172–179.
49. Dalith F (1961) Calcification of the aortic knob: its relationship to the fifth and sixth embryonic aortic arches. *Radiology* **76**: 213–221.
50. Felson B (1973) *Chest Roentgenology*. Saunders, Philadelphia, p. 495.
51. Tehranzadeh J, Kelley MJ (1979) The differential density sign of pericardial effusion. *Radiology* **133**: 23–30.
52. Torrance DJ (1955) Demonstration of subepicardial fat as an aid in the diagnosis of pericardial effusion or thickening. *AJR* **74**: 850–855.
53. Lane EJ, Carsky EW (1968) Epicardial fat: lateral plain film analysis in normals and in pericardial effusion. *Radiology* **91**: 1–5.
54. Chen JTT, Putman CE, Hedlund LW *et al.* (1982) Widening of the subcarinal angle by pericardial effusion. *AJR* **139**: 883–887.
55. Weiss, JM, Spodick DH (1983) Association of left pleural effusion with pericardial disease. *N Engl J Med* **308**: 696–697.
56. MacGregor JH, Chen JTT, Chiles C *et al.* (1987) The radiographic distinction between pericardial and myocardial calcifications. *AJR* **148**: 675–677.
57. Shawdon HH, Dinsmore RE (1967) Pericardial calcification: radiological features and clinical significance in twenty-six patients. *Clin Radiol* **18**, 205–212.
58. Przybojewski JZ (1981) Rheumatic constrictive pericarditis. *S Afr Med J* **59**: 682–686.
59. Bogoch A, Christopherson EF (1950) Calcified cardiac aneurysms. *Ann Intern Med* **32**: 295–308.
60. Schlichter J, Hellerstein HK, Katz LN (1954) Aneurysm of the heart: a correlative study of one hundred and two proved cases. *Medicine* **33**: 43–86.
61. Brean HP, Marks JH, Sosman MC, Schlesinger MJ (1950) Massive calcification in infarcted myocardium. *Radiology* **54**: 33–42.
62. Roberts WC (1986) The senile cardiac calcification syndrome. *Am J Cardiol* **58**: 572–573.
63. Korn D, DeSanctis RW, Sell S (1962) Massive calcification of the mitral annulus: a clinico-pathological study of fourteen cases. *N Engl J Med* **267**: 900–909.
64. Pomerance A (1970) Pathological and clinical study of calcification of the mitral valve ring. *J Clin Pathol* **23**: 354–361.
65. D'Cruz IA, Cohen HC, Prabhu R *et al.* (1977) Clinical manifestations of mitral annulus calcification, with emphasis on its echocardiographic features. *Am Heart J* **94**: 367–377.
66. Shott CR, Kotler MN, Parry WR, Segal BL (1977) Mitral annular calcification: clinical and echocardiographic correlations. *Arch Intern Med* **137**: 1143–1150.
67. Roberts WC, Waller BF (1981) Mitral valve 'anular' calcium forming a complete circle or 'O' configuration: clinical and necropsy observations. *Am Heart J* **101**: 619–621.
68. Hammer WJ, Roberts WC, deLeon AC (1978) 'Mitral stenosis' secondary to combined 'massive' mitral anular calcific deposits and small hypertrophied left ventricles. *Am J Med* **64**: 371–376.

69. Nestico PF, Depace NL, Morganroth J *et al.* (1984) Mitral annular calcification: clinical, pathophysiology, and echocardiographic review. *Am Heart J* **107**: 989–996.
70. Harris A, Davies M, Redwood D *et al.* (1969) Aetiology of chronic heart block: a clinico-pathological correlation in 65 cases. *Br Heart J* **31**: 206–218.
71. Savage DD, Garrison RJ, Castelli WP *et al.* (1983) Prevalence of submitral (anular) calcium and its correlates in a general population-based sample (the Framingham Study). *Am J Cardiol* **51**: 1375–1378.
72. Burnside JW, DeSanctis RW (1972) Bacterial endocarditis on calcification of the mitral anulus fibrosus. *Ann Intern Med* **76**: 615–618.
73. Lewandowski BJ, Winsberg F (1982) Incidence of aortic cusp and mitral annulus calcification as determined by echocardiography: significance and interrelationship. *AJR* **138**: 829–832.
74. Simon MA, Liu SF (1954) Calcification of the mitral valve annulus and its relation to functional valvular disturbance. *Am Heart J* **48**: 497–505.
75. Roberts WC, Perloff JK (1972) Mitral valvular disease: a clinicopathologic survey of the conditions causing the mitral valve to function abnormally. *Ann Intern Med* **77**: 939–975.
76. Gabriele OF, Scatliff JH (1970) Pulmonary valve calcification. *Am Heart J* **80**: 299–302.
77. McCarthey JH, Palmer FJ (1974) Incidence and significance of coronary artery calcification. *Br Heart J* **36**: 499–506.
78. Souza AS, Bream PR, Elliott LP (1978) Chest film detection of coronary artery calcification: the value of the CAC triangle. *Radiology* **129**: 7–10.
79. Aldrich RF, Brensike JF, Battaglini JW *et al.* (1979) Coronary calcification in the detection of coronary artery disease and comparison with electrocardiographic exercise testing. *Circulation* **59**: 1113–1124.
80. Marolis JR, Chen TT, Kong Y *et al.* (1980) The diagnostic and prognostic significance of coronary artery calcification. *Radiology* **137**: 609–616.
81. Waller BF, Roberts WC (1983) Cardiovascular disease in the very elderly: analysis of 40 necropsy patients aged 90 years or over. *Am J Cardiol* **51**: 403–421.
82. Gross BH, Shirazi KK, Slater AD (1983) Differentiation of aortic and mitral valve prostheses based on post operative frontal chest radiographs. *Radiology* **149**: 389–391.
83. Steiner RM, Mintz G, Morse D (1988) The radiology of cardiac valve prostheses. *Radiographics* **8**: 277–298.
84. Sorkin RP, Schuurmann BJ, Simon AB (1976) Radiographic aspects of permanent cardiac pacemakers. *Radiology* **119**: 281–296.
85. Hertzberg BS, Chiles C, Ravin CE (1985) Right atrial appendage pacing: radiographic considerations. *AJR* **145**: 31–33.
86. Steiner RM, Tegtmeyer CJ, Morse D *et al.* (1986) The radiology of cardiac pacemakers. *Radiographics* **6**: 373–399.
87. Wechsler RJ, Steiner RM, Kinori I (1988) Monitoring the monitors: the radiology of thoracic catheters, wires, and tubes. *Semin Roentgenol* **23**: 61–84.

10 Cardiac Catheterization

ANGUS TURNER AND DAVID E. WARD
St George's Hospital, London, UK

Since the first introduction of a cardiac catheter into a human being, when Forssman inserted a catheter into his own right atrium in 1920, the technique has become widespread. The expansion of the procedure came in the 1960s with the development of cardiac surgery requiring accurate preoperative cardiac assessment (1). By introduction of catheters into the arterial and venous systems, information concerning the cardiac chambers, coronary blood supply, valvular apparatus and haemodynamic status of the heart could be obtained.

With the increase in the elderly population (2), coupled with the fact that a significant proportion of these people will suffer from symptomatic coronary artery and valvular disease (3,4), there will be an increase in the number of elderly patients being referred for cardiac catheterization.

The Royal College of Physicians Working Group, 1991, recommended the expansion of cardiological services to accommodate this increasing demand. With this recommendation, the balance between potential risk and expected benefit of catheterization, as well as of the therapeutic interventions arising from the procedure, must be of prime consideration in the elderly patient.

PRACTICAL ASPECTS OF CARDIAC CATHETERIZATION

Cardiac catheterization is a procedure by which catheters can be introduced into the arterial and venous systems to gain information concerning right and left sides of the heart, respectively. This is primarily performed by transducer-measured pressure recordings and injection of radiographic contrast media.

In low-risk cases, the procedure is carried out as a day case and is performed under local anaesthetic, e.g. 2% lignocaine.

The usual catheters used are 7 or 8 French gauge and there is a wide variety of designs available for specific usage (Figure 1). Coronary arteriography is usually carried out using end-hole catheters such as Judkins or Castillo catheters, whereas high-power injections, used in left ventriculography or aortography, are usually administered via side-hole catheters such as a pigtail catheter (which also has an end hole), or an NIH catheter (which has no end hole). The patient is fasted and the use of premedication varies, with light sedation and/or atropine sometimes being given, but often no premedication is used.

Geriatric Cardiology. Principles and Practice. Edited by A. Martin and A.J. Camm
© 1994 John Wiley & Sons Ltd

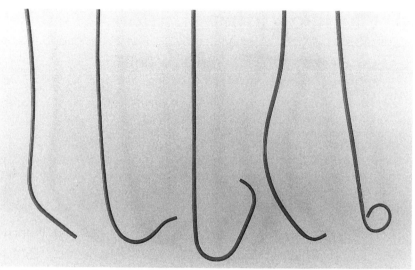

Figure 1. Examples of cardiac catheters. (a) Cournand catheter. (b) Amplatz catheter. (c) Judkins left coronary catheter. (d) Judkins right coronary catheter. (e) Pigtail catheter—note side holes

TECHNIQUES

Left heart catheterization

In this procedure the left ventricle is entered retrogradely across the aortic valve, pressure readings are made and radiographic contrast is injected into the ventricular cavity. Selective coronary angiography is also performed with the aid of specially designed catheters. Left heart catheters are introduced from the femoral or brachial arteries.

Approach

Brachial
The brachial artery is usually performed from the right side where, under sterile conditions, a 1 cm incision is made just below the skin crease of the antecubital fossa. By blunt dissection, the brachial artery is exposed, lying deep to the biceps aponeurosis and lateral to the median nerve. Tapes are introduced under the artery to control bleeding and a 1 mm horizontal incision is made in the vessel. Next, a 0.9 mm straight guide wire is inserted and carefully advanced, allowing the appropriate catheter to be advanced over it. The catheter and the guide wire are advanced into the ascending aorta and the wire withdrawn, allowing the catheter to be connected to pressure-monitoring equipment. Heparin, at a dose of 100 IU/kg, is injected down the catheter at this stage. In the elderly, the branches of the aortic arch are often tortuous and atheromatous; great care

should therefore be taken whilst manipulating the guide wire and catheter in this region. Various J-tipped wires may assist in this regard. At the end of the procedure, the catheter is removed and forward and backward flow in the brachial artery confirmed by release of the appropriate tape. The arteriotomy is then repaired with continuous sutures (6/0 Prolene) and the skin closed with absorbable sutures (2/0 Dexon).

Femoral

With this approach, the right groin is prepared by shaving and the usual aseptic precautions taken. The femoral artery is palpated and the overlying skin and surrounding tissue is infiltrated with 2% lignocaine at a point 1 cm below the inguinal ligament. A 2–3 mm incision is made with a number 11 blade and widened with Spencer–Wells forceps. At this point a 7–8-gauge valved sheath is introduced into the artery using the Seldinger technique, as follows:

An 18-gauge needle (Kimal), connected to a pressure transducer, is inserted through the incision at an angle of 45° and perforates the artery, its entry into the vessel being confirmed by an arterial pressure trace on the transducer. The pressure line is then disconnected and a 0.9 mm guide wire inserted, allowing the needle to be removed. The sheath and introducer are then passed along the wire into the femoral artery and the introducer is removed. Catheters can now be passed down the sheath and into the aorta, ascending retrogradely to the aortic arch.

At the end of the procedure, the sheath is removed and firm pressure is applied over the artery, by hand, for at least 10–15 minutes, or by means of a specially designed clamp, which is slowly released over 1 hour.

Left ventricular angiography

It is usual to record the left ventricular angiogram first; the catheter is therefore manipulated retrogradely across the aortic valve and contrast is power-injected into the left ventricular cavity. A side-hole catheter, such as a pigtail, is used for the power injection, as 30–40 ml contrast is injected over 15–20 seconds. A jet of this velocity through an end-hole catheter may result in an intramyocardial injection, with markedly adverse effects on haemodynamics and cardiac rhythm. For this reason end-hole catheters should not be used for ventriculography.

Two views of the left ventricle are usually obtained, i.e. left anterior oblique and anteroposterior.

Haemodynamics

Before and after left venticulography, information is recorded with respect to the haemodynamic status of the left ventricle and presence or absence of any obstruction in the left ventricular outflow tract.

Once the ventriculography catheter has entered the left ventricle, peak systolic

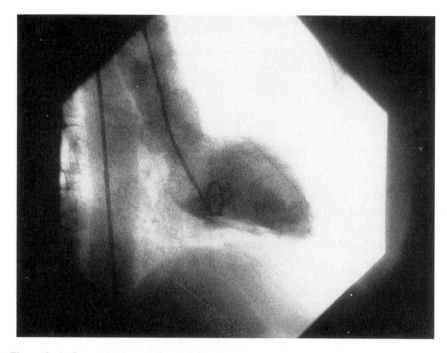

Figure 2. Left ventricular angiogram, anteroposterior view

and end-diastolic measurements are taken. After ventriculography has been performed a repeat peak systolic measurement is recorded and the catheter is then withdrawn across the aortic value and a further peak systolic pressure measurement obtained. A comparison between the two readings reveals any left ventricular outflow tract obstruction.

Coronary angiography

After the pressure measurements are completed the ventriculography catheter is removed and a suitable catheter (e.g. Castillo for brachial and Judkins for femoral approaches) is inserted along the guide wire into the ascending aorta. The catheter is manipulated to engage the left and right coronary arteries in turn, and after a test dose of contrast (1–5 ml) to ensure rapid clearance, and with continuous pressure readings to exclude occlusion of the vessel, angiograms using 5–10 ml of contrast are taken. Six views of the left coronary artery are usually obtained: left anterior oblique (LAO) (Figure 3); LAO with craniocaudal tilt (LAOCC); lateral; anteroposterior; right anterior oblique (RAO); and RAO with craniocaudal tilt (RAOCC). Three views of the right coronary artery are sought: LAO (Figure 4); LAOCC; and RAO. Multiple views are taken in order to open out the major branches and to acquire good views of any lesions in at least two projections.

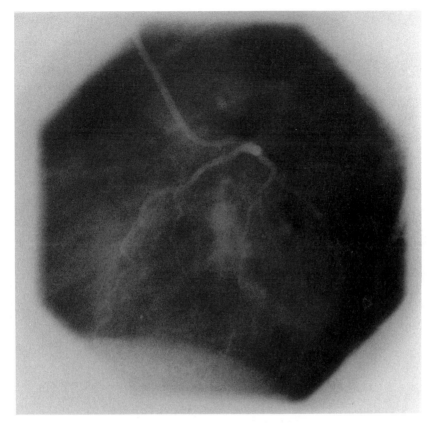

Figure 3. Left coronary angiogram, left anterior oblique view

Aortography

With both approaches, an aortogram may be indicated, e.g. in the presence of aortocoronary bypass grafts or aortic regurgitation. This is performed after withdrawal of the pigtail catheter from the left ventricle, by positioning it 2–3 cm above the aortic valve and power-injecting 40–50 ml of contrast at a rate of 25–30 ml/s. The LAO projection is usually adopted as this provides the best images of grafts and suspected aortic regurgitation. This procedure can also be used, with other views, e.g. RAO, anteroposterior, to investigate suspected aortic pathology such as acute dissection.

Right heart catheterization

This procedure can be carried out via the cephalic vein, using a technique similar to that described for entering the brachial artery (see above), or by percutaneous entry into the formal vein, using the Seldinger method.

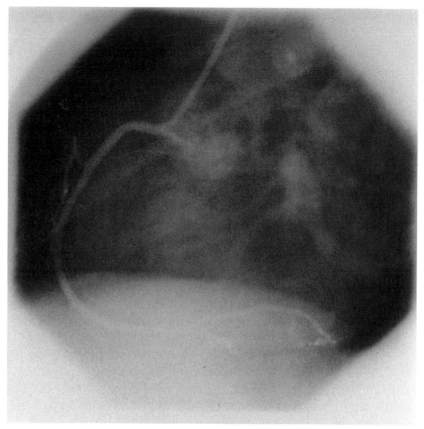

Figure 4. Right coronary angiogram, left anterior oblique view

A catheter (e.g. 7 French gauge Cornand or Goodale–Lubin) is advanced anterogradely into the right atrium, right ventricle and pulmonary artery under fluoroscopic control. Pressure measurements are continuously monitored and venous blood samples may be taken for oxygen saturation measurements. There is also the opportunity to obtain a right ventricular angiogram, if indicated, using a pigtail catheter. The catheter is then advanced down the pulmonary artery until it wedges in one of the smallest arterioles, enabling an indirect measurement of left arterial pressure—the pulmonary artery wedge (PAW) pressure—to be recorded.

THE TRANS-SEPTAL TECHNIQUE

The venous approach can also be used to enter the left side of the heart. A specialized needle (Brockenbrough needle), over which is wrapped a Teflon catheter, is inserted via the femoral vein and positioned in the right atrium. The needle is then pushed through the posterior portion of the inter-atrial septum and the catheter advanced over it. The catheter is then manoeuvred through the mitral valve and into the left ventricle.

This method is used when entry into the left ventricle is difficult by more routine approaches such as the presence of a mechanical aortic valve or severe aortic stenosis. It can be used in conjunction with a catheter in the ascending aorta to give instantaneous pressure recordings across the aortic valve. When both mitral and aortic valves are mechanical, meaningful data can only be obtained by entering the left ventricle by direct percutaneous puncture through the chest wall. This potentially dangerous method is rarely used now that Dopper echocardiography is available.

COMPLICATIONS

Mortality, morbidity and minor transient complications are well-established features of cardiac catherization. The mortality of the procedures is 0.1–0.2% (5,6); other complications occur in approximately 1% of cases.

Assessment of the patient prior to catheterization may identify high-risk cases. Patients with poor left ventricular function, severe aortic stenosis, pulmonary hypertension and widespread peripheral vascular disease have been identified as being at greater risk. Age is an independent risk factor and elderly patients also tend to have more advanced cardiac disease, therefore further increasing the possibility of complications.

The shorter the procedure, the less likely are the chances of complications; this is especially relevant in patients with pre-existing haemodynamic compromise. The duration of the investigation can be shortened by obtaining as much information as possible from non-invasive techniques, such as echocardiography, and therefore identifying specific questions that need answering by catheterization.

Local complications

The comparison of complication rate between brachial and femoral artery approaches is a source of controversy. However, it does seem apparent that the complication rate of either method is directly related to the experience of the operator.

With the brachial approach, trauma to the median nerve can occur during dissection to expose the artery, resulting in immediate pain and a neuropraxia which may persist for some days to weeks. Rarely, the median nerve is mistaken for the brachial artery, and a small 'arteriotomy' made, resulting in permanent neurological deficit. Compromise of the brachial artery may occur, for instance by a small dissection of the vessel caused by the catheter tip, or by inadvertently catching the posterior arterial wall during the arteriotomy repair. Occasionally these problems require specialist surgical intervention.

The femoral approach may result in significant bleeding from the puncture site and subsequent haematoma formation. Occasionally this can develop into a false aneurysm, requiring surgical repair. If the arterial pucture is made above the inguinal ligament, any bleeding will track into the retroperitoneum. This can result in haemodynamically significant blood loss. Damage may also occur to the femoral nerve, resulting in neuropraxia. Rarely, a femoral arteriovenous fistula can be formed (7).

Venous cannulation can result in minor haematomas, but these are seldom of significance.

With all these investigations, adherence to aseptic techniques is required to prevent infective complications.

Emboli

Embolic phenomena occur in approximately 1% of cardiac catheterizations. Emboli can originate from the catheter tip or from areas of atheroma in the brachial artery, femoral artery or aorta. The administration of heparin during the procedure may reduce the risk of this occurrence. The problems arising from emboli are usually minor and short-lived. The most significant complications occur when emboli arise from the ascending aorta, aortic valve or left ventricle and result in embolic cerebrovascular events; these are usually transient but may result in permanent neurological deficit or death.

Embolization of the coronary arteries from the catheter tip or from proximal coronary artery disease may result in transient ischaemic problems and arrhythmias. Again, these events are often transient but serious consequences can occur.

Trauma

Local traumatic complications have already been discussed. Localized dissections of the aorta by the tip of the catheter may occur and are usually managed conservatively, with diligent monitoring of the peripheral pulses distal to the insult. They rarely require active surgical intervention.

The catheter may also cause dissection of the coronary arteries. This occurs in the proximal part of the vessel and the resulting compromise to blood flows results in significant myocardial infarction, arrhythmias and death. Urgent surgical revascularization should be considered.

Occasionally, with right heart catheterization, perforation of the right ventricular wall may occur. The resulting haemopericardium is usually small and observation with repeated echocardiography is all that is required.

The trans-septal method of entering the left side of the heart from the right atrium (see above) can result in the trans-septal needle entering the ascending aorta instead of the left atrium. Again an observational stance can be taken to this occurrence.

Arrhythmias

Arrhythmias usually occur on coronary angiography. Ventricular fibrillation occurs in 0.3–0.6% of patients (5,6) and is easily treated by prompt direct current cardioversion, preceded by immediate withdrawal of the catheter. Ventricular tachycardia may also be seen and is treated along conventional lines; it may be noted when the catheter is in the right ventricular outflow tract. Transient heart block and bradycardias can be detected, especially with right coronary angiograms, or with manipulation of the catheter over the tricuspid valve. Bradycardias can be precipitated by high vagal tone, secondary to intense apprehension and pain. These problems usually respond to prompt catheter withdrawal (where appropriate) and intravenous atropine. Adequate sedation in relevant patients and sufficient local anaesthesia can do much to reduce the effects of vagal hypertonia.

Contrast-related complications

Mild urticarial reactions are common and promptly respond to intravenous antihistamines and hydrocortisone. Major anaphylactic reactions can occur and these demand the use of intravenous adrenaline as well as steroids and antihistamines. Fortunately these potentially fatal complications are rare, with an incidence of one in 40 000 catheterizations (8). In asthmatic patients or those with a known history of atopic reactions, a non-ionic dye (Omnipaque) should be used and prophylactic hydrocortisone given.

During ventriculography, the large volume of contrast given causes transient flushing and vasodilation. This is usually of no consequence but may result in hypotension in patients in whom the ability to increase their cardiac output is compromised, e.g. severe aortic stenosis.

In a standard left heart catheter, between 100 and 150 ml of hypertonic contrast is used. This increases the intravascular volume and may result in acute left ventricular failure and pulmonary oedema in susceptible individuals. The prophylactic use of diuretics immediately after the procedure can be recommended.

Patients with renal disease run the risk of experiencing a deterioration of their renal function following administration of large volumes of contrast material, especially if they suffer from diabetes or dehydration. Established renal failure may result, the risk of which may be reduced by the use of non-ionic contrast dye (8,9).

In order to keep contrast-related complications to a minimum, the smallest amount of dye should be used. Biplanar imaging can be of considerable assistance in achieving this.

INDICATIONS FOR CARDIAC CATHETERIZATION IN THE ELDERLY

Cardiac catheterization can be used to aid diagnosis or to guide management in a variety of cardiac conditions. The former indication should only be considered when non-invasive investigations such as stress testing, thallium perfusion scans and echocardiography have been inconclusive. The major consideration for the latter indication is the appropriateness of further invasive or surgical intervention. This must take into account concomitant risk factors to surgical treatment, the presence or otherwise of significant non-cardiac medical conditions such as diabetes or malignancy, and the informed wishes of the patient.

Coronary artery disease

Elderly patients with symptomatic coronary artery disease which is becoming difficult to control with medical therapy should be considered for cardiac catheterization, when the extent of the disease can be accurately defined and the appropriate management initiated.

The potential risks and expected benefits must be carefully examined prior to catheterization. Significant non-cardiac pathology must be taken into account, not only with respect to cardiac catheterization, but also when considering the ultimate outcome after invasive intervention or surgery. Malignant disease need not be a contraindication to invasive investigation and treatment but there should be a realistic appreciation of the natural history of the condition. The most relevant cardiac factor to be taken into account is the state of the left ventricle. Severely impaired left ventricular function would predispose to complications of cardiac catheterization as well as being an adverse prognostic indicator for cardiac surgery.

Coronary bypass surgery has been shown to result in a marked improvement of symptoms in patients over 65 years of age (10). Favourable results have also been reported with respect to mortality and morbidity (11,12), one study noting an in-hospital mortality of 1.6% (13). Encouraging long-term survival rates have also been demonstrated; in Livesey's study, 95% 1-year and 89% 8-year survival was seen in patients over 65 years of age (14). However, age has been noted by the Coronary Artery Surgery Study (CASS) to be an independent risk factor in surgery, the CASS early mortality figures being 5.2% in the over-65 population (15).

Percutaneous transluminal coronary angioplasty (PTCA) is a widespread technique used to treat suitable lesions identified by cardiac catheterization. It has been shown to be a viable and effective method in the elderly population, with multi-vessel PTCA resulting in 98% overall potency rates (16) and a 3.2% major complication rate. The long-term survival figures are favourable, with a 90% 1-year and a 78% 5-year survival rate (16). The re-stenosis rate is comparable with that of younger patients, being 31% at 6 months in octogenarians (17). The case fatality from coronary artery disease is higher in the elderly population (18). Coronary artery surgery and PTCA also have an increased risk, probably secondary to the greater incidence of poor left ventricular function and the tendency to more extensive disease. The risks of these interventions appear to be outweighed by the potential benefits, and in view of this age itself should not be a barrier to cardiac catheterization in well-selected patients.

Valvular heart disease

With the increased lifespan enjoyed in the Western world, along with the decline in the incidence of rheumatic fever, the spectrum of valvular diseases has changed in the past few decades. Degenerative aortic valve disease is now the most common lesion seen in Western adult practice, whilst over the same period there has been a decline in the number of cases of mitral stenosis (1).

The increasing sophistication of echocardiography has enabled cardiac vascular disease to be identified and assessed to a far greater extent before considering cardiac catheterization. This has enabled specific questions to be answered with catheterization, such as the presence or otherwise of coronary artery disease in a patient being considered for valvular surgery. The commonest conditions requiring cardiac catheterization are aortic and mitral valve disease.

Aortic stenosis

Doppler echocardiography has enabled the gradient across a stenotic aortic valve to be assessed non-invasively, as opposed to the method of passing a catheter retrogradely across the aortic valve and measuring the peak-to-peak difference between the ventricular and aortic systolic pressures on withdrawal. Opinions differ as to the necessity of assessing the aortic valve gradient by cardiac catheter. Both invasive and non-invasive techniques can demonstrate left ventricular function.

Cardiac catheterization is used to outline the anatomy of the coronary arteries with a view to possible bypass surgery in conjunction with aortic valve surgery. This is especially relevant in the elderly population, particularly if angina is present.

Aortic regurgitation

Echocardiography can easily detect the presence of aortic regurgitation and the state of the left ventricle. Cardiac catheterization, however, is required to assess the patency of the coronary arteries prior to surgery and to evaluate the severity of the lesion.

On catheterization, the aortic pulse pressure has a rapid upstroke and downstroke. The left ventricular pressures are normal in early stage of the natural history, but as the disease progresses the end-diastolic pressure rises, and in the late stage the left ventricular end-diastolic pressure rises rapidly in diastole. An aortogram may show a dilated aortic root, and the high blood flow to the dilated and hypertrophied ventricle make the arteries difficult to fill with dye.

Right-sided pressure and the pulmonary artery wedge (PAW) pressure give a further insight into the effects of the regurgitant aortic lesion. Exercising the patient on the catheter table, with a simple set of pedals for instance, may well be relevant as an increase in left ventricular end-diastolic pressure and PAW pressure may be demonstrated, which should correlate with the patient's symptoms.

Rheumatic mitral valve disease

This disease results in a spectrum of conditions from pure mitral stenosis through mixed mitral stenosis and regurgitation, to predominant mitral regurgitation. Cardiac catheterization is indicated to assess the haemodynamic severity of the lesion by measuring the diastolic gradient between the left ventricle and the PAW pressure. Measurement of the right-sided pressures can also give an indication of the haemodynamic compromise and, if the subject is exercised on the table, then marked increases in left atrial pressures (reflected in the PAW pressure) become apparent (up to 35 mmHg).

In mitral stenosis, the PAW pressure trace has a characteristic shape. A dominant 'a' wave is seen if the patient is in sinus rhythm, as a result of left atrial hypertrophy. Because of the obstruction to left atrial filling, the 'y' descent is slow and prolonged. If there is concomitant mitral regurgitation, then a prominent 'v' wave may be seen, although this is not usually as marked as that seen in non-rheumatic mitral regurgitation, unless the regurgitant lesion is markedly dominant.

Again, assessment of the coronary arteries is indicated in patients over the age of 45 years.

Mitral regurgitation

Mitral regurgitation may be the result of rheumatic heart disease or be secondary to other conditions such as mitral valve prolapse. Echocardiography can again provide evidence for the presence and usually the cause of incompetence, but haemodynamic assessment requires cardiac catheterization.

Catheterization of the right side of the heart gives an indication of the severity of secondary pulmonary hypertension. The PAW pressure allows the transmitted systolic 'v' wave to be measured. Both right-sided pressures and the systolic 'v' wave give an indication of the severity of the mitral regurgitation.

Left heart catheterization gives an accurate measure of left ventricular diastolic pressure, and left ventricular angiography will demonstrate evidence of left ventricular dysfunction and will allow the severity of the mitral regurgitation to be visualized. Mitral valve prolapse can be seen on left ventricular angiography; the three-scalloped posterior leaflet is best assessed in the RAO projection and the large, single anterior leaflet is best seen in the LAO view with 30° of craniocaudal tilt.

Assessment of the coronary arteries is also facilitated by catheterization. This is not only relevant with regard to possible bypass grafting but also because significant left ventricular dysfunction associated with ischaemic heart disease may cause abnormal mitral valve closure and mimic non-rheumatic mitral regurgitation.

Surgical considerations

Surgery for valvular heart disease in the elderly has seen some encouraging results. Significant improvement in functional status in successful aortic and mitral valve replacements as well as combined procedures has been reported (19), with patients improving from NYHA grade III/IV preoperatively to NYHA grade I/II postoperatively. The operative mortality of aortic valve replacement has been documented as 5% for the over-65-year age group and 8% for the over-70s, with 88% 1-year and 74% 5-year survival in the combined populations (14). It has been noted that mitral valve replacement and combined aortic and mitral procedures have a higher operative mortality and less favourable prognosis.

In view of the acceptable mortality figures for valvular surgery it is reasonable to take the view that age alone should not be a barrier to invasive investigations in valvular heart disease.

REFERENCES

1. Hall R (1989) Cardiac catheterisation and angiography. In *Diseases of the Heart*, Julian DG, Camm AJ, Fox KM *et al.* (eds). Ballière Tindall, London, p. 363.
2. Lessof MH, Grimely Evans J, Joy MD *et al.* (1991) Cardiological intervention in elderly patients. *J R Coll Physicians London* **25**: 197–205.
3. Wenger NK, Furberg CD, Pitt E (1986) Coronary heart disease in the elderly: review of current knowledge and research recommendations. In *Coronary Heart Disease in the Elderly*, Wenger NK, Furberg CD, Pitt E (eds), Elsevier, New York, pp. 1–7.
4. Mabin TA, Holmes DR, Smith HC *et al.* (1985) Follow-up clinical results in patients undergoing percutaneous transluminal coronary angioplasty. *Circulation* **71**: 754–760.
5. Davies K, Kennedy JW, Kemp HG *et al.* (1979) Complications of coronary angiography from the Collaborative Study of Coronary Artery Surgery. *Circulation* **59**: 1105–1111.
6. Kennedy JW and the Registry Committee of the Society for Cardiac Angiography (1982). Complications associated with cardiac catheterisation and angiography. *Cathet Cardiovasc Diagn* **8**: 5–11.
7. Picus O, Tolly WG (1984) Iatrogenic femoral arterio-venus fistula: evaluation by digital vascular imaging. *Am J Radiol* **142**: 566–570.
8. D'Elia JA, Gleason RE, Alday M *et al.* (1982) Nephrotoxicity from angiographic contrast material: a prospective study. *Am J Med* **72**: 719–725.

9. Eisenberg RL, Bank WO, Hedgecock MW (1980) Renal failure after major angiography. *Am J Med* **68**: 43–46.
10. Gersh BJ, Kronmal RA, Schaff HV *et al.* (1985) Comparison of coronary bypass surgery and medical therapy in patients 65 years of age or older. *N Engl J Med* **313**: 217–224.
11. Gann D, Colin C, Hildner F *et al.* (1977) Coronary artery bypass surgery in patients over seventy years of age and older. *J Thorac Cardiovasc Surg* **73**: 237–241.
12. Stephenson LW, MacVaugh H, Edmunds LH (1978) Surgery using cardiopulmonary bypass in the elderly. *Circulation* **58**: 250–254.
13. Knapp WS, Douglas JS, Craver JM *et al.* (1981) Efficacy of coronary artery bypass grafting in elderly patients with coronary artery disease. *Am J Cardiol* **47**: 923–930.
14. Livesey S, Caine N, Spielghalter D *et al.* (1988) Cardiac surgery for patients aged 65 years and older: a long term survival analysis. *Br Heart J* **60**: 480–484.
15. Gersh BJ, Kronmal R, Frye R *et al.* (1983) Coronary arteriography and coronary artery bypass surgery: morbidity and mortality in patients aged 65 years and older. *Circulation* **67**: 483–491.
16. Bedotto JB, Rutherford BD, McConahay DR *et al.* (1991) Results of multivessel percutaneous transluminal coronary angioplasty in persons aged 65 years and older. *Am J Cardiol* **67**: 1051–1055.
17. Jackman JD, Navetta FI, Smith JE *et al.* (1991) Percutaneous transluminal coronary angioplasty in octogenarians as an effective therapy for angina pectoris. *Am J Cardiol* **68**: 116–119.
18. ISIS-2 (Second International Study of Infarct Survival) Collaborative Group (1988). Randomised trial of intravenous streptokinase, oral aspirin, both or neither among 17,187 cases of suspected acute myocardial infarction: ISIS-2. *Lancet* **ii**: 349–360.
19. Jamieson WR, Dooner J, Munro AI *et al.* (1981) Cardiac valve replacement in the elderly: a review of 320 consecutive cases. *Circulation* **64**: 177–183.

11 Cardiac Nuclear Imaging

ANN C. TWEDDEL
Glasgow Royal Infirmary, Glasgow, UK

As the population grows older, increasingly a larger proportion of patients are seen with degenerative diseases, particularly atherosclerosis. In general, the patients referred for consideration for investigations are among the population of 'free range' elderly, as opposed to those in whom activity is severely limited.

With increasing numbers of patients over 65 years of age being referred for cardiac surgery (1), necessarily there are increasing numbers being referred for assessment and for coronary arteriography. In the last 2 years, 10% of the patients referred to nuclear cardiology in our practice are over the age of 65.

In the elderly, the aspects where nuclear cardiology has something to offer in patient assessment are identical to those of the under-65s, namely non-invasive assessment of left and right ventricular function and the assessment of myocardial perfusion. The one major unresolved problem in dealing with the elderly is the inability to have age-matched controls who are free of coronary disease. Thus, necessarily, our normal control values are drawn from a younger population.

SCAN ACQUISITION

Nuclear cardiology is based on administration of radiopharmaceuticals, which are either taken up in the myocardium or remain within the blood pool. The distribution and intensity of the γ-rays or X-rays emitted by the radiopharmaceutical is imaged using a gamma camera, usually the Anger-type gamma camera. Nowadays, cameras are almost invariably interfaced to digital computers, which acquire and store the images produced by the camera for subsequent analysis.

The basic components of this imaging system comprise the following:

1. *Collimator*: this defines the angle of acceptance of detected gamma rays, and consists of a lead disc with an array of parallel holes. By altering the length of these holes, or by changing the thickness of the septa (the thin sections between the parallel holes), collimators of differing sensitivity and energy can be made to suit the different types of radiopharmaceutical being imaged.

Geriatric Cardiology. Principles and Practice. Edited by A. Martin and A. J. Camm
© 1994 John Wiley & Sons Ltd

2. *Detector*: this is a large-diameter (25–50 cm) single crystal of sodium iodide 9–13 mm thick. When an incident gamma ray meets the crystal, the energy is converted into excited electrons which then fall into inner shells and produce light photons. These are then detected by the photomultipliers.

3. *Photomultiplier array*: this is used to position the event within the crystal, since if the event occurred directly centrally above a photomultiplier this would detect most of the resultant photons, whilst if it was between two photomultiplier tubes then both would detect an equal number of photons, and the event could be located between them. Thus by measuring the amplitude of the signal from each photomultiplier and using suitable positioning circuitry, the coordinates of each event can be recorded.

4. *Camera console*: to check if the detected energy is within the photopeak window, and to perform some energy and uniformity corrections.

5. *Analogue-to-digital converters (ADCs)*: to convert the position and energy signals into a suitable form for the computer system.

6. *Computer system*: to form an image of the gamma ray distribution from the x, y coordinates produced by the ADCs, store it and allow subsequent processing.

There is an extensive range of nuclear medicine computer systems available commercially. Image acquisition should be possible in a 64×64, 128×128 or 256×256 matrix, and all standard imaging-processing routines and methods should be available. In addition, a high-resolution colour and black and white display should be available, since semi-quantitative analysis techniques using colour image display scales can reduce inter- and intra-observer variability in reporting perfusion images. Black and white displays yield better results for assessment of wall motion in gated perfusion imaging or gated blood pool ventriculography.

For nuclear cardiology it is obviously essential for the system to acquire data gated to the electrocardiogram (ECG). Normally the reference signal is taken from the R wave detector of a standard ECG machine, and each R–R interval can be subdivided into a sequence of images (minimum 16, up to 64 frames for some high temporal resolution studies). This can be done in frame mode, as image data are acquired, using fixed, preselected time bins and employing a buffering technique to exclude ectopic beats. Alternatively all the x, y coordinates of each event, along with R wave timing markers and timing pulses, can be stored on a temporary file in the computer, to allow accurate and flexible reconstruction of a representative cardiac cycle of the desired number of frames. This is the listmode technique, and is to be preferred despite the longer processing times required.

7. *Radiopharmaceuticals for nuclear cardiology*: the standard gamma camera is designed to work optimally at the energy of technetium-99m (^{99m}Tc), which is the commonest isotope used in nuclear medicine. In nuclear cardiology it is employed, when labelled to red blood cells, to perform gated blood pool ventriculography—a powerful technique for evaluating right and left ven-

tricular function, both regionally and globally. It has also recently been used as the emitter in the ^{99m}Tc-labelled isonitrile compounds, which are increasingly used as alternatives to thallium-201 (^{201}Tl) for the assessment of myocardial perfusion. This section will describe some of the physical properties of the two isotopes commonly used in nuclear cardiology.

Technetium-99m: this has ideal physical properties for radionuclide imaging due to: its short 6.05-hour half-life; mono-energetic gamma ray emission at 140.6 keV which has a half-value thickness in tissue of ~4.5 cm; ready availability; and the abundance of compounds to which it may be labelled to produce radiopharmaceuticals.

Thallium-201: this has a half-life of 3.05 days and emits X-rays at 70 keV from an electron capture process, with a further emission at 160 keV. In tissue the half-value thickness is ~3.5 cm. Thallium is taken up by all active muscle, resulting in ~4% uptake in the myocardium. Approximately 85% of ^{201}Tl is extracted on the first pass through the coronary arteries, and it therefore allows an assessment of myocardial perfusion. It is commonly administered when the heart is under stress using either dynamic exercise or drugs, to detect areas of lack of perfusion due usually to significant coronary artery disease. The standard activity used is 74 MBq in the UK, although double this is commonly used in the USA.

STRESS TESTING IN THE ELDERLY

The majority of patients seen in cardiology departments are suffering from problems arising from atherosclerotic disease, and such symptoms are only apparent on stress. Stress testing is a method of quantitating these symptoms and their impact on the ability to perform work. In the elderly stress testing can be performed safely and provide useful clinical information. Exercise testing should be performed by medically trained personnel and conditions should conform to those recommended and published in the *European Heart Journal* and *American Journal of Cardiology* (2,3).

EQUIPMENT

Either a bicycle or treadmill may be used and are equally effective, although we find that often elderly women express a preference for the bicycle as this is less frightening and they feel more in control. It has long been argued that the treadmill is 'more physiological' and indeed heart rates and workloads achieved at peak exercise are higher using the treadmill. Using the bicycle, due care must be taken to adjust the seat height, provide toe clips and ensure that isometric exercise is avoided by relaxing the grip on the handlebars. Systolic blood pressure achieved during exercise tends to be higher with the bicycle, thus double product (heart rate × systolic blood pressure), which is an indirect assessment of myocardial oxygen consumption, tends to be very similar in comparison to those achieved with treadmill exercise (4,5).

EXERCISE PROTOCOLS

With age, physical work capacity decreases:

$$\text{Maximum } \dot{V}O_2 = 1.29 \times \frac{L}{H-60} e^{-0.00884T}$$

where $\dot{V}O_2$ = oxygen consumption, L = load in kilopond metres per minute at submaximal work, H = heart rate after 5–6 minutes at L, and T = age in years. Between 35 and 65, the maximal $\dot{V}O_2$ declines from 3.17 l/min to 2.29 l/min (6).

This implies that exercise protocols require adjustment using either the modified Macnaughton protocol on the treadmill or with the bicycle small increments of 10–20 W. In the last 2 years in our laboratory, 190 patients over the age of 65 have been referred for nuclear cardiology assessment on stress. Of these, 29% were over 70 years of age. Only four patients over the age of 70 were unable to perform dynamic exercise. The mean workload achieved was 70 W with a mean exercise heart rate of 106 beats/min (although 94% were on antianginal therapy). Chest pain was the limiting factor in only 29%, leg fatigue in 45% and breathlessness in 22%. Exercise tests were electrocardiographically positive in 31% although all had multiple vessel coronary disease.

PHARMACOLOGICAL ALTERNATIVES TO EXERCISE

Various pharmacological agents have been proposed as alternatives to exercise. These are useful where exercise is impossible, such as in patients limited by severe arthritis, or inadvisable such as in patients with resting lower limb ischaemia, or where exercise testing would be inadequate, such as in patients with peripheral vascular disease.

Dipyridamole

Dipyridamole is the most commonly used pharmacological agent, in a dose usually of 0.56 mg/kg administered as a short intravenous infusion over 4 minutes, followed by a short period of moderate exercise such as a 2-minute walk (7,8). Dipyridamole acts as a potent vasodilator, primarily of the small coronary arterioles. Peak effect occurs at about 7 minutes and lasts approximately 30 minutes. It may be reversed with aminophylline. Side-effects include flushing, headache, nausea, dizziness, vomiting, hypotension, severe chest pain and marked ST–T segment depression. Dipyridamole must be used with care in patients with chronic obstructive airways disease as this may precipitate bronchospasm (9,10). The sensitivity and specificity for the detection of coronary artery disease, in conjunction with thallium imaging, are similar to exercise although the size of inferior defects may be underestimated due to attenuation from subdiaphragmatic uptake (11,12).

Adenosine

Dipyridamole acts by blocking the receptor uptake and transport of adenosine. Adenosine given intravenously therefore acts as a coronary vasodilator, but has a very short duration of action (half-life < 2 seconds). Given as an infusion of 140 μg/kg per minute, it acts as a potent vasodilator and, because of its brief duration of action, side-effects are also of short duration, the commonest being flushing, sensation of breathlessness, chest pain and atrioventricular block. It has been shown that together with thallium imaging, adenosine is safe, well tolerated and an accurate test for the diagnosis of coronary disease (13,14).

Dobutamine

Dobutamine, given as an incremental infusion to a maximum of 400 μg/kg per minute, appears to produce ischaemia predominantly through an increase in inotropic state rather than by increasing heart rate. Arrhythmias may be induced and it must be used with care, but dobutamine stress provides a suitable alternative to exercise (15,16).

VENTRICULAR FUNCTION

Image analysis

Technetium scans

With the *first-pass technique*, 800 MBq of [^{99m}Tc] pertechnetate is rapidly injected intravenously as a compact bolus, usually into an antecubital vein. Complete mixing of this bolus is assumed to have occurred as the technetium enters the left ventricle; thus a time–activity curve from the left ventricular region of interest has cyclical fluctuations, with peaks corresponding to maximal counts and end-diastole, and minimal activity reflects end-systole. Calculations are based on three to four cycles and thus the technique is dependent on obtaining sufficiently high count rates. This is usually best achieved by a multi-crystal camera, which has a higher count rate capacity than the single-crystal camera.

With the *equilibrium technique*, the technetium remains in the vascular space. The cardiac blood pool is imaged and data collected simultaneously with the R wave of the ECG. The R–R interval is subsequently divided into segments (usually 24) by the computer and the counts acquired in these small segments are summated for 300–400 beats. By drawing a region of interest over the left ventricle, and plotting the change in counts, a time–activity curve can be generated (see Figure 1). Images are best obtained in the 40° left anterior oblique view to obtain maximal separation between the right and the left ventricle (Figure 2).

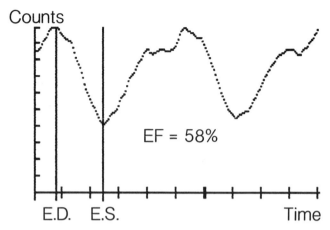

Figure 1. Time–activity curve, demonstrating end-diastole (ED) and end-systole (ES)

End-diastolic and end-systolic frames
These can be identified. The counts within the region of interest drawn around the left ventricle or right ventricle are proportional to the volume. By measuring the activity circulating within the blood and with suitable background subtraction, end-diastolic and end-systolic volumes can be calculated.

Left ventricular ejection fraction
This can be calculated from the formula

$$\frac{(EDC - BC) - (EDS - BC)}{EDC - BC} \times 100\%$$

where EDC = end-diastolic counts, EDS = end-systolic counts, and BC = background activity.

Regional function
By subtracting end-systolic counts from the end-diastolic counts, a stroke volume image can be generated, which represents the regions of the left ventricular wall that move during contraction. Thus, by quantifying the stroke volume image, the extent of regional myocardial dysfunction can be assessed.

By subtracting end-diastolic counts from end-systolic counts, regions that move out of phase with ventricular contraction may be identified; these are usually obviously the atria, but this technique can be used to identify aneurysm formation.

Regional ventricular function may be assessed in many ways, the simplest being the visual analysis of the ventricular wall during the cine display of the ventricular image. Regional ejection fraction measurements are the application

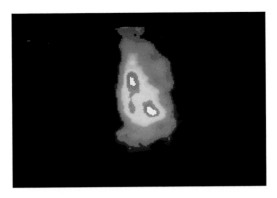

Figure 2. Normal end-diastolic image, technetium scan

(a)

(b)

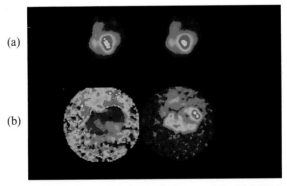

Figure 3. (a) End-diastolic (L) and end-systolic images (R). (b) LHS image, showing an area of delayed phase in green; RHS amplitude image, demonstrating a region of reduced function in the septum

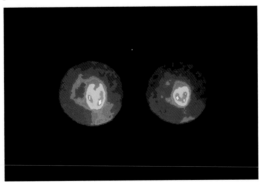

Figure 4. Gated thallium perfusion images. Normal end-diastolic (L) and end-systolic images (R), 40° left anterior oblique projection

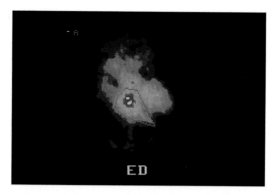

Figure 5. Technetium scan, end-diastolic image, enlarged right ventricle (outlined in red)

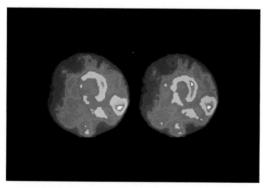

Figure 6. Thallium perfusion images. End-diastolic (**R**) and end-systolic (**L**) images from a patient with a very substantial anterior and inferior perfusion defect, and a dilated left ventricle with poor function

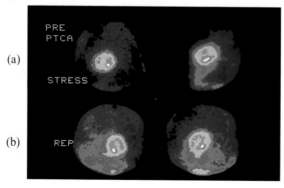

Figure 7. (a) 40° and 70° left anterior oblique projections of thallium images, immediately after stress, showing a small inferior defect. (b) 40° and 70° left anterior oblique projections, showing inferior reperfusion

of the ejection fraction equation to segments around the ventricle. Unfortunately, because the ventricle in contracting not only becomes smaller but is rotated, the apex of the ventricle may rotate out of the region of interest from which the regional ejection fraction is calculated. Perhaps a more accurate method of assessing regional dysfunction is phase analysis. For each pixel which constitutes the image, a time–activity curve is generated and then colour coded so that all pixels at minimum activity at the identical time are the same colour. This permits the representation of the time to minimal activity across the ventricular contraction. Regions of the ventricle where contraction is delayed will therefore be represented as 'phase delay' and will be of a different colour from surrounding regions. Thus the area of delayed phase can be measured (Figure 3).

Analysis of perfusion images

Planar images are usually acquired in three projections: the anterior, 40° left anterior oblique and 70° left anterior oblique. Regions of reduced thallium uptake (or more recently technetium-labelled perfusion agent) within the image can therefore be assigned to differing coronary arteries that usually supply that region. Tomographic images are usually reconstructed into two-dimensional slices but essentially the same system of regional analysis is employed.

Visual analysis

This is the simplest method of analysis and, with experienced observers, is reproducible provided the images are displayed with care and varied to the same extent. By gating the images to the ECG, the pattern of perfusion throughout systole and diastole can be assessed, and this provides a better predictive accuracy for the diagnosis of coronary disease (17) (Figure 4).

Thallium uptake

Thallium uptake within the myocardium and lungs can be measured by simply measuring the syringe pre and post injection and by drawing a region of interest over the heart and lungs and expressing this as a percentage of the injected dose (18). Increased thallium uptake in the lungs is a poor prognostic sign (19).

Statistical analysis

By applying a 'mean normal' image to the patient image, a statistical image can be produced which instantly allows abnormal areas to be identified (20).

Circumferential profiling

By drawing a region of interest around the left ventricular myocardium, this can be divided into multiple sectors. The activity in each sector can be plotted and compared with a normal range. Particularly for tomographic imaging, this method reduces the inter-observer variation (21).

APPLICATIONS

Assessment/angina

The first and most obvious application is in the non-invasive assessment of ventricular function. Where ventricular function is very poor, there may be little point in progressing to angiography as the patient will not be accepted for surgery and is a high-risk candidate for percutaneous transluminal coronary angioplasty (PTCA) (22). However, often breathlessness is an 'angina equivalent' in the elderly and ventricular function may be surprisingly good.

Similarly, it can be useful to assess left ventricular function following cardiac surgery. Regional wall motion abnormalities and reduced function are usually indicative of perioperative or postoperative infarction, often where grafts have been placed on to diseased vessels.

Post infarction

Following myocardial infarction, one of the major determinants of prognosis has been shown to be left ventricular performance (23,24). Radionuclide angiography provides prognostic information—for early mortality and the development of congestive heart failure. In addition to assessing global ventricular function, the extent and location of regional wall motion abnormalities and abnormalities in right ventricular performance can be measured. The combination of right ventricular with left ventricular dysfunction carries a very grave prognosis (Figure 5). In 100 consecutive patients admitted with chest pain to our coronary care unit (prior to the era of thrombolysis), 83 were subsequently proved to have sustained a myocardial infarction. With a left ventricular ejection fraction (LVEF) below 30% being considered poor left ventricular function and a right ventricular ejection fraction (RVEF) below 35% poor right ventricular function, twenty-five patients were considered to have biventricular involvement. At a mean follow-up time of 18 months, 44% were dead as compared with 33% of those with left ventricular dysfunction alone (11/45) and 0/19 patients with solely right ventricular dysfunction.

Assessment of breathlessness

In the elderly, breathlessness is often an 'angina equivalent' and it may be more appropriate to perform a myocardial perfusion scan to assess the extent of myocardial involvement. A resting blood pool scan will demonstrate left ventricular function and end-diastolic, and end-systolic volume may be calculated. It should be remembered that end-diastolic volume increases with age (25) and this should be recognized when commenting on scans.

Blood pool scans, performed during and immediately post exercise, can give variable information with respect to the development of new wall motion abnormalities and their extent (26). These studies need to be performed with care, making sure that the chest does not move in relation to the gamma camera and thus avoiding motion artefact and blurring of the image. Several pharmacological alternatives are available, of which dipyridamole is the most commonly used during echocardiography.

Right ventricular function is important in the assessment of breathlessness. In our population, maturity-onset asthma or coexistent obstructive lung disease is common. The right ventricle, being normally a 'low-pressure system', as the pulmonary pressures increase so the right ventricle dilates and becomes less efficient. In patients with chronic obstructive lung disease, where the RVEF is less than 30% on exercise, pulmonary vascular resistance tends to rise with a further decrease in right ventricular function, reflected mainly by an increased end-systolic volume (27).

PERFUSION IMAGING

Rest imaging

Using ^{201}Tl, a rest image (acquired in 15–20 minutes) can allow an assessment of the extent of scar tissue from previous myocardial infarction, and obviously the extent of the myocardium receiving a blood supply at rest.

Rest imaging performed acutely, on admission to coronary care, can accurately assess infarct size and thus provides important information for subsequent prognosis (the development of cardiogenic shock, congestive heart failure, etc.) (28,29) (Figure 6).

Antimyosin imaging

Indium-labelled antimyosin is a monoclonal antibody that bonds to cardiac myosin, which is exposed during myocardial cell death. By performing dual imaging with ^{111}In-labelled antimyosin and ^{201}Tl, infarct size and the percentage of infarcted myocardium can be accurately assessed, and viable and necrotic tissue may be differentiated. However, images can only be obtained reliably at 48 hours post infarction, which obviates any opportunity to intervene acutely (e.g. with streptokinase) (30).

Stress perfusion imaging

There is very little value in using stress thallium imaging in the elderly as a diagnostic tool, as the incidence of coronary artery disease in this population is high. It does, however, have the ability to provide clinically useful information as to the extent and site of ischaemia, and by differentiation of 'viable' and infarcted myocardium.

Extent and site of ischaemia

In our laboratory the predictive accuracy of thallium imaging for the detection of coronary artery disease in a younger population (mean age 52) is 90%. Both false negative and false positive results may occur; false negative images may be due to the size of the defects being below the limit of resolution of the camera, the influence of collateral supply which may be particularly effective in long-standing ischaemia, diffuse ischaemia (analysis is a relative differentiation between normal/abnormal) and inadequate levels of exercise (31).

Viable and infarcted myocardium

Abnormalities on stress images may be indicative either of areas of myocardium where the blood flow is impaired during stress, but adequate at rest, or of areas of infarction. Conventionally, differentiation of these two conditions is made by performing images 3–4 hours after stress—redistribution images (Figure 7). In a small proportion of patients 'ischaemia' is not reversed by 3–4 hours and this may be overcome by either delayed imaging (at 24 hours), by injecting a further small dose of thallium or by performing a rest perfusion image on a separate day. The strategy used is dependent on the practicalities of the situation (e.g. if the patient has travelled a distance it would be inconvenient to attend for 24-hour imaging) (32,33).

Several studies have shown the superiority of stress thallium as a predictor of future cardiac events. In patients without previous myocardial infarction, the extent of reversible thallium perfusion defects was the best predictor of future cardiac events (angina pectoris, infarction and cardiac death) (34,35).

Similarly, post infarction, where the ECG is already abnormal, ^{201}Tl stress scintigraphy was able to differentiate patients with a fixed defect, with a low subsequent complication rate (6%), and those with reversible defects or multiple perfusion defects (perfusion defects outside the infarct site) who were at risk of future events (81%) (36).

The identification of reversible ischaemia, and the extent of this, is also useful when patients are being assessed for general anaesthetic to perform other procedures such as repair of aortic aneurysms (37,38).

Perfusion imaging is also useful as a method of assessing the efficacy of mechanical interventions, such as angioplasty or coronary surgery. In patients with recurrent angina, following intervention, by identifying regions of reversible ischaemia, this provides an indication as to whether this is in the region of the intervention or in a distant myocardial region.

REFERENCES

1. Elyada MAA, Hall RJ, Gray AG *et al.* (1984) Coronary revascularisation in the elderly patients. *J AM Coll Cardiol* **3**: 1398–1402.
2. Schlant R, Blomquist CG, Brandenburg RO *et al.* (eds) (1986) Guidelines for exercise

testing (a report of the Joint American College of Cardiology/American Heart Association Task Force on assessment of cardiovascular procedures). *Circulation* **74** (3), 653A–667A.

3. Löllger H, Ulmer HV, Crean P (1988) Recommendations and standard guidelines for exercise testing. *Eur Heart J* **9** (Suppl K): 3–37.

4. Bruce RA (1974) Methods of exercise testing: step tests, bicycle, treadmill, isometrics. *Am J Cardiol* **33**: 715–720.

5. Nagle FJ, Balke B, Naughton JP (1965) Graduational step tests for assessing work capacity. *J Appl Physiol* **20**: 745–748.

6. von Dobelin W, Astrand I, Bergstrom A (1967) Analysis of age and other factors related to maximal oxygen uptake. *J Appl Physiol* **22**: 934–938.

7. Gould KL (1978) Noninvasive assessment of coronary stenosis by myocardial perfusion imaging during pharmacologic coronary vasodilation. 1. Physiologic basis and experimental validation. *Am J Cardiol* **41**: 267–278.

8. Laarman GI, Bruschke AVG, Verzijhergen JF et al. (1990) Thallium 201 scintigraphy after dipyridamole infusion with low level exercise. II: quantitative analysis vs visual analysis. *Eur Heart J* **11**: 162–172.

9. Homma S, Gilliland Y, Guiney TE et al. (1987) Safety of intravenous dipyridamole for stress testing with thallium imaging. *Am J Cardiol* **59**: 152–154.

10. Ranhosky A, Kempthorne-Rawson J and the Intravenous Dipyridamole-thallium Imaging Study Group (1990) The safety of intravenous dipyridamole thallium perfusion imaging. *Circulation* **81**: 1205–1209.

11. Laarman GI, Bruschke AVG, Verzijibergen JF et al. (1988) Efficacy of intravenous dipyridamole with exercise in thallium-201 myocardial perfusion scintigraphy. *Eur Heart J* **9**: 1206–1214.

12. Leppo J, Boucher RA, Okado RD et al. (1982) Serial thallium-201 myocardial imaging after dipyridamole infusion: diagnostic utility in detecting coronary stenosis and relationship to regional wall motion. *Circulation* **66**: 649–657.

13. Verani MS, Matimerian JJ (1991) Myocardial perfusion scintigraphy during maximal coronary artery vasodilation with adenosine. *Am J Cardiol* **67**: 12D–17D.

14. Iskandrian AS, Heo J, Nguyen T et al. (1991) Assessment of coronary artery disease using single-photon emission computed tomography with thallium-201 during adenosine-induced coronary hyperaemia. *Am J Cardiol* **67**: 1190–1194.

15. Mason, JR, Palae RT, Freeman ML et al. (1984) Thallium scintigraphy during dobutamine infusion: non exercise dependent screening test for coronary disease. *Am Heart J* **107**: 481–485.

16. Mannering D, Cripps T, Leech G et al. (1988) The dobutamine stress test as an alternative to exercise testing after acute myocardial infarction. *Br Heart J* **59**: 521–526.

17. Martin W, Tweddel A, McGhie AI, Hutton I (1987) Gated thallium scintigraphy in patients with coronary artery disease: an improved planar imaging technique. *Clin Phys Physiol Meas* **8**: 343–354.

18. Tweddel AC, Martin W, McGhie I, Hutton I (1988) Improved detection of coronary artery disease by estimated myocardial thallium uptake. *Eur J Nucl Med* **15**: 336–340.

19. Kahn JK, Carry MM, McGhie I et al. (1989) Quantitation of post exercise lung thallium-201 uptake during single photon emission computed tomography. *J Nucl Med* **30**: 288–294.

20. Martin W, Tweddel AC, McGhie AI, Hutton I (1989) An automated analysis technique for thallium images. *Clin Phys Physiol Meas* **10**: 259–266.

21. Maddahi J, Garcia EV, Berman DS et al. (1981) Improved noninvasive assessment of coronary artery disease by quantitative analysis of regional stress myocardial distribution and washouts of thallium-201. *Circulation* **64**: 924–925.

22. Pryor DB, Harrell FE, Lee KL *et al.* (1984) Prognostic indications from radionuclide angiography in medically treated patients with coronary artery disease. *Am J Cardiol* **53**: 18–22.
23. Morris KG, Palmeri Califf RM *et al.* (1985) Value of radionuclide angiography for predicting specific cardiac events after acute myocardial infarction. *Am J Cardiol* **55**: 318–324.
24. Ong L, Green B, Reiser P, Morrison J (1986) Early prediction of mortality in patients with acute myocardial infarction: a prospective study of clinical and radionuclide risk factors. *Am J Cardiol* **57**: 33–38.
25. Levy D, Garrison RJ, Savage D *et al.* (1989) Left ventricular mass and incidence of coronary heart disease in an elderly cohort: the Framingham Heart Study. *Ann Int Med* **110**: 101–107.
26. Iskandrian AS, Hakki AH, Schwartz JS *et al.* (1984) Prognostic implications of rest and exercise radionuclide ventriculography in patients with suspected or proven coronary heart disease. *Int J Cardiol* **6**: 707–718.
27. Tweddel A, Martin W, Neilly B *et al.* (1987) Right ventricular function and haemodynamics in chronic obstructive airways disease at rest and exercise. In *Proceedings of the European Nuclear Meeting. Nuklearmedizin*, Schmidt HAE, Emrich D (eds). Schattauer Verlag, pp. 124–125.
28. Tamaki S, Kambara H, Kaddla K *et al.* (1984) Improved detection of myocardial infarction by emission computed tomography with thallium-201: relation to infarct size. *Br Heart J* **52**: 621–627.
29. Silverman KJ, Becker LC, Bulkley RH *et al.* (1980) Value of early thallium-201 scintigraphy for predicting mortality in patients with acute myocardial infarction. *Circulation* **61**: 996–1003.
30. Johnson LL, Seldin DW, Keller AM *et al.* (1990) Dual isotope thallium and indium antimyosin SPECT imaging to identify acute infarct patients at further ischaemic risk. *Circulation* **81**: 37–45.
31. Limitations of exercise thallium-201 myocardial imaging. In *Nuclear Cardiology and Cardiac Magnetic Resonance*, van der Wall EE (ed.). Hans Soto, The Netherlands, pp. 73–75.
32. Dilsizian V, Rocco TP, Freedman NMT *et al.* (1990) Enhanced detection of ischaemic but viable myocardium by the reinjection of thallium after stress redistribution imaging. *N Engl J Med* **323**: 141–146.
33. Kiat H, Bermans DS, Maddahi J *et al.* (1988) Late reversibility of tomographic myocardial thallium-201 defects: an accurate marker of myocardial viability. *J Am Coll Cardiol* **12**: 1456–1463.
34. Brown KA, Boucher CA, Okada RD *et al.* (1983) Prognostic value of exercise thallium-201 imaging in patients presenting for evaluation of chest pain. *J Am Coll Cardiol* **i**: 994–1001.
35. Ladenheim MI, Pollock BH, Rozanski A *et al.* (1986) Extent and severity of myocardial hypoperfusion as predictors of prognosis in patients with suspected coronary artery disease. *J Am Coll Cardiol* **7**: 464–471.
36. Gibson RS, Watson DD, Craddock GB *et al.* (1983) Prediction of cardiac events after uncomplicated myocardial infarction, prospective study comparing pre discharge exercise thallium-201 scintigraphy and coronary angiography. *Circulation* **68**: 321–336.
37. Boucher CA, Brewster DC, Darling RC *et al.* (1985) Determination of cardiac risk by dipyridamole-thallium imaging before peripheral vascular surgery. *N Engl J Med* **312**: 389–394.
38. Leppo JA, Plaza J, Gronec M *et al.* (1987) Non invasive evaluation of cardiac risk before elective vascular surgery. *J Am Coll Cardiol* **9**: 269–276.

12 Cardiac Magnetic Resonance Imaging

DAVID J. DELANY AND JOHN HERBETKO
Southampton University Hospital, Southampton, UK

The clinical applications of magnetic resonance (MR) imaging has continued to increase across and within the medical specialties. One rapidly expanding area of usage and research is in cardiac imaging. The ability of MR to extract information from both normal and pathological tissues based on the magnetic properties of their nuclei and the surrounding molecular environment has allowed the production of detailed high-resolution images with good tissue contrast. Initial long scanning times made static structures, in particular the head and extremities, the obvious and easiest areas to target for imaging. More recently improved computing software with newer imaging sequences (in particular electrocardiogram (ECG) gated techniques) has allowed highly detailed anatomical and functional information to be obtained from moving structures and in particulart the heart, great vessels and the circulating blood pool. Cardiac MR has now evolved to such a level as to provide definitive diagnoses in diseases of the myocardium, pericardium and great vessels in addition to characterizing mass lesions both within the heart and involving the pericardiac structures. Its accepted safety and proven efficacy make it particularly advantageous in investigating certain cardiac diseases in the elderly. It does not have the disadvantage of angiographic contrast media; patients are not exposed to harmful radiation; it provides broader anatomical information than can be seen on echocardiography (and no imaging window is required); and images can be obtained in any plane. In addition, myocardial perfusion imaging is now evolving with MR, and its greater spatial resolution compared to isotope imaging may eventually prove to be a strong competitor.

However, the cost of MR remains its greatest detraction from more frequent usage. Decreased scan times have reduced financial cost proportionally but, with an average cardiac scan taking 30 minutes, patient throughput is limited. Awareness of the advantages of cardiac MR imaging and of its limitations will allow appropriate patient selection. For example there are certain prosthetic implant devices that are absolute contraindications to MR scanning. These include cardiac pacemakers which may be induced to stimulate arrythmias or lose their preprogrammed memories and aneurysm or haemostatic clips which

Geriatric Cardiology. Principles and Practice. Edited by A. Martin and A.J. Camm
© 1994 John Wiley & Sons Ltd

may be dislodged. Surprisingly, most other metallic implants are not contraindications to scanning, although locally induced field changes by ferrous implants may prevent easy image acquisition and interpretation. With most metallic cardiac valve implants the forces of magnetic deflection are considerably less than the mechanical stresses placed upon these by cardiac pulsation. One exception to this is the Starr–Edwards pre-6000 series valve. A full list of over 250 metallic implants/materials and their safety for MR scanning has been provided by Shellock and Curtis (1). It is also important to have at least some insight into what an MR scan entails for the patient. This will allow informed reassurance to be given, thus decreasing the chances of a non-completed study. There are several parts of the examination with which patients feel particularly uncomfortable. Claustrophobia results in failed scans in about 5% of adult cardiac patients. The enclosed scanning space of an MR scanner is considerably smaller than that of a computed tomographic (CT) scanner. Similarly, examination duration is significantly longer. It is also worth mentioning the noise factor of MR scanners. Imaging necessitates a repetitive loud tapping sound within the scanner. The use of earphones is possible in most scanners and provides comfort and distraction to most patients. Patients who are told to expect a similar investigation to CT consider they have been misled by this explanation (2). In addition to these general considerations there are more specific problems associated with cardiac MR imaging. Limitations on resolution (the ability to see small structures) makes coronary artery imaging unreliable, with the exception of detecting patency of proximal or graft vessels in most patients. Many arrhythmias may prevent adequate cardiac gating, and high jet flow velocities associated with stenotic valvular disease can lead to problems assessing lesion severity. However, if the present rate of improvement of MR imaging capabilities continues, the next decade should see many of these difficulties resolved.

GENERAL PRINCIPLES

Whilst a detailed knowledge of the underlying physical principles of MR is unnecessary, some understanding of the descriptive terminology will allow better communication and image interpretation for the clinician. The following section is meant to provide only a broad outline of these. The Appendix is a slightly more detailed review of the physics of MR but there are many comprehensive radiological and physics textbooks available for those requiring further insight.

The essential components of any MR imager include a larger superconducting coil magnet, smaller gradient, transmitter and receiver coils and considerable computing software. The field strength of the main magnet in clinically utilized machines are of the order of 0.5–1.5 tesla (the latter figure being 15 000 times the magnetic field of the earth). To attain this strength and the uniformity required for useful images, magnets need to be of small diameter, long enough to encompass a large volume of the patient, and are usually supercooled, adding considerably to their running costs. Patients are subjected to a sequential barrage of low-strength radio-frequency (RF) pulses. These stimulate hydrogen nuclei (small magnets in their own right) which then emit their own RF echoes. These received pulses are measured and eventually computed to form an image. By varying the magnetic field strength at any point in the region of the patient under study, spatial localization of signals received is possible. The significant number of signals required to form an image necessitates long scanning times and requires considerable patient cooperation to maintain a fixed relaxed position on the scanning table. T1, T2 and relative proton density refer to inherent tissue characteristics dependent on molecular structure and environment. Specific RF pulse sequences can produce images more dependent on one of these values than the other two (T1 weighted, T2 weighted, proton density images). These intrinsic tissue parameters can be altered with the use of paramagnetic contrast agents such as gadolinium detoxified by binding this to other molecules such as diethylenetriaminepentaacetic acid (DTPA). Spin echo (SE) and inversion recovery (IR) pulse sequences refer to two of the most commonly utilized pulse sequences in generating an image. Many others exist. In particular, gradient echo (GRE) sequences allow rapid image acquisitions at some cost to image clarity. All of these techniques rely on 'flipping' the direction of induced magnetic vectors within local tissues by small (GRE) or large (SE and IR) amounts. Even more complex manipulations are possible when information relating to flowing blood is required.

CLINICAL APPLICATION

Most cardiac MR imaging now utilizes ECG-gated techniques. Adjacent cross-sectional cardiac images can be built up over many cardiac cycles largely using SE techniques. However, the rapid imaging capability of GRE sequences (with some loss of image differential contrast and resolution) allow images to be obtained at regular time intervals throughout the cardiac cycle, located in this case in a single cross-sectional position. These images can then be viewed individually or as a rapid real-time dynamic study (cine loop). In addition these sequences can be repeated in different planes including axial, long-axis, short-axis or oblique orientations for major vessel or other stucture profiling. These two techniques are complementary, one providing predominantly anatomical information (Figure 1a, b), the other providing predominantly functional information (Figure 2), and are the basic imaging requirements for most cardiac MR examinations. Unfortunately flowing blood can produce complex signals, and additional dedicated scan sequences may be required for complete angiographic characterization.

ISCHAEMIC HEART DISEASE

At present adequate MR imaging of coronary vessels beyond their first branch points is not yet possible and the role of MR in ischaemic heart disease (IHD) or

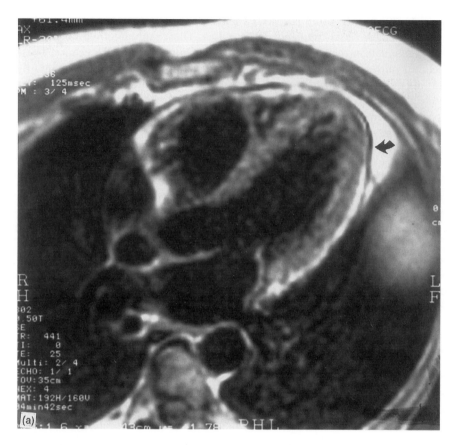

Figure 1. (a) Transverse spin echo image through the left ventricle in diastole. The small black arrow shows the position of the pericardium. (b) (opposite) Same patient at the same level in systole with the mitral valve closed (black arrow)

following myocardial infarction (MI) is predominantly to identify those secondary complications of left ventricular dysmotility, left ventricular aneurysm formation and to detect the presence of intraventricular mural thrombus. Although MR may provide information relating to areas of myocardial ischaemia or infarction, this has yet to be one of its major functions. Since coronary arteries vary in diameter between 3 and 4 mm, to detect a 50% stenosis would require resolution in three dimensions of less than 1 mm, which is below the present capabilities of MR. Whilst the proximal left and right native coronary arteries can be identified (Figure 3), this is not true of their distal branches, where atherosclerotic plaques are more frequent (3,4). MR can identify the presence of both saphenous and internal mammary coronary artery bypass grafts and usefully assess their patency with relative accuracy (3,5–7).

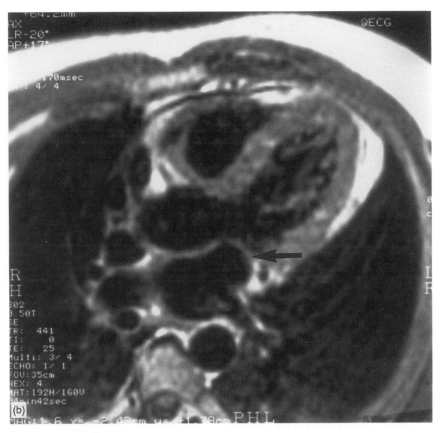

However, patency does not exclude significant stenosis, which will remain undiagnosed with MR in these cases.

The relatively uniform signal intensity of the normal myocardium is clearly visualized sandwiched between the contrasting signals of intraventricular blood and epicardial tissue and pericardium (Figure 1). This allows assessment of both focal and generalized myocardial damage on SE images in addition to visualizing focal areas of dysmotility (8), including that associated with left ventricular aneurysm (9) using GRE cine sequences (Figure 4). Multi-planar capabilities allow clear definition of these areas since they can be assessed in profile. MR thus has the advantage of identifying myocardial contractility (and viability) and this is further assisted by comparing end-systolic and end-diastolic wall thicknesses (10,11). In areas of previous infarction, myocardial thinning can be detected and in addition decreased signal on T2 weighted images may be seen (12). With acute infarction this T2 signal initially increases but often proves difficult to detect due to longer signal acquisition times for T2 weighted images (13). The use of intravenous gadolinium DTPA (Gd-DTPA) allows the detection of increased signal in areas of acute infarction using T1 weighted sequences. Since these

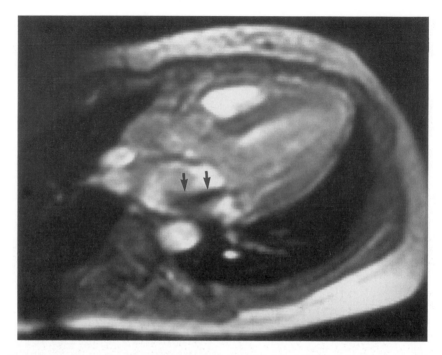

Figure 2. Gradient echo image through the long axis of the left ventricle, showing narrow jet of mitral incompetence (black arrows) and grey shadow of flowing blood into aortic root

images have greater clarity and are more rapidly acquired, Gd-DTPA may be advantageous (14). Gd-DTPA may also provide information on the reversibility of ischaemic myocardium following reperfusion (15–17).

Whilst echocardiography is highly sensitive in detecting left ventricular thrombus, false positive or technically difficult scans are not uncommon (18). The clinical value of MR in detecting intracardiac thrombus in patients with equivocal or inadequate findings on echocardiography has been well demonstrated (19,20). SE imaging has good sensitivity and specificity in detecting left ventricular thrombi (21) but problems of image interpretation due to the varying signal intensities of this thrombus and difficulty differentiating this from flowing blood may still be encountered. This can be resolved to some extent by using GRE images (22).

CARDIOMYOPATHIES

Echocardiography, isotope studies and left ventricular angiography provide the mainstay of investigations in patients with cardiomyopathy, and MR is an adjunct to these. The presence, distribution and severity of hypertrophic cardiomyopathy can accurately be defined with MR and this has proven

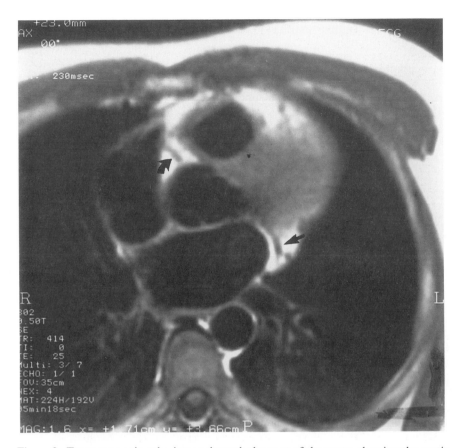

Figure 3. Transverse spin echo image through the root of the aorta, showing the aortic valve cusps and the origin of the right (small curved arrow) and circumflex coronary arteries (small straight arrow)

particularly valuable in midventricular or apical variants (23). The resulting mechanical interference of increased muscle bulk during systolic contraction can clearly be visualized on long- and short-axis cine MR imaging allowing preoperative surgical planning.

Postpharmacological or postoperative interventional treatment can be assessed in patients with hypertrophic cardiomyopathy, and in a similar way the effectiveness of antihypertensive treatment in hypertensive cardiac hypertrophy has been demonstrated (24).

In congestive cardiomyopathies, wall thickness, ventricular dilatation and mural thrombi can all be visualized (25) and cardiac output calculated.

With restrictive cardiomypathies, left ventricular end diastolic pressure is increased and has been shown to cause a relative stasis of blood within the atria. This results in an increase in the signal from intra-atrial blood throughout the

248

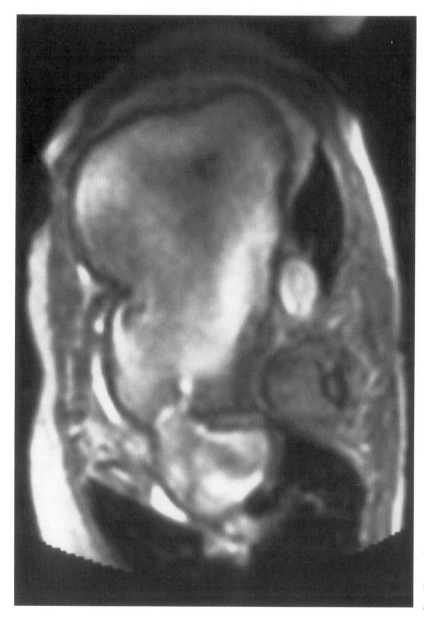

Figure 4. Gradient echo transverse image of gross left ventricular aneurysm which has expanded to fill the whole left hemithorax. Note the extremely thin myocardial shell around the aneurysm

cardiac cycle (16). The clear visualization of the pericardium provides the distinction between constrictive pericarditis (thickened pericardium and areas of low pericardial signals from the presence of fibrosis or calcification) and restrictive cardiomyopathy (normal pericardium) (10,26).

Alterations in the signal characteristics of myocardium have been reported sporadically in certain infiltrative cardiomyopathies, including sarcoidosis (increased T2 signal) (27), amyloid heart disease (increased signal on short tau inversion recovery sequence (STIR)) (23) and systemic lupus erythematosis (increased T1 signal in active disease) (29) and in haemochromatosis, although this appears as a late event compared to deposition in the liver and spleen (30).

THE PERICARDIUM

The normal pericardium is clearly imaged on MR due to the low signal of its predominantly fibrous make-up, contrasting clearly with the high signals of pericardial and epicardial fat (Figure 1). It has uniform thickness measuring up to 3 mm and even postoperatively has been reported as measuring less than 3.4 mm (31,32). In one of these series (31), in all patients with proven pericardial constriction the pericardium exceeded 3.3 mm. The converse is not true in that thickened pericardium does not necessarily imply constriction, although the presence of fibrinous adhesions seen on MR suggests subacute constrictive pericarditis (33). Additional features suggesting constriction include a decrease in the size of the right ventricle, tubular configurations of both ventricles and concavity of the right ventricular free wall (28). As previously mentioned, the finding of a normal pericardium with restrictive cardiomyopathies allows its differentiation from constriction. Focal areas of thickening may suggest malignant pericardial infiltration, and MR is extremely sensitive in imaging pericardial involvement by mediastinal malignancies. In this respect it is more sensitive than echocardiography or CT (16,33,34), and more generally this is true for visualization of the anterior portion of the pericardium. MR likewise has advantages in being extremely good at detecting small or focal loculated pericardial effusions—important if diagnostic tapping is required in suspected disease not seen on echocardiography. It has also proved useful in differentiating exudates with their increased signal intensity relative to myocardium from transudates which have lower signal strength compared to myocardium (10).

Whilst echocardiography may have problems differentiating pericardial haematoma or some pericardial masses from fluid, this has not been reported as a problem with MR. Dynamic MR imaging in all of these diseases allows their functional effect on cardiac contractility to be assessed.

TUMOURS AFFECTING THE HEART AND GREAT VESSELS

Patients with equivocal findings of an intracardiac mass on echocardiography have been shown to be ideal subjects for MR imaging. Many cases can be

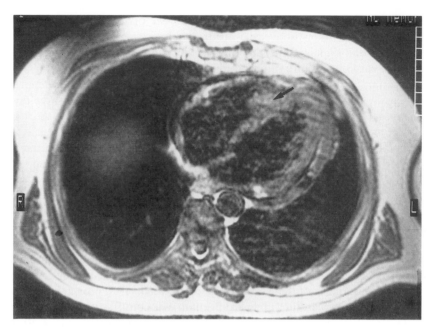

Figure 5. Transverse spin echo image through the interventricular septum, showing sessile tumour on the right ventricular aspect (arrow). The lesion was a metastasis from squamous carcinoma of the lung

resolved this way by the demonstration of a definite mass, an anatomical variant or artefact from areas of calcification giving the appearance of a mass on echocardiography. Alternatively the findings of normal cardiac anatomy and chambers will exclude the presence of a mass (19).

Intracardiac tumours are well shown with MR (Figure 5). Signal characteristics have helped identify specific tissue pathologies. In particular, lipomas have high signal intensity on T1 imaging and fibromas have low signal intensity on T2 weighted images. This low signal is also seen in areas of calcification (19). Whilst myxomas are well visualized as pedunculated tumours usually arising from the intra-atrial septum or from the posterior wall of the left atrium, they do not produce characteristic or diagnostic signals. It is not always possible to distinguish between small intracardiac tumours and mural thrombus, since both may have similar signal characteristics. In addition, slow-flowing blood can also cause confusion with clot on T1 weighted images, but GRE cine MR will show alteration in the signal from slow-flowing blood during the cardiac cycle not seen with clot. Alternatively, presaturation techniques are also able to make this distinction (35). Dynamic studies have the additional advantage of demonstrating atrial myxomas which interfere with normal mitral valve function resulting in reflux. Paracardial masses are clearly imaged with MR. Precise relationships of tumours to the myocardium, pericardium, great vessels or extracardiac structures can be evaluated. By orientating the plane of imaging along and perpendicular to specific structures, presurgical planning may be facilitated (36). Extension into the pericardium, aorta, pulmonary artery or other mediastinal structures is useful preoperative information.

THORACIC AORTA AND PULMONARY ARTERY

MR of the thoracic aorta is particularly valuable in patients with suspected or known aortic dissection and has been shown to be superior to echocardiography, CT and angiography in this respect (37,38). Distinguishing between dissections involving the ascending aorta or arch requiring urgent surgical intervention and those distal to the left subclavian artery treated medically is of prime importance. The former are associated with a high incidence of involvement of the aortic valve (insufficiency), coronary arteries (myocardial infarction) or rupture into the pericardial space (tamponade). The intimal flap is clearly seen on ECG-gated MR images since at any phase of the cardiac cycle the flap will return to a similar position as on subsequent heart beats. In addition, differing signal strengths between flowing blood, the intimal flap and the aortic wall exaggerated by unequal flow rates (and further signal changes) within the true and false lumen provide excellent inherent contrast. The signal from slow-flowing blood within the false lumen can be identified on SE imaging but at low velocities this may be indistinguishable from thrombus. This may prevent identification of the flap on some images but can be resolved using cine MR, velocity mapping techniques or multi-echo sequences (39). Other advantages of the multi-planar imaging capability of MR include the ability to identify the extent of the tear in addition to the points of entry and exit of blood flowing through the false lumen (40), and the relationship of the dissection to the major aortic branch vessels. Unfortunately it is not often possible to assess the relationship of the coronary arteries to the false lumen, which is important information since the dissection may extend into these. Evaluation of patients who develop complications following surgical repair of their dissection is a particularly useful role of MR. This avoids potentially large doses of angiographic contrast agents. In addition, metallic valve prostheses and dense boluses of contrast in the superior vena cava (SVC) result in considerably more artefactual image degradation with CT than is seen with MR, although MR has its own specific artefacts related to imaging aortic dissections. Motion artefact in the phase encoding direction and artefacts resulting from normal anatomical structures are seen particularly at the origins of the arch branch vessels, the point of contact of the left brachiocephalic vein with the arch, or where the superior pericardial recess lies behind the ascending aorta. These usually appear on a single image but examination of contiguous slices seldom fails to clarify these cases (41).

In addition to its role in aortic dissection, MR has proven useful in distinguishing thrombus from moving blood in aortic aneurysms (42). Since thrombus is not imaged on angiography (only the patent aortic lumen is seen)

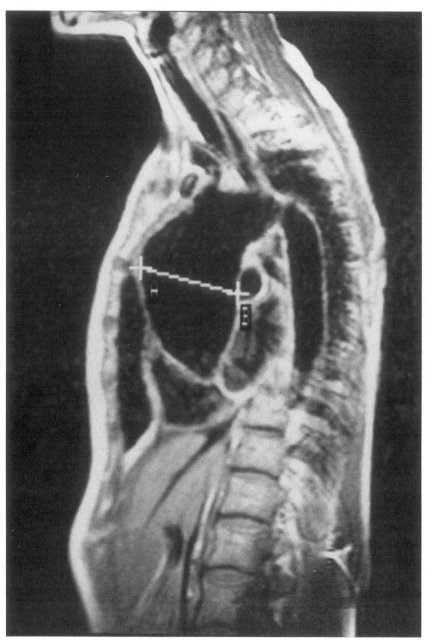

Figure 6. Oblique sagittal spin echo image of patient with cystic medial necrosis affecting the ascending aorta. The diameter of the aneurysm is measured as shown

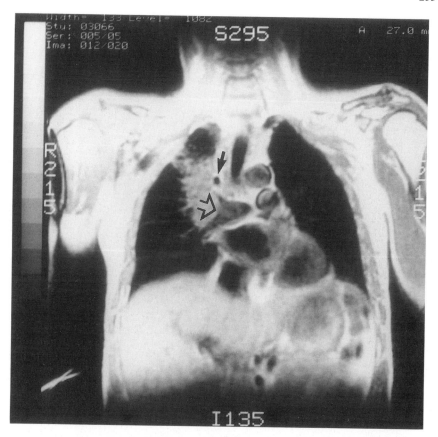

Figure 7. Coronal spin echo image through the thorax of a patient with squamous carcinoma of the right upper lobe invading the right hilum. The patent azygos vein is shown (straight arrow). The open arrow shows tumour invading the bifurcation of the right pulmonary artery

aneurysms can be missed or their size underestimated unless calcium is present in the aortic wall. Since saccular aneurysms have a greater tendency to rupture, MR imaging can accurately locate their origin in several planes. Acccurate, non-invasive interval studies can be made for any aortic disorder (Figure 6).

Once again malignant infiltration of the aortic wall or the main pulmonary vessels is important information provided by MR when surgical resection is being considered (Figure 7).

One of the more serious complications of bacterial endocarditis of the aortic valve is the consequential formation of perivalvular infectious pseudo-aneurysms. The presence of a prosthetic aortic valve hinders echocardiographic interpretation of the region of the perivalvular ring. Diagnosis is essential and considered an indication for surgical intervention in most cases. MR has been shown to be particularly useful in detecting these cases (43,44). Since these

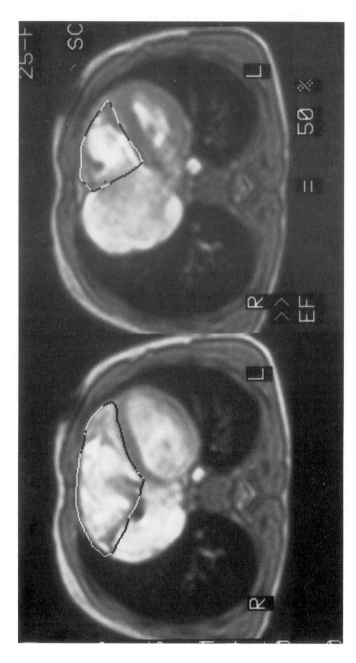

Figure 8. Gradient echo transverse images through the right ventricle in diastole on the left and systole on the right, with planimetered outlines representing a stage in the volumetric analysis of the chamber

pseudo-aneurysms drain into the ventricular or aortic lumen they contain moving blood and appear as low signal intensity anatomical out-pouchings. Their exact positions can be determined along with their relationships to other cardiac chambers preoperatively. This remains the case even in the presence of a prosthetic aortic valve, which is not usually visualized on MR. When the use of echocardiography with or without angiography remains inconclusive in cases of suspected pseudo-aneurysm, utilization of MR should be considered.

FUNCTIONAL STUDIES

In addition to visualizing the physiological motion of anatomical structures and in particular the cardiac chambers, myocardium and cardiac valves, MR has the ability to image blood flow directly without the need for intravascular contrast agents. Sequences in which signal from the myocardium appears distinctly different from that of blood within the atria and ventricles allow analysis of cardiac chamber volumes. Left ventricular volume is calculated by summating slice volumes on contiguous sections usually in the short-axis scan encompassing the whole ventricular chamber. Ten 1 cm slices are usually sufficient for most normal left ventricles. These stacked images do not depend on geometric models used in angiography. Ejection fraction can be calculated using ECG-gated images at end-systole and end-diastole. With cine images good reproducibility of left ventricular function has been demonstrated in normal subjects (45,46). Establishing reproducibility now allows treatment response studies in myocardial or valvular disease. Right ventricular ejection fraction can similarly be measured (Figure 8) and in patients with single regurgitant valves regurgitant volumes are calculated from the difference between right and left ventricular ejection fractions. There are alternative MR imaging methods for calculating regurgitant jet volumes and severity. Cine MR depicts regurgitant jets from mitral (Figure 2) and aortic valves as areas of signal void within the left atrium and left ventricle. Volumes of signal void can be calculated and related to the severity of reflux as determined by echocardiographic findings with good correlation (47,48). At present similar calculation using poststenotic signal voids in valvular stenoses have revealed only moderately good correlation with valvular pressure gradients (49). More recently, newer modified velocity mapping techniques have shown promise in evaluating stenoses (50).

MAGNETIC RESONANCE SPECTROSCOPY

Clinical MR spectroscopy is an extension of MR imaging which allows metabolic information to be obtained from diseased tissues and compared to that from healthy ones. The nucleus of phosphorus-31 (^{31}P) has attracted most attention for research as it is only present in a few selected biological molecules and represents the only form of naturally occurring phosphorus. Additionally many of the molecules of energy production or consumption involve ^{31}P. Many other molecules can also be studied, including hydrogen (^{1}H), carbon (^{13}C) and sodium (^{23}Na) (51). It is the detection of small alterations in resonant frequencies of these nuclei dependent upon their chemical environment that is the physical basis of MR spectroscopy. Spectroscopic analysis of signals spatially localized in the myocardium have allowed the characterization and detection of certain disease states (52), including ischaemic cardiac muscle (differentiating between reversible and irreversible ischaemic damage), cardiomyopathies, cardiac transplant rejection and Adriamycin cardiotoxicity. It has also been used to study the metabolic effects of certain drugs on the myocardium (51). At the present time MR spectroscopy remains an area of specialized research. Clinical utilization is hampered by several logistical problems. Clinical MR machines need specific software and hardware additions to allow good spectroscopic studies. High-quality coils are a necessity for good analysis, and higher magnetic field strengths even above 1.5 tesla allow better interpretation of signal data. Spectroscopic MR of the heart remains some way from everyday clinical usage.

SUMMARY

Whilst the complete role of MR imaging in the investigation of cardiac disease is still evolving, newer imaging sequences, the use of paramagnetic contrast agents and spectroscopy ensure that this will continue to expand. It is difficult to imagine that the difficulties presently encountered in producing adequate images of the coronary arteries will not eventually be overcome. Whilst this does not appear imminent (16) its potential non-invasive role in diagnosing ischaemic heart disease would then be second to none.

APPENDIX: MAGNETIC RESONANCE PHYSICS

The hydrogen nucleus with its single proton and its abundance in animal tissues is an ideal element for MR imaging. Whilst both protons and neutrons act as small magnetic dipoles owing to their rapid axial spins, magnetic cancellation occurs when these are paired in the same nucleus. Like all magnets, the proton will experience a torque when placed within another magnetic field and will attempt to line itself up in the same direction, similar to a spinning top attempting to align itself with the vertical gravitational force. While spinning on its own axis, the top also rotates about the vertical axis. This also occurs for the hydrogen nucleus, which 'precesses' around the direction of the magnetic field. This rate of precession is predetermined by the strength of the applied magnetic field and the molecular make-up of that tissue. However, the total magnetization of any collection of protons will be along the externally applied magnetic field. When an excitatory external radio frequency pulse is applied this magnetization vector can be made to 'flip' $90°$ into a plane (xy) perpendicular to the magnetic field (z). The xy plane is usually the axial plane of the patient. When the RF pulse ends, this magnetization vector will return to the z plane, releasing energy as an RF emission which can be measured. This forms the basis of all MR imaging. If the body is thought of as consisting of multiple tiny volumes of tissue (voxels) each with its own differing magnetization vector depending on the proton density and molecular structure amongst other intrinsic parameters, a cross-sectional image of signal strengths represents the MR image. This magnetization vector, whilst decaying in the xy plane (T2 = the time taken to decay by 63% in the xy plane), will increase in size along the z axis (T1 = the time taken to return to 63% of initial strength along the z axis). These variable T1, T2 are further independent intrinsic parameters.

It is not possible to detect the initial magnetization vector in the xy plane, and an 180° refocusing RF pulse needs to be applied (this builds up the signal once more in the xy plane) such that measurement can take place. This is the basis of the most commonly used SE imaging. The time taken for these echoes to occur from the initial 90° pulse is the time to echo (TE) and the repetition time (TR) is the time between each 90° pulse. Both TR and TE can be varied independently to obtain images of differing tissue contrast, e.g. T1 weighted, T2 weighted, or for rapid-accumulation GRE imaging using angles less than 90°. These GRE images are rapidly acquired (seconds) although at some cost to image clarity. Further refinements to detect flowing blood or to differentiate this from thrombus are also necessary. How are the differing signals localized to each voxel? By using small magnetic field gradients superimposed on the main field magnet in the z, x and y directions (x and y directions are called phase- and frequency-encoding gradient directions) each voxel magnetic vector will have its own individual rate of spin (frequency) and direction (phase) and can thus be localized in space (x, y, z).

Finally, paramagnetic contrast agents alter the local chemical environments of the protons and consequently alter the intrinsic tissue values of T1 and T2, etc. In the case of cardiac imaging the natural contrast between blood and myocardial tissue is usually sufficient not to necessitate the use of these agents.

REFERENCES

1. Shellock FG, Curtis JS (1991) MR imaging and biomedical implants, materials and devices: an updated MR review. *Radiology* **180**: 541–550.
2. Quirk ME, Letendre AJ, Ciottone RA, Lingley JF (1989) Anxiety in patients undergoing MR imaging. *Radiology* **170**: 463–466.
3. Gomes AS, Lois JF, Drinkwater DC, Corday SR (1987) Coronary artery bypass grafts: visualization with MR imaging. *Radiology* **162**: 175–179.
4. Cassidy MM, Schiller NB, Botvinick EH *et al.* (1989) Assessment of coronary artery imaging by gated magnetic resonance: an evaluation of the utility and potential of the currently available imaging method. *Am J Cardiac Imaging* **3**: 100–107.
5. White RD, Caputo GR, Mark AS *et al.* (1987) Coronary artery bypass graft patency: noninvasive evaluation with MR imaging. *Radiology* **164**: 681–686.
6. Aurigemma GP, Reichek N, Axel L *et al.* (1989) Noninvasive determination of coronary artery bypass graft patency by cine magnetic resonance imaging. *Circulation* **80**: 1595–1602.
7. White RD, Pflugfelder PW, Lipton MH, Higgins CB (1988) Coronary artery bypass

grafts: evaluation of patency with cine MR imaging. *AJR* **150**: 1271–1274.

8. Edelman RR, Mattle HP, Atkinson DJ, Hoogewoud HM (1990) MR angiography. *AJR* **154**: 937–946.

9. McNamara M, Higgins CB (1986) Magnetic resonance imaging of chronic infarcts in man. *AJR* **146**: 315–320.

10. Pettigrew RI (1989) Dynamic cardiac MR imaging. *Radiol Clin North Am* **27**: 1183–1203.

11. Pflugfelder PW, Sechtem UP, White RD *et al.* (1988) Quantification of regional myocardial function by rapid cine MR imaging. *AJR* **150**: 523–529.

12. McNamara MT, Higgins CB (1984) Magnetic resonance imaging of chronic myocardial infarcts in man. *AJR* **143**: 1135.

13. Aisen AM, Buda AJ, Zotz RJ, Buckwalter KA (1987) Visualization of myocardial infarction and subsequent coronary reperfusion with MRI using a dog model. *Magn Reson Imaging* **5**: 399–404.

14. Nishimura T, Kobayashi H, Ohara Y *et al.* (1989) Serial assessment of myocardial infarction by using gated MR imaging and Gd-DTPA. *AJR* **153**: 715–720.

15. McNamara MT, Tscholakoff D, Revel D *et al.* (1986) Differentiation of reversible and irreversible myocardial injury by MR imaging with and without gadolinium-DTPA. *Radiology* **158**: 765–769.

16. Higgins CB (1986) Overview of MR of the heart—1986. *AJR* **146**: 907–918.

17. Johns JA, Leavitt MB, Newell JB *et al.* (1990) Quantitation of acute myocardial infarct size by nuclear magnetic resonance imaging. *J Am Coll Cardiol* **15**: 143–149.

18. Stratton JR, Lighty GW, Pearlman AS, Ritchie JL (1982) Detection of left ventricular thrombus by two dimensional echocardiography: sensitivity, specificity and causes of uncertainty. *Circulation* **66**: 156–166.

19. Winkler M, Higgins CB (1987) Suspected intracardiac masses: evaluation with MR imaging. *Radiology* **165**: 177–122.

20. Gomes AS, Lois JF, Brown K, Batra P (1987) Cardiac tumours and thrombus: evaluation with MR imaging. *AJR* **49**: 895–899.

21. Sechtem U, Theissen P, Heindel W *et al.* (1989) Comparison of magnetic resonance imaging, computed tomography, echocardiography and angiography in the diagnosis of left ventricular thrombi. *Am J Cardiol* **64**: 1195–1199.

22. Jungehulsing M, Sechtem U, Theissen P *et al.* (1992) Left ventricular thrombi: evaluation with spin echo and gradient echo MR imaging. *Radiology* **182**: 225–229.

23. Higgins CB, Byrd BF, Stark D (1985) Magnetic resonance imaging of hypertrophic cardiomyopathy. *Am J Cardiol* **55**: 1121–1125,

24. Eichstadt HW, Felix R, Langer M *et al.* (1987) Use of nuclear magnetic resonance imaging to show regression of hypertrophy with Ramipril treatment. *Am J Cardiol* **59**(10): 98D–103D.

25. Dooms GC, Higgins CB (1986) MR imaging of cardiac thrombi. *J Comput Assisted Tomogr* **10**: 415–420.

26. Soulen R, Stark DD, Higgins CB (1985) Magnetic resonance imaging of constrictive pericardial disease. *Am J Cardiol* **55**: 480–484.

27. Reidy K, Fisher MR, Belic N, Koenigsberg DI (1988) MR imaging of myocardial sarcoidosis. *AJR* **151**: 915–916.

28. Hartnell G (1991) Clinical applications of cardiac MRI. In *Clinical MRI*, Vol. I, No. 2, Goddard P, Hartnell G (eds). Clinical Press, Bristol, pp. 51–64.

29. Been M, Thomson BJ, Smith MA *et al.* (1988) Myocardial involvement in systemic lupus erythematosus detected by magnetic resonance imaging. *Eur Heart J* **9**: 1250–1256

30. Johnston DL, Rice L, Vick GW *et al.* (1989) Assessment of tissue iron overload by nuclear magnetic resonance imaging. *Am J Med* **87**: 40–47.

31. Hartnell CG, Papouchado M, Rozkovec A *et al.* (1990) Magnetic resonance imaging

of pericardial disease (Abstract). *Br Heart J* **64**: 99–100.
32. Sechtem U, Tscholakoff D, Higgins CB (1986) MRI of the normal pericardium. *AJR* **147**: 239–244.
33. Sechtem U, Tscholakoff D, Higgins CB (1986) MRI of the abnormal pericardium. *AJR* **147**: 245–252.
34. Mulvagh SL, Rokey R, Vick W, Johnston DL (1989) Usefulness of nuclear magnetic resonance imaging for evaluation of pericardial effusions and comparison with two-dimensional echocardiography. *Am J Cardiol* **64**: 1002–1009.
35. Ehman RL, Felmlee JP, Julsrud PR *et al.* (1987) Technique for eliminating flow artifacts and for improving the depiction of vascular anatomy in MRI. *Magn Reson Imaging* **5** (Suppl. 1): 33.
36. Lund JT, Ehman RL, Julsrud PR *et al.* (1989) Cardiac masses: assessment by MR imaging. *AJR* **152**: 469–473.
37. Pernes JM, Grenier P, Desbleds MT, de Brux JL (1987) MR evaluation of chronic aortic dissection. *J Comput Assisted Tomogr* **11**: 975–981.
38. White RD, Higgins CB (1989) Evaluation of thoracic aortic disease with CT and MRI: appraisal of the imaging procedure of choice. In *New Concepts in Cardiac Imaging 1989*, Pohost GM, Higgins CB, Nanda NC *et al.* (eds). Year Book Publications, Chicago.
39. Bogren HG, Underwood SR, Firmin DN *et al.* (1988) Magnetic resonance velocity mapping in aortic dissection. *Br J Radiol* **61**: 456–462.
40. Amparo EG, Higgins CB, Hricak H, Solitto R (1985) Aortic dissections: magnetic resonance imaging. *Radiology* **155**: 399–406.
41. Solomon SL, Brown JJ, Glazer HS *et al.* (1990) Thoracic aortic dissection: pitfalls and artifacts in MR imaging. *Radiology* **177**: 223–228.
42. Duke RA, Barrett MR, Payne SD *et al.* (1987) Compression of left main bronchus and left pulmonary artery by thoracic aortic aneurysm. *AJR* **149**: 261–263.
43. Atkins EW, Slone RM, Wiechmann BN *et al.* (1990) Perivalvular pseudoaneurysm complicating bacterial endocarditis: MR detection in five cases. *AJR* **156**: 1155–1158.
44. Winkler ML, Higgins CB (1986) MRI of perivalvular infectious pseudoaneurysms. *AJR*: **147**: 253–256.
45. Semelka RC, Tomei E, Wagner S *et al.* (1990) Normal left ventricular dimensions and function: interstudy reproducibility of measurements with cine MR imaging. *Radiology* **174**: 763–768.
46. Sechtem U, Pflugfelder PW, Gould RG *et al.* (1987) Measurement of right and left ventricular volumes in healthy individuals with cine MR imaging. *Radiology* **163**: 697–702.
47. Pflugfelder PW, Landzberg JS, Cassidy MM *et al.* (1989) Comparison of cine MR imaging with Doppler echocardiography for the evaluation of aortic regurgitation. *AJR* **152**: 729–735.
48. Pflugfelder PW, Sechtem UP, White RD *et al.* (1989) Non-invasive evaluation of mitral regurgitation by analysis of left atrial signal loss in cine magnetic resonance. *Am Heart J* **117**: 1113–1119.
49. Mitchell L, Jenkins JP, Watson Y *et al.* (1989) Diagnosis and assessment of mitral and aortic valve disease by cine-flow magnetic resonance imaging. *Mag Reson Med* **12**: 181–197.
50. Kilner PJ, Firmin DN, Rees RSO *et al.* (1991) Valve and great vessel stenosis: assessment with MR jet velocity mapping. *Radiology* **178**: 229–235.
51. Higgins CB, Saeed M, Wendland M, Chew WM (1989) Magnetic resonance spectroscopy of the heart: overview of studies in animals and man. *Invest Radiol* **24**: 962–968.
52. Brown JJ, Mirowitz SA, Sandstrom JC, Perman WH (1990) MR spectroscopy of the heart. *AJR* **155**: 1–11.

Part III

PATHOPHYSIOLOGY OF AGEING

13 Cardiovascular Pathology in Old Age

JESSICA M. MANN AND MICHAEL J. DAVIES

St George's Hospital Medical School, London, UK

Life expectancy has increased significantly in the twentieth century, although the maximum possible lifespan remains essentially the same. The actual expected survival in the UK is 73 years for men and 78 for women. However, there are well-documented instances of people living to reach 110 years or more (1), although isolated reports of individuals aged over 130 years have not been proven. On the other hand, the number of elderly people as a percentage of the general population continues to increase. Between 1981 and 1989, the percentage of people aged 74–85 years increased by 16% in the UK, and for those aged 85 and above it increased by 39% (2). This age group tends to include a large proportion of disabled people (up to 60%) (2), and, although they do not constitute more than 12% of the population, they consume up to one-third of health system resources (3). The increase in life expectancy has led to an increased awareness of elderly people and the physiological changes that occur, and to efforts to define the frontiers between 'normal ageing' and pathological changes.

This chapter will deal exclusively with the 'normal' ageing changes that can be observed in hearts from elderly subjects.

HEART WEIGHT

Elderly people tend to have bigger hearts. Several reports in the literature (4.5) have shown that heart weight increases with age, at a rate of 1–1.5 g per year from the age of 30 onwards. This increase in heart weight could be partly due to the increase in subepicardial fat, as well as to the increased frequency of systemic hypertension, leading to left ventricular hypertrophy, in the ageing population. On the other hand, it is well known that physical activity is decreased in elderly people, and this fact could be responsible for a decrease in total heart weight. The final heart weight probably reflects the interaction between all these factors. Kitzman *et al.* (5) analysed heart weight as a function of body weight in a group of 765 necropsy patients aged from 30 to 99 years, and found that between the third and seventh decades the heart weight increased in women but remained

Geriatric Cardiology. Principles and Practice. Edited by A. Martin and A.J. Camm
© 1994 John Wiley & Sons Ltd

stable in men. However, it decreased in both men and women between the seventh and tenth decades of life.

FAT CONTENT

The amount of subepicardial fat is increased in the hearts of elderly people, mainly over the anterior surface of the right ventricular wall and the atrioventricular sulci (Figure 1). Another area of the heart that shows increased adipose tissue is the interatrial septum, constituting the so-called 'lipomatous hypertophy of the atrial septum'. Its importance lies in the fact that it has occasionally been related to the presence of atrial arrhythmias.

ATRIAL SIZE

Although the total size of the heart tends to decrease with advanced age, the size of the left atrial cavity increases. This may be partly due to the presence of systemic hypertension, but also to the increased work required of the left atrium (atrial 'kick') in order to maintain cardiac output.

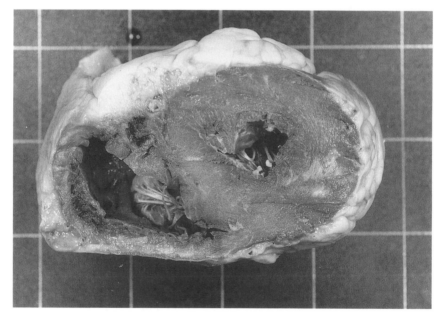

Figure 1. Transverse cut of both ventricles of the heart of a 96-year-old woman. Epicardial fat is increased over the anterior aspect of the heart

VENTRICULAR SEPTUM: 'THE SIGMOID SHAPE'

In many elderly hearts, the basal portion of the ventricular septum bulges into the left ventricular outflow tract. This is mainly due to the relative increase in left atrial size as well as to the dilatation and shift to the right of the ascending aorta, leading to a 'sigmoid' configuration of the ventricular septum. The thickness of the ventricular septum has been reported to increase from the seventh decade of life (5), resulting in a septum-to-free-wall thickness ratio greater than 1.3. The importance of this sigmoid configuration lies in the fact that it can be mistaken echocardiographically for asymmetric septal hypertrophy, and lead to a false diagnosis of hypertrophic cardiomyopathy.

LEFT VENTRICULAR CAVITY

In normal elderly hearts, the left ventricular cavity tends to decrease with age, mainly in the long-axis plane. This is probably a reflection of the decrease in cardiac output noted with age, and its consequence is the relative increase in left atrial size in order to increase the 'atrial kick' contribution to the forward stroke volume.

MYOCARDIUM

Brown atrophy

The term 'brown atrophy' describes the increase in lipofuscin observed in elderly hearts. It has been well documented that the amount of lipofuscin in the myocardium increases with age. Histologically, lipofuscin appears in the form of yellow-brown intracytoplasmic granules. It is thought to be derived from dead lysosomes. The accumulation of lipofuscin has not been found to have any clinical or functional consequences.

Basophilic degeneration

Basophilic degeneration is a very common finding in the elderly heart. It is due to the accumulation of a periodic acid–Schiff (PAS)-positive material in the cytoplasm of the myocardial fibres. This material is probably a glycan, and its presence has not been associated with any functional impairment.

Amyloid deposits

Cardiac involvement is a constant feature in primary amyloidosis and in myeloma-associated amyloidosis, as well as a leading cause of sudden death. In contrast, senile cardiac amyloidosis is a benign condition, generally asymptomatic, seen in patients over 65 years of age. Hodkinson and Pomerance (6) have shown an increase in frequency of senile cardiac amyloidosis related to age, affecting over 50% in a population of 244 patients aged over 65. Other reports in the literature (7,8) report a frequency ranging from 10% to 70%, probably due to differences in sampling and to differences in histochemical staining methods.

Macroscopically, amyloid can occasionally be seen on the left atrial surface as small translucent nodules. Histologically, it ranges from small deposits around small vessels to broad bands of amorphous material compressing myocardial fibres. The diagnosis is confirmed by special stains such as Congo Red and polarization to obtain the typical salmon pink–apple green birefringence. The clinical consequences of atrial amyloid have not yet been well defined: small atrial deposits are thought to be of no clinical significance; however, larger deposits have been related to the presence of atrial arrhythmias. Amyloid has not been shown to infiltrate the conducting system.

Cornwell et al. (9) screened the hearts and the aortae of 85 patients over the age of 80, and found biochemical differences between the amyloid substance in the aorta and that in the left atrium. Senile amyloid with diffuse involvement was found in the inner third of the aortic media in 100% of these patients; this type of amyloid contained tryptophan and the amyloid fibril protein ASc1; extracardiac involvement was present in most of the patients. Isolated atrial amyloid was observed in 78% of their population; it did not contain any tryptophan or ASc1, and extracardiac involvement was very unusual.

Amyloid deposits have occasionally been shown on cardiac valves, being relatively more frequent on the atrioventricular valves than on the semilunar valves (10).

CARDIAC VALVES

Aortic valve

Ageing changes in the cardiac valves can be viewed as the result of a degenerative 'wear-and-tear' process.

In the aortic valve, this degenerative process involves the valve cusps themselves, leading to calcium deposition. These calcium deposits start at the base and extend into the body of the cusps, but rarely, if ever, reach the free edge. They are symmetrical and involve all three cusps. This feature, together with the absence of commissural fusion, makes the differential diagnosis with rheumatic involvement of the aortic valve relatively easy. Histological examination of these valves shows calcium in the valve fibrosa, but no thickening of the vessels or any signs of prior inflammatory process (11). Viewed from the aortic side, the aortic valve orifice has a typical Y-shape (Figure 2).

The lack of commissural fusion has been held responsible for the 'spraying' of the blood flow into the ascending aorta, giving rise to a less intense systolic murmur at the base than that of rheumatic aortic stenosis. Also, the lack of fusion of the cusps may allow them to vibrate, resulting in a musical systolic murmur (12).

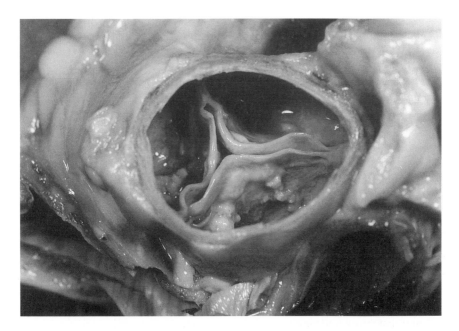

Figure 2. View from the aortic side of a three-cuspid aortic valve in a 92-year-old man. All three valve cusps show calcific deposits which are C-shaped and do not involve the free edge. No commissural fusion is seen

Most elderly aortic valves will show no haemodynamic abnormality due to calcium deposition on the valve cusps, but a small percentage of patients will have symptomatic and/or severe aortic stenosis, requiring surgical treatment. In their review of 40 patients over the age of 90, Waller and Morgan (13) found that 55% had macroscopically visible calcific deposits in at least one of the aortic valve cusps, although two of these 22 patients had haemodynamically significant aortic valve stenosis. Lie and Hammond (3), in a review of 237 hearts from individuals aged between 90 and 105 years, found calcification of the aortic valve in approximately 40% of their population, of which only a third had haemodynamically significant aortic stenosis. In a study of more than 100 hearts with aortic stenosis, Pomerance (14) showed that congenitally bicuspid calcified aortic valves were the most common cause for aortic stenosis between the ages of 60 and 75, and that degenerative three-cuspid aortic stenosis was the most common aetiology in patients over 75. Aortic stenosis due to 'degenerative' changes has been reported as the most frequent valvular lesion requiring surgical treatment in elderly patients (15).

Elderly cardiac valves also have fatty 'degeneration' of the collagen of the valve, leading to a yellow discoloration at the base of the aortic valve cusps. The same phenomenon can be observed on the anterior mitral leaflet. Histological examination shows lipid droplets in the fibrosa.

Kitzman *et al.* (5) studied 765 normal hearts from patients aged between 20 and 99 years. They found a progressive increase in valve circumference with increasing age; this increase was more marked in the semilunar than in the atrioventricular valves. The aortic valve was the most affected, showing progressive dilatation, reaching the pulmonary valve circumference by the fourth decade, and the mitral valve circumference by the tenth decade. The ratio of aortic to pulmonary valve circumference increased throughout life, with the aortic valve circumference exceeding the pulmonary in elderly patients. When comparing the aortic to the mitral valve circumference, the ratio was close to 1 in patients aged over 90 years. This age-dependent dilatation should be taken into account when evaluating annuloaortic ectasia in elderly patients.

Mitral valve

Mitral annulus calcification has been considered as the hallmark of the aged heart (Figure 3). The calcific deposits usually tend to involve the mitral annulus, and only rarely the mitral valve itself. These calcific deposits tend to grow and form large C- or J-shaped masses, leading to mitral regurgitation because of valvular distortion and rigidity of the annulus. Sometimes, if the calcific deposits are predominantly subvalvular, they may lead to a haemodynamically stenotic mitral valve. The mass of calcium may occasionally undergo central necrosis, and it may be mistaken for an abscess.

Mitral annular calcification is a disease of the elderly heart: most of the patients are over the age of 70 years. Female predominance (4:1) is obvious (3,11). There is an established association between mitral annular calcification and conduction disturbances, ranging from bundle branch block to complete atrioventricular block (16,17), the latter instance being known as Rytand's syndrome (16).

Mitral valve prolapse has been found in hearts of up to 17% of women and 13% of men between the ages of 90 and 105 (3). Tricuspid valve prolapse is an occasional finding (Figure 4), always in association with mitral valve prolapse; the incidence reported by Lie and Hammond is around 10% (3). Davies *et al.* (18) have shown that the frequency of mitral valve prolapse increases with age. The mitral valve cusps become white, opaque and thickened, with the redundant valvular tissue prolapsing into the left atrium and producing mitral regurgitation. The changes are more marked in the posterior mitral leaflet, which increases significantly in depth, sometimes becoming larger than the anterior mitral leaflet. The chordae tendineae are elongated and translucent. In the presence of significant mitral regurgitation, the left atrium is dilated, and jet lesions are evident on the atrial endocardium.

The biochemical abnormality consists of a decrease in type III collagen, and an increase in collagen precursors but not in mature collagen.

Whenever a prolapsing mitral valve becomes haemodynamically regurgitant,

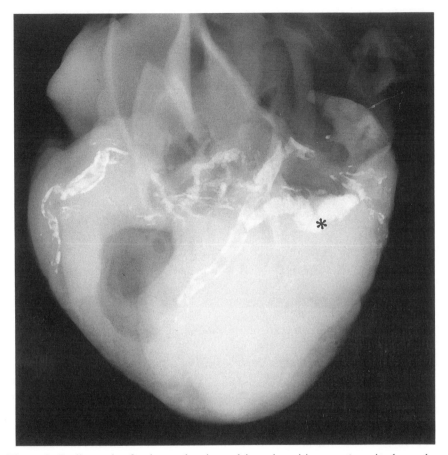

Figure 3. Radiograph of a heart showing calcium deposition on the mitral annulus (asterisk) as well as on the aortic valve and the epicardial coronary arteries

there is an increased risk of infective endocarditis, which can lead to acute mitral regurgitation requiring emergency mitral valve replacement. Sudden spontaneous chordal rupture is another mechanism leading to abrupt mitral regurgitation. Mitral valve prolapse has also occasionally been reported as a cause of sudden cardiac death (18).

CONDUCTION SYSTEM

Sinus node

The sinus node contains small specialized myocytes scattered within the collagen, around the nodal artery. These myocytes are called 'P' (pacemaker) cells. With increasing age, and generally after the age of 70, there is a sharp decrease in the

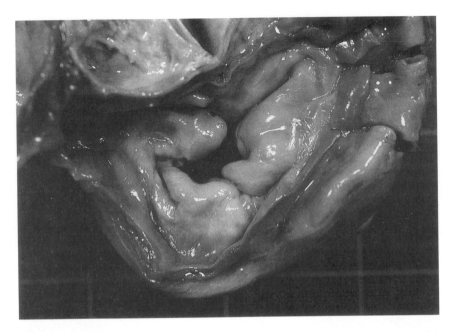

Figure 4. Atrial view of the tricuspid valve, showing prolapse of all cusps into the right atrium

number of 'P' cells in the sinus node, sometimes falling below 10% (19). The decrease in the number of 'P' cells does not bear any relationship to the presence or absence of arteriosclerosis. Sometimes, amyloid deposits can be found in the sinus node area. Fat infiltration also increases with age.

This depletion of 'P' cells is responsible for the 'sick sinus syndrome' (sinus bradycardia, sinus arrest, or bradycardia–tachycardia syndrome) in the elderly age group. It is currently thought that, in the absence of amyloid deposits in the nodal area, the decrease in 'P' cells can be ascribed to 'ageing': this decrease would probably also explain why atrial fibrillation can be triggered so easily in elderly people.

Atrioventricular node

The atrioventricular node seems quite resistant to the effects of ageing, showing only a mild degree of loss of atrioventricular myocytes. The atrioventricular bundle, however, is much more susceptible to the increase in collagen and fibrous tissue observed in the upper part of the ventricular septum, seen mainly in hypertensive patients. This process is known as 'sclerosis of the cardiac skeleton'. Concomitant arteriosclerosis of the small vessels is also partially responsible for the loss of conduction fibres. Atherosclerotic coronary artery disease resulting in infarction of the septal area may also lead to atrioventricular block (30% of cases) (19).

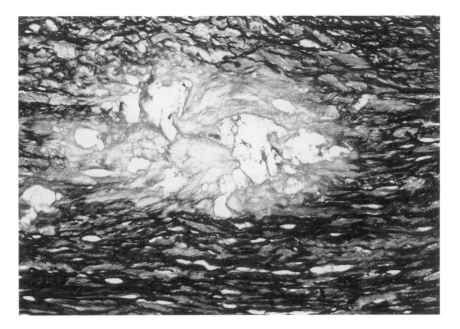

Figure 5. Photomicrograph from the ascending aorta in a 97-year-old woman. The elastic laminae are fragmented, and 'cystic' areas are present (elastic haematoxylin and eosin stain)

AORTA

The ascending aorta together with the supra-aortic ridge dilates with age. Dilation is associated with thinning and fragmentation of the elastic laminae and with a decrease in medial smooth muscle, so that the media becomes more collagenous. This may cause some aortic regurgitation, and is certainly responsible for the widening of the aortic arch observed on chest radiographs.

A more severe degree of medial damage, including the appearance of cystic change (Figure 5), may occur in younger people and be a cause for aortic regurgitation. The relationship of this to age-related changes is uncertain (20).

In old age, a specific form of inflammatory aortitis can be seen: giant cell aortitis. The elastic laminae become necrotic, triggering a granulomatous inflammatory reaction. Some cases are seen in association with temporal arteritis or polymyalgia rheumatica. Aneurysm formation is quite common.

REFERENCES

1. Leaf A (1979) Search for the oldest people: every day is a gift when you are over 100. *Natl Geogr* **34**: 94–97.
2. Evans JG (1991) Challenge of aging. *Br Med J* **303**: 408–409.

3. Lie JT, Hammond PI (1988) Pathology of the senescent heart: anatomic observations on 237 autopsy studies of patients 90 to 105 years old. *Mayo Clin Proc* **63**: 552–564.
4. Waller BF, Roberts WC (1983) Cardiovascular disease in the very elderly: analysis of 40 necropsy patients aged 90 years or over. *Am J Cardiol* **51**: 403–421.
5. Kitzman DW, Scholz DG, Hagen PT *et al.* (1988) Age-related changes in normal human hearts during the first 10 decades of life. Part II (Maturity): a quantitative anatomic study of 765 specimens from subjects 20 to 99 years old. *Mayo Clin Proc* **63**: 137–146.
6. Hodkinson HM, Pomerance A (1977) The clinical significance of senile cardiac amyloidosis: a prospective clinicopathological study. *Q J Med* **46**: 381–387.
7. Cohen AS (1967) Amyloidosis. *N Engl J Med* **277**: 574–583.
8. Katenkamp D, Stiller D (1971) Histotopographische Untersuchungen zur senilen Herzamyloidose. *Pathol Eur* **6**: 109–123.
9. Cornwell GG, Murdoch WL, Kyle RA *et al.* (1983) Frequency and distribution of senile cardiovascular amyloid: a clinicopathologic correlation. *Am J Med* **75**: 618–623.
10. Smith TJ, Kyle RA, Lie JT (1984) Clinical significance of histopathologic patterns of cardiac amyloidosis. *Mayo Clin Proc* **59**: 547–555.
11. Pomerance A (1981) Cardiac pathology in the elderly. *Cardiovasc Clin* **12**: 9–54.
12. Tresch DD (1987) Atypical presentations of cardiovascular disorders in the elderly. *Geriatrics* **42**: 31–46.
13. Waller BF, Morgan R (1987) The very elderly heart. *Cardiovasc Clin* **18**: 361–410.
14. Pomerance A (1972) Pathogenesis of aortic stenosis and its relation to age. *Br Heart J* **34**: 569–574.
15. Rahimtoola SH, Cheitlin MD, Hutter AM (1987) Valvular and congenital heart disease. *J Am Coll Cardiol* **10** (Suppl. A): 60A–62A.
16. Rytand DA, Lipsitch LS (1946) Clinical aspects of calcification on the mitral annulus fibrosus. *Arch Intern Med* **78**: 544–564.
17. Fulkerson PK, Beaver BM, Auseon JC, Grabler HL (1979) Calcification of the mitral annulus: etiology, clinical associations, complications and therapy. *Am J Med* **66**: 967–977.
18. Davies MJ, Moore BP, Braimbridge MV (1978) The floppy mitral valve: study of incidence, pathology and complications in surgical, necropsy and forensic material. *Br Heart J* **40**: 468–481.
19. Davies MJ (1988) The pathological basis of arrhythmias. *Geriatr Cardiovasc Med* **1**: 181–183.
20. Schlatmann TJM, Becker AE (1977) Histologic changes in the normal aging aorta: implications for dissecting aortic aneurysm. *Am J Cardiol* **39**: 13–20.

14 Changes in the Autonomic Nervous System

KEITH G. LURIE[a] AND JANICE B. SCHWARTZ[b]

[a] *University of Minnesota Medical School, Minnesota, USA*
[b] *University of California, San Francisco, California, USA*

Age-dependent changes in the autonomic nervous system have far-reaching effects on the regulation of cardiovascular function. Nearly every process which regulates the interactions between the sympathetic and parasympathetic nervous system and the cardiovascular response to normal physiological stresses is altered with ageing. These changes are particularly important clinically since what is considered to be a normal cardiovascular response in a young patient is not necessarily a normal response in an elderly patient.

There is a large body of literature evaluating the influence of age on the autonomic nervous system and its relationship to the cardiovascular system. Here we review some of the changes which occur during the ageing process in relationship to the anatomy, physiology and pharmacology of cardiovascular function. Discussion is focused on changes which occur during the transition from adulthood to senescence. In the final section specific disease states are addressed.

ANATOMY

Changes in contractile muscle

β-Adrenergic nervous system modulation of cardiac function decreases with age. Anatomical studies in animals as well as humans have demonstrated that there is a decrease in tissue noradrenaline (norepinephrine) content with ageing (1,2). In people, progressive adrenergic axonal degeneration occurs beginning by the fifth decade (2). In animal models of ageing, there is a loss of the number of viable nerves innervating the heart but the amount of noradrenaline in the remaining nerves remains constant (2). Electrically induced release of noradrenaline from cardiac sympathetic nerves is significantly reduced in older rat hearts, probably secondary to a defect in neuronal calcium channels which develops with ageing (3).

Geriatric Cardiology. Principles and Practice. Edited by A. Martin and A. J. Camm
© 1994 John Wiley & Sons Ltd

Changes in conduction elements

Within the cardiac conduction system the anatomical changes which occur with senescence are striking. Sinus nodal axonal degeneration progresses with ageing. There is a decrease in the number of sinus nodal cells, an increase in the transverse diameter of the remaining cells, and increased irregularity of sinus nodal morphology (4–6). Cell drop-out occurs especially after the age of 60 years. Lev and others found that fatty infiltration accounts for much of this change (7). Fatty infiltration in humans occurs earlier than cell drop-out.

In addition to fatty infiltration, the sinus node undergoes progressive fibrosis (6). Nodal cells become stretched and encapsulated with collagen (4,5). Yet, despite these changes, the correlation between fibrosis and sinus node function is poor (8,9). By age 75 only approximately 10% of the original cells may remain. Nonetheless, pacemaker activity is most often normal in patients of this age group (10).

Compared to the sinoatrial node, where the decrease in muscle cells and the increases in collagen are striking after age 70 years, muscle drop-out and increases in collagen in humans occur to a lesser extent in the remainder of the conduction system (10). There is some reduction in the number of specialized conduction cells, particularly within the left and right bundle branches (10). In the Fischer 344 rat model of ageing there is some increase in collagen in the AV nodal region and an even more pronounced increase in collagen content in the bundle branches (11). Regulation of this collagen deposition process remains poorly understood. However, it is unlikely that impaired blood supply is primarily causal, at least in the sinus node, where sinus nodal artery luminal size is usually adequate and even increased with ageing (4).

Changes in blood vessels

Within the vasculature multiple age-related alterations have also been described in humans and other species (12,13). Endothelial cells become irregular in size and shape. In addition, there is an increase in the number of multinucleated giant cells. Within the subendothelial layers there is an increase in connective tissue, with calcification and lipid deposition near the internal elastic lamina. In pure-bred beagles, a well-characterized animal model of ageing displaying β-adrenergic changes similar to those in man and a species essentially devoid of atherosclerosis, wall thickness and the wall/lumen ratio of epicardial vessels increases with age while the overall size of the capillary bed decreases (14).

Although a number of distinct changes in the anatomy of cardiac muscle and cardiac conductive elements have been described (4,15), particularly in the older literature, much less is known about the anatomical changes which occur in the innervation of the heart with ageing. This is most likely due to the difficulty in obtaining fresh samples from senescent hearts. Even with fresh samples, localization of catecholamines and study of neuronal elements can be difficult. Such studies are nearly impossible in postmortem hearts.

PHYSIOLOGY

In contrast to the relationship between the autonomic nervous system and anatomical changes in the heart with ageing, more is known about changes in cardiovascular function in relation to the autonomic nervous system. Distinct changes have been observed in contractile muscle function, the electrophysiological properties of muscle and conduction system elements, and vascular responsiveness. As outlined in Table 1, the modulatory effects of the autonomic nervous system on all of these processes are significantly altered with ageing.

Changes in contractile muscle

Although the correlation between myocyte drop-out with ageing and the decreased responsiveness of the myocardium to catecholamines and adrenergic agonists has not been clearly established, cardiac contractile and conductive tissues have a decreased response to β-adrenergic stimulation as the ageing process progresses (16–23). There is general agreement that with advancing age there is an increase in resting levels of circulating noradrenergic and an even larger difference in responses to stress (24–27). In addition, the regulation of catecholamine release by prejunctional α-adrenergic receptors may be altered with ageing. In particular, animal studies suggest that with ageing there is enhanced neuronal uptake of noradrenaline (28), perhaps in response to increased circulating catecholamines.

Plasma noradrenaline response to upright posture and isometric exercise increases linearly with age (26,27,29). In contrast to observations that older subjects have higher basal blood pressures than younger subjects and demonstrate greater increases in blood pressure in response to stress, myocardial contractile and electrophysiological properties showed decreased responses to β-adrenergic stimulation, while α-adrenergic vascular responses appear relatively unaffected by age (30,31). There appears to be a generalized 'down-regulation' of β-adrenergic cardiac contractile and electrophysiological responsiveness in the cardiovascular system with increasing age (20,22,23,31).

In this regard, many efforts to date have centred on trying to elucidate the mechanism underlying the consistent alterations in response to β-adrenergic stimulation with ageing (20,23,32–34). Nonetheless, the decreased inotropic and chronotropic responsiveness of the heart to adrenergic agonists observed with increasing age is not fully understood. There are differences of opinion whether these age-related changes are due to myocardial β-adrenergic receptor number and affinity changes or changes in the β-adrenergic effector pathway at some point distal to the receptor (32,34). It is likely, however, that age-related alterations in response to β_1-adrenergic agonists cannot be explained simply by a reduction in the density of β_1-receptor binding sites (32,34). It is probable that the affinity of the β-receptor to adrenergic agonists decreases with age. Reduced β-adrenergic receptor-stimulated adenylate cyclase activity has been observed in

Table 1. Sympathetic alterations with ageing

Cardiac noradrenaline stores	Decreased (1,2)
Plasma noradrenaline	
Resting	Probably increased (24,25,27)
Standing	Increased (26,75)
Exercise	Increased (26,29)
β-Adrenergic	
Isoproterenol	Blunted heart rate response (19,23,25,33,34,39)
	Blunted AV nodal conduction response (11,59,60)
	Blunted contractility response (19,20,33)
β_1-Receptor number	
Non-cardiac	Decreased (25,32,35,37,39,91)
Myocardium	Decreased/unchanged (19,33,37)
AV node	Probably decreased (62)
β_1-Receptor affinity	Decreased (32,34)
β_2 Vasodilation	Decreased (31,36,64)
β_2-Receptor number	
(polymorphonuclear leucocytes)	Probably decreased (63)
α-Adrenergic	
α_1 Response to phenylephrine	Probably unchanged (66)
α_1 Vasoconstrictor response	Probably unchanged (31,65,66)
α_2 Prejunctional sensitivity	Decreased (animal data) (78,79)
Baroreceptor reflexes and	
cardiopulmonary reflexes	
Sensing	Decreased (72,73,92)
Processing	Unknown
Response	Complex, parasympathetic withdrawal (64,72,74)
	Heterogeneous sympathetic response
Clinical findings	
Heart rate response to stress	Decreased (26,75)
Maximal achievable heart with exercise	Decreased (26,75)
Heart rate response to propranolol	Decreased (23)
Blood pressure at rest	(Systolic) probably increased (65)
Blood pressure during stress	(Systolic) probably increased (65)

human lymphocytes with ageing as well as in hearts from senescent animals (25,32,35). Interestingly, in the rat model, the decreased sensitivity of the vasculature to β_2-adrenergic stimulation observed with senescence can be reversed with thyroid treatment (36).

The cause for decreased responsiveness to β-agonists may be multifactorial and not only include changes in adrenergic receptor affinity but also changes in neuronal uptake of catecholamines, alterations in protein kinase activation or a decreased ability of catecholamines to increase intracellular calcium available for contraction (19,20,28,32,33,37–39). In addition to a reduction in the acute effects of β_1-adrenergic stimulation on heart rate, prolonged exposure to β-agonists in older people produces a more profound tolerance when compared to a younger population (40). β_2-Adrenergic receptor-mediated vascular relaxation decreases with ageing, and the overall ability to increase or decrease surface adrenergic receptor number is decreased with age (31). However, although many studies demonstrate a decreased responsiveness of the myocardium to infusion of β-adrenergic agonists with ageing, these observations must be interpreted with caution since much of the control of cardiovascular function is neuronal rather than humoral, especially in the resting state (22).

Changes in the specialized conduction system: electrophysiological consequences of ageing

The electrophysiological changes which occur in the cardiac conduction system with ageing are clinically important and are outlined in Table 2. The sinus node, atrioventricular (AV) node, the His and bundle branches all manifest significant changes in function. In the sinus node, all electrophysiological measurements of intrinsic nodal function demonstrate a progressive and significant prolongation

Table 2. Effects of ageing on cardiac electrophysiology

Sinus node		Increased sinus node dysfunction (41,43,44)
Heart rate	Resting	No change or decreased (27,43,44,75)
	Response to exercise	Decreased (23)
	R–R variability	Decreased (52–55)
Conduction velocity	Sinoatrial conduction	Decreased (41,44,45)
	A–H interval	Probably decreased (9,42,58–61)
	H–V interval	Unknown (45,61)
Refractory periods	Atrial	Increased (41,45)
	AV nodal	Increased (45)
	Ventricular	Increased (45)
Ectopy	Atrial	Increased APCs (43,56,57)
		Increased atrial fibrillation and flutter (43,56,57)
	Ventricular	Increased VPCs (43,56,57)
		Increased incidence of couplets and non-sustained ventricular tachycardia (43,56,57)

APCs = atrial premature contractions; VPCs = ventricular premature contractions with increasing age. The heart rate slows progressively, and the corrected sinus node recovery time as well as the sinoatrial conduction time increase in duration with ageing (41–45). Despite these changes only approximately 2/1000 patients develop clinical symptoms of sinoatrial dysfunction that require pacemaker therapy (41). One consequence of the decrease in heart rate is that ventricular end-diastolic volume and stroke volume increase so that overall cardiac output does not decrease with ageing (46).

Although the neuronally mediated sympathetic activity which helps to modulate sinus nodal function is thought to remain unchanged throughout life, there is a progressive parasympathetic tone withdrawal with increasing age (44). With the vagolytic agent atropine, younger people develop a pronounced tachycardia. In senescent subjects the increase in heart rate with vagolysis is markedly attenuated (47). Similar effects are observed with vagolytic agents when assessing sinus node recovery times and atrial conduction times. In rat models of ageing, both increased and decreased sinus node responsiveness to vagal stimulation and acetylcholine have been reported (48,49). Thus, with ageing, parasympathetic effects, which predominate in the young, decrease and the sympathetic and parasympathetic influences on sinus node function become more balanced (50). As a result the basal properties of the sinus node remain relatively stable throughout life.

With exercise or infusion of β-adrenergic agonists, such as isoproterenol, the responsiveness of the sinus node decreases significantly with age (23). This is a well-established observation in humans and animal models of ageing (51). Furthermore, studies which examine variations in sinus cycle length demonstrate a decrease in R–R variability with ageing (52–55). This is thought to be secondary to both central and cardiac-mediated decreases in sympathetic and parasympathetic influence on nodal cell automaticity.

In the absence of detectable ischaemia, atrial and ventricular ectopy increase with age (43,56). The incidence of atrial fibrillation increases with age (43,56,57). In one study of 98 people aged 60–85 years without detectable cardiac ischaemia, supraventricular tachyarrhythmias were found in one-third of the subjects and 15% had ventricular couplets or short bursts of non-sustained ventricular tachycardia (56). Others have confirmed these results (43,57). In contrast, bradyarrhythmias of any variety are uncommon (43).

In patients with organic heart disease, there is an age-related increase in AV conduction times and in the incidence of complete heart block (42). However, in the absence of organic heart disease, the relationship between AV nodal function and age is less clear (9,42,58). Some have found no linear relationship between progression to spontaneous AV block with age (42,59). Others have reported that in normal patients, ranging in age from 18 to 73 years old, there is an age-dependent increase in atrial effective refractoriness, AV nodal effective refractoriness and ventricular effective refractoriness, but no age-related changes in resting sinus cycle length, the P–R interval, the QRS duration, the A–H interval, the H–V interval, or the corrected sinus node recovery time (45,60). In contrast, many larger population studies suggest a modest increase in P–R intervals on electrocardiogram (ECG) with increasing age.

Studies using high-fidelity surface ECGs in normal senescent subjects without any evidence of heart disease revealed that only the A–H conduction time increases with ageing, while the H–V interval is constant (61). This was a small group of normal subjects but the results that the A–H interval increases with ageing are similar to the findings of others (45). In symptomatic patients with sinus node dysfunction, in the absence of concomitant cardiac disease, the development of new AV block is 1% per year (41). Our own data in rats suggest that decreased β-adrenergic receptor density in the AV node may contribute to increased AV conduction time (62). Although AV conduction intervals probably prolong with physiological ageing in humans the mechanisms underlying this process remain to be further elucidated.

Changes in vascular responsiveness

Relatively little is known about how ageing affects the vascular responsiveness to α- and β-adrenergic stimulation. In humans, there appears to be a selective decline in β_2-adrenergic-mediated arterial and venous relaxation with ageing (63). Using the response to intra-arterial isoproterenol on changes in forearm blood flow in young and older subjects, some data suggest that there is an age-related decline in β_2-adrenergic receptor-mediated vasodilation (64).

Hemodynamic studies in young and older subjects reveal that heart rate and systolic blood pressure increase with ageing while diastolic blood pressure decrease. There is little change in the mean arterial blood pressure (65). Some have reported a decreased pressor potency of the α_1-selective agonist phenyl-ephrine with ageing (66) while others report no change in response to arterial or venous α-adrenergic tone with ageing (31,65). One concludes from these studies that the overall vascular responsiveness to α_1-adrenergic receptor-mediated vasoconstriction appears to remain relatively constant with increasing age.

Less data are available regarding the parasympathetic regulation of the vasculature with age. The vasodilatation observed with acetylcholine may be reduced in older patients (67). Similar findings were not observed in senescent rats (68).

One area of control of vascular tone which has received a recent resurgence of interest concerns age-related changes in arterial baroreflexes and cardiopulmon-ary reflexes. With ageing the arterial baroreflex undergoes progressive impair-ment. This impairment involves not only baroreceptor reflexes which reflexively modulate heart rate when stimulated by changes in blood pressure but also baroreceptor reflexes that help maintain vascular tone (66,69,70). Angiotensin and phenylephrine infusions are frequently used to assess baroreceptor function (63,69,71). Baroreceptor sensitivity is determined by plotting the decrease in R–R interval versus the increase in blood pressure. Age-related changes observed with these agents involve a decreased ability to sense change in blood pressure and a decreased ability to respond normally to blood pressure alterations. In patients with a history of myocardial infarction, there is a significant reduction in baroreflex sensitivity with ageing(71).

The cardiopulmonary reflexes (64,72,73), like arterial baroreceptors, also play a large role in cardiovascular regulation. The ability of volume receptors located in the cardiopulmonary region to control circulation reflexively is markedly depressed in the elderly. There is a reduced ability to sense and respond normally to changes in volume. Little is known about the age-related changes in sensing shifts in volume status, the changes in the processing of the sensed events, or the altered response observed with ageing. The depressed response involves both the blood pressure and blood volume control of the reflex (74). Although the mechanism is not fully known, it is likely that the impairment of the cardiopulmonary reflex in older people is due to a reduced ability of central blood volume to stretch cardiac volume receptors and thereby sense changes in volume. Consequently, reflex-mediated noradrenaline release is diminished and blood pressure regulation becomes impaired. Thus, in the case of the decreased cardiopulmonary reflexes with ageing, there is a complex interaction which is altered between the 'senescent' hearts which are hypertrophied and less distensible, the inability of the cardiac volume receptors to 'sense' changes in volume, and the subsequent cardiopulmonary reflex-mediated release of neurotransmitters (74). This reflex is even more complicated in that plasma renin activity is markedly depressed in elderly people. The lower renin levels further potentiate this decreased ability to adjust for changes in volume. Consequently, despite a nearly twofold increase in vascular resistance with ageing, the combination of altered arterial baroreflexes and altered cardiopulmonary reflexes result in a decreased ability rapidly to adjust for shifts in volume (79). These impaired reflexes may play an important role in orthostatic hypotension observed in elderly patients.

PHARMACOLOGY

Pharmacokinetics at the sympathetic neuroeffector junction

As stated earlier, higher average circulating noradrenaline and adrenaline levels are seen in elderly versus younger subjects (22,27). This may result from increased production/release or decreased clearance of circulating catecholamines. In humans, greater increments (released) accompany equivalent levels of exercise or stress (22,26,29,75) in older individuals, and clearance from the circulation is diminished (76). Age-related differences in neuronal reuptake of noradrenaline have not been found in studies in man (77). Analogously, in animal models studies of evoked neuronal noradrenaline release, stimulation from the rat tail artery has been shown to increase with age (78), while no age-related change in neuronal uptake or metabolism is seen.

Neuronal noradrenaline release is modulated by presynaptic/prejunctional

α_2-adrenergic receptors. An age-related decline in the sensitivity of prejunctional α_2-adrenergic receptors of the rat peripheral vasculature to both agonists and antagonists has been demonstrated (78,79), but the mechanism responsible for this change remains unclear and may involve competition for substrate uptake, or age-related differences in α_2 subtypes in the peripheral vasculature. Similarly, no age-related changes have been detected during prejunctional dopamine D_2 activation (78).

These age-related changes in neuronal noradrenaline release and α_2-adrenergic function, however, may be limited to the peripheral vasculature, since it has been suggested that electrically stimulated cardiac neuronal noradrenaline release decreases with age (3), while noradrenaline uptake may increase with ageing (28). A potential explanation is that the neuronal calcium channels regulating intracardiac neuronal noradrenaline release are altered with ageing (3). Data from both rat peripheral vasculature and hearts are in agreement that the functional neuronal transmitter pool size does not change with age.

To summarize, most data available today regarding the neuroeffector junction have been obtained in animal models of ageing. These models demonstrate that changes in the peripheral vasculature may not reflect changes in the cardiac adrenergic bed. Furthermore, higher circulating noradrenaline levels are seen in elderly versus younger individuals in all models but the mechanisms for this increase is multifactorial and not completely elucidated.

Systemic pharmacology: pharmacokinetics

Ageing from maturity to senescence is accompanied by changes in age-dependent alterations in pharmacokinetics. Most of the current evidence leads to the conclusion that drug metabolism is reduced in the elderly. Physiological changes that influence cardiac drug metabolism include: (i) decreased gastric acid secretion, reduced splanchnic blood flow and gastrointestinal motility and possibly decreased absorptive changes in capacity of enterocytes leading to small changes in drug absorption. Potential age-related changes in transdermal, rectal or transbronchial drug absorption have not been definitively determined. (ii) Declines in total body weight due to decreases in fat and lean body mass in the very elderly (> 75 years of age) and changes in plasma proteins lead to minor to modest decreases in drug volume of distribution in the very old years. Finally, the most important and consistent changes seen with ageing are (iii) decreases in organ drug clearance. Currently available drugs are largely eliminated by one of two routes: renal or hepatic. Perhaps the most consistent alteration in drug elimination with ageing is seen in renal clearance, as originally shown for glomerular filtration (22). This leads to a decrease in excretion of both endogenous (creatinine) and exogenous (drug) compounds eliminated by the kidney. Changes in creatinine clearance are of the order of a decline in 10% per decade after the age of 20 but can be estimated by the method of Cockcraft and Gault (80), where:

$$\text{creatinine clearance} = \frac{(140 - \text{age}) \ (\text{weight} \ (\text{kg}))}{72 \times \text{serum} \ \text{creatinine} \ (\text{mg})}$$

in males. For females, multiply by 0.85. Renal tubular secretion and reabsorption also decrease with age to a slightly lesser extent (approximately 7% per decade) and changes in one may offset the other.

Hepatic drug metabolism changes with ageing are more variable. While a trend for decreased drug metabolism in humans appears to be present for drugs undergoing oxidative drug elimination or biotransformation (cytochrome P_{450}), alcohol dehydrogenase activity or metabolism of drugs by glucuronidation may not demonstrate age-related decrements. In general, clearance for most cardiac drugs can be assumed to decrease with ageing (81). For age-related changes in the pharmacokinetics of autonomic agents, see Table 3.

CARDIOVASCULAR DISEASE STATES IN THE ELDERLY

Sinus node dysfunction

Sinus node disease increases in a unimodal distribution with increasing age (41). The incidence of sinus node dysfunction peaks around age 70 years old. Intrinsic

Table 3. Age-related changes in autonomic drug clearance

Drug	Organ or clearance	Age-related alteration
β-Adrenergic blockers		
Atenolol	Renal	Some decrease
Nadolol	Renal	Some decrease
Pindolol	Hepatic	Decrease
Propranolol	Hepatic	Decrease
Metoprolol	Hepatic	Some (small) decrease
α-Adrenergic blockers		
Clonidine	Renal + hepatic	Decrease
Prazosin	Hepatic	Some (small) decrease
Terazosin	Hepatic, renal	? Decrease
α-Methyldopa	Renal	Decrease
β-Agonists		
Isoproterenol	Liver and COMT[a] in other tissues	? (No change)
Adrenaline	Liver (and other tissues) COMT and MAO[a]	?
Noradrenaline	Liver, COMT and MAO	?
Terbutaline	Renal	?
Dopaminergic agonists		
Dopamine	Hepatic and COMT, MAO, intraneuronal	?
Dobutamine	Hepatic	? Decrease

[a]COMT = Catechol-*o*-methyltransferase, MAO = monoamine oxidase.

sinus node disease is caused by multiple factors, including ischaemia to the sinus node and loss of sinus nodal cells secondary to infiltration of collagen and other infiltrative processes. Evaluation of the autonomic control of the sinus node has potential relevance in the assessment of patients who have sinus node dysfunction. For example, the appropriateness of the transient bradycardic response to carotid sinus massage, valsalva manoeuvre or pharmacologically induced hypertension (by the administration of phenylephrine), or alternatively the tachycardic response to exercise, upright tilt or pharmacologically induced hypotension, all shed light on the appropriateness of sinus node function. (Refer to references 41 and 82 for extensive review.) Chronotropic incompetence can lead to symptoms of exertional fatigue, dizziness, change in mental status, or syncope. Although the aetiology for sinus node dysfunction is multifactorial and poorly understood, the bradyarrhythmias and tachyarrhythmias produce a wide range of symptoms. In patients with extrinsic sinus node dysfunctions, causes such as abnormalities in thyroid hormone levels, electrolyte abnormalities or drug therapies must be considered. Diagnosis is made by correlating symptoms with Holter or continuous-loop 'event' recorders, telemetry, ECG or with electrophysiology testing.

Atrioventricular nodal and Hisian dysfunction

Changes which occur with ageing in the AV node and His bundle are often associated with concomitant disease states, including coronary artery disease and cardiomyopathy. However, idiopathic bilateral bundle branch fibrosis remains the most common cause of Stokes–Adams attacks (83). Pathologists have differentiated diseases of the central portion of the conduction system into two different types. Lev described a very focal fibrosis which occurs in the proximal portion of the conduction system (7,83). In contrast, Lenègre described a more diffuse disease process which affects middle and distal portions of the bundle branches (84). Both processes occur with increased frequency in elderly persons. The pathological basis for both processes is poorly understood. However, Lev and others speculate that some sort of traumatic event may be an initiating trigger.

Age-related muscle dysfunction

Although it is difficult to separate the 'pure' age-related changes in cardiac muscle function from those secondary to atherosclerosis, there appears to be general agreement that with ageing and the associated myocyte drop-out the heart becomes less distensible, stiffer, larger, and responds more poorly to β-adrenergic stimulation (21). Thus, although multiple co-morbid conditions may modulate the impact of ageing on cardiac function, it has become increasingly clear that as the mean age of the population increases the number of patients with clinical heart failure has also increased dramatically. Although the treatment of elderly patients with heart failure is similar to treatment of younger patients with heart failure, it is important to recognize that the response to drugs that affect the autonomic nervous system in elderly patients may be altered (85).

Syncope

There are multiple reasons why the incidence of syncope is increased in elderly patients. Some of the reasons are described above and relate to changes in arterial baroreflexes and pulmonary volume reflexes with ageing. Although it is beyond the scope of this review to discuss in detail the multiple causes of syncope in the elderly (43,52,86–88), there are some important differences in the approach to syncope in the elderly. With ageing there is an increase in syncope secondary to postural hypotension and sinus node dysfunction. Evaluation of syncopal disorders is the same in the elderly population as in younger patients, although the incidence of ventricular arrhythmias is increased with age (43). Diagnostic interventions include Holter monitoring, continuous-loop event recordings, electrophysiological studies, head-up tilt table testing and adjustment of vasoactive medications.

Intolerance to medical therapy for syncope is often increased in the elderly population. This is particularly true for therapies directed towards the treatment of orthostatic hypotension and neurally mediated vasovasal syncope. For example, fluorocortisone may exacerbate heart failure, β-blockers may also worsen heart failure or produce profound bradycardia, disopyramide may not be tolerated due to the anticholinergic effects of this drug, and less commonly used drugs such as scopolamine and ephedrine may be similarly difficult to use in the elderly patient. Fortunately there are no significant age-related increases in problems associated with pacemaker implantation. However, although the role of pacemakers in the treatment of bradycardia is well established, use of pacemakers in treatment of neurally mediated syncope should be reserved for patients who have been demonstrated to benefit from pacing during head-up tilt-testing protocols or during carotid sinus massage (89,90).

CONCLUSIONS

Although it is difficult to separate co-morbid diseases from the natural process of ageing, the changes which occur in the autonomic nervous system during the senescent process can profoundly alter cardiac function. Despite a lack of understanding at a fundamental mechanistic level of many of the age-related changes in the autonomic control of heart rate, blood pressure and susceptibility to the development of arrhythmias, the clinical importance of the changes with ageing in the heart is well described. The clinical manifestations of the gradual decline in autonomic regulatory control of cardiovascular function with ageing should be well understood if therapies directed towards the treatment of the elderly are to be maximally effective.

REFERENCES

1. Martinez JL, Vasquez BJ, Messing RB *et al.* (1981) Age-related changes in the catecholamine content of peripheral organs in male and female F344 rats. *J Gerontol* **36**: 280–284.
2. McLean MR, Goldberg PB, Roberts J (1983) An ultrastructural study of the effects of age on sympathetic innervation and atrial tissue in the rat. *J Moll Cell Cardiol* **15**: 75–92.
3. Almquist A, Gornick CC, Benson DW Jr *et al.* (1985) Carotid sinus hypersensitivity: evaluation of the vasodepressor component. *Circulation* **71**: 927–937.
4. Davies MJ (1976) Pathology of the conducting system. In *Cardiology in Old Age*, Caird FI, Dall JLC, Kennedy RD (eds). Plenum, New York, p. 57.
5. Davies MJ, Pomerance A (1972) Quantitative study of ageing changes in the human sinoatrial node and internodal tracts. *Br Heart J* **34**: 150–152.
6. Inoue S, Shinohara F, Niitani H, Gotoh K (1986) A new method for the histological study of aging changes in the sinoatrial node. *Jpn Heart J* **27**: 653–660.
7. Lev M (1984) Aging changes in the human sinoatrial node. *J Gerontol* **9**: 1–9.
8. Simms HS, Berg BN (1957) Longevity and the onset of lesions in male rats. *J Gerontol* **12**: 244–252.
9. Thery C, Gosselin B, Lekieffre J, Warembourg H (1977) Pathology of sinoatrial node: correlations with electrocardiographic findings in 111 patients. *Am Heart J* **93**: 735–740.
10. Fujino M, Okada R, Arakawa K (1983) The relationship of aging to histological changes in the conduction system of the normal human heart. *Jpn Heart J* **24**: 13–20.
11. Schmidlin O, Bharati S, Lev M, Schwartz JB (1992) Effects of physiological aging on cardiac electrophysiology in perfused Fischer 344 rat hearts. *Am Physiol Soc* **262**: H97–H105.
12. Cotton R, Wartman WB (1961) Endothelial patterns in human arteries, their relationship to age, vessel site, and atherosclerosis. *Arch Pathol* **2**: 15–24.
13. Gerrity RG, Cliff WJ (1972) The aorta tunica intima in young and aging rats. *Exp Mol Pathol* **16**: 382–402.
14. Tomanek RJ, Aydelotte MR, Torry RJ (1991) Remodelling of coronary vessels during aging in purebred beagles. *Circ Res* **69**: 1068–1074.
15. Erickson EE, Lev M (1952) Aging changes in the human atrioventricular node, bundle, and bundle branches. *J Gerontol* **7**: 1–12.
16. Anversa P, Palackal T, Sonnenblick EH *et al.* (1990) Myocyte cell loss and myocyte cellular hyperplasia in the hypertrophied aging rat heart. *Circ Res* **67**: 871–885.
17. Anversa P, Hiler B, Ricci R *et al.* (1986) Myocyte cell loss and myocyte hypertrophy in the aging rat heart. *J Am Coll Cardiol* **8**: 1441–1448.
18. Klausner SC, Schwartz AB (1985) The aging heart. *Clin Geriatr Med* **1**: 119.
19. Lakatta EG, Gerstenblith G, Angell CS *et al.* (1975) Diminished inotropic response of aged myocardium to catecholamines. *Circ Res* **36**: 262–269.
20. Lakatta EG (1983) Determinants of cardiovascular performance: modification due to aging. *J Chron Dis* **36**: 15–30.
21. Olivetti G, Melissari M, Capasso JM, Anversa P (1991) Cardiomyopathy of the aging human heart: myocyte loss and reactive cellular hypertrophy. *Circ Res* **68**: 1560–1568.
22. Rowe JW, Troen BR (1980) Sympathetic nervous system and aging in man. *Endocr Rev 1980* **1**: 167–179.
23. Vestal RE, Wood AJJ, Shand DG (1979) Reduced β-adrenoreceptor sensitivity in the elderly. *Clin Pharmacol Ther* **26**: 181–186.
24. Christensen NJ (1973) Plasma noradrenaline and adrenaline in patients with thyrotoxicosis and myxoedema. *Clin Sci Mol Med* **45**: 163.

25. Krall JF, Connelly M, Weisbart R, Tuck ML (1981) Age-related elevation of plasma catecholamine concentration and reduced responsiveness of lymphocyte adenylate cyclase. *J Clin Endocrinol Metab* **52**: 863–867.
26. Palmer GP, Ziegler MG, Lake CR (1978) Response of norepinephrine and blood pressure to stress increases with age. *J Gerontol* **33**: 482–487.
27. Ziegler MG, Lake CR, Kopin IJ (1976) Plasma noradrenaline increases with age. *Nature* **261**: 333–335.
28. Kreider MS, Goldberg PB, Roberts J (1984) Effect of age on adrenergic neuronal uptake in rat heart. *J Pharmacol Exp Ther* **231**: 367–372.
29. Fleg JL, Tzunkoff SP, Lakatta EG (1985) Age-related augmentation of plasma catecholamines during dynamic exercise in healthy males. *J Appl Physiol* **59**: 1033–1039.
30. Kotchen JM, McKean HE, Kotchen TA (1982) Blood pressure trends with aging. *Hypertension* **4** (Suppl. III): 128–134.
31. Pan NYM, Hoffman BB, Perske RA, Blaschke TF (1986) Decline in β-adrenergic receptor-mediated vascular relaxation with aging in man. *J Pharmacol Exp Ther* **239**: 802–807.
32. Feldman RD, Limbird LE, Nadeau J *et al.* (1984) Alterations in leukocyte β-receptor affinity with aging: a potential explanation for altered β-adrenergic sensitivity in the elderly. *N Engl J Med* **310**: 815–819.
33. Lakatta EG, Yin FCP (1982) Myocardial aging: functional alterations and related cellular mechanisms. *Am J Physiol* **242**: H927–H941.
34. Scarpace PJ (1988) Decreased receptor activation with age: can it be explained by desensitization? *Geriatr Biosci* **36**: 1067–1071.
35. Abrass IB, Scarpace PJ (1982) Catalytic unit of adenylate cyclase: reduced activity in aged human lymphocytes. *J Clin Endocrinol Metab* **55**: 1026–1028.
36. Tsujimoto G, Hashimoto K, Hoffmana BB (1987) Effects of thyroid hormone on β-adrenergic responsiveness of aging cardiovascular systems. *Am J Physiol* **252**: H513–H520.
37. Guarnieri T, Filburn CR, Zitnik G *et al.* (1980) Contractile and biochemical correlates of β-adrenergic stimulation of the aged heart. *Am J Physiol* **239**: H501–H508.
38. Kelly J, O'Malley K (1984) Adrenoceptor function and aging. *Clin Sci* **66**: 509–515.
39. Montamat SC, Davies AO (1989) Physiological response to isoproterenol and coupling of beta-adrenergic receptors in young and elderly human subjects. *J Gerontol Med Sci* **44**: M100–105.
40. Zahniser NR, Wiser A, Cass WA *et al.* (1992) Terbutaline-induced desensitization of polymorphonuclear leukocyte β_2-adrenergic receptors in young and elderly subjects. *Clin Pharmacol Ther* **51**: 432–439.
41. Benditt DG, Milstein S, Goldstein M *et al.* (1990) Sinus node dysfunction: pathophysiology, clinical features, evaluation and treatment. In *Cardiac Electrophysiology: From Cell to Bedside*, Zipes DP, Jalife J (eds). Saunders, Philadelphia, p. 708.
42. Bhat PK, Watanabe K, Luisada AA (1974) Conduction defects in the aging heart. *J Am Geriatr Soc* **22**: 517–520.
43. Camm AJ, Evans KE, Ward DE, Martin A (1981) The rhythm of the heart in active elderly subjects. *Am Heart J* **99**: 598–603.
44. De Marneffe M, Jacobs P, Haardt R, Englert M (1986) Variations of normal sinus node function in relation to age: role of autonomic influence. *Eur Heart J* **7**: 662–672.
45. Kavanagh KM, Wyse G, Mitchell LB, Duff HJ (1989) Cardiac refractoriness: age-dependence in normal subjects. *J Electrocardiol* **22**: 221–225.
46. Rodeheffer RJ, Gerstenblith G, Becker LC *et al.* (1984) Exercise cardiac output is

maintained with advancing age in healthy human subjects: cardiac dilatation and increased stroke volume compensate for a diminished heart rate. *Circulation* **69**: 203–213.

47. Dauchot P, Gravenstein JS (1971) Effects of atropine on the electrocardiogram in different age groups. *Clin Pharmacol Ther* **12**: 274–280.
48. Ferrari AU, Daffonchio A, Gerosa S, Mancia G (1991) Alterations in cardiac parasympathetic function in aged rats. *Am Physiol Soc* **260**: H647–H649.
49. Kelliher GJ, Conahan ST (1980) Changes in vagal activity and response to muscarinic receptor agonists with age. *J Gerontol* **45**: 842–849.
50. Pfeifer MA, Weinberg CR, Cook D *et al.* (1983) Differential changes of autonomic nervous system function with age in man. *Am J Med* **75**: 249–258.
51. Yin FCP, Spurgeon HA,Greene HL *et al.* (1979) *Mech Ageing Dev* **10**: 17–25.
52. Camm AJ, Lau CP (1988) Syncope of undetermined origin: diagnosis and management. *Prog Cardiol* **1**: 139–156.
53. Schwartz JB, Gibb WJ, Tran T (1991) Aging effects on heart rate variation. *J Gerontol* **46**: M99–106.
54. Simpson DM, Wicks R (1988) Spectral analysis of heart rate indicates reduced baroreceptor-related heart rate variability in elderly persons. *J Gerontol Med Sci* **43**: M21–M24.
55. Waddington JL, MacCulloch MJ, Sambrooks JE (1979) Resting heart rate variability in man declines with age. *Experientia* **35**: 1197–1198.
56. Fleg JL, Kennedy HL (1982) Cardiac arrhythmias in a healthy elderly population: detection by 24-hour electrocardiography. *Chest* **81**: 302–307.
57. Kantelip JP, Sage E, Duchene-Marullaz P (1986) Findings on ambulatory electrocardiograpic monitoring in subjects older than 80 years. *Am J Cardiol* **57**: 398–401.
58. Sims BA (1972) Pathogenesis of atrial arrhythmias. *Br Heart J* **34**: 336–340.
59. Dhingra RC, Whyndham C, Deedwania PC *et al.* (1980) Effect of age on atrioventricular conduction in patients with chronic bifascicular block. *Am J Cardiol* **45**: 749–756.
60. Michelucci A, Padeletti L, Fradella GA *et al.* (1984) Ageing and atrial electrophysiologic properties in man. *Int J Cardiol* **5**: 75–81.
61. Fleg JL, Das DN, Wright J, Lakatta EG (1990) Age-associated changes in the components of atrioventricular conduction in apparently healthy volunteers. *J Gerontol Med Sci* **45**: M95–100.
62. Schwartz JB, Lurie K, Dutton J, Capili H (1992) Decreased beta-adrenergic receptor density in the atrioventricular node with aging. *Clin Res* **40**: 195A.
63. Rutledge DR, Steinberg JD (1991) Effect of age on lymphocyte beta$_2$-adrenergic responsiveness. *Ann Pharmacother* **25**: 532–538.
64. Van Brummelen P, Buhler FR, Kiowski W, Amann FW (1981) Age-related decrease in cardiac and peripheral vascular responsiveness to isoprenaline: studies in normal subjects. *Clin Sci* **60**: 571–577.
65. Klein C, Hiatt WR, Gerber JG, Nies AS (1987) The balance between vascular alpha- and beta-adrenoceptors is not changed in the elderly. *Clin Pharmacol Ther* **42**: 260–264.
66. Elliot HL, Sumner DJ, McLean K, Reid JL (1982) Effect of age on the responsiveness of vascular α-adrenoceptors in man. *J Cardiovasc Pharmacol* **4**: 388–392.
67. Hollenberg NA, Adams DF, Solomon HS *et al.* (1974) Senescence and the renal vasculature in normal man. *Circ Res* **34**: 309–316.
68. Fleisch JH (1980) Age-related changes in the sensitivity of blood vessels to drugs. *Pharmacocl Ther* **8**: 477–480.
69. Gribbin V, Pickering TG, Sleight P, Peto R (1971) Effect of age and high blood pressure on baroreflex sensitivity in man. *Circ Res* **29**: 424–431.

70. Haidet G (1992) Effect of age on cardiovascular responses to static muscular contraction in beagles. *J Appl Physiol* **73**: 2320–2327.
71. La Rovere MT, Specchia G, Mortara A, Schwartz RJ (1988) Baroreflex sensitivity, clinical correlates and cardiovascular mortality among patients with a first myocardial infarction. *Circulation* **78**: 816–824.
72. Duke PC, Wade JG, Hickey RF, Larson CP (1976) The effects of age on baroreceptor reflex function in man. *Can Anaesth J* **23**: 111–124.
73. Randall O, Esler M, Culp B *et al.* (1978) Determinants of baroreflex sensitivity in man. *J Lab Clin Med* **91**: 514–519.
74. Cleroux J, Giannattasio C, Bolla G *et al.* (1989) Decreased cardiopulmonary reflexes with aging in normotensive humans. *Am J Physiol* **257**: H961–H968.
75. Young JB, Rowe JW, Pallotta JA *et al.* (1980) Enhanced plasma norepinephrine response to upright posture and oral glucose administration in elderly human subjects. *Metabolism*.
76. Veith RC, Featherstout JA, Leonard OA, Halter JB (1986) Age differences in plasma norepinephrine kinetics in humans. *J Gerontol* **44**: 319–324.
77. Stromberg JS, Linares OA, Supiano MA *et al.* (1991) Effect of desipramine on norepinephrine metabolism in humans with aging. *Am J Physiol* **261**: R1484–R1490.
78. Buchholz J, Tsai H, Friedman D, Duckles SP (1991) Influence of age on control of norepinephrine release from the rat tail artery. *J Pharmacol Exp Ther* **2**: 722–727.
79. Docherty JR, O'Malley K (1985) Aging and α-adrenoceptors. *Clin Sci* **68**: 133s–136s.
80. Cockcraft DW, Gault MH (1976) Prediction of creatinine clearance from serum creatinine. *Nephron* **16**: 31–41.
81. Roberts J, Goldberg PB (1979) Changes in responsiveness of the heart to drugs during aging. *Fed Proc* 1927–1932.
82. Gautschy B, Weidemann P, Gnadinger MP (1986) Autonomic function tests as related to age and gender in normal man. *Klin Wochenschr* **64**: 499–505.
83. Waller BF (1990) Clinicopathological correlations of the human cardiac conduction system. In *Cardiac Electrophysiology. From Cell to Bedside*, Zipes DP, Jalife J (eds). Saunders, Philadelphia, pp. 249–269.
84. Lenègre J (1964) Etiology of bilateral bundle branch fibrosis in relation to complete heart block. *Prog Cardiovasc Dis* **6**: 317.
85. Abrams WB (1990) Cardiovascular drugs in the elderly. *Chest* **98**: 980–986.
86. Lipsitz LA, Wei JY, Rowe JW (1985) Syncope in an elderly, institutionalized population: prevalence, incidence, and associated risk. *Q J Med* **55**: 45–54.
87. Lipsitz LA, Marks ER, Koestner J *et al.* (1989) Reduced susceptibility to syncope during postural tilt in old age: is beta-blockade protective? *Arch Intern Med* **149**: 2709–2712.
88. Lipsitz LA (1983) Syncope in the elderly. *Ann Intern Med* **99**: 92–105.
89. Almquist A, Goldenberg IF, Milstein S *et al.* (1989) Provocation of bradycardia and hypotension by isoproterenol and upright posture in patients with unexplained syncope. *N Engl J Med* **320**: 346–351.
90. Strasberg B, Sagie A, Erdman S *et al.* (1989) Carotid sinus hypersensitivity and the carotid sinus syndrome. *Prog Cardiovasc Dis* **31**: 379–391.
91. Schocken DD, Roth GS (1977) Reduced beta-adrenergic receptor concentrations in aging man. *Nature* **267**: 856–858.
92. Smyth HS, Sleight P, Pickering GW (1969) Reflex regulation of arterial pressure during sleep in man: a quantitative method of assessing baroreflex sensitivity. *Circ Res* **24**: 109–121.

15 Pharmacological Aspects of Cardiac Drug Treatment in the Elderly

LIONEL H. OPIE
University of Cape Town Department of Medicine, Cape Town, South Africa

THE PATIENT

How old age modifies cardiac drug therapy

Besides pharmacokinetic changes to be considered in the next section, there are many aspects altering cardiac drug therapy in the elderly. In general, elderly patients constitute a group in whom diseases are 'creeping up'. While some elderly patents behave as if they are much younger from the physiological point of view, others are incapacitated by a multitude of illnesses, each often only relatively minor, and yet the sum total of many small disabilities wears them down physically and psychologically. Diseases such as uraemia or anaemia may contribute to fatigue. Against such a background, it is often difficult to assess the cardiac contribution to symptoms such as dyspnoea, fatigue and palpitations. In short, before cardiac drug therapy comes cardiac diagnosis, and before cardiac diagnosis comes the assessment of the patient as a whole. Particular attention must be paid to renal and hepatic function, as well as to the state of the circulation, which are among the major factors which can influence pharmacokinetics in the elderly.

The other major factor is that elderly patients, for a variety of reasons not always clear, are often treated with a host of drugs including mood-altering agents, which can interact with the cardiac drugs. Polypharmacy, therefore, may breed multiple drug interactions which may be more serious because of pre-existing degrees of impairment of function of kidney, liver and heart.

In general, besides changes in renal, hepatic and cardiac function as well as changes in receptor sensitivity, it should be considered that absorption of the drug may be decreased by, for example, decreased splanchnic blood flow, and the distribution may be altered by decreased lean body mass, decreased total water and decreased serum albumin (1).

Renal function governs the dose of commonly used drugs which are excreted by

Geriatric Cardiology. Principles and Practice. Edited by A. Martin and A. J. Camm
© 1994 John Wiley & Sons Ltd

the kidneys and not metabolized by the liver, such as digoxin and atenolol. Renal impairment also governs the ultimate excretion of some drugs that undergo prior hepatic metabolism, such as antiarrhythmics, several β-blockers and methyldopa.

Hepatic function governs the clearance of these drugs which undergo hepatic metabolism. The trend to a decreased liver blood flow in the elderly means that such drugs can accumulate in the blood with, for example in the case of propranolol, the potential for serious central nervous side-effects.

Sometimes *malnutrition* occurs in the elderly, and there are low plasma protein concentrations which in turn can alter the pharmacokinetics of plasma-bound β-blockers (propranolol and pindolol), so that lower doses are required for the same effective blood levels.

Finally, *tissue sensitivity* to a drug can fall as, for example, β-receptor density decreases.

PHARMACOKINETICS OF SPECIFIC DRUGS

The general pharmacokinetic rule is that the tendency is towards a decreased drug clearance, higher effective blood levels, and therefore a greater chance of side-effects. In general, drug doses may be lower in the elderly, although not as low as commonly supposed (an example is the tendency to give elderly patients digoxin at half the normal adult dose even though their renal function may only be minimally impaired; such a low dose is relatively ineffective).

Digoxin

Even before considering pharmacokinetic changes with age, the major point to evaluate is whether digoxin really is needed in any given elderly patient. Diastolic dysfunction is increasingly recognized as a cause of early heart failure; sometimes it may not even be accompanied by systolic failure. In elderly patients, there is a cardiomyopathy, often associated with hypertension with prominent diastolic dysfunction, in which the appropriate therapy is β-blockade or verapamil, but not digoxin (2).

The major indication for digoxin remains the combination of left ventricular (LV) failure and atrial fibrillation. Secondly, in overt LV systolic failure, digoxin is also often used together with diuretics and angiotensin-converting enzyme (ACE) inhibitors. Among the many points to consider concerning digoxin pharmacokinetics in the elderly (Table 1) is that the same dose of digoxin tends to give higher blood concentrations and a longer blood half-life in the elderly, due to the smaller body size and decreased renal excretion (3). Digoxin clearance is linearly related to the creatinine clearance but not to the creatinine plasma level (creatinine clearance can decrease over 50% before there is a significant rise in plasma creatinine concentration). It follows that ideally renal function should be established by means of creatinine clearance or glomerular filtration rates (GFR) before instituting digoxin in elderly subjects.

Table 1. Digoxin pharmacokinetics and effects in the elderly

Process	Effect of age	Reference
Absorption	Slight delayed	(9)
Distribution to tissue	Decreased distribution volume	(3)
Protein binding (20%)	Unchanged	(10)[a]
Binding to receptor	Probably normal	(11)[a]
Inotropic effect	Decreased	(11)[a], (12)
Toxic arrhythmias	Unchanged	(12)
Plasma half-life	Increased	(5)
Renal excretion	May be decreased	(3)

From Opie, Mabin and Meiring (48), with permission.
[a]Animal studies.

Another important aspect of digoxin usage is the tendency to toxic effects, probably made more marked by the greater tendency to myocardial ischaemia in the elderly with a consequent greater risk of arrhythmias. Hence, in elderly patients receiving digoxin, toxicity should be considered as an important risk (4). The symptoms of digoxin toxicity in the elderly are often diffuse and difficult to diagnose.

A simple table showing the relation between creatinine clearance and the daily dose of digoxin in the elderly has been proposed by Whiting *et al.* (5). It should be noted that the 'traditional' half-tablet of digoxin daily for the elderly patient is only justified if the creatinine clearance falls below 25 ml/min, which implies significant renal impairment.

β-Blockers

β-Blockade is, in fact, a permissible form of therapy for the elderly hypertensive. Propranolol has specific problems stemming from the low cardiac output and its poor renal perfusion, with a diminished first-pass effect and hence with an unexpected accumulation in the blood. This may compensate for a decreased β-receptor density (Table 2), but there is also risk of hepatic interaction with other drugs that might be used in the elderly.

A simple pharmacokinetic pattern without hepatic metabolism is less likely to cause unexpected variations in blood levels of β-blocking agents and to have fewer risks of interactions with other drugs, including nicotine. Renal-excreted β-blockers, such as atenolol, nadolol and celiprolol, with high-water and low-lipid solubility, would seem to be the preferred agents. The doses need downward adjustment when GFRs fall, but the fall has to be severe to alter drug excretion rates. Thus, GFR should fall below 25–30 ml/min before the dose of water-soluble β-blockers needs reduction. β-Blockers such as celiprolol and pindolol are more likely to maintain a normal cardiac output in the elderly and, therefore, to avoid the effects of poor hepatic blood flow. However, these assumptions need confirmation and testing.

Table 2. Propranolol pharmacokinetics in the elderly

Process	Effect of age	Reference
Absorption	Probably delayed	—
Hepatic metabolism	Diminished metabolism	(13)
Bioavailability	Increased	(14)
Receptor sensitivity	Decreased	(14)
Lymphocyte receptor density	Decreased	(15)

Table 3. Effect of age on pharmacokinetics of calcium antagonists

Drug	Effect	Recommendation	Reference
Amlodipine	Clearance decreased	Modest dose decrease	(16), (17)
Diltiazem	Clearance decreased	Decrease dose	(18)
Isradipine	Clearance decreased or unchanged	Dose unchanged or decreased[a]	(19), (20), (21)
Nicardipine	Clearance decreased or unchanged	Dose unchanged or decreased[a]	(22), (23)
Nifedipine	Clearance decreased	Decrease dose	(24), (25)
Verapamil	Clearance decreased	Decrease dose	(26), (27)

[a]In 'young' elderly.

Calcium antagonists

The major effect of ageing on the kinetics of the calcium antagonists is shown in Table 3. It should be noted that in general calcium antagonists are lipid-soluble agents which are highly metabolized in the liver and, therefore, with age they are likely to accumulate unless the dose is somewhat reduced. Very much depends on whether one is dealing with the 'young elderly' who seem to have normal clearance rates, or the 'truly elderly' in whom the clearance rates are reduced and the doses should also be reduced. Although data are not available on all calcium antagonists, it is clear that the trend shown in Table 3 indicates that clearance of the calcium antagonist is very likely to be decreased, so that a dose reduction may be required. The magnitude of the dose reduction may vary from patient to patient and is a matter of dose titration while observing the antihypertensive effect and the side-effects.

Angiotensin-converting enzyme inhibitors

In general, these agents have reduced clearance because they are metabolized by the liver and the products of metabolism excreted by the kidneys. There are basically three types of agents.

First, captopril is an agent already in the active form which undergoes metabolism in plasma to mixed disulphides (6). Captopril and its disulphides are excreted chiefly (75%) by the kidneys and the rest (16%) in faeces. Captopril is actively secreted by the kidneys, with renal clearance values more than double those of the GFR. In the elderly, there are no special changes in the pharmacokinetics (7) in patients with relatively well-preserved renal function. In case of severe renal impairment, dose reduction would be required.

Second, prodrugs like enalapril are converted in the liver to active forms such as enalaprilat. Such active diacids are then excreted by the kidney, so that if there is renal impairment associated with ageing the blood concentration of the active form tends to increase. An exception is fosinoprilat—the active form of fosinopril—which is dually excreted by bile and urine, so that dose reduction in the elderly is not needed for this agent.

Third, agents like lisinopril undergo no metabolism, are water soluble, and are excreted by the kidneys in relation to the creatinine clearance. Therefore, if renal function falls with age, a corresponding dose reduction is required.

Thus, in general, excretion of active forms of ACE inhibitors is by the kidneys, so that the dose of ACE inhibitors in elderly subjects may either be unchanged or decreased depending on renal function (Table 4).

Antiarrhythmic agents (Table 5)

In general, such agents should be used only when there are specific indications such as life-threatening symptomatic arrhythmias. Most antiarrhythmic agents are metabolized in the liver and then excreted in the urine. A reduced cardiac output with reduced hepatic blood flow or decreased renal function could change the pharmacokinetic patterns and lead to dose reduction. There appear to be few changes that occur simply as the result of the ageing process itself.

Effects of ageing on other drugs

These are shown in Table 6. In general, doses should be lower to allow for various kinetic changes with age. In the case of the β_2-agonists, dose reduction may be required because of an increased vasodilator response (8).

Drug interactions

As in younger patients, drug interactions can occur. Because such interactions are the result of complex pharmacokinetic interactions or added pharmacodynamic effects, there is a somewhat greater risk of drug interactions in the elderly. When the interactions do occur, they are also likely to be more serious. Hence, greater caution with multiple drug therapy is required in the elderly than in younger patients.

Table 4. Pharmacokinetics of ACE inhibitors in the elderly

Drug	Change	Recommendation	Reference
1. *Captopril*			
Captopril	Small fall in renal clearance	No change in dose, or slight reduction	(7)
2. *Prodrugs*			
Cilazapril	Reduced clearance; higher plasma levels	Usually no change; may need small dose reduction	(28)
Enalapril	Reduced clearance	Check renal function; check hepatic function; may need dose reduction	(29), (30)
Fosinopril	None (small 11% increase in area under the curve)	No change in dose	Manufacturer's data
Perindopril	Reduced clearance, increased area under the curve, higher perindoprilat values; increased bioavailability	Reduce dose by half	(31)
Ramipril	Reduced clearance; higher ramiprilat values	Reduce dose	(32)
3. *Lisinopril-like agents* (water-soluble, not metabolized)			
Lisinopril	Reduced renal clearance in relation to creatinine clearance	Check renal function; may need dose reduction	(33)

SUMMARY

In summary, for most of the drugs there is a potential dose reduction in elderly patients. This is largely dependent on decreases in hepatic and renal blood flow and function. However, it should be borne in mind that many 'younger' elderly patients have normal hepatic and renal haemodynamics and therefore require normal doses. Often dose reduction is automatically applied in elderly patients without considering whether such a reduction is appropriate. Conversely, if dose reduction is not applied when it should be applied, there is a risk of cardiac or other toxicity. Therefore, it is wise to obtain indices of hepatic and renal function, as well as to estimate the cardiovascular status of elderly patients before giving them drugs which are metabolized by liver or kidney. The simplest drugs to use are those which do not undergo hepatic metabolism and primarily depend on renal excretion, such as digoxin, atenolol or lisinopril.

Table 5. Pharmacokinetics of antiarrhythmic agents in the elderly

Antiarrhythmic agent	Change	Recommendation	Reference
Class 1A			
Quinidine	Decreased renal and total clearance	Dose reduction	(34), (35)
Procainamide	Decreased renal excretion of procainamide; increased blood levels	Dose reduction	(11)
Disopyramide	Half the drug is excreted in the unchanged form in the urine	Dose reduction if renal impaired	(36), (37)
Class 1B			
Lidocaine	Decreased clearance with age	Dose reduction	(35), (38)
Tocainamide	40% excreted unchanged in the urine; elimination half-life may be increased	Consider dose reduction	—
Phenytoin	Decreased rate of hepatic metabolism with increased plasma concentration	Consider dose reduction	(39)
Moricizine	Undergoes liver metabolism followed by renal excretion; these processes may be impaired in the elderly	Dose reduction may be considered	Manufacturer's information (40)
Mexiletine	High rate of hepatic metabolism; may accumulate in blood if output reduced	Consider dose reduction	
Class 1C			
Propafenone	High rate of hepatic metabolism in dominant genetic phenotype is followed by renal excretion of metabolites; there are no special age-related changes	Dose usually unchanged	USA package insert
Encainide	Predominant hepatic metabolism; no special changes in the elderly	Dose unchanged or reduced	(41)
Flecainide	About one-third excreted unchanged in kidneys with rest metabolized in liver; should therefore be safe in the elderly	Dose unchanged	(42)
Class 2			
Propranolol	Increased plasma levels due to depressed rate of hepatic metabolism; refer to Table 1		
Class 3			
Amiodarone	If decreased renal function, iodine may accumulate with risk of hypothyroidism	Dose reduction	(41)
Sotalol	Water-soluble, high rate of renal excretion, therefore plasma levels will increase if there is renal failure	Consider dose reduction	(43)
Class 4			
Verapamil	Decreased clearance due to decreased liver blood flow	Dose reduction	(26), (27), (44)

Table 6. Effects of ageing on other drugs

Drug	Effect of age	Reference
β_1-Agonists	Decreased chronotropic response	(45), (46)
	Decreased inotropic response	(46), (12)
β_2-Agonists	Increased vasodilator response	(8)
Nitroprusside	Greater fall in blood pressure during infusion	(1)
Warfarin	Greater depression of clotting factors	(47)

REFERENCES

1. Ouslander JG (1981) Drug therapy in the elderly. *Ann Intern Med* **95**: 711–722.
2. Topol EJ, Nicklas JM, Kander MH *et al.* (1988) Coronary revascularization after intravenous tissue plasminogen activator for unstable angina pectoris: results of a randomized, double-blind placebo-controlled trial. *Am J Cardiol* **62**: 368–371.
3. Ewy GA, Kapadia GG, Yao L (1969) Digoxin metabolism in the elderly. *Circulation* **39**: 449–453.
4. Dall JLC (1970) Maintenance digoxin in elderly patients. *Br Med J* **2**: 705–706.
5. Whiting B, Wandless I, Summer DJ, Goldberg A (1978) A computer-assisted review of digoxin therapy in the elderly. *Br Heart J* **40**: 8–13.
6. Punzi HA, Zusman RM (1990) Specific angiotensin-converting enzyme inhibitors. In *Cardiovascular Drug Therapy*, Messerli FH (ed.). Saunders, Philadelphia, pp. 770–791.
7. Creasey WA, Funke PT, McKinstry DN, Sugerman AA (1986) Pharmacokinetics of captopril in elderly healthy male volunteers. *J Clin Pharmacol* **26**: 264–268.
8. Kendall MJ, Woods KL, Wilkins MR, Worthington DJ (1982) The effects of age are cardioselective. *Br J Clin Pharmacol* **14**: 821–826.
9. Causack B, Kelly J, O'Malley K *et al.* (1979) Digoxin in the elderly: pharmacokinetic consequences of old age. *Clin Pharmacol Ther* **25**: 772–776.
10. Berman W Jr, Musselman J (1979) The relationship of age to the metabolism and protein binding of digoxin in sheep. *J Pharmacol Exp Ther* **208**: 263–266.
11. Gerstenblith G, Spurgeon HA, Froehlich JP *et al.* (1979) Diminished inotropic responsiveness to ouabain in aged rat myocardium. *Circ Res* **44**: 517–523.
12. Guarnieri T, Spurgeon HA, Froehlich JP *et al.* (1979) Diminished inotropic responses but unaltered toxicity to acetylbrophanthidin in the senescent beagle. *Circulation* **60**: 1548–1554.
13. Castleden CM, George CF (1979) The effect of ageing on the hepatic clearance of propranolol. *Br J Clin Pharmacol* **7**: 49–54.
14. Vestal RE, Wood AJ, Shand DG (1979) Reduced beta-adrenoceptor sensitivity in the elderly. *Clin Pharmacol Ther* **26**: 181–186.
15. Schocken DD, Roth GS (1977) Reduced beta-adrenergic receptor concentrations in ageing man. *Nature* **267**: 856–858.
16. Elliott HL, Meredith PA, Reid JL, Faulkner JK (1988) A comparison of the disposition of single oral doses of amlodipine in young and elderly subjects. *J Cardiovasc Pharmacol* **12** (Suppl. 7): S64–S66.
17. Abernethy DR, Gutkowska J, Winterbottom LM (1990) Effects of amlodipine, a long-acting dihydropyridine calcium antagonist in aging hypertension: pharmacodynamics in relation to disposition. *Clin Pharmacol Ther* **48**: 76–86.
18. Echizen H, Eichelbaum M (1986) Clinical pharmacokinetics of verapamil, nifedipine

and diltiazem. *Clin Pharmacokinet* **11**: 425–449.

19. Schran HF, Jaffe JM, Gonasun LM (1988) Clinical pharmacokinetics of isradipine. *Am J Med* **84** (Suppl. 3B): 80–89.
20. Rowe JW (1988) Approach to the treatment of hypertension in older patients: preliminary results with isradipine. *Am J Med* **84** (Suppl. 3B): 46–50.
21. Chellingsworth MC, Willis JV, Broadfoot D *et al.* (1988) Pharmacokinetics and pharmacodynamics of israpidine (PN 200–110) in young and elderly patients. *Am J Med* **84** (Suppl. 3B): 72–79.
22. Forette F, Bellet M, Henry JF *et al.* (1985) Effect of nicardipine in elderly hypertensive patients. *Br J Clin Pharmacol* **20** (Suppl. 1): 125S–129S.
23. Brown ST, Freedman D, DeVault GA *et al.* (1985) Elderly Multicenter Study Group: safety, efficacy and pharmacokinetics of nicardipine in elderly hypertensive patients. *Br J Clin Pharmacol* **22** (Suppl.): 289S–295S.
24. Scott M, Castleden CM, Adam HK *et al.* (1988) The effect of ageing on the disposition of nifedipine and atenolol. *Br J Clin Pharmacol* **25**: 289–296.
25. Robertson DRC, Waller DG, Renwick AG *et al.* (1988) Age-related changes in the pharmacokinetics and pharmacodynamics of nifedipine. *Br J Clin Pharmacol* **25**: 297–305.
26. Storstein L, Larsen A, Midtbo K *et al.* (1983) Pharmacokinetics of calcium blockers in patients with renal insufficiency and in geriatric patients. *Acta Med Scand* (Suppl. 681): 25–30.
27. Cox JP, O'Boyle CA, Mee F *et al.* (1988) The antihypertensive efficacy of verapamil in the elderly evaluated by ambulatory blood pressure measurement. *J Hum Hypertens* **2**: 41–47.
28. Williams PEO, Brown AN, Rajaguru S *et al.* (1989) A pharmacokinetic study of cilazapril in elderly and young volunteers. *Br J Clin Pharmacol* **27**: 211S–215S.
29. Hockings N, Ajayi LAA, Reid JL (1985) The effects of age on the pharmacokinetics and dynamics of the angiotensin converting enzyme inhibitors enalapril and enalaprilat. *Br J Clin Pharmacol* **20**: 262P–263P.
30. Lees, KR, Reid JL (1987) Age and the pharmacokinetics and pharmacodynamics of chronic enalapril treatment. *Clin Pharmacol Ther* **41**: 597–602.
31. Lees KR, Green ST, Reid JL (1988) Influence of age on the pharmacokinetics and pharmacodynamics of perindopril. *Clin Pharmacol Ther* **44**: 418–425.
32. Gilchrist WJ, Beard K, Manhem P *et al.* (1987) Pharmacokinetics and effects on the renin–angiotensin system of ramipril in elderly patients. *Am J Cardiol* **59**: 28D–32D.
33. Gautam PC, Vargas E, Lye M (1987) Pharmacokinetics of lisinopril (MK 521) in health young and elderly subjects and in elderly patients with cardiac failure. *J Pharm Pharmacol* **39**: 929–931.
34. Ochs HR, Greenblatt DJ, Woo E, Smith TW (1978) Reduced quinidine clearance in elderly persons. *Am J Cardiol* **42**: 481–485.
35. Drayer DE, Hughes M, Lorenzo B, Reidenberg M (1980) Prevalence of high (3*S*)-3-hydroxyquinidine/quinidine ratios in serum, and clearance of quinidine in cardiac patients with age. *Clin Pharmacol Ther* **27**: 72–75.
36. Burk M, Peters U (1983) Disopyramidine kinetics in renal impairment: determinants of interindividual variability. *Clin Pharmacol Ther* **34**: 331–340.
37. Garrett ER, Hinderling PH (1975) Pharmacokinetics of disopyramide in healthy human subjects (Abstract). *Clin Pharmacol Ther* **17**: 234.
38. Nation RI, Triggs EJ, Selig M (1977) Lignocaine kinetics in cardiac patients and aged subjects. *Br J Clin Pharmacol* **4**: 439–448.
39. Bauer LA, Blouin RA (1982) Age and phenytoin kinetics in adult epileptics. *Clin Pharmacol Ther* **31**: 301–304.
40. Prescott LF, Pottage A, Clements JA (1977) Absorption, distribution and elimination

of mexiletine. *Postgrad Med J* **53** (Suppl. 1): 50–55.

41. Schneeweiss A (1990) Cardiovascular therapy in the elderly. In *Cardiovascular Drug Therapy*, Messerli FH (ed.). Saunders, Philadelphia, pp. 140–180.

42. Singh BN, Opie LH, Marcus FI (1991) Antiarrhythmic agents. In *Drugs for the Heart*, 3rd edn, Opie LH (ed.). Saunders, Philadelphia, pp. 180–216.

43. Ishizaki T, Hirayama H, Tawara K *et al.* (1980) Pharmacokinetics and pharmacodynamics in young normal and elderly hypertensive subjects: a study using sotalol as a model drug. *J Pharmacol Exp Ther* **212**: 173–181.

44. Freedman SB, Richmond DR, Ashley JJ, Kelly DT (1981) Verapamil kinetics in normal subjects and patients with coronary artery spasm. *Clin Pharmacol Ther* **30**: 644–652.

45. Yin FCP, Spurgeon HA, Raizes GS *et al.* (1976) Age-associated decrease in chronotropic response to isoproterenol (Abstract). *Circulation* **54**: II–167.

46. Cokkinos DV, Tsartsalis GD, Heimonas ET, Gardikas CD (1980) Comparison of the inotropic action of digitalis and isoproterenol in younger and older individuals. *Am Heart J* **100**: 802–806.

47. Shepherd AM, Hewick DS, Moreland TA, Stevenson IH (1977) Age as a determinant of sensitivity to warfarin. *Br J Clin Pharmacol* **4**: 315–320.

48. Opie LH, Mabin TA, Meiring P de V (1984) Medical treatment of cardiovascular disease in the elderly. In *Cardiovascular Disease in the Elderly*, Messerli F (ed.). Kluwer Academic, Boston, 3rd Ed, pp. 473–497.

Part IV

SYSTEMATIC DISEASES

16 Hypertension in the Elderly

JOHN F. POTTER AND MARTIN D. FOTHERBY
Leicester General Hospital, Leicester, UK

EPIDEMIOLOGY: BLOOD PRESSURE CHANGES WITH AGE

In Westernized populations blood pressure (BP) rises with increasing years, although this cannot be accepted as a normal corollary of ageing as no such changes are seen in secluded or more primitive societies, where BP tends to remain constant or even show a decline with advancing age (1)

Cross-sectional studies from the UK (2) and USA (3,4) have shown a near-linear rise in systolic blood pressure (SBP) with age up to 80 years, men tending to have lower values than women after the age of 50 years (see Figure 1). For diastolic blood pressure (DBP) a similar trend is seen although the peak values tend to occur earlier and, for males over the age of 60 years, DBP plateaus and then declines. Longitudinal studies of the Framingham cohort revealed a different pattern, with DBP for men being consistently higher (by about 5 mmHg) than that for women for all age groups. Systolic blood pressure, however, showed a similar increase for both sexes, there being little difference in age-related values. Whilst the sex differences in DBP may be explained by selective mortality (higher mortality rates occurring in those with higher BPs, especially in males) resulting in an under-representation of those with initially elevated BPs in the older age groups, longitudinal studies have shown similar BP changes with age. Thus the plateauing of DBP over the age of 60 is probably a real effect and the continued rise in SBP in both sexes probably just reflects the decrease in arterial compliance with age.

PREVALENCE

Any definition of 'hypertension' or 'old age' is completely arbitrary as both are continuous variables, there being no clear cut-off point for defining a sudden change in risk. In the Framingham study the prevalence of definite hypertension (defined as SBP > 160 mmHg and/or DBP > 95 mmHg or on antihypertensive treatment) for the age range 65–94 years was 39% for men and 48% for women (5). The distribution of elderly hypertensives between those defined as having combined (BP > 160/95 mmHg), isolated systolic and isolated diastolic hyperten-

Geriatric Cardiology. Principles and Practice. Edited by A. Martin and A. J. Camm
© 1994 John Wiley & Sons Ltd

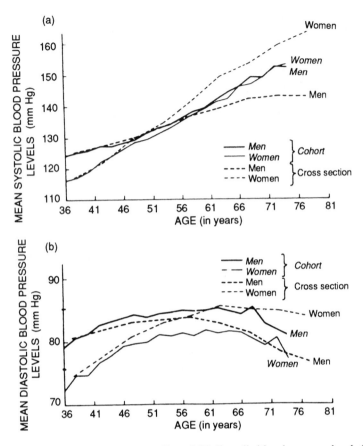

Figure 1. Average age trends in (a) systolic and (b) diastolic blood pressure levels for men and women based on cross-sectional (dotted lines) and longitudinal (cohort, unbroken lines) data on participants in the Framingham study. Reproduced from Volkonas *et al.* (5) with permission from *Current Science*

sion (SBP < 160 mmHg; DBP > 95 mmHg) in the Framingham study is shown in Figure 2. Similar figures have been obtained in the UK; a large general practice screening study of 10 732 persons aged 60–79 years found 44% had a SBP > 160 mmHg and/or a DBP > 90 mmHg (6).

When BP is remeasured on further examinations higher values tend to fall and estimates of 'definite' sustained hypertension are therefore lower; values of about 13% for men and 16% for women over the age of 65 years have been reported (7).

Isolated systolic hypertension

The rise with age in SBP is greater than that for DBP, and isolated systolic hypertension (ISH) (defined as SBP > 160 mmHg and DBP < 90–95 mmHg)

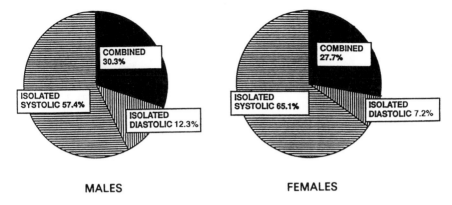

MALES   FEMALES

Figure 2. Distribution of hypertensives (65–89 years). From Kannel (8) with permission

accounts for more than half the cases of hypertension in males and two-thirds in females over the age of 65 years (8). The results of a recent meta-analysis of 12 studies (9) assessing the prevalence of ISH in the general population is shown in Figure 3. After repeated BP measurements the prevalence of ISH in those over 60 years decreases from 14.1% to 9.5% (10) and on ambulatory BP measurements an even greater decline in prevalence is found (11). It has been suggested that the prevalence of ISH is falling in the elderly with time; for women aged 65–74 years in the NHANES study there has been a reduction from over 23% in 1961 to just under 14% in 1972, with a similar trend being found in men (12). A more recent retrospective analysis did not find a decrease in the prevalence of ISH over the last two decades, however (9).

RISKS OF HYPERTENSION IN THE ELDERLY

Total mortality

Cardiovascular disease is the most common cause of mortality in persons over the age of 65 years. The 1979 Blood Pressure Study using insurance data demonstrated a positive and independent relationship between mortality, SBP and DBP for both sexes and in all age groups studied (13).

Overall mortality rates obtained from the Framingham data were more than doubled and cardiovascular mortality tripled for those aged >65 years with definite hypertension compared to an age/sex-matched normotensive group (8). However, for the very old (>80 years), the adverse effects of an elevated BP on mortality are not so convincing, some studies even reporting an inverse relationship between SBP, DBP and mortality (14–16).

Cardiovascular disease

A recent meta-analysis of prospective observational studies of individuals aged 25–84 years found a positive and almost linear relationship between casual DBP

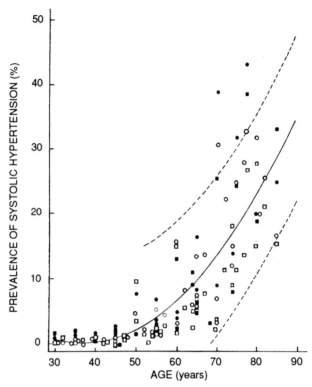

Figure 3. Prevalence of isolated systolic hypertension by the mid-point of the age classes reported in various studies. The 95% confidence interval for the prediction of individual points is presented for the age range 50–90 years. □, white males; ■, black males; ○, white females; ●, black females. Reproduced from Staessen *et al.* (9) with permission from *Current Science*

and the risk of stroke and coronary heart disease (CHD), with no evidence of a threshold effect for DBP levels down to 75 mmHg (17). A 5 mmHg increase in DBP has been shown to be associated with a 34% increase in stroke and a 21% increase in CHD risk. Similarly for SBP the Framingham study showed that the risk of cardiovascular events increased progressively with SBP levels, with no threshold effect (5).

   Although the age-adjusted risk ratio for cardiovascular events is lower in elderly hypertensives, because cardiovascular disease is so prevalent in this age group the absolute risk is greater (see Figure 4). It has been shown from Framingham data that the risk of developing congestive heart failure is closely associated with hypertension, being six times greater in hypertensive than normotensive subjects, the absolute risk increasing with age (18). After age, hypertension is the main predisposing factor for stroke, particularly athero-thrombotic brain infarction, for all age groups from 45 to 74 years (19).

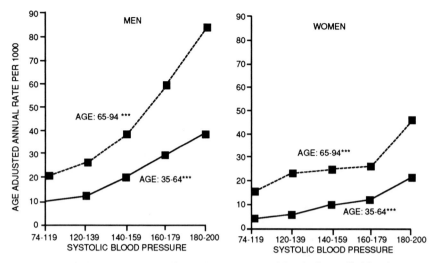

Figure 4. Risk of cardiovascular disease by age, sex and level of systolic blood pressure, from a 30-year follow-up in the Framingham study. ***$p < 0.001$ (Wald statistic for logistic regression analysis). Reproduced from Volkonas *et al.* (5) with permission from *Current Science*

Hypertensive subjects in the Chicago Stroke Study aged 65–74 years showed a significant increased incidence of stroke, the 3-year incidence in those with SBP > 179mmHg being three times greater than in those with SBP < 130 mmHg (20).

It has been estimated that hypertension in the elderly is responsible for 33% of all cases of cardiac disease, 42% of strokes in elderly men and 70% of strokes in elderly women.

Risk of isolated systolic hypertension

Mortality

Although both SBP and DBP predict cardiovascular risk in the elderly, the relationship is much stronger for systolic than diastolic BP (21). A study of Dutch civil servants aged 40–65 years showed total mortality for men with ISH to be more than twice that for normotensive subjects after 25 years of follow-up (22). Similar results were obtained from the Framingham cohort in a 20-year follow-up, with a twofold increase in total mortality for men and women with ISH compared to normotensives, most of this excess being due to cardiovascular disease (23). Results from several other studies suggests mortality from cardiovascular disease is between five and seven times higher in subjects with ISH compared to normotensives (24). Garland *et al.* (25) found that males with ISH had an excess risk of death from stroke (relative risk 4.0) and the Chicago Stroke

Study found a 2.5 times greater incidence of stroke in those with ISH compared to normotensives (20).

BENEFITS OF ANTIHYPERTENSIVE THERAPY IN THE ELDERLY

Clinical trials

Evidence abounds that hypertension is a risk factor for cardiovascular morbidity and mortality in the elderly, although this does not necessarily infer that treatment of an elevated BP will be beneficial. There are in fact many anecdotal reports of antihypertensive therapy having serious adverse effects in this age group (26). It is only relatively recently that the results of trials specifically assessing the effects of antihypertensive treatment in the elderly have been published. Up until then the only data available were from subgroup analysis of larger studies which were not directly aimed at the 65 + age group and therefore based on very small numbers.

Randomized intervention trials in the elderly

Five major randomized intervention trials wholly consisting of persons over the age of 60 years will be considered in addition to four other trials which included subjects over 60 years.

The prospective study of the Treatment of Mild Hypertension in the Aged by Kuramoto et al. enrolled 91 patients, mean age 76 years, who were followed for up to 4 years (27). After randomization to placebo or thiazide, BP differences after 2 years between the groups were small (5/2 mmHg). Only when eight placebo group patients who were withdrawn from the study as their BP exceeded 200/110 mmHg were included in the analysis of fatal and non-fatal cardiovascular events was there a statistically significant benefit seen with active treatment.

Sprackling et al.'s open randomized trial of methyldopa in the elderly enrolled 120 subjects (DBP > 100 mmHg), mostly female with a mean age of 80 years, into an observed only or a treated group (28). Antihypertensive treatment did not decrease mortality or non-fatal cardiovascular events. There are many statistical problems in interpreting these two studies as both were small and the number of trial end-points few, limiting the likelihood of demonstrating a statistically significant effect of antihypertensive treatment.

In 1985 the results of the European Working Party in Hypertension in the Elderly (EWPHE Trial) became available; 840 patients aged over 60 years (mean age 72 years, range 60–80 + years) were entered if sitting SBP was between 160 and 239mmHg and DBP between 90 and 119mmHg (29). Subjects initially received hydrochlorothiazide plus triamterene or matching placebo in a double-blind randomized fashion. After 3 years BP fell in the active treatment group from 183/101 to 149/85 mmHg (placebo group BP fell from 182/101 to 172/94 mmHg). After a $4\frac{1}{2}$-year follow-up period the actively treated group showed a significant reduction in cardiovascular mortality (-27%, $p = 0.037$), mainly due to a 60% reduction in deaths from myocardial infarction, but a non-significant reduction in overall mortality (-9%, $p = 0.41$) and cerebrovascular deaths (-32%, $p = 0.16$). Cardiovascular mortality rose with increasing baseline SBP but not DBP. The main benefits of active treatment were seen in patients under 80 years of age, but were independent of sex and cardiovascular complications at randomization. However, as most patients were recruited from hospital outpatient clinics, results may not be applicable to the elderly population in general.

Coope and Warrender, in their trial of Hypertensive Elderly Patients (HEP) in general practice, randomized 884 patients aged 60–79 years (SBP > 170 mmHg or DBP > 105 mmHg on two occasions) to either treatment (atenolol with or without bendrofluazide) or an observation group (30). During the $4\frac{1}{2}$ years of follow-up there was an average BP difference of 18/11 mmHg between the groups. Those actively treated had a significant reduction in fatal and total strokes, but not myocardial infarction, with a trend to lower total and cardiovascular mortality, but this did not reach statistical significance.

The Systolic Hypertension in the Elderly Project (SHEP) is the first trial to test the efficacy of antihypertensive drug treatment on clinical endpoints for persons with ISH (31). It recruited subjects over 60 years with SBP > 160 mmHg and DBP < 90 mmHg into a double-blind randomized trial of chlorthalidone 12.5 mg daily or placebo. Of the 447 921 screened, just over 1% (4736) were recruited. The 5-year mean reduction in BP in the treated versus placebo group was 12/4 mmHg. Active treatment reduced the incidence of stroke by 36% and on an intention-to-treat basis the 5-year cumulative stroke rates were 5.2 per 100 participants in the actively treated group and 8.2 per 100 for placebo. The benefit of treatment may be even greater than suggested as 35% of the placebo group received antihypertensive drugs during the trial. Treatment was equally effective in those over or under 80 years of age, unlike the results of the EWPHE study. Overall mortality was reduced by 13% in the treated group but this difference was not statistically significant. Fatal and non-fatal cardiovascular events were reduced by 32% in the active treatment group, with a 5-year absolute benefit of 55 events per 1000 participants. Total CHD events were reduced by 25% but total cardiovascular mortality was not significantly affected, in contrast to the EWPHE study where it was significantly reduced by 38%.

The Swedish Trial in Old Patients with Hypertension (STOP-Hypertension) recruited 1627 patients aged 70–84 years with an SBP > 180 mmHg and DBP 90–105 mmHg and randomized them to treatment with a β-blocker and/or thiazide diuretic compared to placebo (32). After 4 years the mean difference in blood pressure between the active and placebo groups was 27/10 mmHg, with a mean duration of follow-up of 25 months. The actively treated group showed significant reduction in cardiovascular and total mortality (-43%), stroke events (-46%) and cardiovascular events (-40%) but no significant reductions in myocardial infarction (-13%) or sudden death (-50%) rates. It was estimated that 14 elderly hypertensive patients would need treatment for 5 years to prevent one stroke and one death.

The Medical Research Council trial of treatment of hypertension in older adults enrolled 4396 patients from general practices aged 65–74 years with SBP 160–204 mmHg and DBP < 115 mmHg (33). They were randomized to atenolol 50 mg daily, hydrochlorothiazide 25 mg or 50 mg plus amiloride 2.5 mg or 5.0 mg, or placebo, and followed up for an average of 5.8 years. Blood pressure in the active group fell by 15/6 mmHg compared to the placebo group. Actively treated subjects had a 25% reduction in stroke ($p = 0.04$) and a 17% reduction in all cardiovascular events ($p = 0.03$). There was a non-significant reduction in coronary events of 19%. On treatment analysis showed those treated with diuretic had a significant reduction in stroke (31%; $p = 0.04$), coronary events (44%; $p < 0.001$) and all cardiovascular events (35%; $p < 0.001$) compared with placebo. Those treated with β-blocker showed no significant reduction in fatal stroke or total coronary events, or in all cardiovascular events or death. It was also found that the reduction in strokes in the actively treated subjects was confined to non-smokers.

The following trials also included elderly subgroups as part of larger studies.

The Veterans Administration Cooperative Study of mild to moderate hypertension (DBP 90–114 mmHg) recruited men under 75 years of age to a double-blind randomized trial using hydrochlorothiazide, reserpine and hydralazine (33A). After a 3.3 years' follow-up of the 81 subjects aged 60–75 years, 38 of whom received active treatment, there was a significant 54% reduction in all cardiovascular events, due mainly to a reduction in left ventricular failure, but not in the incidence of myocardial infarction or sudden death. Those with the highest blood pressure and a previous history of cardiovascular disease benefited the most from treatment.

The Hypertension Stroke Cooperative Study (HSCS) recruited 452 stroke survivors under 75 years (mean age 59 years) to a reserpine/thiazide combination or placebo (34). After 3 years of follow-up in the 200 subjects aged over 60 years, total stroke recurrence and total cardiovascular endpoints were similar in the two groups. Overall, treatment reduced the incidence of congestive cardiac failure in stroke survivors but did not affect the risk of stroke recurrence, despite BP being 25/12 mmHg lower in the actively treated group.

The Hypertension Detection and Follow-up Programme (HDFP) (35) was not a placebo-controlled trial, but compared the effects of antihypertensive treatment (chlorthalidone) in a group receiving specialized care (Stepped Care—SC) with a group using normal facilities (Referred Care—RC). In the group aged 60–69 years 1204 subjects were in the SC group and 1172 in the RC group. The percentage reduction in 5-year mortality for the SC group (who had better control of their hypertension) compared to the RC group was 25.3% in those of 50–59 years and 16.4% for those in the 60–69 year age group. Total strokes were significantly reduced in the SC group compared to the RC group, with the 60–69 year age group having the greatest reduction in stroke rate.

In the Australian Therapeutic Trial in Mild Hypertension (DBP 95–109 mmHg and SBP < 200 mmHg) a subgroup of 582 men and women aged 60–69 years with average blood pressure 166/101 mmHg were randomized to placebo or chlorothiazide, with methyldopa, β-blocker or vasodilator being added as required (36). The mean DBP difference between the active and placebo-treated groups was 7 mmHg. After 4 years' follow-up, trial endpoints (death and cardiovascular disease) were significantly reduced by 39% in the actively treated group, mainly due to a reduction in ischaemic heart disease and stroke.

Meta-analysis of trials in elderly hypertensives

A recent meta-analysis (37) of all trials up to 1986 of anti-hypertensive therapy involving the elderly showed that overall treatment was beneficial with respect to reducing total cardiovascular mortality and morbidity, cerebrovascular events and incidence of congestive cardiac failure (see Table 1). In absolute terms treatment benefit increased with increasing age, baseline BP and presence of cardiovascular complications at entry. The results of the trials suggest that treating 100 elderly hypertensive patients for 5 years would prevent a cardiovascular event in at least 10 individuals.

PATHOPHYSIOLOGY

The predominant vascular changes seen with age are loss of the elastic lamina in the aorta and major vessels, increased atherosclerosis of the large and medium-sized arteries and hyaline degeneration of the arterioles, resulting in a decreased wall-to-lumen ratio. These changes result in a loss of arterial compliance and an increase in peripheral vascular resistance. Hyaline degeneration also occurs in the carotid and aortic baroreceptors, which may explain the age-related decrease in baroreceptor sensitivity (BRS), the greater BP variability

Table 1. The effects of antihypertensive therapy in elderly patients on various trial endpoints: results of a meta-analysis (excluding SHEP, STOP-hypertension and MCR trials). A negative sign indicates a reduction with treatment

Outcome	Difference in mortality with treatment		Difference in fatal and non-fatal events with treatment	
Cardiovascular	−28%	$p = 0.016$	41%	$p < 0.001$
Cerebrovascular	−41%	$p = 0.03$	−40%	$p < 0.001$
Coronary	−28%	n.s.	−7%	n.s.
Total	−14%	n.s.		

Reproduced from Staessen et al. (37).

Table 2. Pathophysiological changes in elderly hypertensives

---

1.   Vascular changes
      Large and medium-sized arteries: loss of elastic lamina atheroma
      Arterioles: hyaline degeneration leading to
      ↓ arterial compliance
      ↑ systemic vascular resistance
      ↓ baroreceptor sensitivity
2.   ↓ cardiac output
3.   ↓ intravascular volume
4.   ↓ renal blood flow
5.   ↑ renal vascular resistance
6.   ↓ plasma renin activity
7.   ↑ plasma noradrenaline levels
8.   ↓ β-adrenoceptor activity
    ?↓ α-adrenoceptor activity

---

and increased susceptibility to postural hypotension in the elderly hypertensive. However, although the effect of a rise in BP on BRS is well documented, definitive evidence for the independent effects of age are lacking.

The characteristic pathophysiological differences between young and old essential hypertensives (defined as DBP > 90 mmHg (38)) are shown in Table 2. Such differences also exist between young and elderly patients with ISH, the elderly demonstrating a lower cardiac index, left ventricular ejection rate and plasma volume but a higher vascular resistance than their younger counterparts (39). As SBP is determined by left ventricular stroke volume, peak ejection rate and distensibility of the arterial wall, it is not surprising that a greater rise in systolic than diastolic BP is seen with age.

Plasma renin levels and renal blood flow decrease with age; the fall in plasma resin activity (PRA) has been found to be more marked in elderly hypertensives than normotensives. The PRA response to sodium depletion, postural change and diuretics also decreases with age. The reasons for the decrease in PRA with increasing years is still unclear but may be related to a decrease in renal mass, hyaline degeneration of the afferent renal arterioles and a decrease in juxtaglomerular β-adrenergic receptor numbers and/or response. There is an age-related rise in muscle sympathetic activity and plasma noradrenaline (NA) levels, although there is little difference between plasma NA values found in elderly normotensive and hypertensive individuals. The reasons for the age-associated increase in plasma NA concentration have not been fully elucidated but are probably the result of increased spillover into the plasma rather than as a result of reduced NA clearance. Increasing age has been said to increase, decrease or not alter plasma adrenaline levels. We and others have found plasma adrenaline but not NA levels to be directly related to BP levels in the elderly (40).

Much controversy exists concerning the changes in adrenoreceptor function with age (41). Although it is accepted that β_1 and β_2-adrenoceptor activity decreases with age, the evidence for this has been questioned. It appears that

β-adrenoceptor density is probably unchanged with age but there is a decrease in postsynaptic response to β-adrenoceptor stimulation, probably resulting from multiple changes in the molecular and biochemical nature of the receptor coupling and postreceptor mechanisms. Similarly, data on the chronological changes in α-adrenoreceptor are scant but it appears that α_1 activity is probably unchanged although α_2 responsiveness may decrease.

DIAGNOSIS AND EVALUATION

As over one-third of the elderly population may be classified as hypertensive if only one BP reading is taken, it is essential that an accurate assessment of not only BP, but also evidence of target organ damage is made before treatment is started.

Blood pressure variability

BP levels vary on a short-, medium- and long-term basis. Minute-to-minute BP variations occur due to respiratory and vasomotor tone changes (42); over the 24-hour period BP changes are related to factors such as mental and physical activity (43), postprandial changes (44) and sleep (45). Seasonal variations also occur and are more marked in the old, BP levels being approximately 5 mmHg higher during the winter months (46). Hypertensive patients have a greater absolute BP variability (as measured by the standard deviation of the difference between hourly daytime BPs), although there is no difference compared to normotensive individuals when variability is related to baseline BP levels (47).

For an individual patient substantial variations between BPs taken during a clinic visit, as well as between clinic visits, are often encountered (48). A trend for an elevated BP to decrease with time has been noted in many placebo phases of intervention trials, e.g. 3 months after randomization in the EWPHE study BP fell in the placebo group by a mean of 7/3 mmHg, this effect being more pronounced in the older patients. The tendency for high BPs to fall with time is probably related mainly to two factors: regression to the mean, and familiarity with the surroundings and procedure of BP measurement. This emphasizes the need to take the BP on at least three occasions before thinking of initiating therapy in the majority of patients.

Blood pressure is often higher when taken in the clinic than away from it (49), and higher when taken by a doctor than another health worker (50). This alerting or pressor reaction, termed the 'white coat effect', occurs in both young and elderly patients (51,52), is not predictable (53) or related to anxiety levels (54) and is unaffected by antihypertensive treatment (55). The use of home BP or ambulatory BP monitoring may help distinguish between those who have high clinic BP due to the 'white coat' phenomenon and those who have sustained high BP both in and away from the clinic (56).

The standard deviation of the difference (as a measure of BP variability)

Table 3. Clinic and 24-hour ambulatory blood pressure (ABP) variability in elderly hypertensive subjects (mean age 76 years, $n = 22$) on repeating measurements after a median period of 9.9 weeks (range 4–43 weeks). SDD = standard deviation of the difference; CV = coefficient of variation; CR = coefficient of reproducibility

	Visit 1	Visit 2	Diff.	(SDD)	Cr (mmHg)	CV%
A SBP (mmHg)	151.3	151.7	−0.5	6.3	12.6	4.2
A DBP (mmHg)	86.1	84.8	1.3	4.8	9.6	5.6
C SBP (mmHg)	178.4	178.7	−0.3	17.4	34.8	9.7
C DBP (mmHg)	95.5	93.9	1.6	7.0	14.8	7.4

Table 4. Comparison of clinic and 24-hour blood pressure variability between younger (< 55 years, $n = 24$) and older (> 55 years, $n = 26$) patients with hypertension. Variability as defined as the standard deviation of all readings obtained during the 24-hour period

	Younger patients	Older patients
Casual SBP (mmHg)	143 ± 3	153 ± 3
Mean 24-hour SBP (mmHg)	135 ± 3	136 ± 3
Variability of SBP (mmHg)	15.2 ± 0.7	18.1 ± 0.8*
Casual DBP (mmHg)	96 ± 3	94 ± 2
Mean 24-hour DBP (mmHg)	89 ± 2	87 ± 2
Variability of DBP (mmHg)	12.5 ± 0.5	13.7 ± 0.6

Reproduced from Drayer *et al.* (57) with permission from the *American Journal of Medicine*.
*$p < 0.01$ young versus old.

between two 24-hour ambulatory blood pressure monitoring (ABPM) recordings in an elderly, mild to moderate hypertensive group compared to that of clinic BPs is shown in Table 3. ABPM gives a more precise and quicker means of establishing an individual's actual BP levels if at least 20 readings are obtained throughout the day. With advancing age the disparity between ambulatory and clinic pressures increases (see Table 4), but in general 80% of patients with suspected hypertension will have lower ambulatory than clinic BPs (57,58).

Twenty-four-hour BP profiling may also be of use in assessing aspects of cardiovascular risk. A recent study has shown that elderly hypertensive patients without a nocturnal fall in BP have a higher incidence of cardiovascular disease than those in whom BP falls during sleep (59). More prospective studies are, however, needed to confirm this finding.

However, intervention studies so far in elderly hypertensives have been based on clinic BP rather than ABPM values and as yet there are no set criteria for diagnosing hypertension in this age group on ABPM levels. This, along with the expense of the equipment, makes it difficult to recommend its routine use in clinical practice, although the procedure is well tolerated by the elderly.

Confirming hypertension

Further sources of variation or error in BP measurement can stem from the measurer. Initial measurements should be taken with the subject sitting (or supine) after at least 10 minutes' rest and in both arms, as 10% of the elderly may have a between-arm difference of > 10 mmHg. Blood pressure should also be taken after 2 minutes' standing as nearly all patients who are going to experience a significant and symptomatic orthostatic fall in BP will do so by this time. A cuff of adequate size is required; the width should be equal to about two-thirds of the distance from the axilla to the antecubital fossa, with the bladder placed over the brachial artery and encircling at least 80% of the arm. Using too small a cuff will lead to falsely elevated blood pressure readings. Palpating for disappearance of the radial pulse on cuff inflation provides an estimate of the systolic pressure, which should be exceeded by 10–20 mmHg before deflation at about 2 mmHg/s to allow determination of phases 1 and 5 Korotkoff sounds.

Pseudo-hypertension refers to falsely high readings caused by a rigid artery resisting collapse until high pressures are reached. Its incidence in a non-selected elderly population has been found to be very low (< 2%) (60).

In general for an asymptomatic patient with mild to moderate elevations of BP and no evidence of end organ damage, at least two readings plus a standing measurement should be taken on a minimum of three occasions over 2–3 months. If BPs are gradually settling more measurements can be taken over a further 3–6 months.

INVESTIGATIONS

Initial investigations of an elderly hypertensive patient should be similar to those conducted in younger persons. Blood tests should include a full blood count, plasma urea, creatinine, electrolytes, uric acid and glucose; an electrocardiogram (ECG) and chest radiograph should also be obtained. Estimation of serum cholesterol levels, echo-determined left ventricular mass and microalbuminuria may help management but cannot at present be considered routine investigations; they are discussed further below. Reversible secondary causes of hypertension are uncommon and further investigations are rarely justified. Atherosclerotic renal artery stenosis, the most frequent secondary cause, is considered later.

Assessment of target organ damage

The eyes, heart, brain and kidneys are the organs most vulnerable to the effects of hypertension, although it is often difficult to separate the effects of ageing from those of mild hypertension on these organs.

Eyes

Fundoscopic changes seen in mild hypertension are indistinguishable from those of ageing. It appears that fundoscopy is of no use in the assessment of mild to moderate hypertension. However, fundoscopy is important to identify flame-shaped haemorrhages, soft exudates and papilloedema indicating the presence of 'malignant' hypertension, and should be performed in the initial assessment of all patients with hypertension. Concomitant diabetic retinopathy will also therefore not be missed.

Cardiovascular system

In addition to congestive cardiac failure (CCF) and CHD, hypertension is the main precursor of left ventricular hypertrophy (LVH), there being a stronger relationship of LVH to SBP than DBP (61). The prevalence of ECG-determined LVH increases steeply with age from <2% in subjects aged 49–54 years to 10% in those aged 75–82 years (62). There is no decline in the relationship between ECG-diagnosed LVH and cardiovascular risk with age; 5-year mortality rates of 50% for men and 35% for women have been reported in the elderly (62).

Echocardiography is a more sensitive method than the ECG for detecting the presence of LVH. In the Framingham study there was a strong positive association between echo-diagnosed LVH and age, increasing from 6% in those under 30 years to 43% in the 70+ year age group, this relationship being independent of BP levels and obesity. In elderly hypertensives the prevalence of LVH on echo has been estimated to be as high as 60% (63).

Echo-determined LVH may identify a high-risk group benefiting from more aggressive therapy; unfortunately because of pulmonary disease, obesity and other technical factors, adequate echoes can only be obtained in about 60–70% of elderly patients (64).

Elderly hypertensives are at an increased risk of peripheral arterial disease, atheromatous renal artery stenosis, aortic dissection and fusiform abdominal aortic aneurysm. Palpation of peripheral pulses and abdomen and auscultation of major arteries, epigastrium and flanks for bruits should be undertaken in all elderly hypertensive patients.

Renal function

It can be difficult to determine whether hypertension has caused renal disease or has primarily arisen because of it, especially as the kidney in essential hypertension shows changes suggestive of an acceleration of the normal physiological ageing process (65).

Atheromatous renovascular hypertension (RVH) is the only major cause of secondary hypertension in the elderly. It must be suspected in those with abrupt onset or rapid progression of existing hypertension particularly in smokers and also in patients in whom BP is difficult to control with conventional therapy, especially in those with evidence of atherosclerotic diseases such as peripheral vascular and coronary artery disease (66). There are several screening tests available—abdominal ultrasound (looking for inequality of renal size) and intravenous urography along with more specific tests, including captopril isotope renography (67), peripheral vein renin response to single-dose captopril and, perhaps most helpful, intravenous digital subtraction angiography combined with differential renal vein renin determinations (68,69). If these tests suggest RVH, arteriography should be considered with a view to angioplasty.

Glomerular filtration rate (GFR) has been found to be maintained for a considerable period in hypertensive patients (65). The placebo group of the EWPHE study had stable serum creatinine levels over the 5-year follow-up period, while those in the treated group suffered more renal-related mortality and morbidity and had a significant increase in serum creatinine levels (70). Overall, the effects of mild essential hypertension on the ageing kidney do not appear to lead to major changes in serum creatinine levels (71,72). However, particularly in the elderly, a 'normal' serum creatinine level can be maintained despite GFR being reduced to 40% of normal.

Proteinuria detected by the dipstick method is a significant and independent risk factor for cardiovascular disease in hypertensive patients (73). Low-level albuminuria (microalbuminuria 20–200 μg/min) is strongly positively correlated with BP and in cross-sectional studies has been found to be associated with CHD and peripheral vascular disease (74). Whether microalbuminuria is a sensitive and early marker of elevated blood pressure levels and hypertension-induced renal and cardiovascular disease in the elderly is not yet known. A recent study from Denmark showed urinary microalbumin levels to be directly related to mortality in the elderly, along with male gender, serum creatinine levels and the presence of hypertension (75).

Other cardiovascular risk factors

In the overall assessment of a hypertensive patient it is important to take account of other cardiovascular risk factors and diseases present and current medications. Smoking remains a risk factor for cardiovascular mortality in the elderly (relative risk (RR) 2.0 for men and 1.6 for women), and the benefits of stopping in terms of total and cardiovascular mortality probably continue in those over 65 years (76,77).

The value of serum cholesterol levels in predicting cardiovascular or total mortality in elderly hypertensive persons has not been established. Serum cholesterol levels rise with age and remain a significant independent predictor of CHD mortality in elderly men (few studies have enrolled women) although no clear link with stroke has been established (78). Although the relative risk of serum cholesterol for CHD may decline with age the absolute risk will rise because of the increasing prevalence of CHD in the elderly. Follow-up data from the Whitehall Study suggest serum cholesterol measurement in middle age is a better predictor of death up to 80 years than is a level taken in later years (79). In the EWPHE study there was a negative association between serum total cholesterol and mortality (80). Even if elevated plasma cholesterol values did predict mortality, there is no evidence yet that reducing these plasma levels decreases the risk of cardiovascular morbidity or mortality. Therefore the value of measuring serum cholesterol levels in elderly hypertensive persons remains a debatable point.

Assessment of obesity, daily exercise taken, alcohol and dietary electrolyte intake (sodium and potassium) are required in order for non-pharmacological advice to be tailored to the individual. The strength of the association between obesity, measured as body mass index (BMI) (weight/[height]2) and hypertension declines with age (RR 5.6 for 20–45-year-olds; 1.9 for 45–75-year olds (81)). However, an increasing waist-to-hip ratio, as a measure of abdominal fat, is more strongly related to hypertension and is a better predictor of stroke and ischaemic heart disease than BMI (82). The relationship between dietary electrolyte intake and hypertension seems to increase with age (83). It has been estimated that for a 100 mmol per 24-hour increase in sodium intake mean BP increases 5 mmHg in those aged 19 years, but is double this in 60–69-year-olds.

TREATMENT

What level to treat

No rigid criteria should be given for starting antihypertensive drug treatment as circumstances vary from patient to patient. As a guideline the following is suggested. For an asymptomatic elderly person with established uncomplicated mild hypertension (SBP 160–185 mmHg, DBP 95–110 mmHg) non-pharmacological treatment should be commenced. If after a further 3–6 months of follow-up DBP remains > 90 mmHg and/or SBP > 60 mmHg antihypertensive drug treatment may for some patients be indicated along with non-pharmacological methods. For higher BPs drug treatment can be started earlier. If standing BPs are significantly lower than sitting or supine pressures, they should guide treatment to try and reduce symptoms of orthostatic hypotension.

What age to treat

Again, as biological ageing is very variable, no rigid criteria can be given. The EWPHE trial showed no benefit of hypotensive treatment after 80 years although the SHEP and STOP-Hypertension trials did. In general treatment is indicated up to the age of 80 years and, for those who are biologically young, treating until the mid-80s is reasonable.

Those with conditions aggravated by hypertension such as congestive cardiac failure or angina should have antihypertensive treatment at any age.

Special groups

Isolated systolic hypertension

Benefits of treating beyond 80 years of age have been shown for those with isolated systolic hypertension (ISH) (SBP > 160, DBP < 90 mmHg) (31). Non-pharmacological methods should be tried for 4–6 months in the first instance before resorting to drug therapy.

Stroke

There is good evidence that antihypertensive therapy reduces the incidence of primary stroke, although this is not the case for stroke recurrence where hypertension does not appear to be such a strong risk factor. The Hypertension Stroke Cooperative Study (34) found no significant difference in stroke recurrence between active treatment and placebo groups despite active treatment lowering SBP by 12 mmHg. A smaller study also found no benefit of antihypertensive treatment on stroke recurrence in subjects over 65 years, although stroke recurrence was reduced by 50% in those under 65 years on treatment (84).

For the first few days after a stroke BP often rises to high levels (85) although treatment is rarely indicated unless hypertensive encephalopathy is present. BP levels tend to fall spontaneously over the following few days although baseline levels may not be reached for 1–2 weeks. Antihypertensive treatment immediately following a stroke, particularly if it leads to rapid lowering of BP, can be disastrous (86). A chronic rise in BP is associated with an upward shift in the autoregulation of cerebral blood flow, leading to cerebral hypoperfusion if BP drops rapidly, even though the BP may still be in the 'normal range' (87). Following stroke regional blood flow and its regulation are further impaired, with the possibility of causing infarct extension if BP is lowered too quickly (88).

Non-pharmacological treatment

There are few studies which have examined the effect of non-pharmacological therapy on BP in the elderly. On theoretical grounds, and extrapolating from studies performed mostly in younger subjects, it is likely that the elderly will respond well to such measures.

Salt restriction

The BP fall to a given degree of salt restriction appears to increase with age. In subjects aged 50–59 years BP fell by 5–7 mmHg after a 50 mmol dietary sodium reduction (89). An overview of trials in all age groups found a BP reduction of 5/3 mmHg in hypertensive subjects with varying degrees of salt restriction (90). A reduction in sodium intake of 50 mmol/day can be achieved by avoiding salty foods and by not adding salt in cooking or at the table. Reducing salt added to processed foods, in addition to the above measures, would make even greater reductions.

Increasing dietary potassium intake

A recent trial in elderly untreated hypertensive patients (mean age 75 years) found that potassium supplementation of 60 mmol per day lowered clinic BP by 10/6 mmHg and 24-hour ambulatory BP by 6/2 mmHg (91). An overview of trials of potassium supplementation in hypertensives found an average fall in clinic BP of 8/5 mmHg (92). In addition to lowering BP higher potassium intakes may protect against stroke (93). The average intake of potassium in this country is 60–70 mmol per day; an intake of 100–110 mmol per day could be achieved by increasing the consumption of fresh fruit, vegetables and fruit drinks.

Weight reduction

Hypertensive patients have been shown to have initial BP reductions of 4/3 mmHg per kilogram weight loss (94). Ambulatory BP monitoring has shown that moderate weight loss (5% of BMI) in mild hypertensive patients reduces BP by 4/5 mmHg (95). On withdrawal of antihypertensive medications 60% of a middle-aged weight reduction group (mean weight loss 4.5 kg) maintained normotension compared to 35% of a control group not on a weight-reducing programme (96). The hypotensive effect appears to be independent of concurrent dietary changes such as reduction of sodium or energy intake and is additive to the effects of sodium restriction (97). However, the risk of obesity and benefits of weight reduction are less clear in the elderly. In the EWPHE study a U-shaped relationship between BMI and cardiovascular disease was noted; interestingly non-cardiovascular mortality decreased with increasing BMI (98). Other studies in the elderly have shown a similar association (99). It was suggested that weight reduction should be recommended to those with a BMI > 29 kg/m².

Alcohol

Alcohol consumption has been shown to have a pressor effect, both clinically and epidemiologicaly (100). This relationship is not linear, however, in most epidemiological studies, taking a J- or U-shaped form, with the lowest incidence of hypertension being seen in occasional or light drinkers (101). The effect of reducing alcohol consumption has mainly been studied in short-term trials where significant falls, especially in SBP, have been found (100,102). Larger reductions in BP following alcohol abstention have been reported in elderly alcoholics (aged 70–74 years) where BP was found to fall by 19/10 mmHg (102). As there appears to be a protective effect of mild alcohol intake on CHD, up to 2 units per day would appear to be a reasonable upper limit.

Exercise

Modest decreases in BP have been reported in older people taking mild aerobic exercise. After 1 year of an exercise programme in subjects aged 50–74 years involving brisk walking for a minimum of 30 minutes, 3 days per week, 24-ambulatory SBP fell by 6–7 mmHg, although DBP did not change (104). The BP changes after 6 months were not significantly reduced from baseline levels. Other studies based on casual BP measurements have shown greater hypotensive effects of exercise, with a 20/11 mmHg drop in BP being reported after 9 months of low-intensity exercise in a group with a mean age of 64 years (105). Low-intensity aerobic exercise seems to have an equal or greater hypotensive action than more strenuous exercise and is of a similar magnitude in old and young subjects. However, not all studies have shown a significant hypotensive effect (106). In addition to dietary changes daily exercise has been shown to be feasible and effective in subjects over 70 years old. Isotonic or aerobic exercises such as swimming, cycling or brisk walking can be recommended to most patients.

PHARMACOLOGICAL THERAPY

Thiazide diuretics

Most intervention studies showing benefit from antihypertensive therapy in the elderly have used thiazide diuretics, and they remain an effective, popular and cheap treatment in the elderly. Their mode of action has not been fully resolved but is due in part to a lowering of total peripheral resistance and a decrease in intravascular volume (107,108). In ISH they are also effective, lowering SBP by approximately 25 mmHg without causing significant symptomatic postural hypotension (109,110). The adverse metabolic profiles of thiazide diuretics and other side-effects are well known (see Table 5). Thiazides may initiate or aggravate pre-existing diabetes, gout, urinary incontinence, prostatism or impotence. However, in the SHEP pilot study only one case of gout occurred in approximately 500 patients treated for 1 year (110), and in the EWPHE trial the main determinants of uric acid levels were gender and renal function, not

Table 5. Adverse metabolic effects of thiazide diuretics

Hypokalaemia
Hypomagnesaemia
Hyponatraemia
Decreased glucose tolerance
Increased serum uric acid
Increased creatinine levels
Adverse effect on lipids (increased low-density lipoprotein cholesterol)

diuretics (111). Serum electrolytes should be checked a month after starting treatment to assess the need for potassium-sparing diuretics.

The adverse affect of thiazides on plasma lipids (112) could increase cardiovascular morbidity and mortality in the elderly, although this is, as yet, unproven. However, the long-term use may have a favourable effect in reducing hip fractures (113). Low-dose thiazide diuretics have a similar hypotensive effect as previously used higher doses, with fewer metabolic side-effects (114,115). If their hypotensive action is inadequate the dose should not be doubled but another class of drug substituted or added instead. Thiazide diuretics remain one of the first-line agents in treating the elderly hypertensive because of their proven efficacy, their cost and once-daily dosing regime aiding compliance.

β-Adrenoceptor blockers

Theoretically β-blockers would appear unsuitable for treating hypertension in the older age groups because of the age-related decreases in β-adrenoceptor responsiveness (116) and plasma renin levels and the reduction in cardiac output and increased peripheral resistance (117) associated with their use. However, Coope and Warrender's trial (30) found atenolol to be an effective and well-tolerated hypotensive agent in the elderly. Other studies have shown no definite age-related decrease in the hypotensive effect of β-blockers and they reduce BP to a similar extent as thiazides, calcium antagonists and angiotensin-converting enzyme (ACE) inhibitors (118–120). They should be avoided in patients with congestive heart failure, chronic obstructive airways disease, asthma, peripheral vascular disease, heart block and perhaps diabetes mellitus. However, those with angina, recent myocardial infarction and certain arrhythmias may benefit.

Increased fatigue, tiredness and depression have been reported in elderly hypertensives receiving β-blockers. The lipophilic β-blockers, in particular propranolol and metoprolol, have also been reported to cause sleep disturbance and adversely effect mental performance such as alertness and memory (121–123), although studies in elderly hypertensives have not shown this to be a significant problem (124). β-Blockers with intrinsic sympathomimetic activity such as pindolol may theoretically offer advantages by maintaining cardiac output and preserving LV function, although whether they offer any advantage in practice is unclear (125). Third-generation β-blockers, such as celiprolol, have weak vasodilating properties, lowering peripheral resistance with little effect on resting cardiac output or heart rate, and having similar antihypertensive efficacy as other β-blockers (126); their benefits over other β-blockers in the elderly hypertensive have yet to be shown. The use of β-blockers as first-line agents in the treatment of elderly hypertensives has been brought into question following the recent publication of the MRC study (33) which showed atenolol, unlike diuretics, did not reduce the rates of fatal stroke or decrease overall cardiovascular events and mortality.

Calcium channel blockers

These are effective hypotensive agents and acceptable to elderly hypertensives. They reduce smooth muscle tone causing vasodilatation and a reduction in peripheral vascular resistance without inducing a reflex tachycardia or impairing renal blood flow (127). They have neutral effects on lipids, do not adversely affect renal function and are well tolerated. They can cause headache, constipation, flushing and ankle oedema, although newer calcium channel blockers (CCB) such as amlodipine have been reported to have fewer side-effects. They can be safely used in those who also have peripheral vascular disease, diabetes and obstructive airways disease.

α-Adrenoceptor blockers

Stimulation of postsynaptic α_1-adrenoreceptors results in vacoconstriction and a rise in blood pressure. α-Adrenocoptor blockers reduce peripheral vascular resistance but non-selective agents will also cause a reflex tachycardia. While the α_1-selective blocker prazosin avoids this, unfortunately first-dose syncope and orthostatic hypotension, probably due to venous dilation, have limited its use (128). Newer α_1-blocking drugs such as doxazosin and terazosin have been shown to be effective antihypertensive agents but with less reported effect on postural hypotension (129). No adverse effects on renal function or on pre-existing renal impairment have been found. Favourable effects on serum lipids and symptoms of prostatic hypertrophy have also been reported and may be of some advantage in older persons.

Angiotensin-converting enzyme inhibitors

These are effective antihypertensive agents in the young and old and may be particularly useful when CCF is also present (130,131). Marked first-dose hypotension may occur, particularly in those who are hypovolaemic, hyponatraemic or taking diuretics. It is advisable to stop any existing diuretic therapy for a few days before introducing ACE inhibitors and to prescribe a low starting dose, e.g. captopril 6.25 mg daily or enalapril 2.5 mg daily. This dose can be initially given at night, reducing the problem of orthostatic hypotension. Because ACE inhibitors lead to reduced secretion of aldosterone, potassium levels may rise; addition of potassium-sparing diuretics may therefore lead to dangerous hyperkalaemia. Problems of renal failure have been reported with ACE inhibitors particularly in older patients taking non-steroidal anti-inflammatory drugs (NSAIDs), diuretics or in those who have pre-existing renal impairment (132). Renal failure may also be precipitated in those with bilateral renal artery stenosis or unlateral renal stenosis to a solitary kidney (133). It is recommended to check serum urea and electrolytes before starting therapy and at regular intervals afterwards.

No adverse effects on serum lipids or glucose intolerance have been reported (134); however, cough is a not infrequent side-effect which may be severe enough to lead to treatment withdrawal. ACE inhibitors eliminated by the kidney (e.g. enalapril, lisinopril) may accumulate in the elderly owing to the age-related decline in renal function or to pre-existing renal impairment. Low maintenance doses only may therefore be required.

Changes in homeostatic mechanisms and drug handling dictate that low doses of drugs should be used in the elderly. Low-dose thiazides, e.g. bendrofluazide, 2.5 mg, calcium channel antagonists, e.g. nifedipine SR 10 mg b.d. or β-blockers, e.g. atenolol 25 mg, can be recommended as first-line antihypertensive treatment.

How far to lower blood pressure

There has been concern that reducing BP too far can increase mortality particularly in those with pre-existing ischaemic heart disease. Analysis of the Framingham data showed that patients with a previous history of myocardial infarction demonstrated a U-shaped relationship between DBP and CHD death, with the lowest mortality in the DBP range 79–94 mmHg whether treated or untreated (135). Others have found a similar relationship (136). In the elderly, who are likely to have some degree of ischaemic heart disease, it would seem wise not to reduce DBP much below 70 mmHg. Indications for target SBP levels are less clear although it is unlikely that reducing SBP below 140 mmHg will confer much additional benefit (137).

A prospective study using ambulatory monitoring suggested that 50% of a group with clinic DBP >95 mmHg on treatment had ABP<90 mmHg and intensifying therapy based on the clinic readings resulted in over-treatment with no real gain in BP control (138).

Withdrawal of treatment

It may be possible and desirable to withdraw antihypertensive treatment in those whose BP is well controlled on monotherapy provided regular follow-up is undertaken. The results of several studies of treatment withdrawal in well-controlled hypertensives indicate that between 15% and 50% can maintain normotension for sustained periods (139). By using non-pharmacological methods the number successfully withdrawn from drug treatment increases: 35–60% of previously drug-treated hypertensive patients could successfully remain off treatment for between 1 and 4 years, compared to 5–35% of a group withdrawn from treatment but not given dietary advice (140,141). Patients' age does not seem to affect the success rate although high pretreatment BP levels, obesity, short duration of treatment and LV hypertrophy make successful withdrawal of treatment less likely (139).

Quality of life

In most trials adverse reactions to antihypertensive drugs have resulted in withdrawal rates of 16–33% (142). However, many more patients may experience mild side-effects and psychological changes that do not lead to drug withdrawal. The concept of quality of life aims to cover these areas—not only physical well-being but emotional well-being, sexual and social functioning and cognitive ability. Thiazide diuretics have been reported to cause no adverse affects on cognitive function or behaviour (144,145) although their use is associated with male sexual dysfunction and urinary problems in the elderly (146). In short-term trials, compared to placebo, β-blockers show no adverse affects on mental performance (147) or psychological distress (148) although, when compared to other antihypertensives such as ACE inhibitors, thiazide diuretics or calcium channel blockers, they compare poorly on tests of memory performance (149,150). Hydrophilic cardioselective β-blockers may have a better quality-of-life profile than lipophilic agents (151). ACE inhibitors compare well with other antihypertensive drugs in quality-of-life studies (152). No adverse affects have been shown regarding fatigue, memory or cognitive impairment, depression or sexual dysfunction (153,154), although there are little data specific to the elderly. Again little data are available on the effects of calcium channel blockers, particularly the newer agents, on quality of life, although sustained-release diltiazem and amlodipine have similar quality-of-life profiles to other antihypertensive agents (155). However, nifedipine has been reported to have an adverse affect on cognitive function (156,157). Patients' relatives may be more likely to report adverse psychological changes than patients or physicians!

Compliance

Estimates of compliance with antihypertensive drug therapy suggest that only 50% of subjects comply with at least 80% of their medication (158). Regarding medication in general the elderly appear to be as compliant or more so than the young (159). This is surprising, as many factors affecting compliance such as poor memory, impaired concentration, poor eyesight and inability to open containers are more common in the elderly. Non-compliance increases with the number of drugs prescribed, when the dosing frequency increases and when side-effects cause problems (160). Clearly the simpler the drug regime and the fewer the side-effects the greater the compliance, particularly if the patient is motivated by discussion of the condition and the aims of treatment with the doctor or practice nurse.

CONCLUSIONS

There is now encouraging evidence that treating hypertension in subjects aged up to at least 80 years of age reduces cardiovascular morbidity and mortality, whether patients have an elevated SBP and DBP or ISH. However, selecting the patients who are going to benefit most from treatment remains a problem. In particular, blood pressure variability and the 'white coat' effect make identifying the elderly person with true, sustained hypertension difficult. Only through repeated measurements over several visits can casual BP measurements identify such people, although ambulatory BP measurements may in the future make this process easier and quicker, if not more expensive. Other than 'routine' tests, further investigations to uncover a cause for hypertension should rarely be embarked upon. Once diagnosed, sustained SBP levels of > 160 mmHg or DBP > 90 mmHg should lead to most patients initially receiving non-pharmacological advice before considering drug treatment. A wide range of antihypertensive agents are now available, with low-dose diuretics probably being the first-line treatment of choice, although β-blockers and calcium channel blockers have been shown to be effective antihypertensive agents in this age group. Those with concomitant heart failure may benefit from ACE inhibitors. If a patient has been well controlled on a simple treatment regime for several years a trial period off treatment can be tried, together with reinforcement of non-pharmacological advice.

REFERENCES

Epidemiology

1. Lowenstein WG (1961) Blood pressure in relation to age and sex in the tropics and subtropics. *Lancet* i: 389.
2. Miall WE, Brennan PJ (1981) Hypertension in the elderly: the South Wales Study. In *Hypertension in the Young and Old*, 1st edn, Onesti G, Kim KE (eds). Grune & Stratton, New York, p. 277–283.
3. Roberts J, Maurer K (1977) Blood pressure levels of persons 60–74 years, United States, 1971–1974. National Center for Health Statistics **11**: 1.
4. Gordon T, Shurtleff D (1977) Section 29: means at each examination and inter-examination variation of specified characteristics: Framingham Study, Exam 1 to Exam 10. In *The Framingham Study: An Epidemiological Investigation of Cardiovascular Disease*, Kannel WB, Gordon T (eds). US DHEW (National Institutes of Health), Washington DC, pp. 74–78.
5. Volkonas PS, Kannel WB, Cupples LA (1988) Epidemiology and risk of hypertension in the elderly: the Framingham Study. *J Hypertens* **6** (Suppl. 1): S3–S9.
6. Miall WE, Chinn S. (1974) Screening for hypertension: some epidemiological observations. *Br Med J* **2**: 595.
7. Bulpitt CJ (1989) Definition, prevalence and incidence of hypertension in the elderly. In *Handbook of Hypertension, Vol. 12: Hypertension in the Elderly*, Amery A, Staessen J (eds). Elsevier, Amsterdam, pp. 153–169.
8. Kannel WB (1991) Epidemiology of essential hypertension: the Framingham experience. *Proc R Coll Phys Edinb* **21**: 273–287.
9. Staessen J, Amery A, Fagard R (1990) Isolated systolic hypertension in the elderly. *J Hypertens* **8**: 393–405.
10. Staessen J, Fagard R, Joosens JV *et al.* (1988) Salt intake and blood pressure in the general population: a controlled intervention trial in 2 towns. *J Hypertens* **6**:

965–973.

11. Silagy CA, McNeil JJ, McGrath BP (1990) Isolated systolic hypertension: does it really exist on ambulatory blood pressure monitoring? *Clin Exp Pharmacol Physiol* **17**: 203–206.

12. Uedak S, Onass T, Hasuo Y, Kiyohaua Y (1989) Impact of high blood pressure on morbidity and mortality. In *Handbook of Hypertension, Vol. 12: Hypertension in the Elderly*, Amery A, Staessen J (eds). Elsevier, Amsterdam, pp. 174–185.

13. Society of Actuaries and Association of Life Insurance Medical Directors of America (1980) *Blood Pressure Study: 1979*, p. 197.

14. Mattila K, Haavisto M, Rajala S, Heikinheimo R (1988) Blood pressure and five year survival in the old. *Br Med J* **296**: 887–889.

15. Agnar E (1983) Predictive valve of arterial blood pressure in old age. *Acta Med Scand* **214**: 285–294.

16. Heikinheimo R, Haavisto Kaarela R, Kanto A *et al.* (1990) Blood pressure in the very old. *J Hypertens* **8**: 361–367.

17. MacMahon S, Peto R, Cutler J *et al.* (1990) Blood pressure, stroke and coronary heart disease. Part 1, prolonged differences in blood pressure: prospective observational studies corrected for the regression dilution bias. *Lancet* **335**: 765–774.

18. Kannel W, Castelli WP, McNamara PM *et al.* Role of blood pressure in the development of congestive heart failure: the Framingham Study. *N Engl J Med* **287**: 781–787.

19. Kannel W, Dawber TR, Sorlie P, Wolf PA *et al.* (1976) Components of blood pressure and risk of atherothrombotic pain infarction: the Framingham Study. *Stroke* **7**: 327–331.

20. Ostfeld A, Shekelle RB, Klawans ML, Tufo HM *et al.* (1974) Epidemiology of stroke in an elderly welfare population. *Am J Public Health* **64**: 450–458.

21. Birkenhager W, de Leeuw P (1988) Impact of systolic blood pressure on cardiovascular prognosis. *J Hypertens* **6** (Suppl. 1): S21–S24.

22. Van Den Ban GJE, Kampman E, Schouten EG *et al.* (1989) Isolated systolic hypertension in Dutch middle aged and all cause mortality: 25 year prospective study. *Int J Epidemiol* **18**: 95–99.

23. Kannel W, Dauber T, McGee D (1980) Perspectives on systolic Hypertension: the Framingham Study. *Circulation* **61**: 1179–1182.

24. Silagy CA, McNeil JJ (1992) Epidemiologic aspects of isolated systolic hypertension and implications for future research. *Am J Cardiol* **69**: 213–218.

25. Garland C, Barrett-Connor E, Suarez L, Criqui MH *et al.* (1983) Isolated systolic hypertension and mortality after age 60 years. *Am J Epidemiol* **118**: 365–376.

26. Jackson G, Mahon W, Pierscianowski TA, Cordon J (1976) Inappropriate antihypertensive therapy in the elderly. *Lancet* **ii**: 1317–1319.

27. Kuramoto K, Matsushita S, Kuwajima I, Murakami M (1981) Prospective study on the treatment of mild hypertension in the aged. *Jpn Heart J* **22**: 75–85.

28. Spackling ME, Mitchell JRA, Short AH, Watt E (1981) Blood pressure reduction in the elderly: a randomised controlled trial of methyldopa. *Br Med J* **283**: 1151–1153.

29. Amery A, Birkenhager W, Brixko P *et al.* (1985) Mortality and morbidity results from the European Working Party on High Blood Pressure in the Elderly Trial. *Lancet* **i**: 1349–1354.

30. Coope J, Warrender TS (1986) Randomised trial of treatment of hypertension in elderly patients in primary care. *Br Med J* **293**: 1145–1151.

31. SHEP Co-operative Research Group (1991) Prevention of stroke by antihypertensive drug treatment in older persons with isolated systolic hypertension. *JAMA* **265**: 3255–3264.

32. Dahlof B, Lindholm LH, Hansson L *et al.* (1991) Morbidity and mortality in the

Swedish Trial in Old Patients with Hypertension (STOP-Hypertension). *Lancet* **338**: 1281–1284.

33. MRC Working Party (1992) Medical Research Council trial of treatment of hypertension in older adults: principal results. *Br Med J* **304**: 405–412.

33A. Veterans Administration Co-operative Study Group on Anti-Hypertensive Agents (1972) Effects of treatment on morbidity in hypertension. III. Influence of age, diastolic pressure and prior cardiovascular disease. *Circulation* **45**: 991–1004.

34. Hypertension Stroke Co-operative Study Group (1974) Effect of anti-hypertensive treatment on stroke recurrence. *JAMA* **229**: 409–418.

35. Hypertension Detection and Follow-Up Programme Co-operative Group (1979) Five year findings of the hypertension detection follow-up programme. II. Mortality by race, sex and age. *JAMA* **242**: 2572–2577.

36. Australian Therapeutic Trial in Mild Hypertension (1981) The Management Committee. Treatment of mild hypertension in the elderly. *Med J Aust* 1981; **68**: 398–402.

37. Staessen J, Fagard R, Van Hoof R, Amery A (1988) Mortality in various intervention trials in elderly hypertensive patients: a review. *Eur Heart J* **9**: 215–222.

38. Messerli FH, Sundgaard-Riise K, Ventura H *et al.* (1983) Essential hypertension in the elderly: haemodynamics, intravascular volume, plasma renin activity and circulating catecholamine levels. *Lancet* **ii**: 983–986.

39. Adamopoulos P, Chrysanthakapoulis S, Frohlich ED (1975) Systolic hypertension: nonhomogeneous disease. *Am J Cardiol* **36**: 697–701.

40. Stern N, Beahm E, McGinty D *et al.* (1985) Dissociation of 24 hr catecholamine levels from blood pressure in older men. *Hypertension* **7**: 1023–1029.

41. O'Malley K, Docherty J, Kelly JG (1988) Adrenoceptor status and cardiovascular function in ageing. *J Hypertens* **6** (Suppl. 8): s1–s7.

Diagnosis and evaluation

42. Dornhorst AC, Howard P, Leathart GL (1952) Respiratory variations in blood pressure. *Circulation* **6**: 553–558.

43. Harshfield GA, Pickering TG, Kleinert HD *et al.* (1982) Situational variation of blood pressure in ambulatory hypertensive patients. *Psychosom Med* **44**: 237–245.

44. Lipsitz LA, Nyquist RP, Wey JY, Rowe JW (1983) Post prandial reduction in blood pressure in the elderly. *N Engl J Med* **309**: 81–83.

45. Athanassiadis D, Draper GJ, Honour AJ, Cranstone WI (1969) Variability of automatic blood pressure measurements over 24 hour periods. *Clin Sci* **36**: 147–156.

46. Brennan PJ, Greenburg G, Miall WE, Thompson SG (1982) Seasonal variations in arterial blood pressure. *Br Med J* **285**: 919–923.

47. Watson RDS, Stallard TJS, Flinn RM, Littler WA (1980) Factors determining direct arterial pressure and its variability in hypertensive man. *Hypertension* **2**: 333–341.

48. Watson RDS, Lumb R, Young MA *et al.* (1987) Variation in cuff blood pressure in untreated outpatients with mild hypertension: implications for initiating anti-hypertensive treatment. *J Hypertens* **5**: 207–211.

49. James GD, Pickering TG, Yee LS *et al.* (1988) The reproducibility of average ambulatory, home and clinic pressure. *Hypertension* **11**: 545–549.

50. Mancia G, Parati G, Pomidossi G *et al.* (1987) Alerting reaction and rising blood pressure during measurement by physician and nurse. *Hypertension* **9**: 209–215.

51. Sokolow M, Perloff D, Cowan R (1980) Contribution of ambulatory blood pressure to the assessment of patients with mild to moderate elevations of office blood pressure. *Cardiovasc Rev Rep* **1**: 295–303.

52. Shimada K, Ogan H, Kawamoto A *et al.* (1990) Non-invasive ambulatory blood pressure monitoring during clinic visit in elderly hypertensive patients. *Clin Exp Hypertens Theory Pract* **A12** (2): 151–170.

53. Porchet M, Bussian JP, Waeber B *et al.* (1986) Unpredictability of blood pressures recorded outside the clinic in the treated hypertensive patient. *J Cardiovasc Pharmacol* **8**: 332–335.

54. Gerardi RJ, Blanchard EB, Andrasik F (1985) Psychological dimensions of office hypertension. *Behav Res Ther* **23**: 609–612.

55. Corcoran AC, Dustan HP, Page IH (1955) The evaluation of anti-hypertensive procedures, with particular reference to their effects on blood pressure. *Ann Intern Med* **43**: 1161–1177.

56. Torriani S, Waeber B, Antoine P *et al.* (1988) Ambulatory blood pressure monitoring in the elderly hypertensive patient. *J Hypertens* **6** (Suppl. 1): S25–S27.

57. Drayer JIM, Waeber MA, Young JL, Wyle FA (1982) Circadian blood pressure patterns in ambulatory hypertensive patients: effects of age. *Am J Med* **73**: 493–499.

58. Kaplan NM (1987) Misdiagnosis of systemic hypertension and recommendations for improvement. *Am J Cardiol* **60**: 1303–1386.

59. Kobrin I, Oigman W, Kuman A *et al.* (1984) Diurnal variation of blood pressure in elderly patients with essential hypertension. *J Am Geriatr Soc* **312**: 896–899.

60. Kuwajima I, Hoh E, Suzuki Y *et al.* (1990) Pseudo-hypertension in the elderly. *J Hypertens* **8**: 429–432.

61. Kannel WB (1976) Some lessons in cardiovascular epidemiology from Framingham. *Am J Cardiol* **37**: 269–282.

62. Kannel WB, Dannenberg AL, Levy D (1987) Population implications of electrocardiographic left ventricular hypertrophy. *Am J Cardiol* **60**: 85–93.

63. Messerli FH, Ventura HO, Glade LB *et al.* (1983) Essential hypertension in the elderly: haemodynamics, intravascular volume, plasma re-inactivity and circulating catecholamine levels. *Lancet* **ii**: 983–986.

64. Savage DD (1987) Considerations of the use of echocardiography in epidemiology: the Framingham Study. *Hypertension* **9**: II-40–II-44.

65. Bauer JH, Reams GP, Wu Z (1991) The aging hypertensive kidney: pathophysiology and therapeutic options. *Am J Med* **90** (Suppl. 4B): 21S–27S.

66. Pickering TG (1990) Renovascular hypertension medical evaluation and non-surgical treatment. In *Hypertension Pathophysiology, Diagnosis and Management*, Laragh JH, Brenner BN (eds). Raven Press, New York, p. 1548.

67. Muller FB, Seeley JE, Case CB *et al.* (1986) The Captopril tests for identifying renovascular disease in hypertensive patients. *Am J Med* **80**: 633–644.

68. Smith CW, Winfield AC, Price RR *et al.* (1982) Evaluation of digital venous angiography for diagnosis of renovascular hypertension. *Radiology* **144**: 51.

69. Couch NP, Sullivan J, Crane C (1976) The predictive accuracy of renal vein renin activity in the surgery of renovascular hypertension. *Surgery* **79**: 70.

70. de Leeuw PW (1991) Renal function in the elderly: results from the European Working Party on High Blood Pressure in the Elderly Trial. *Am J Med* **90** (Suppl. 3A): 45S–49S.

71. Rosansky SJ, Hoover DR, King L, Gibson J (1990) The association of blood pressure levels with change in hypertensive and non-hypertensive subjects. *Arch Intern Med* **150**: 2072–2076.

72. Rostand SG, Brown G, Kirk K *et al.* (1989) Renal insufficiency and treated essential hypertension. *N Engl J Med* **320**: 684–688.

73. Kannel WB, Stanpfer MJ, Castelli WP, Verter J (1984) The prognostic significance of proteinuria: the Framingham Study. *Am Heart J* **108**: 1347–1352.

74. Yudkin JS, Forest RD, Jackson CA (1988) Microalbuminaria as predictor of

vascular disease in non-diabetic subjects. Islington Diabetes Survey. *Lancet* **ii**: 530–533.

75. Dausgaard EM, Froland A, Jargensen OD, Mogensen CE (1990) Microalbuminuria as predictor of increased mortality in elderly people. *Br Med J* **300**: 297–300.

76. Kannel WB, Higgins AM (1990) Smoking and hypertension as predictors of cardiovascular risk in population studies. *J Hypertens* **8** (Suppl. 5): S3–S8.

77. La Croix AZ, Lang J, Scherr P *et al.* (1991) Smoking and mortality among older men and women in three communities. *N Engl J Med* **324**: 1619–1625.

78. Gordon DJ, Rifkind BN (1989) Treating high blood cholesterol in the older patient. *Am J Cardiol* **63**: 48H–52H.

79. Shipley MJ, Pocock SJ, Marmot MG. Does plasma cholesterol concentration predict mortality from coronary heart disease in elderly people? 18 year follow-up in Whitehall Study. *Br Med J* **303**: 89–92.

80. Fagard R (1991) Serum cholesterol levels and survival in elderly hypertensive patients: analysis of data from the European Working Party on High Blood Pressure in the Elderly. *Am J Med* **90** (Suppl. 3A): 62S–63S.

81. Van Itallie TB (1985) Health implications for overweight and obesity in the United States. *Ann Intern Med* **103**: 983–988.

82. Larsson B, Svardsudd K, Welin L *et al.* (1984) Abdominal adipose tissue distribution, obesity, and risk of cardiovascular disease and death: 13 year follow-up of participants in the study of men born in 1913. *Br Med J* **288**: 1401–1404.

83. Law MR, Frost CD, Wold NJ (1991) By how much does dietary salt reduction lower blood pressure? I. Analysis of observational data among populations *Br Med J* **302**: 811–815.

84. Barham Carter A (1970) Hypotensive therapy in stroke survivors. *Lancet* **i**: 485–489.

85. Wallace JD, Levy LL (1981) Blood pressure after stroke. *JAMA* **246**: 2177–2180.

86. Britton M, deFaire V, Helmers C (1980) Hazards of therapy for excessive hypertension in acute stroke. *Acta Med Scand* **207**: 253–257.

87. Strandgaard S (1976) Autoregulation of cerebral blood flow in hypertensive patients: the modifying influence of prolonged antihypertensive treatment on the tolerance to acute, drug induced hypotension. *Circulation* **53**: 720–727.

88. Yatsu FM, Zivin J (1985) Hypertension in acute ischaemic strokes: not to treat. *Arch Neurol* **42**: 999–1000.

89. Law MR, Frost CD, Wald MJ (1991) By how much does salt restriction lower blood pressure? III: Analysis of data from trials of salt reduction. *Br Med J* **302**: 819–824.

90. Cutler JA, Follmann D, Elliott P, Suh I (1991) An overview of randomised trials of sodium reduction on blood pressure. *Hypertension* **17** (Suppl. 1): I-27–I-33.

91. Fotherby MD, Potter JF (1991) Potassium supplementation reduces clinic and ambulatory blood pressure in elderly hypertensive subjects. *J Hypertens* **10**: 1403–1408.

92. Cappucio FP, MacGregor A (1991) Does potassium supplementation lower blood pressure? A meta-analysis of published trials. *J Hypertens* **9**: 465–473.

93. Khaw KT, Barrett Connor E (1987) Dietary potassium and stroke associated mortality. *N Engl J Med* **316**: 235–240.

94. Schotte DE, Stunkard AJ (1990) The effects of weight reduction on blood pressure on 301 obese patients. *Arch Intern Med* **150**: 1701–1704.

95. Scherrer U, Nussberger J, Torriani S *et al.* (1991) Effect of weight reduction in moderately overweight patients on recorded ambulatory blood pressure and free cytosolic platelet calcium. *Circulation* **83**: 552–558.

96. Langford GH, Blaufox MD, Oberman A *et al.* (1985) Dietary therapy slows the return of hypertension after stopping prolonged medication. *JAMA* **253**: 657–669.

97. Weinsier RL, James LD, Darnell, B *et al.* (1991) Obesity related hypertension:

evaluation of the separate effects of energy restriction and weight reduction on haemodynamic and neuroendocrine status. *Am J Med* **90**: 460–468.

98. Tuomilehto J (1991) Body mass index and prognosis in elderly hypertensive patients: a report from the European working party on high blood pressure in the elderly. *Am J Med* **90** (Suppl. 3A): 34S–41S.

99. Rajala SA, Kanto AJ, Haavisto MV *et al.* (1990) Body weight and three year prognosis in very old people. *Int J Obes* **14**: 997–1003.

100. Potter JF, Beevers DG (1984) Pressor effect of alcohol in hypertension. *Lancet* **i**: 119–122.

101. Friedman GD, Klatsky AL, Siegelaub AB (1983) Alcohol intake in hypertension. *Ann Intern Med* **98**: 846–849.

102. Puddey IB, Beilin LJ, Vandongen R (1987) Regular alcohol use raises blood pressure in treated hypertensive subjects. *Lancet* **i**: 647–651.

103. Schnall C, Weiner JS (1958) Clinical evaluation of blood pressure in alcoholics. *Q J Stud Alcohol* **19**: 432–446.

104. Seals DR, Reiling MJ (1991) Effects of regular exercise on 24 hour arterial pressure in older hypertensive humans. *Hypertension* **18**: 583–592.

105. Hagburg JM, Montain SJ, Martin WH, Ehsani AA (1989) Effect of exercise training in 60–69 year old persons with essential hypertension. *Am J Cardiol* **64**: 348–353.

106. Blumenthal JA, Seigel WC, Appelbaum M (1991) Failure of exercise to reduce blood pressure in patients with mild hypertension. *JAMA* **266**: 2098–2104.

107. Lund-Johansen P (1970) Haemodynamic changes in long term diuretic therapy of essential hypertension. *Acta Med Scand* **187**: 509–518.

108. DeCarvalho JGR, Dunn FG, Lohmoller G, Frohlich ED (1977) Haemodynamic correlates of prolonged thiazide therapy: the comparison of responders and non-responders. *Clin Pharmacol Ther* **22**: 875–880.

109. Niarchos AP, Weinstein DL, Laragh JH (1984) Comparison of the effects of diuretic therapy and low sodium intake in isolated systolic hypertension *Am J Med* **77**: 1061–1068.

110. Hulley SB, Furberg CD, Gerland B *et al.* (1985) Systolic hypertension in the elderly programme (SHEP): antihypertensive efficacy of chlorthalidone. *Am J Cardiol* **56**: 913–920.

111. Staessen J *et al.* (1991) The determinants and prognostic significance of serum uric acid in elderly patients of the European Working Party on high blood pressure in the elderly trial. *Am J Med* **90** (Suppl. 3A): 3A-60S–3A-61S.

112. Weinberger M (1985) Antihypertensive therapy and lipids: evidence, mechanisms and implications. *Arch Intern Med* **145**: 1102–1105.

113. La Croix AZ, Wienpahl J, White LR *et al.* (1990) Thiazide diuretics agents and the incidence of hip fractures. *N Engl J Med* **322**: 286–290.

114. Matterson BJ, Cushman WC, Goldstein G *et al.* (1990) Treatment of hypertension in the elderly: results of a department of veterans affairs co-operative study, parts 1 and 2. *Hypertension* **15**: 348–369.

115. Carlsen JE, Kober L, Torp-Pedersen C, Johansen P (1990) Relation between dose of Bendrofluazide, antihypertensive effect and adverse biochemical effects *Br Med J* **300**: 975–978.

116. Vestal RE, Wood AJJ, Shand DG (1979) Reduced beta adrenoceptor sensitivity in the elderly. *Clin Pharmacol Ther* **26**: 181–186.

117. Tarazi RC, Dustan HP (1972) Beta adrenoceptor blockade in hypertension: practical and theoretical implications of long term haemodynamic variations. *Am J Cardiol* **29**: 633–640.

118. Wigstrand J, Westerglen G, Berglan G *et al.* (1986) Antihypertensive treatment with metoprolol or hydrochlorothiazide in patients aged 60–75 years: report from a

double blind international multi-centre study. *JAMA* **255**: 1304–1310.

119. Jackson G, Roland M, Adam G *et al.* (1986) A placebo controlled double blind randomised cross over trial of atenolol, hydrochlorothiazide and amiloride and the combination in patients over 60 years of age. *Br J Clin Pract* **40**: 230–234.

120. The Treatment of Mild Hypertension Research Group (1991) The treatment of mild hypertension study: a randomised, placebo controlled trial of a nutritional hygienic regimen along with various drug monotherapies. *Arch Intern Med* **151**: 1413–1423.

121. Westerland A (1985) Central nervous system side effects with hydrophilic and lipophilic beta blockers. *Eur J Clin Pharmacol* **28S**: 73–76.

122. Lichter I, Richardson PJ, Wyke MA (1986) Differential effects of atenolol and enalapril on memory during treatment for essential hypertension. *Br Med J Pharmacol* **21**: 641–645.

123. Betts TA, Alford C (1983) Beta blocking drugs and sleep: a controlled trial. *Drugs* **25** (Suppl. 2): 268–272.

124. Gengo FM, Fagan SC, DePadova A *et al.* (1988) The effects of beta blockers on mental performance on older hypertensive patients. *Arch Intern Med* **148**: 779–784.

125. Man In't Veld AJ, Schalekamp MADH (1984) Haemodynamics of beta blockers. In *Beta Blockers in the Treatment of Cardiovascular Disease*, Costis JB, De Felice EA (eds). Raven Press, New York, pp. 229–251.

126. Anonymous (1991) Celiprilol: theory and practice. *Lancet* **338**: 1426–1427.

127. Van Zwieten PA, Blauw GJ, Vann Brummelen P (1989) Calcium antagonists (calcium entry blockers): general considerations. In *Handbook of hypertension, Vol. 12: Hypertension in the Elderly*, Amery A, Staessen J (eds). Elsevier, Amsterdam, pp. 245–257.

128. Westerman RF, Schouten JA, Hengeveld WL (1985) Prazosin once or twice daily? *Eur J Clin Pharmacol* **28**: 11–15.

129. Cox DA, Leeder P, Milson JA, Singleton W (1986) The antihypertensive effects of doxazosin: a clinical overview. *Br J Clin Pharmacol* **21** (Suppl. 1): 83S–90S.

130. Baker SL (1988) A study of the use of captopril in elderly hypertensive patients. *Age Ageing* **17**: 17–20.

131. Cox JP, Duggan J, Oboyle CA *et al.* (1989) A double blind evaluation of captopril in elderly hypertensives. *J Hypertens* **7**: 299–303.

132. Verbeelen DL, DeBoel S (1984) Reversible acute or chronic renal failure during captopril treatment. *Br Med J* **289**: 20–21.

133. Hricik DE, Browning PJ, Coppleman RI *et al.* (1983) Captopril induced functional renal insufficiency in patients with bilateral renal artery stenosis or renal artery stenosis in a solitary kidney. *N Engl J Med* **308**: 373–376.

134. Groel JT, Tadros SS, Dreslinski GR, Jenkins AC (1983) Longterm antihypertensive therapy with captopril. *Hypertension* **5**: III-145–III-151.

135. D'Agostino RB, Belander AJ, Kannel WB, Cruickshank JM (1991) Relation of low diastolic blood pressure to coronary heart disease in the presence of myocardial infarction: the Framingham study. *Br Med J* **303**: 385–389.

136. Farnett L, Mulrow CD, Linn WD *et al.* (1991) The J curve phenomenon and the treatment of hypertension: is there a point beyond which pressure reduction is dangerous? *JAMA* **265**: 489–495.

137. Cruickshank JM, Higgins TJC, Pennert K *et al.* (1987) The efficacy and tolerability of antihypertensive treatment based on atenolol in the prevention of stroke and the regression of left ventricular hypertrophy. *J Hum Hypertens* **1**: 87–93.

138. Waeber B, Scherrer U, Petrillo A *et al.* (1987) Are some hypertensive patients overtreated? Results of a prospective study of ambulatory blood pressure recording. *Lancet* **ii**: 732–734.

139. Fletcher AE, Franks PJ, Bulpitt CJ (1988) The effect of withdrawing antihyperten-

sive therapy: a review *J Hypertens* **6**: 431–436.
140. Langford HG, Blaufox MD, Oberman A *et al.* (1985) Dietary therapy slows the return of hypertension after stopping prolonged medication. *JAMA* **253**: 657–664.
141. Stamler R, Stamler J, Grim R *et al.* (1987) Nutritional therapy for high blood pressure: final report of a four year randomised controlled trial—the hypertension control programme. *JAMA* **257**: 1484–1491.
142. Curb JD, Borhani NO, Blaszkowski TP *et al.* (1985) Long term surveillance for adverse effects of antihypertensive drugs. *JAMA* **253**: 3263–3268.
143. Bird AS, Blizzard RA, Mann AH (1990) Treating hypertension in the older person: and the evaluation of the association of blood pressure level and its reduction with cognitive performance. *J Hypertens* **8**: 147–152.
144. Curb JD, Schnider K, Taylor JO *et al.* (1988) Antihypertensive drug side effects in the hypertension detection and follow up programme. *Hypertension* **11** (Suppl. II): II-51–II-55.
145. Chang SW, Fine R, Siegel D *et al.* (1991) The impact of diuretics therapy on reported sexual function. *Arch Int Med* **151**: 2402–2408.
146. Kline LE, German PS, Levine DM *et al.* (1984) Medication problems among outpatients: a study with emphasis on the elderly. *Arch Int Med* **144**: 1185–1188.
147. Gengo FM, Fagin SC, De Padova A *et al.* (1988) The effects of beta blockers on mental performance of older hypertensive patients. *Arch Int Med* **148**: 779–784.
148. Wassertheil-Smoller S, Blaufox MD, Oberman A *et al.* (1991) Effect of antihypertensives on sexual function and quality of life: the TAIM study. *Am Int Med* **114**: 613–620.
149. Blumenthal JA, Ekelund LG, Emery CF (1990) Quality of life among hypertensive patients with a diurectic background who are taking atenolol and analopril. *Clin Pharmacol Ther* **48**: 447–454.
150. Lichter I, Richardson PJ, Wyke MA (1986) Differential effects of atenolol and analopril on memory during treatment for essential hypertension. *Br J Clin Pharmacol* **21**: 641–645.
151. Steiner SS, Friedhoff AJ, Wilson BL *et al.* (1990) Antihypertensives and quality of life: a comparison of atenolol, captopril, analopril and propanolol. *J Hum Hypertens* **4**: 217–225.
152. Croog SH, Levene S, Testa MA *et al.* (1986) The effects of antihypertensive therapy on the quality of life. *N Engl J Med* **314**: 1657–1664.
153. Fletcher AE Bulpitt CJ, Hawkins CM *et al.* (1990) Quality of life and antihypertensive therapy: a randomised double blind controlled trial of captopril and antenolol. *J Hypertens* **8**: 463–466.
154. Richardson PJ, Wyke MA (1988) Memory function: effects of different antihypertensive drugs. *Drugs* **35** (Suppl. 5): 80–85.
155. Applegate WB, Phillips HL, Schnaper H *et al.* (1991) A randomised controlled trial of the effects of three antihypertensive agents on blood pressure control and quality of life in older women. *Arch Int Med* **151**: 1817–1823.
156. Fletcher AE, Chester PC, Hawkins CMA *et al.* (1989) The effects of verapamil and propranolol on quality of life in hypertension. *J Hum Hypertens* **3**: 125–130.
157. Palmer A, Fletcher AE, Hamilton G *et al.* (1990) A comparison of verapamil and nifedipine on quality of life. *Br J Clin Pharmacol* **30**: 365–370.
158. Sackett DL, Haynes RB (eds) (1976) *Compliance with Therapeutic Regimens*. Johns Hopkins University Press, Baltimore.
159. Kline LE (1987) Compliance and blood pressure control. *Hypertension* **11** (Suppl. II): II-61–II-64.
160. Morgan TO, Nowson C, Murphy J, Snowden R (1986) Compliance and the elderly hypertensive. *Drugs* **31** (Suppl. 4): 174–183.

17 Ischaemic Heart Disease in the Elderly

ANDREW T. ELDER[a] **AND KEITH A. A. FOX**[b]
[a] Eastern General Hospital, Edinburgh, UK
[b] Royal Infirmary, Edinburgh, UK

In both elderly and younger populations, ischaemic heart disease may manifest as stable or unstable angina pectoris, myocardial infarction, heart failure or sudden 'cardiac' death. The most common underlying cause of these clinical syndromes is coronary artery disease characterized by atheromatous intimal and medial damage which, in association with coronary arterial spasm or intraluminal thrombus formation, can cause partial or complete luminal obstruction and consequent impairment of myocardial blood supply. Myocardial ischaemia can also occur in the absence of any recognizable coronary vascular disease, for example when significant ventricular hypertrophy or profound anaemia is present, and in rare cases may be secondary to spasm of the epicardial coronary arteries, functional impairment of the coronary microvasculature ('syndrome X') or non-atheromatous but obstructive coronary disease such as arteritis. In the following discussion, the term 'ischaemic heart disease' applies only to ischaemia caused by atheromatous, obstructive coronary arterial disease.

THE EPIDEMIOLOGY OF ISCHAEMIC HEART DISEASE IN THE ELDERLY

Our knowledge of the epidemiology of ischaemic heart disease in elderly populations is derived from autopsy and clinical studies, hospital activity statistics and national and international mortality and morbidity statistics.

Autopsy studies

Atheromatous lesions increase in extent and severity with age in all systemic arterial systems including the coronary tree (1), and it has been estimated that some 2% of the coronary intimal surface is affected at the age of 20 years compared to 20% at the age of 60 years (2). Although males tend to have more severe disease than females at all ages, the difference is least in the oldest age groups. In one study 41% of males and 12% of females aged 30–49 years had at

Geriatric Cardiology. Principles and Practice. Edited by A. Martin and A. J. Camm
© 1994 John Wiley & Sons Ltd

least one stenosis occluding more than 75% of a coronary artery, and similar disease was found in 81% of males and 43% of females aged 60–69 years. In those over 70 years of age only 72% of males but 54% of females were similarly affected (3). Endogenous oestrogens appear to exert a cardioprotective influence in premenopausal women via their effects on lipoprotein metabolism (4,5) and some evidence suggests that the rise in the incidence of postmenopausal ischaemic heart disease may be reduced by hormone replacement therapy (5,6). Despite the higher prevalence of coronary artery disease in elderly individuals, it should not be considered an inevitable consequence of ageing, and elderly individuals with normal coronary arteries and good left ventricular function are frequently found in both autopsy and clinical studies. Although coronary artery stenoses can be demonstrated at autopsy their relationship to clinical syndromes of ischaemic heart disease is indirect, the only direct evidence of pre-existent ischaemic heart disease being transmural or subendocardial myocardial infarction or ventricular aneurysm. Other pathological lesions such as myocardial fibrosis have been interpreted as evidence of previous myocardial ischaemia (7), but such changes are not pathognomic and may be associated with ageing *per se* (8,9). Importantly, significant coronary artery disease is often found at autopsy in individuals in whom no pathological evidence or clinical history of ischaemic heart disease exists. Epidemiological studies which define the prevalence of ischaemic heart disease by the presence of coronary artery disease, or vice versa, are therefore potentially prone to error. The discrepancy between the prevalence of coronary disease at autopsy and the prevalence of antemortem ischaemic heart disease exists in all age groups, but is most marked in the elderly. Among those aged over 65 years, 60% have coronary artery disease of severity apparently sufficient to cause ischaemia (3) but only 20–30% exhibit clinical evidence of ischaemic heart disease (10–15). In an autopsy study of patients aged over 90 years (16), 60% of those with significant coronary disease had no pertinent clinical history; the prevalence of apparently asymptomatic coronary artery disease therefore appears to increase with age. This occurs despite age-related changes in myocardial and circulatory pathophysiology that theoretically make ischaemia more likely to occur. These include amyloid deposition (17) and left ventricular hypertrophy (18) which may be associated with reduced left ventricular compliance (19) and diastolic dysfunction (20) and a consequent decline in myocardial and subendocardial blood flow (21). Ischaemia is made even more likely by increased aortic impedance and peripheral vascular resistance (22).

Clinical studies

Attempts to define the presence, extent and severity of coronary artery disease in large populations during life are hindered by the absence of sensitive yet specific non-invasive markers. Calcified coronary plaques on the plain chest X-ray may suggest the presence of coronary artery disease (23), but this abnormality is

Table 1. Prevalence of ischaemic heart disease in older individuals

Reference	n	Age	Criteria for IHD	Prevalence (%)
(16)	501	>65	Rose questionnaire angina Documented history of MI Minnesota coded Q/QS items	11 4.5 10
(17)	2254	>65	Minnesota coded Q/QS items 'Exertional chest pain' History of MI	6 12 3
(18)	487	>62	Rose questionnaire angina Minnesota coded Q/QS items	10 6
(19)	1500	>65	Angina questionnaire	14–17
(20)	—	>65	Survey of nitrate prescriptions	4–7
(29)	8359	>65	Rose questionnaire angina	3–6
(14)	708	>62	Angina/history MI/ECG change	30
(28)	259	>65	Rose questionnaire angina	11

IHD = ischaemic heart disease; MI = myocardial infarction.

insensitive and has poor specificity in older age groups (16). Clinically, coronary artery disease can only be demonstrated unequivocally by coronary arteriography, the invasive nature of which precludes widespread use for research purposes. In the future, techniques such as transoesophogeal echocardiography (24), high-resolution magnetic resonance imaging (25) and ultrafast computed tomography (CT) scanning (26) may prove useful, but currently the existence of coronary artery disease is frequently inferred, without definitive anatomical proof, from the presence of one of the clinical syndromes of ischaemic heart disease.

Table 1 summarizes the findings of prevalence studies of ischaemic heart disease among elderly populations, which are invariably based on 12-lead electrocardiography and the Rose Angina Questionnaire (27). Several large longitudinal studies have demonstrated an age-related increase in the incidence of ischaemic heart disease (28–34), and if all clinical indices of the presence of ischaemic heart disease are considered the estimated prevalence among the elderly is approximately 20–30% (10–12,14,35–38)—substantially lower than the 60% prevalence of significant coronary artery disease in a population of similar age (3). How can this difference between the prevalence of ischaemic heart disease and significant coronary disease be explained? Restricted physical activity and the 'physiological β-blockade' that accompanies ageing and modifies the cardiovascular response to exercise or emotional stress (20) may make ischaemia less likely to occur. Alternatively, myocardial ischaemia may occur but pass undetected. Ambulatory electrocardiograph (ECG) monitoring can document transient, episodic ST segment depression concurrent with angina pectoris, or occurring in the absence of symptoms—so-called 'silent ischaemia'—and in one study of elderly individuals the prevalence of ischaemic heart disease increased from 30% to 38% when this technique was added to conventional methods (39). Myocardial ischaemia may also occur in association with atypical symptoms or 'anginal equivalents' such as exertional breathlessness or fatigue (40), and both silent and atypical ischaemia become more common with increasing age (28,39,41,42). Additionally, altered pain perception may alter the classical description of angina (41,42) and lead to misdiagnosis and under-recognition. Elderly patients also tend to under-report their symptoms and all or any of these factors may explain the apparently low prevalence of ischaemia.

Alternative diagnostic techniques have been used to investigate the possible occurrence of less overt ischaemia in elderly individuals. In one study, a large elderly population was investigated with exercise thallium scintigraphy, which demonstrates defects in myocardial perfusion induced by exercise. Among those over 70 years of age the prevalence of ischaemic heart disease was estimated by conventional methods to be approximately 22%, but positive thallium tests increased the estimated prevalence to 54% (43), which is closer to the estimated prevalence of significant coronary disease in a population of this age (3).

The response of left ventricular ejection fraction to exercise, assessed by isotope ventriculography, has also been studied as a possible index of myocardial ischaemia. Although exercise cardiac output is apparently maintained in healthy older individuals (44) the ejection fraction falls in up to 95% of those aged over 70 years without overt ischaemic heart disease (45), and as this is in excess of the prevalence of coronary artery disease in this age group (3) the technique is not sufficiently specific to be of value in the screening of asymptomatic populations.

Table 2 shows the incidence of each of the manifestations of ischaemic heart disease in males and females at different ages. The incidence of angina pectoris and sudden death among males declines with age but the incidence of all manifestations of ischaemic heart disease increases among females. In those aged

Table 2. Annual age- and sex-specific incidence rates (per 10 000 population) for ischaemic heart disease and its manifestations in the Framingham Heart Study

Age (years)	MI		SD		Angina		All IHD	
	M	F	M	F	M	F	M	F
55–64	93	18	27	4	75	58	209	98
65–74	116	34	13	14	56	65	202	127

Adapted from Margolis et al. (30) with permission from the *American Journal of Cardiology*.
MI = myocardial infarction; SD = sudden death; IHD = ischaemic heart disease.

over 65 years, angina occurs more frequently in females than in males and, in those over 75 years of age, the overall prevalence of ischaemic heart disease is almost equal in males and females (14). These changes and the longer lifespan of females account for the larger proportions of female patients found in clinical series among the elderly.

Given the limitations of mortality statistics discussed below there is less certainty regarding the incidence of sudden cardiac death in the very old, although the increasing prevalence of apparently inexplicable death at autopsy (46) may suggest that it increases. In the Framingham study the incidence of sudden cardiac death increased with age in those of either sex without known coronary disease, but only in women with previously recognized coronary disease (47). Similarly, sudden death became an increasingly prevalent first manifestation of coronary artery disease. Some evidence suggests that the incidence of sudden death may currently be declining (29).

Heart failure becomes more prevalent with increasing age (48) and several studies have demonstrated that significant coronary artery disease is found more frequently in those dying of heart failure than those dying from other causes (49–52). Although the prevalence of heart failure associated with angina or previous myocardial infarction therefore appears to increase with age, there is no evidence to suggest that heart failure becomes a more common initial manifestation of ischaemic heart disease.

The relationship between asymptomatic coronary artery disease, ischaemic heart disease and arrhythmia in the elderly is imprecisely defined. In one study a history of ischaemic heart disease was not associated with atrial or ventricular arrhythmias (53). The incidence of sinus node disease appears to peak in the seventh decade (54) but a substantial proportion of these patients do not have evidence of disease of the sinus node artery (55). Chronic atrioventricular block is usually associated with degenerative pathology but acute cases can complicate acute myocardial infarction. Bundle branch block becomes more common with age but there is no evidence to incriminate coronary artery disease as the major cause.

Mortality statistics

Mortality statistics for ischaemic heart disease among elderly populations must be interpreted with caution. The accuracy of clinical diagnosis of major and coexistent pathologies, and hence death certificate information, declines markedly with age (56) and confirmatory postmortem examinations are performed less frequently in older age (46). At autopsy some 30% of deaths in the over-85s can be ascribed to no particular pathological cause (46)—a proportion far in excess of those certified as due to old age, or indeed to sudden cardiac death—and attempts at diagnostic precision after death may therefore lead to inaccuracy if no autopsy is performed. In addition mortality statistics derived from death certificates assess not only the incidence of a condition but also the case fatality

Table 3. Mortality rate (%) for hospitalized patients with myocardial infarction: Scotland 1985

Age (years)	Male	Female
25–44	3.3	5.5
45–64	8.1	10.7
65–74	19.7	22.9
75 and over	38	39.5
All	15.7	24.9

Adapted from Scottish Hospital In-patient Statistics (57).

rate. Death certificate information therefore over-exaggerates the increase in incidence of myocardial infarction with age as the case fatality rate in elderly individuals is much higher. This is shown in the mortality rates for myocardial infarction in Scottish hospitals in 1985 in Table 3 (57).

Ischaemic heart disease is a major cause of mortality in the UK. In England and Wales in 1988, 30.2% of all male deaths and 23.5% of all female deaths were certified as due to ischaemic heart disease (ICD codes 410–414), with 60% of these deaths due to myocardial infarction (58). Among those dying before 65 years of age, 34.4% of male and 15.6% of female deaths were due to ischaemic heart disease, with 30.1% of males and 25.1% of females aged over 65 years similarly classified.

Figure 1 shows the proportion of deaths due to ischaemic heart disease in different age groups and Figure 2 the death rate from ischaemic heart disease by age. Although the death rate rises progressively with age, ischaemic heart disease becomes proportionately less common as a cause of death among the oldest

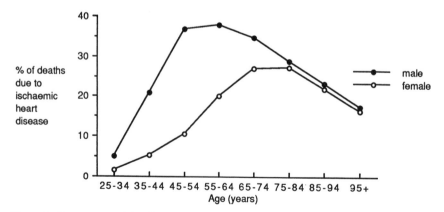

Figure 1. Percentage of deaths due to ischaemic heart disease at different ages. Adapted from Mortality Statistics (58) with permission from the Controller of Her Majesty's Stationery Office

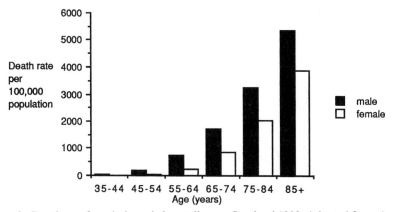

Figure 2. Death rate from ischaemic heart disease: Scotland 1989. Adapted from Annual Report, Registrar General for Scotland (1989) with permission from the Controller of Her Majesty's Stationery Office

Table 4. Deaths from ischaemic heart disease (IHD) and myocardial infarction (MI) at different ages: England and Wales 1988

	All ages		Under 65 years		Over 65 years		65–74 years		Over 75 years	
	n		%		%		%		%	
	IHD	MI	IHD	MI	IHD	MI	IHD	MI	IHD	MI
Male	84 880	54 240	26	26	74	74	33	34	41	40
Female	68 204	42 164	9	9	91	91	22	25	69	66
Total	153 084	94 404	18	17	82	83	29	30	53	53

Adapted from Mortality Statistics (58) with permission from the Controller of Her Majesty's Stationery Office.

patients. The majority of all deaths from ischaemic heart disease do, however, occur among the elderly. Of 153 084 ischaemic heart disease deaths in 1988, 82% occurred in those aged over 65 years, and 53% in those over 75 years. Table 4 shows the number of individuals dying from ischaemic heart disease and myocardial infarction in 1988, and the percentage of the deaths that occurred in each age group. Total mortality rates from ischaemic heart disease have declined in many countries in recent years (59) in both younger and elderly populations (60), with the greatest decline observed in younger age groups.

Health service activity statistics

Hospital or health service data based on the demand for, or use of, services may underestimate the prevalence of many conditions among the elderly as a result of under-reporting of illness. Additionally the tendency to conservative manage-

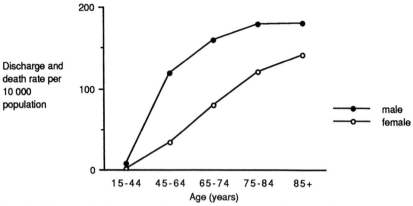

Figure 3. Hospital discharge and death rate from ischaemic heart disease: England and Wales 1984. Adapted from Hospital Inpatient Enquiry (61) with permission of the Controller of Her Majesty's Stationery Office

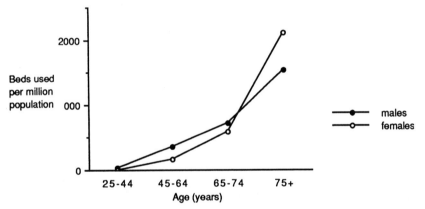

Figure 4. Rate of bed use by patients with ischaemic heart disease: Scotland 1985. Adapted from Scottish Hospital Inpatient Statistics (62)

ment and relative, and often appropriate, under-investigation of older patients may lead to diminished accuracy of diagnosis and be reflected in discharge coding.

Figure 3 shows the discharge (including death) rate for ischaemic heart disease in England and Wales in 1984 (61), and Figure 4 the bed occupancy rate for ischaemic heart disease in Scotland in 1985 (62). Although hospitalization rates and length of stay due to ischaemic heart disease increase with age, the proportion of admissions attributed to ischaemic heart disease declines in older age, from 15% in those aged 45–64 years to 8% in those over 75 years of age (62).

In primary care consultation rates for ischaemic heart disease also increase with age, although angina pectoris is slightly less commonly seen in those over 75 years (63).

The number of elderly patients undergoing coronary arteriography, angio-plasty and bypass surgery has greatly increased in the past 10 years. In the USA 30–40% of those investigated are over 65 years (64,65), but in the UK the limited information available suggests that this proportion is substantially smaller (66). In the USA the elderly comprise 25–35% of those undergoing angioplasty (64,65) and the proportion of elderly coronary bypass patients has increased from 2–8% in the 1970s to 17–30% in the 1980s (64,67,68) and is currently as high as 45% in some centres (65).

Epidemiology and demographic change

The total number of individuals aged over 65 years in the UK will increase in the next 20 years (68), with numbers of the very elderly (aged over 80 years) projected to rise from approximately 1.8 million to 2.6 million by the year 2010 (69). Will the already high prevalence of ischaemic heart disease have changed among these individuals? In recent years the incidence of death from ischaemic heart disease has fallen in all age groups, with the relative reduction smaller among the elderly (59), and this may be associated with the decline in prevalence of several of the known risk factors for coronary disease recorded over the same period (33). If large-scale population prevention strategies are successfully implemented, age *per se* may become a relatively more powerful risk factor for ischaemic heart disease, and presentation may be more frequently delayed into older age. Additionally, the use of more aggressive interventional and surgical treatments of ischaemic heart disease in younger patients may improve prognosis and delay death until older age is reached. The death rate from coronary disease in the oldest age groups might therefore be expected to increase, as 'rectangularization' of our population's survival curve occurs, and the burden of morbidity imposed by coronary artery disease will also be further extended into old age. Indeed, the limited data currently available on the morbidity, functional impairment and disability caused by ischaemic heart disease (59) do not demonstrate a decline commensurate with that seen in mortality in recent years.

Adequate prediction of the needs of elderly individuals with angina and the resources required for their care in coming years will therefore require the development of databases with which the changing incidence of ischaemic heart disease and the impact of interventional strategies can be accurately monitored.

Prognosis of coronary artery disease

Any discussion of the prognosis of disease in elderly individuals must take into account the prognosis imposed by old age itself. Life table analysis (1982) demonstrates that the average survival for a 70-year-old is 11 years for a male and 14 years for a female. A man of 79, or a woman of 82, has a 50% chance of surviving a further 5 years (70). How does the presence of coronary artery disease or its manifestations affect these figures?

In the CASS Registry patients aged over 65 years with angina and three-vessel coronary disease had a 47% 5-year survival and those with poor left ventricular function (left ventricular ejection fraction under 35%) had a 31% survival rate over a similar period. The 5-year survival rates for younger patients with similar disease were 67% and 56%, respectively, and for elderly patients with chest pain but normal coronary arteries and good left ventricular function 86% (71).

As absolute survival declines with age in healthy populations, it is not surprising that absolute survival also declines with age among patients with angina (31,72). The relative survival, or ratio of observed to expected survival, provides a measure of the excess mortality imposed by angina and is no greater in older than younger populations (72). This may suggest that age *per se* is a much less powerful predictor of mortality than the extent of coronary disease or degree of impairment of left ventricular function.

The presence of angina pectoris is associated with a two- to threefold increase in risk of death in older age (38), although if the resting 12-lead ECG is normal no excess mortality may be detected (73). Electrocardiographic abnormalities compatible with ischaemia are associated with excess mortality from coronary disease, irrespective of the presence of chest pain (10,12,74). Similarly, evidence of left ventricular hypertrophy on the ECG (75,76) or echocardiography (77), or cardiomegaly on chest X-ray (78), is associated with increased risk but regression of abnormal electrocardiographic appearances may be associated with an improved prognosis (79).

The occurrence of myocardial infarction, whether occult or recognized, is followed by a 60% 4-year risk of further coronary events and death (28,80,81), although total mortality may not be increased in those over 75 years of age (13).

Among elderly patients with clinically recognized coronary artery disease, echocardiographic evidence of impaired left ventricular function (82), transient asymptomatic ST segment depression during Holter monitoring (39,83) and positive thallium scanning (84) all predict an increased risk of further clinical events.

RISK FACTORS FOR CORONARY ARTERY DISEASE

In clinical practice, it is frequently assumed that coronary artery disease is an inevitable accompaniment of ageing, and the importance of potentially remediable risk factors may therefore be overlooked. Management decisions may concentrate on the relief of symptoms rather than improvement of prognosis, even among the younger elderly whose life expectancy may exceed 15 years (70).

However, as the greatest reductions in absolute risk should be anticipated from treating those with the highest probability of developing disease, older individuals may still benefit from strategies designed to prevent coronary disease. The high prevalence of anatomically significant but clinically silent disease in older individuals cannot, however, be overlooked and may account for the strong association between age and the probability of developing clinical manifestations of coronary artery disease even in individuals with no identifiable risk factor. The factors that may promote transition from the asymptomatic to the symptomatic state therefore require further study.

In general, factors that predict the risk of developing ischaemic heart disease among younger populations, such as systolic blood pressure, plasma glucose, body mass index and total serum cholesterol are more highly prevalent in older age and all retain some association with the incidence of future ischaemic heart disease (76). The demonstration of such association does not, however, necessarily imply that intervention will confer benefit to an individual. The effects of treating the following risk factors in elderly populations have been investigated.

Hypertension

As both systolic and diastolic blood pressure increase with age, the prevalence of hypertension is high in the elderly (85), and data from the Framingham study suggest that it is a more potent predictor of both relative and absolute risk than in younger age groups (75). Elevated systolic and diastolic pressure are both associated with increased risk although the predictive value of diastolic pressure loses power in older women (14,86). Isolated systolic hypertension (systolic blood pressure > 160 mmHg, diastolic blood pressure < 90 mmHg) is present in approximately 20% of elderly men and women (87) and also appears to confer increased cardiovascular risk (86–88).

Studies of primary prevention with antihypertensive agents in the elderly have demonstrated variable reductions in cardiovascular and total mortality, but beneficial effects on the incidence of ischaemic heart disease have been found, at least for those under the age of 80 years (89,90). The benefits of treating isolated systolic hypertension have recently been established, even for those aged over 80 years (91). Currently, we suggest treatment if systolic pressure is above 160 mmHg or diastolic pressure above 90 mmHg, especially in the presence of ischaemic heart disease.

Hypercholesterolaemia

The relationship between serum cholesterol level and the incidence of ischaemic heart disease in the elderly is controversial and requires further investigation (92). Total serum cholesterol remains a risk factor for death from ischaemic heart disease mortality in older age groups in both sexes (14,76,93,94) although the predictive value declines among men. If the level of high- and low-density lipoprotein cholesterol fractions are considered, predictive value is restored (14,75,86,95) and there is also limited evidence that triglyceride levels predict risk among elderly populations (14).

Should hypercholesterolaemia in an elderly individual be treated? Although it has been demonstrated that cholesterol can be successfully lowered in this age group, the absence of controlled trials to demonstrate clear evidence of benefit of such treatment on total mortality in the elderly suggests that widespread drug treatment is not indicated (96–98).

Obesity

Obesity is associated with hypertension and hyperlipidaemia and appears to retain an independent association with the incidence of ischaemic heart disease in older individuals (86). All older patients who are obese should be advised of the potential beneficial effects of weight loss, particularly if they are hypertensive or diabetic, are already suffering from angina or are prospective surgical candidates.

Diabetes mellitus

Although diabetes mellitus and hyperglycaemia are powerful predictors of risk of ischaemic heart disease in the elderly (86), there is no evidence that improved control of hyperglycaemia reduces the incidence of future coronary events. Hyperinsulinaemia and 'insulin resistance' have recently been identified as risk factors in younger individuals (90).

Physical inactivity

Regular, vigorous, physical activity improves many patients' feeling of well-being and can reduce blood pressure, body weight and serum low-density lipoprotein and increase high-density lipoprotein (100). The improved conditioning of skeletal muscle that results is associated with haemodynamic changes that particularly benefit individuals with heart failure, and there is evidence that exercise may also be associated with a decreased risk of coronary events in those over 65 years of age (86,101–103).

Cigarette smoking

Cigarette smoking is associated with an increased risk of death from ischaemic heart disease in older individuals (104,105) although the relationship of smoking status with other indices of coronary artery disease is less clearly defined (76,86). Coronary mortality declines if smoking is stopped (104,106) and, given the additional association of cigarette smoking with peripheral and cerebrovascular disease, chronic obstructive airways disease and pulmonary neoplasia, even elderly smokers should be encouraged to stop.

ANGINA PECTORIS: DIAGNOSIS, INVESTIGATION AND TREATMENT

The successful management of ischaemic heart disease is primarily dependent on the recognition of myocardial ischaemia, typically in the form of angina pectoris. In community studies of the elderly between 10% and 15% are found to have angina (10–12,36) but such studies probably underestimate the true prevalence in older patients (107) as communication difficulties may make history taking difficult and the description (41) or recollection of symptoms may be vague or incomplete. A history of chest pain or myocardial infarction, admitted in one interview, may be denied at the next (12). A more sedentary lifestyle may protect the elderly patient from exertional ischaemia and postprandial or nocturnal symptoms may consequently become more prominent. The character and site of anginal discomfort is frequently different in older patients (41), and coexistent conditions, such as gastroesophogeal reflux, may mask or mimic the pain. 'Anginal equivalents' such as exertional dyspnoea or fatigue are more common in the elderly (40), and are thought to relate to ischaemic left ventricular and papillary muscle dysfunction, mitral regurgitation and dysrhythmia, but their prevalence and functional significance have not been studied.

Despite these difficulties, an accurate history remains of great value, as the presence of typical angina pectoris is as highly predictive of the presence of significant coronary artery disease as in younger patients, and of greater predictive value than atypical or non-specific chest pain (108) (Figure 5).

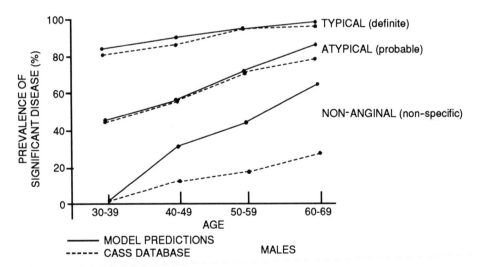

Figure 5. Influence of clinical assessment of chest pain on prevalence of significant coronary artery disease. Reproduced from Pryor *et al.* (108) with permission from the *American Journal of Medicine*

Symptoms may have been present for many years but in some the history is brief, although even in such cases coronary disease is frequently found to be more extensive than in younger patients with a similarly short history.

How does angina affect the lives of elderly people? Unfortunately, few studies have investigated the impact of angina on independence, function and quality of life in elderly individuals, although an association between angina and disability has been suggested (36). Studies of patients undergoing coronary arteriography (66,109) or coronary artery bypass surgery (127,128) suggest that older patients tend to have more severe or unstable symptoms than do younger patients. The prevalence of coexistent diabetes, hypertension, heart failure, pulmonary disease, cerebrovascular disease and renal impairment are also higher (127,128) but this may simply reflect varying selection policies for these procedures rather than true differences between age groups. Accurate information regarding the clinical and functional characteristics of elderly individuals with angina is of importance, as current predictions of future resource requirements for the management of angina are based predominantly on population projections and prevalence data which take no account of the severity of symptoms or their effect on function. Equally, many elderly patients with angina may be disabled by other major system disease which not only minimizes the effect of their angina but may also preclude interventional treatment.

Investigation

In many elderly individuals the diagnosis of angina pectoris can be made confidently from the history. Physical examination is most helpful in these cases where ischaemia is caused or exacerbated by valvular disease or complicated by heart failure and may also demonstrate other cardiac, vascular or major system disease that might compromise the patient's capacity to undergo invasive investigation or treatment.

The high prevalence of abnormalities found in the resting 12-lead ECG, even in asymptomatic elderly populations (11), and the recognition that a normal appearance does not exclude ischaemic heart disease limits its diagnostic value, but a routine trace does provide a baseline with which future recordings, particularly those obtained during pain, may be usefully compared. Anaemia and hyperthyroidism should be excluded.

Once identified angina pectoris should be considered only as a symptom of underlying myocardial ischaemia. Commonly the cause is a fixed coronary artery stenosis but occasionally excessive demands imposed on a normal coronary circulation by a hypertrophied left ventricle in patients with aortic stenosis, hypertrophic cardiomyopathy or hypertensive heart disease can produce identical symptoms and can be simply excluded by clinical examination and echocardiography. Additional non-cardiac investigations may be indicated if alternative causes of atypical pain such as gastro-oesophageal reflux are considered likely.

Most elderly patients can be successfully managed without recourse to any further investigations. If the history is atypical, or symptoms are poorly controlled by antianginal drugs and intervention is feasible, or it is thought that prognosis should be more precisely established, the following investigations may be indicated.

Exercise testing

Several investigations share the principle that an increase in cardiac work, usually induced by isotonic exercise, may provoke myocardial ischaemia or dysfunction not observed at rest and be detected by 12-lead electrocardiography, echocardiography, radionuclide ventriculography or thallium scintigraphy. These tests permit objective assessment of functional capacity, the correlation of symptoms to objective evidence of ischaemia, risk stratification, and definition of the location and extent of ischaemia.

The value of any investigation which requires the patient to undertake exercise declines with age. Lack of fitness or coexistent neurological, peripheral vascular or musculoskeletal disease may limit or preclude exertion, and exercise capacity declines with age even in fit individuals. Only a limited number of elderly individuals can therefore perform exercise sufficient to raise their heart rate to 75–85% of the predicted value—a prerequisite for accurate interpretation of results. Furthermore maximum achievable heart rate declines with age and even those who attain such 'target' heart rates may not therefore achieve an increase in cardiac work sufficient to induce ischaemia.

In addition to these problems in performance, the diagnostic utility of these investigations is limited by the high prevalence of coronary artery disease in the general elderly population. This, according to Bayesian probability, will influence the diagnostic value of any test for the index disease. In particular the predictive value of a negative test declines (110). In addition, the presence of typical angina in an elderly patient is associated with a high pretest probability of significant coronary disease that will be little altered by further non-invasive investigations (108). Despite these limitations each of the following techniques may be useful in selected patients.

Exercise electrocardiography

Exercise electrocardiography remains the most simple, non-invasive and widely employed investigation. A variety of exercise protocols are used, employing treadmill, bicycle or rarely isotonic arm exercise alone. The Bruce and modified Bruce treadmill protocols are most suited to elderly individuals but all such testing must be particularly closely supervised and conducted in accordance with recognized guidelines (111).

In elderly individuals with interpretable baseline ECG traces who can exercise to a workload sufficient to raise heart rate to 85% of the predicted maximal (usually over 5 metres), the sensitivity of exercise electrocardiography is higher than in younger individuals (i.e. false negatives decrease) but specificity falls (i.e. false positives increase) (112,113). A high prevalence of multi-vessel disease, as is found in elderly populations, will also increase the sensitivity of the exercise test (112) but multivariate analysis suggests that other, undetermined factors are responsible for the rise in sensitivity that occurs with age (112). Exercise duration is, however, often brief in unselected elderly populations and, as false negative tests become more frequent with shortening duration of exercise, sensitivity may be significantly curtailed.

Thallium scintigraphy

The addition of thallium scintigraphic imaging to standard exercise electrocardiography permits further assessment of the extent and location of induced ischaemia. The limited information available on its value as a diagnostic test in elderly patients suggests that sensitivity and specificity are not significantly different than in younger patients (114). Some studies suggest that thallium scintigraphy (84,115,116) may predict prognosis more accurately than standard exercise electrocardiography (117).

Radionuclide ventriculography

This technique is used to evaluate changes in left ventricular function during exercise. Although a decline in ejection fraction with exercise may not be specific for coronary artery disease in apparently healthy older patients (45), studies of elderly individuals with chest pain suggest that the sensitivity and specificity in detecting significant coronary artery disease are similar to those aged under 60 years (118).

The possibility of inducing ischaemia without performing exercise holds obvious attractions for the investigation of the elderly. Dipyridamole, dobutamine, adenosine, isoprenaline (119) cardiac pacing or cold-water hand immersion have all been investigated, as have alternative forms of exercise such as arm ergometry and isometric handgrip exercise (120). Dipyridamole thallium scintigraphy holds most promise, provided its safety in the elderly can be confirmed, and initial experience suggests that sensitivity is retained in the elderly (121) and that important prognostic information can be obtained (122). Dobutamine, dipyridamole and adenosine echocardiography (123,124) are also being investigated in younger patients, although the poor acoustic window found in some elderly patients may limit their use.

Coronary arteriography

The standard for the diagnosis of coronary artery disease in life is coronary arteriography. The anatomical extent of coronary artery disease can be conclusively demonstrated, but as such disease is highly prevalent in the general elderly population (3) caution must be employed in the interpretation of arteriographic appearances. Ideally the functional effect of a stenosis should also be demonstrated, if possible by one of the methods discussed above, although in practice those elderly patients who undergo arteriography frequently have symptoms of such severity that exercise testing is prohibited. Coronary arteriography is therefore rarely employed as a diagnostic test in elderly patients but is routinely used to assess suitability for treatment by coronary surgery or angioplasty. Although complications occur more frequently than in younger patients, most are minor and transient, and the overall rate is low (109). The severity and extent of coronary disease and associated left ventricular dysfunction demonstrated at coronary angiography differ in elderly and younger populations. Among those referred for angiography more older patients are found to have three-vessel or left main stem disease and to have impaired left ventricular function (109) but there is no evidence that age *per se* is associated with an increased frequency of diffuse disease of the distal vessels. Such differences might be anticipated from the postmortem data reviewed earlier, but may be exaggerated by the selection policies for arteriography applied to older patients, who are more likely than younger patients to have severe and long-standing symptoms when investigation is undertaken (66).

Treatment

The principal aim of treatment of elderly patients with angina is the control of symptoms, although for an increasing number of fit older individuals management should include some consideration of prognosis and its modification by interventional treatment.

General measures and advice

Education and explanation are important, with emphasis given to the cause and significance of the chest discomfort. If angina occurs at rest, or persists for more than 30 minutes, the patient should seek urgent medical attention. Some patients with exertional angina may be prepared, and able, to modify their activities in order to reduce the frequency of symptoms. The patient should know that if modification of activity and drug treatment prove unsatisfactory further investigation and interventional treatment is not precluded by age alone. Patients should be persuaded to discontinue smoking; many units will only refer non-smokers for coronary surgery. Exacerbating conditions such as hypertension, thyrotoxicosis, anaemia, heart failure, paroxysmal tachycardia and obesity should be sought and treated.

Drug treatment

Aspirin in doses from 75 to 300 mg affords protective benefit to individuals with angina. True aspirin intolerance is unusual and minor gastric irritation may be reduced by use of enteric coated preparations. Most elderly patients will require treatment with at least one antianginal drug, all of which have the capacity to cause side-effects. Drug treatment should be titrated, beginning with lower dosages, and compliance may be improved by the use of once-daily formulations, although perceived efficacy and adverse effects are more important determinants of this.

Sublingual or buccal nitrates in tablet or spray form remain the cornerstone of symptomatic treatment and may be taken to relieve discomfort or before precipitating activities. Headache and lightheadedness may be ameliorated if the patient sits. On many occasions more than one tablet or spray will be required, and fears that this may cause addiction or loss of effect must be allayed. If glyceryl trinitrate (GTN) tablets are used the supply must be renewed every 6 weeks.

Frail patients or those with very occasional symptoms may be managed with GTN and aspirin alone but all other patients should commence treatment with a prophylactic antianginal agent such as a β-blocker, calcium antagonist, or long-acting nitrate to attempt to reduce the detrimental effects of repetitive minor ischaemia on left ventricular function. β-Blockers may be contraindicated by the presence of asthma, chronic obstructive airways disease, peripheral vascular disease, heart failure or disease of the atrioventricular node, but remain effective in suitable older patients. A cardioselective β-blocker such as metoprolol or atenolol should be used but adverse effects such as tiredness and cold extremities may still be disabling and should not be dismissed.

If symptoms continue a calcium antagonist should be added. The combination of a β-blocker with verapamil or diltiazem can cause symptomatic bradycardia or atrioventricular block, and nifedipine is therefore preferred in this situation. In the absence of β-blockade, verapamil or diltiazem are the agents of choice as they do not cause reflex tachycardia. All calcium antagonists can cause hypotension and flushing, and nifedipine may cause peripheral oedema and verapamil constipation.

The frequent presence of cardiac failure in the elderly can further complicate the treatment of angina as β-blockers, verapamil and diltiazem have significant negative inotropic properties. Some patients may tolerant nifedipine or alternatively a nitrate may be effective. The efficacy of nitrates is, however, variable and may decrease after 4–6 weeks of treatment due to the development of nitrate tolerance. A 'nitrate-free' period is therefore recommended and may be achieved by using once-daily preparations, a short-acting preparation twice daily, or removing any transcutaneous preparation at night. In some patients, an agent from each of the three classes may be required before symptoms are controlled. The principles of management of angina in older patients are summarized in Figure 6.

Interventional treatment: coronary artery bypass surgery and coronary angioplasty

Most elderly patients obtain adequate symptom control from antianginal therapy. Those who do not should be advised of the possibility of treatment by

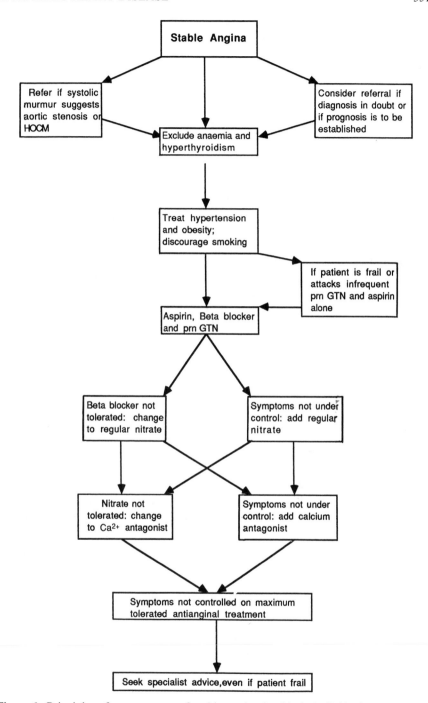

Figure 6. Principles of management of stable angina in elderly individuals

coronary angioplasty or coronary artery surgery. Some patients are too frail to be considered or choose not to undergo investigation and may achieve further symptom control by further modification of activity, weight loss or treatment of hypertension. The extent and severity of coronary artery disease and degree of left ventricular dysfunction can be determined by coronary arteriography, and these factors and the presence of any significant non-cardiac disease are the primary determinants of suitability for coronary artery surgery or angioplasty. Some elderly patients are found to be unsuitable for either treatment following catheterization, particularly if extensive, diffuse disease is demonstrated in the distal portions of the coronary arteries.

Until recently, percutaneous transluminal coronary angioplasty was preferred if single-vessel disease was demonstrated. However, developments in angioplasty technique and the recognition that symptoms in a patient with multi-vessel disease may be attenuated or abolished by dilatation of a single 'culprit lesion' may further extend the use of angioplasty in the elderly (126). Restenosis and myocardial infarction occur more frequently than in younger patients, particularly if the procedure is performed urgently (126) but overall risk is lower than for coronary surgery. Although emergency surgery may be required if occlusion complicates the attempted dilatation, many centres are now prepared to attempt angioplasty in severely symptomatic elderly patients who are fit for neither emergency nor elective surgery. Adoption of such a policy requires careful assessment of the likely benefits and risks in each individual patient but could greatly extend the potential application of the technique in elderly populations. Severe left main stem disease, which is found more frequently than in younger patients (109), is not, however, safely treated by angioplasty at any age.

The efficacy of coronary artery bypass surgery for the relief of angina in elderly patients has been clearly demonstrated in numerous studies (127–130). At present most elderly patients selected to undergo coronary artery surgery are highly symptomatic, often requiring urgent surgery, and have a greater prevalence of three-vessel or left main stem coronary disease, impaired left ventricular function and other major system disease than is found in younger patients (109,130). As several of these factors are associated with increased operative risk in surgical patients of any age (131) operative mortality is predictably higher than in younger patients (109) and, although age is undoubtedly an independent risk factor for mortality, the overall rate should be considered as surprisingly low rather than prohibitively high. The associated morbidity, length of hospital stay and hospital costs are also higher (132,133), but despite severe disease the symptomatic result is as good as that seen in younger patients, and long-term survival equals that of the age-matched population in general (71). These results might be further improved if elderly patients were referred for investigation before their symptoms become critical, as is commonly the case for younger patients.

Relatively few studies have assessed the effect of surgery on the quality of life of elderly patients or explored the possibility that 'minor' complications such as

impaired sternal wound healing or the more subtle neuropsychological consequences of bypass procedures have a prolonged detrimental functional effect.

The presence of coronary artery disease and any accompanying left ventricular
impairment is associated with a shortened lifespan at all ages. In patients aged
over 65 years with normal coronary arteries, 6-year survival is 80% but this falls
to 40% if all three major coronary vessels are diseased and 30% if left ventricular
function is poor (71). In patients under 65 years of age coronary artery bypass
surgery can increase life expectancy if left main stem disease or three-vessel
disease combined with moderate ventricular impairment is present (134,135) but
the studies that demonstrated this effect included few patients over 65 years of
age. Non-randomized studies of elderly patients with angina suggest that surgical
treatment is associated with an improved survival in some subgroups (127)
despite the increased operative mortality that is experienced. It is not yet known
whether angioplasty confers benefit on long-term survival in any age group.

As the severity of symptoms correlates poorly with the extent of underlying
coronary artery disease, many younger patients with mild symptoms undergo
exercise testing or coronary arteriography to assess disease severity and establish
prognosis. Should more elderly patients be managed in this way and be referred
for coronary surgery if severe disease is found? The implementation of such a
policy would incur resource demands that could not be met by the current British
health care system. In the future, the increasing knowledge and expectations of
our elderly patients may provoke further consideration of this issue. A strategy
for the investigation and management of elderly patients with angina is shown in
Figure 7.

Unstable angina

The prevalence of unstable angina may decline with age (136) but elderly patients
comprise a substantial proportion of those reported in large series of unstable
angina. Unstable symptoms are frequently the first to bring elderly individuals to
the attention of hospital physicians although many may have a long history of
stable angina. Management should differ little from that of younger patients but
intolerance of drugs may be more common and interventional strategies less
frequently feasible.

MYOCARDIAL INFARCTION

The incidence and prevalence of acute myocardial infarction increases with age
(30,32) and over half of all those who die from myocardial infarction in the UK
are aged over 75 years of age (Table 4). The prevalence of myocardial infarction
among the elderly is dependent on the age group studied and the diagnostic
criteria applied and varies between 10% and 25% (11,13,137–139). One-third to
one-half of these infarcts are clinically unrecognized or 'silent' (13,28).

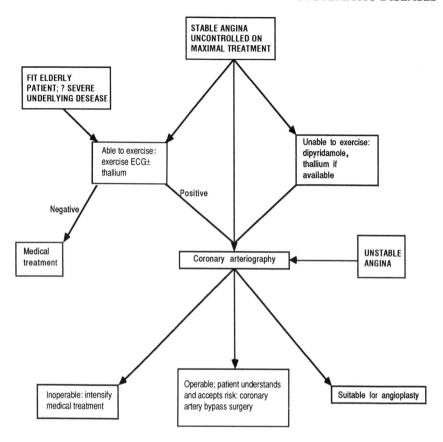

Figure 7. Strategy for investigation and interventional treatment in elderly patients with angina

Clinical features

The diagnosis of acute myocardial infarction in the elderly is based on the same criteria as are applied to younger patients: history, electrocardiographic change and cardiac enzyme abnormality. The evaluation of each, however, poses particular problems among elderly patients which make diagnostic delay more likely and hence potentially reduce the efficacy of thrombolytic therapy.

A wide variation in the presentation of acute myocardial infarction in the elderly has been described (140) with the reported prevalence of 'atypical infarction' varying between 12% (141) and 81% (142). This variation may be explained by differing referral patterns and admission policies between study centres, with studies from coronary care or acute medical beds often demonstrating a higher incidence of 'classical' presentation than those from geriatric units (142,143), residential homes (144) or populations of older elderly (145). Atypical

Table 5. Prevalence (%) of symptoms of myocardial infarction at different ages

Symptom (%)	Age (years)					
	65–70	70–74	75–79	80–84	85+	All (n = 777)
Chest pain	76	79	68	51	37	66
Dyspnoea	38	43	41	47	43	42
Sweating	36	32	27	17	14	27
Vomiting	18	21	18	17	16	18
Syncope	9	8	15	21	18	13
Weakness	7	7	8	6	10	7
Giddiness	6	7	4	5	5	5
Palpitation	4	2	2	1	1	2
Confusion	3	3	8	8	19	7
Stroke	2	2	5	9	7	4
Embolus	1	1	0	0	0	0.5

Adapted from A. J. Bayer, J. S. Chadha, R. R. Farag and M. S. J. Pathy, Changing presentation of myocardial infarction with increasing old age, *Journal of the American Geriatrics Society*, **34**, 263–266, 1986, © by the American Geriatric Society.

presentations are undoubtedly more common in the elderly, and are partially accounted for by communication difficulties, including cognitive impairment (146), and altered pain perception (42) although diabetes mellitus does not appear to be causally associated with this feature (147). Pain may become a less commanding feature, and its site and character differ. Autonomic accompaniments such as sweating and nausea may predominate or, conversely, be absent. Breathlessness or overwhelming fatigue may be the dominant symptom and some patients present with delayed complications such as arrhythmia, stroke or peripheral arterial embolism. Table 5 shows the prevalence of symptoms of myocardial infarction in one large study of the elderly (148).

In the Multicenter Chest Pain Study (149) some 'typical' features of myocardial infarction, such as radiation of pain to the neck or pain of a 'pressing' character, occurred less frequently in elderly patients presenting with acute chest pain, but others were observed more frequently, particularly prolonged pain which was more severe than the patient's usual angina. However, those patients who were subsequently found not to have sustained an infarct were noted to have generally more 'typical' symptoms. This feature and the high prevalence of abnormal baseline ECGs and past history of angina or infarction in the population studied was thought to explain the observation that elderly patients with chest pain were more likely to be admitted to hospital but less likely to have sustained an infarction (149). Beyond the age of 85 years atypical presentations predominate (148) and diagnosis from the history alone is sufficiently unreliable to make 12-lead electrocardiography mandatory in the assessment of any elderly individual with acute illness.

The high prevalence of resting electrocardiographic abnormalities, in particular left bundle branch block and pre-existent q waves, can further compound diagnostic difficulty, but there is no evidence that the evolution of electrocardiographic abnormalities in elderly patients with transmural infarction is different from that seen in younger populations. Subendocardial infarction is more frequently encountered (32) and the development of ST segment or T wave changes in sequential traces without Q wave formation should not be overlooked. The possibility that elevated enzyme titres are spurious should be considered in the frail elderly, as a significant rise in titre may follow skeletal muscle injury, such as that caused by a fall (150). If possible, myocardium-specific isoenzymes such as CK-MB should be measured. Infarct size is generally smaller (32,81), but there is no difference in observed prevalence of infarct site (136).

Mortality and morbidity

Both recognized and silent myocardial infarction are associated with a higher fatality rate in the elderly than is found in younger individuals (13,28,32,151–154), with those aged over 75 years experiencing an in-hospital mortality rate seven times higher than those under 55 years (32). The absolute mortality in the period after hospital discharge is also higher in older individuals (32), with those over 75 years of age having at least a twofold risk of death (32) compared to younger infarct patients and elderly patients without infarction. Although age *per se* remains a powerful predictor of mortality in multivariate analysis (32,155), elderly patients with myocardial infarction display several additional characteristics that partially account for their higher mortality. The prevalence of pre-existent heart failure, myocardial infarction, angina, hypertension and diabetes are all higher (81,156), as is underlying multi-vessel coronary disease (81). The relative excess of females among the elderly (32) and the less active treatment that some elderly individuals receive (32) may also be of importance. Age-related admission policies will also influence the patient characteristics documented in some studies. In many centres only elderly patients with specific complications of definite infarction are admitted to coronary care. Similarly, many elderly patients with uncomplicated or 'small' myocardial infarction may not be referred to hospital. Mortality statistics derived from such studies may therefore reflect the outcome for a particularly sick group of elderly patients.

The management of myocardial infarction

In recent years, discussions regarding the management of elderly patients with acute myocardial infarction have centred on two issues: the benefits of admission to hospital, and the use of thrombolytic treatment.

Admission to hospital, and ideally to a coronary care unit, permits prompt identification and treatment of arrhythmia and heart failure, and administration of specific therapies designed to limit infarct size and improve prognosis. In addition symptoms can be effectively monitored and controlled. If an elderly patient is significantly disabled by physical or psychiatric illness and such active management is felt inappropriate, hospital admission may not be justified provided symptoms can be adequately controlled. The majority of elderly individuals are not, however, disabled to such a degree and as the mortality of myocardial infarction is higher than in younger patients (13,32,151–154) and the outcome of thrombolysis and treatment of ventricular fibrillation as good (157,158), their potential to benefit from admission and active treatment is at least equivalent to younger patients (159). Do they receive such treatment? In a survey of coronary care units in the UK, 20% and 33% operated age-related policies for admission and thrombolysis, respectively, although the upper age limit for thrombolysis ranged from 75 to 95 years (160). Although these figures suggest that most coronary care units are prepared to treat older individuals, concern remains that patients are frequently excluded from treatment on the grounds of their age alone (68,161,162,190).

General management

Immediate attention should be given to the relief of the common symptoms of pain, anxiety, nausea and breathlessness. The dose of some drugs, including opiates and antiarrhythmics such as lignocaine, may require reduction. Continuous electrocardiographic monitoring is required if the patient is to be resuscitated in the event of a cardiac arrest. The risks of bed rest increase in the old, and early mobilization should be encouraged in uncomplicated infarction. Subcutaneous heparin or support stockings may be used to inhibit deep venous thrombosis. Complications including pulmonary oedema (157), atrial fibrillation (81), conduction disturbances, cardiogenic shock and hypovolaemia (32) are all more commonly encountered. Stroke occurs more commonly than in younger populations and is found in 1.4–1.6% of older individuals (163,164).

In uncomplicated cases discharge can occur between 5 and 7 days. The mean length of hospital stay following myocardial infarction is greater in the elderly and this may relate to specific complications of the infarct itself and age-related problems such as chest and urinary infection, premorbid dependency and social problems. The early intervention of a team skilled in the rehabilitation of the elderly can therefore minimize such difficulties and shorten the length of hospital stay.

Exercise testing may be employed following myocardial infarction as a means of identifying those with a poor prognosis (165) and may be performed in selected elderly patients if surgical treatment would be feasible and acceptable to the patient. Many elderly patients are, however, considered ineligible for predischarge exercise testing and this characteristic *per se* has been identified as a risk factor for mortality in the first year following myocardial infarction (166). Risk factors for further events should be identified, and selected elderly patients may benefit from treatment of hypertension and hyperlipidaemia.

Table 6. Mortality in relation to age in major studies of thrombolysis

	Age	Mortality rate (%)		Mortality reduction	
		Treatment	Placebo	%	Lives saved/1000
GISSI (151)	<60	5.7	7.7	26	20
(SK alone)	65–75	16.6	18.1	8	15
	>75	28.9	33.1	13	42
ISIS-2 (153)	<60	4.2	5.8	28	16
(SK alone)	60–69	10.6	14.4	26	38
	>70	18.2	21.6	16	34
ISIS-2	<60	4.5	5.5	18	10
(aspirin alone)	60–69	10.9	14.0	22	31
	>70	17.6	22.3	21	47
ISIS-2	<60	3.7	6.2	40	25
(SK plus aspirin)	60–69	9.1	16.1	43	70
	>70	15.8	23.8	34	80
AIMS (153)	<65	5.2	8.5	38	33
(anistreplase)	>65	12.2	30.2	60	180
ASSET (154)	56–65	6.5	7.9	18	14
(TPA)	66–75	10.8	16.4	34	56

SK = streptokinase; TPA = tissue plasminogen activator.

Thrombolytic treatment

Treatment with thrombolytic drugs is associated with a substantial reduction in the immediate and longer-term mortality of patients with myocardial infarction (151–154). Although elderly patients were specifically excluded from several large trials of thrombolysis, sufficient numbers of younger elderly (under 75 years) have now been studied to permit an analysis of efficacy and safety.

Table 6 compares the early (30-day) mortality rate in older and younger individuals in the GISSI, ISIS-2, AIMS and ASSET studies (151–154). The relative reduction in mortality varies between studies but the effect on absolute mortality (lives saved per 1000 treated) is consistently higher in elderly patients, as might be anticipated from the higher case fatality rate in this group. The beneficial effects of treatment with aspirin alone should not be overlooked, particularly in those elderly patients who are managed outside coronary care units. Maximum benefit from thrombolysis is dependent on prompt administration, which should ideally be within 6 hours of onset of symptoms, and the delayed presentation (167) and diagnostic difficulties encountered in the elderly may result in treatment being considered later than in younger patients. Some survival benefit can, however, follow treatment administered up to 24 hours from the onset of symptoms (151).

Concern has surrounded the risk of haemorrhagic complications of thrombolytic therapy in the elderly, for although major events such as intracerebral haemorrhage are rare they are often catastrophic. The GISSI study demonstrated an increased risk of stroke with age in both treated (1.7% in those over 75 years) and placebo (1.1% in those over 75 years) groups but the excess of strokes occurring in the older patients treated with streptokinase was no greater than in younger patients (163). Studies with other thrombolytic agents have provided conflicting evidence of an association between age and an increased incidence of major haemorrhagic complications (168,169). As many of these complications relate to sites of vascular access, they are potentially avoidable and it appears that the elderly are exposed to no greater increase in risk with thrombolytic treatment than are younger patients (153). The contraindications to thrombolytic treatment are more highly prevalent in the elderly and are shown in Table 7.

The demonstrated efficacy and safety of thrombolytic treatment have led to increasing awareness of the need to promote their use in the elderly (68,161,170,171), particularly as they currently appear to be frequently excluded from such treatment (162). The elderly patients who participated in the studies of thrombolysis were, however, highly selected and it remains to be seen whether efficacy and safety are equivalent in more widespread clinical use. Although absolute mortality reductions are greater in elderly patients treated with thrombolysis, the effect of this treatment on alternative endpoints such as symptoms, function and dependence must be assessed in elderly patients. An

Table 7. Contraindications to thrombolytic treatment in elderly patients

---

Absolute
History of significant gastrointestinal haemorrhage within past 6 months
Documented peptic ulcer within past 3 months
Stroke or documented transient ischaemic attack within past 6 months
Trauma, head injury or major surgery within past 6 weeks
Bleeding diathesis
Chronic liver disease

Relative
Systolic blood pressure > 200 mmHg or diastolic pressure > 110 mmHg
Cardiopulmonary resuscitation lasting over 1 minute
Diabetic proliferative retinopathy
Non-compressible arterial puncture within past 14 days
Dental extraction within past 14 days
Oral anticoagulant treatment
Malignant disease
Significant premorbid functional impairment
Previous treatment with streptokinase or anistreplase—risk of allergy (use TPA)

TPA = tissue plasminogen activator.

improvement in survival following myocardial infarction is of arguable value to elderly patients if their subsequent quality of life is poor. In addition, if the use of thrombolysis in this age group is to be rational, elderly patients must have equal access to any diagnostic or therapeutic procedures that are subsequently required. Although recent studies suggest that invasive investigation following thrombolytic treatment is not routinely required (172), a substantial proportion of patients have recurrent symptoms and require investigation and subsequent revascularization by surgery or angioplasty. It is not known if the proportion of elderly patients experiencing this outcome is greater, or if the early benefits on mortality will be offset by a greater requirement for subsequent interventional treatment of relatively high risk (173).

β-Blockade

The demonstrated reduction in mortality associated with β-blockade following myocardial infarction may relate to a decrease in the incidence of ventricular rupture (174). This complication is more common in the elderly (175,176), who might therefore be expected to receive particular benefit.

Elderly individuals were excluded from the majority of studies of β-blockade following myocardial infarction, but in studies of timolol (177), metoprolol (178) and propranolol (179) 3-month mortality was reduced by up to 45% in 65–75-year-olds and beneficial longer-term effects often of greater magnitude than in younger patients were also observed. The use of these drugs in elderly patients may be limited as they are less well tolerated (178) and heart failure is a more frequent complication of infarction (32).

Coronary angioplasty

Although this technique is feasible following myocardial infarction, results in elderly patients have been variable and often disappointing (180,181). As early routine arteriography and angioplasty following acute myocardial infarction are not of benefit (172,182), use should be restricted to those elderly patients with severe, unstable or continuing symptoms following myocardial infarction in whom the risks of surgery are prohibitive.

Cardiopulmonary resuscitation

Primary ventricular fibrillation occurs less frequently in older patients with myocardial infarction (157), and the outcome of defibrillation is equal to that of younger patients (158). Asystolic arrest is associated with a poor outcome in all age groups. Age has not been identified as an independent predictor of poor outcome in hospital series of cardiopulmonary resuscitation (183,184) but long-term survival among elderly patients resuscitated out of hospital is lower than in younger patients, despite similar initial response rates (185). The desirability and appropriateness of attempted resuscitation of an elderly patient should be based on consideration of each individual's premorbid functional ability and health, the prognosis of their current condition, the likely outcome of resuscitation and knowledge of any wishes previously documented by the patient. 'Resuscitation policies' based on age alone cannot be justified. We believe that a decision regarding attempted resuscitation should be made as soon as possible after admission to hospital before any acute event precipitates unconsidered and perhaps inappropriate treatment or inactivity.

Rehabilitation

Significant physical and psychological disability can follow myocardial infarction. Rehabilitation programmes designed to ameliorate these consequences have focused on younger individuals and have often operated specific exclusion criteria for those over 65 years of age. Return to work—a convenient means of assesing benefit in younger people—is obviously invalid in elderly populations but more sophisticated indices of function, quality of life and perception of well-being have recently been developed.

Functional impairment following myocardial infarction in the elderly is probably under-recognized and under-treated. A substantial decline in psychological indices of well-being and in ability to perform basic activities of daily living has been demonstrated in such patients (186) and lack of improvement of these indices in the first 3 months following discharge was a predictive factor for mortality in the next 3 years (187). The relative contribution of specific medical problems such as heart failure or angina or of other factors such as psychological state to such disability in the elderly has not been defined. The value of simple measures, including advice on returning to social and household activities and education regarding the patient's condition and the benefits of exercise, stopping smoking and weight reduction, should not be overlooked. Exercise training has been evaluated in limited numbers of selected elderly patients and improvements in haemodynamic and functional parameters similar to those seen in younger patients observed (188). Currently, supervised cardiac rehabilitation of this nature is not widely available for elderly patients in the UK.

REFERENCES

1. McGill HC, Arias-Stella J, Carbonnel LM *et al.* (1968) General findings of the International Atherosclerosis Project. *Lab Invest* **18**: 498–502.
2. Eggin DA, Solberg LA (1968) Variation of atherosclerosis with age. *Lab Invest* **18**: 571–579.
3. Elveback L, Lie JT (1984) Continued high prevalence of coronary artery disease at autopsy in Olmstead County Minnesota 1950–1979. *Circulation* **70**: 345–349.
4. Hazzard WR (1984) Atherosclerosis and aging: a scenario in flux. *Am J Cardiol* **63**: 20H–24H.
5. Barrett-Connor E, Bush TL (1991) Estrogen and coronary heart disease in women

JAMA **265**: 1861–1867.

6. Vandenbroucke JP (1991) Postmenopausal oestrogen and cardioprotection. *Lancet* **337**: 833–834.

7. Pomerance A (1981) Cardiac pathology in the elderly. In RJ Noble and DA Rothbaum (Eds.) *Geriatric Cardiology*, Noble RJ, Rothbaum DA (eds). Davis, Philadelphia, pp. 9–54.

8. Schwartz CJ, Mitchell JRA (1962) The relation between myocardial lesions and coronary artery disease. *Br Heart J* **24**: 761–786.

9. Kilma M, Burns TA, Chopra A (1990) Myocardial fibrosis in the elderly. *Arch Pathol Lab Med* **114**: 938–942.

10. Kennedy RD, Andrews GR, Caird FI (1977) Ischaemic heart disease in the elderly. *Br Heart J* **39**: 1121–1127.

11. Campbell A, Caird FI, Jackson TFM (1974) Prevalence of abnormalities of the electrocardiogram in old people. *Br Heart J* **36**: 1005–1011.

12. Kitchin AH, Milne JS (1977) Longitudinal survey of ischaemic heart disease in a randomly selected sample of the older population. *Br Heart J* **39**: 889–893.

13. Nadelmann J, Frishman WH, Ooi WL *et al.* (1990) Prevalence, incidence and prognosis of recognised and unrecognised myocardial infarction in persons aged 75 years or older: the Bronx Aging Study. *Am J Cardiol* **66**: 533–537.

14. Aronow WS, Herzig AH, Etienne F *et al.* (1989) 41 month follow up of risk factors correlated with new coronary events in 708 elderly patients. *J Am Geriatr Soc* **37**: 501–506.

15. Lernfelt B, Landahl S, Svanborg A (1990) Coronary heart disease at 70, 75 and 79 years of age: a longitudinal study. *Age Ageing* **19**: 297–303.

16. Waller BF, Roberts WC (1983) Cardiovascular disease in the very elderly: analysis of 40 necropsy patients aged 90 years or over. *Am J Cardiol* **51**: 403–421.

17. Hodkinson HM, Pomerance A (1977) *Q J Med* **46** 381–387.

18. Gerstenblith G, Frederiksen J, Yin FCP *et al.* (1977) Echocardiographic assessment of a normal adult aging population. *Circulation* **56**: 273–278.

19. Fleg JL, Lakatta EG (1985) Aging of the normal cardiovascular system. In *Geriatric Heart Disease*, Coodley EL (ed.). PSG, Littleton, MA, pp. 35–92.

20. Morley JE, Reese SS (1989) Clinical implications of the ageing heart. *Am J Med* **86**: 77–86.

21. Hachamovitch R, Wicker P, Capasso J, Anversa P (1989) Alterations of coronary blood flow and reserve with aging in Fischer 344 rats. *Am J Physiol* **256**: H66–H73.

22. Nichols WW, O'Rourke MF, Avoalio AP *et al.* (1985) The effects of age on ventricular–vascular coupling. *Am J Cardiol* **55**: 1179–1184.

23. Tampas JP, Soule AB (1966) Coronary artery calcification: incidence and significance in patients over 40 years of age. *Am J Roentgenol* **97**: 369.

24. Yoshida K, Yoshikawa J, Hozumi T *et al.* (1990) Detection of left main coronary artery stenosis by transoesophogeal colour Doppler and two-dimensional echocardiography. *Circulation* **81**: 1271–1276.

25. Mohiaddin RH, Firmin DN, Underwood SR *et al.* (1989) Chemical shift magnetic resonance imaging of atheroma. *Br Heart J* **62**: 81–89.

26. Anonymous (1991) Ultrafast CT scanning for coronary calcification. *Lancet* **337**: 1449–1450.

27. Rose GA (1962) The diagnosis of ischaemic heart pain and intermittent claudication in field surveys. *Bull WHO* **27**: 645–658.

28. Kannel WB (1984) Incidence and prognosis of unrecognized myocardial infarction. *N Engl J Med* **311**: 1144–1147.

29. Elveback LR, Connoly DC, Kurland LT (1981) Coronary heart disease in residents of Rochester, Minnesota. II: Mortality, incidence and survivorship, 1950–1975.

Mayo Clinic Proc **56**: 665–672.

30. Margolis JR, Gillum RF, Feinleib M *et al.* (1976) Community surveillance for coronary heart disease: the Framingham Cardiovascular Disease Survey; comparisons with the Framingham Heart Study and previous short term studies. *Am J Cardiol* **37**: 61–67.

31. Weinblatt E, Frank CW, Shapiro S, Sager RV (1968) Prognostic factors in angina pectoris: a prospective study. *J Chron Dis* **21**: 231–245.

32. Goldberg RJ, Gore JM, Gurwitz JH *et al.* (1989) The impact of age on the incidence and prognosis of initial acute myocardial infarction: the Worcester heart attack study. *Am Heart J* **117**: 543–549.

33. Kannel WB, Vokonas PS (1986) Primary risk factors for coronary heart disease in the elderly: the Framingham Study. *Coronary Heart Disease in the Elderly*, Wenger NK, Furberg CD, Pitt E (eds). Elsevier, New York, pp. 83.

34. Gillum RF, Folsom A, Luepker RV *et al.* (1983) Sudden death and acute myocardial infarction in a metropolitan area 1970–1980: the Minnesota Heart Survey. *N Engl J Med* **309**: 1353–1358.

35. Dewhurst G, Wood DA, Walker F *et al.* (1991) A population survey of cardiovascular disease in elderly people. *Age Ageing* **20**: 353–360.

36. Vetter NJ, Ford D (1990) Angina among elderly people and its relationship with disability. *Age Ageing* **19**: 159–163.

37. Cannon PJ, Connell PA, Stockley IH *et al.* (1988) Prevalence of angina as assessed by a survey of the prescription of nitrates. *Lancet* **i**: 979–981.

38. La Croix AZ, Guralnik JM, Curb JD *et al.* (1990) Chest pain and coronary heart disease mortality among older men and women in three communities. *Circulation* **81**: 437–446.

39. Aronow WS, Epstein S (1988) Usefulness of silent myocardial ischaemia detected by ambulatory electrocardiographic monitoring in predicting new coronary events in the elderly. *Am J Cardiol* **62**: 1295–1296.

40. Nejat M, Greif E. The ageing heart: a clinical review. *Med Clin North Am* **60**: 1059–1078.

41. Mukerji V, Holman A, Alpert M (1989) The clinical description of angina pectoris in the elderly. *Am Heart J* **117**: 705.

42. Miller PF, Sheps DS, Bragdon EE *et al.* (1990) Aging and pain perception in ischaemic heart disease. *Am Heart J* **120**: 22.

43. Gerstenblith G, Frederiksen J, Yin FCP *et al.* (1980) Stress testing redefines the prevalence of coronary artery disease in epidemiologic studies (Abstract). *Circulation* **62**: (II) III-308.

44. Rodeheffer RJ, Gerstenblith G, Becker LC *et al.* (1984) Exercise cardiac output is maintained with advancing age in healthy human subjects: cardiac dilatation and increased stroke volume compensate for a diminished heart rate. *Circulation* **69** (2): 203–213.

45. Port S, Cobb FR, Coleman RE, Jones RH (1980) Effect of age on the response of the left ventricular ejection fraction to exercise. *N Engl J Med* **303**: 1133–1137.

46. Kohn RR (1982) Cause of death in very old people. *JAMA* **247**: 2793–2797.

47. Kannel WB, Schatzkin A (1985) Sudden death: lessons from subsets in population studies. *J Am Coll Cardiol* **5**: 141B–149B.

48. McKee PA, Castelli WP, McNamara PM, Kannel WB (1971) The natural history of congestive heart failure: the Framingham study. *N Engl J Med* **285**: 1441–1446.

49. Pomerance A (1982) Cardiac pathology in the elderly. *Cardiovasc Clin* **12**: 9–54.

50. Pomerance A (1965) Pathology of the heart with and without cardiac failure in the aged. *Br Heart J* **27**: 697–710.

51. Klainer LM, Gibson TC, White KL (1965) The epidemiology of cardiac failure.

   J Chron Dis **18**: 797–814.
52. Rose GA, Wilson RR (1959) Unexplained heart failure in the aged. *Br Heart J* **21**: 511–517.
53. Camm AJ, Evans KE, Ward DE, Martin A (1980) The rhythm of the heart in active elderly subjects. *Am Heart J* **99**: 598–603.
54. Rubenstein JJ, Schulman CL, Yurchak PM, DeSanctis RW (1972) Clinical spectrum of the sick sinus syndrome. *Circulation* **46**: 5–13.
55. Engel TR, Meister SG, Feitosa GS *et al.* (1975) Appraisal of sinus node artery disease. *Circulation* **52**: 286–291.
56. Cameron HM, McGoogan E (1981) A prospective study of 1152 hospital autopsies I. Inaccuracies in death certification. *J Pathol* **133**: 273–283.
57. Published Table 2:270, Scottish Hospital In-patient Statistics (1985) Information Services Division, Scottish Health Services. Common Services Agency, Edinburgh.
58. Mortality Statistics: Cause. England and Wales (1988) Office of Population Censuses and Surveys, Series DH2 no 15. HMSO, London.
59. Uemara K (1988) International trends in cardiovascular disease in the elderly. *Eur Heart J* **9** (suppl. D): 1–8.
60. Simons LA (1989) Epidemiologic considerations in cardiovascular diseases in the elderly: international comparisons and trends. *Am J Cardiol* **63**: 5H–8H.
61. Hospital In Patient Enquiry: Summary Tables (1984) Office of Population Censuses and Surveys, Series MB4 no. 24. HMSO, London.
62. Published Table 2:27. Scottish Hospital In-Patient Statistics (1985) Information Services Division; SHS. Common Service Agency, Edinburgh.
63. Morbidity statistics from general practice (1981–2) OPCS General Practice morbidity series M85 no. 1. HMSO, London.
64. Stason WB, Sanders CA, Smith HC (1987) Cardiovascular care of the elderly: economic considerations. *J Am Coll Cardiol* **10**: 18A–21A.
65. Weintraub WS, Jones EL, King SB *et al.* (1990) Changing use of coronary angioplasty and coronary bypass surgery in the treatment of chronic coronary artery disease. *Am J Cardiol* **65**: 183–188.
66. Elder AT, Shaw TRD, Turnbull CM, Starkey IR (1991) Coronary arteriography in patients older and younger than 70 years *Br Med J* **303**: 950–3.
67. Grondin CM, Thornton JC, Engle JC *et al.* (1989) Cardiac surgery in septuagenarians: is there a difference in morbidity and mortality? *J Thorac Cardiovasc Surg* **98**: 908–914.
68. Royal College of Physicians (1991) Report of joint working group on cardiological intervention in elderly patients. RCP, London.
69. Thompson J (1987) Ageing of the population: contemporary trends and issues. *Population Trends 50*. OPCS HMSO, London.
70. English Life Tables. No. 14 (1980–1982) OPCS HMSO, London, pp. 8–11.
71. Gersh BJ, Kronmal RA, Schaff HV *et al.* (1983) Long term (5 year) results of coronary bypass surgery in patients aged 65 years or older. *Circulation* **68** (suppl. II). II-190–II-199.
72. Richards D (1956) *J Chron Dis* **4**: 423–433.
73. Connoly DC, Elveback LR, Oxman HA (1984) Coronary heart disease in residents of Rochester Minnesota. IV. Prognostic value of the resting electrocardiogram at the time of the initial diagnosis of angina pectoris. *Mayo Clin Proc* **59**: 247–250.
74. Caird FI, Campbell A, Jackson TFM (1974) Significance of abnormalities of the electrocardiogram in old people. *Br Heart J* **36**: 1012–1018.
75. Castelli WP, Wilson PWF, Levy D, Anderson K (1989) Cardiovascular risk factors in the elderly. *Am J Cardiol* **63**: 12H–19H.
76. Harris T, Cook EK, Kannel WB, Goldman L (1988) Proportional hazards analysis

of risk factors for coronary heart disease in individuals aged 65 or older. *J Am Geriatr Soc* **86**: 1023–1028.

77. Levy D, Garrison RJ, Savage DD *et al.* (1989) Left ventricular mass and incidence of coronary heart disease in an elderly cohort: the Framingham heart study. *Ann Intern Med* **110**: 101–107.

78. Nadelmann J, Tepper D, Greenberg S *et al.* (1991) Prognostic implications of cardiomegaly in the old old: the Bronx longitudinal aging study (Abstract). *J Am Coll Cardiol* **17**: 293A.

79. Frishman W, Wolfson S, Ooi WL *et al.* (1991) Prognostic implications of left ventricular hypertrophy and its regression in the old old: the Bronx longitudinal aging study (Abstract). *J Am Coll Cardiol* **17** (2): 293A.

80. Aronow WS (1989) New coronary events at four year follow up in patients with recognised and unrecognised myocardial infarction. *Am J Cardiol* **63**: 621–622.

81. Tofler GH, Muller JE, Stone PH *et al.* (1988) Factors leading to shorter survival after acute myocardial infarction in patients aged 65 to 75 years compared with younger patients. *Am J Cardiol* **62**: 860–867.

82. Aronow WS, Epstein S, Koenigsberg M, Schwartz KS (1988) Usefulness of echocardiographic left ventricular ejection fraction, paroxysmal ventricular tachycardia and complex ventricular arrythmias in predicting new coronary events in patients over 65 years of age. *Am J Cardiol* **61**: 1349–1351.

83. Aronow WS, Epstein S, Koenigsberg M (1990) Usefulness of echocardiographic left ventricular ejection fraction and silent myocardial ischaemia in predicting new coronary events in elderly patients with coronary artery disease or systemic hypertension. *Am J Cardiol* **65**: 811–812.

84. Iskandrian AS, Heo J, Decoskey G *et al.* (1988) Use of exercise thallium-201 imaging for risk stratification in elderly patients with coronary artery disease. *Am J Cardiol* **61**: 269–272.

85. Amery A, Hansson L, Andrew L *et al.* (1981) Hypertension in the elderly. *Acta Med Scand* **210**: 221–229.

86. Kannel, WB, Vokonas PS (1986) Primary risk factors for coronary heart disease in the elderly: the Framingham Study. In *Coronary Heart Disease in the Elderly*, Wenger NK, Furberg CD, Pitt E (eds). Elsevier, New York, p. 81.

87. Kannel WB, Dawber TR, McGee DL (1980) Perspectives on systolic hypertension: the Framingham study. *Circulation* **61**: 1179–1182.

88. Garland C, Barret-Connor E, Suarez L, Criqui MH (1983) Isolated systolic hypertension and mortality after age 60. *Am J Epidemiol* **118**: 365–376.

89. Amery A, Birkenhager W, Brixco P *et al.* (1985) Mortality and morbidity results from the European Working Party on High Blood Pressure in the Elderly Trial. *Lancet* **i**: 1349–1354.

90. Hypertension Detection and Follow-up Program Cooperative Group (1979) Five-year findings of the Hypertension Detection and Follow-up Program. *JAMA* **242**: 2562–2571.

91. SHEP Cooperative Research Group (1991) Prevention of stroke by antihypertensive drug treatment in older persons with isolated systolic hypertension. *JAMA* **265**: 3255–3264.

92. Beaglehole R (1991) Coronary heart disease and elderly people. *Br Med J* **303**: 69–70.

93. Benfante R, Reed D (1990) Is elevated serum cholesterol a risk factor for coronary heart disease in the elderly? *JAMA* **263**: 393–396.

94. Shipley MJ, Pocock SJ, Marmot MG (1991) Does plasma cholesterol predict mortality from coronary heart disease in elderly people? 18 year follow up in the Whitehall study. *Br Med J* **303**: 89–92.

95. Nikkila M, Heikkinen J (1990) Serum cholesterol, high density lipoprotein cholesterol and five year survival in elderly people. *Age Ageing* **19**: 403–408.

96. Kaiser FE, Morley JE (1990) Cholesterol can be lowered in elderly persons—should we care? *J Am Geriatr Soc* **38**: 84–85.

97. Denke MA, Grundy SM (1990) Hypercholesterolaemia in elderly persons: resolving the treatment dilemma. *Ann Int Med* **112**: 780–792.

98. Kafonek SD, Kwiterovich PO (1990) Treatment of hypercholesterolaemia in the elderly. *Ann Int Med* **112**: 723–725.

99. Yudkin JS (1991) Hypertension and non-insulin dependent diabetes. *Br Med J* **303**: 730–732.

100. Larsson B, Renstrom P, Svardsudd K *et al.* (1984) Health and aging characteristics of highly physically active 65 year old men. *Eur Heart J* **5** (Suppl. E): 31–35.

101. Donahue RP, Abbott RD, Reed DM, Yano K (1988) Physical activity and coronary heart disease in middle aged and elderly men: the Honolulu heart program. *Am J Publ Health* **78**: 683–685.

102. Paffenberger RS, Wing AL, Hyde RT (1978) Physical activity as an index of heart attack risk in college alumni. *Am J Epidemiol* **108**: 161–175.

103. Posner JD, Gorman KM, Gitlin LN *et al.* (1990) Effects of exercise training in the elderly on the occurrence and time to onset of cardiovascular diagnoses. *J Am Geriatr Soc* **38**: 205–210.

104. Jajich CL, Ostfeld AM, Freeman DH (1984) Smoking and coronary heart disease mortality in the elderly. *JAMA* **252**: 2831–2834.

105. LaCroix AZ, Lang J, Scherr P *et al.* (1991) Smoking and mortality among older man and women in three communities. *N Engl J Med* **324**: 1619–1625.

106. Hermanson B, Omenn GS, Kronmal RA *et al.* (1988) Beneficial six year outcome of smoking cessation in older men and women with coronary artery disease. *N Engl J Med* **319**: 1365–1369.

107. Milne JS, Hope K, Williamson J (1969) Variability in replies to a questionnaire on symptoms of physical illness. *J Chron Dis* **22**: 34–41.

108. Pryor DB, Harrell FE, Lee KL *et al.* (1983) Estimating the likelihood of significant coronary artery disease. *Am J Med* **75**: 771–780.

109. Gersh BJ, Kronmal RA, Frye RL *et al.* (1983) Coronary arteriography and coronary artery bypass surgery: morbidity and mortality in patients aged 65 years or over. *Circulation* **67**: 483–491.

110. Epstein SE (1980) Implications of probability analysis on the strategy used for noninvasive detection of coronary artery disease. *Am J Cardiol* **46**: 491–499.

111. Royal College of Physicians of London (1974) The place of exercise testing in cardiac patients. *J R Coll Phys Lond* **9**: 318–324.

112. Hlatky MA, Pryor DB, Harrell FE *et al.* (1984) Factors affecting sensitivity and specificity of exercise electrocardiography. *Am J Med* **77**: 64–71.

113. Gaul G (1984) Stress testing in persons above the age of 65 years: applicability and diagnostic value of a standard maximal symptom-limited testing protocol. *Eur Heart J* **5** (Suppl. E): 51–53.

114. Cobb FR, Higginbotham M, Mark D (1986) Diagnosis of coronary disease in the elderly. In *Coronary Heart Disease in the Elderly*, Wenger NK, Furberg CD, Pitt E (eds). Elsevier, New York, pp. 303–319.

115. Pollock SG, Beller GA, Watson DD, Kaul S (1991) The value of exercise thallium-201 testing in the elderly (Abstract). *J Am Coll Cardiol* **17** (2): 151A.

116. Hilton T, Shaw L, Goodgold H *et al.* (1991) Prognostic value of exercise thallium scintigraphy in the elderly (Abstract). *J Am Coll Cardiol* **17** (2): 236A.

117. Glover DR (1984) Diagnostic exercise testing in 104 patients over 65 years of age. *Eur Heart J* **5**: (Suppl.) 59.

118. Cobb FR, Higginbotham M, Mark D (1986) Diagnosis of coronary disease in the elderly. In *Coronary Heart Disease in the Elderly*, Wenger NK, Furberg CD, Pitt E (eds.). Elsevier, New York, pp. 315–316.
119. Fujita T, Ajisaka R, Matsumoto R *et al.* (1986) Isoproterenol infusion stress two dimensional echocardiography in diagnosis of coronary artery disease in elderly patients. *Jpn Heart J* **27**: 287–297.
120. Stratmann HG, Kennedy HL (1989) Evaluation of coronary artery disease in the patient unable to exercise: alternatives to exercise stress testing. *Am Heart J* **117**: 1344–1365.
121. Lam JY, Chaitman BR, Glaenzer M *et al.* (1988) Safety and diagnostic accuracy of dipyridamole thallium imaging in the elderly *J Am Coll Cardiol* **11**: 585–589.
122. Shaw L, Hilton T, Kong B *et al.* (1991) Dipyridamole thallium imaging for prognosis in elderly patients (Abstract). *J Am Coll Cardiol* **17** (2): 226A.
123. Picano E, Lattanzi F (1991) Dipyridamole echocardiography. *Circulation* **83** (Suppl. III): III-19–III-26.
124. Previtali M, Lanzarini L, Ferrario M *et al.* (1991) Dobutamine versus dipyridamole echocardiography in coronary artery disease. *Circulation* **83** (Suppl. III): III-27–III-31.
125. Imburgia M, King TR, Soffer AD *et al.* (1989) Early results and long term outcome of percutaneous transluminal coronary angioplasty in patients aged 75 years or older. *Am J Cardiol* **63**: 1127–1129.
126. Thompson RC, Holmes DR, Gersh BJ *et al.* (1991) Percutaneous transluminal coronary angioplasty in the elderly: early and long-term results. *J Am Coll Cardiol* **17**: 1245–1250.
127. Gersh BJ, Kronmal RA, Schaff HV *et al.* (1985) Comparison of coronary artery bypass surgery and medical therapy in patients aged 65 years or older: a nonrandomized study from the Coronary Artery Surgery Study (CASS) Registry. *N Engl J Med* **313**: 217–224.
128. Loop FD, Lytle BW, Cosgrove DM *et al.* (1988) Coronary artery bypass graft surgery in the elderly. *Cleve Clin J Med* **55**: 23–34.
129. Naunheim KS, Kern MJ, McBride LR *et al.* (1987) Coronary artery bypass surgery in patients aged 80 years or older. *Am J Cardiol* **59**: 804–807.
130. Acinapura AJ, Rose DM, Cunningham JN *et al.* (1988) Coronary artery bypass in septuagenarians: Analysis of mortality and morbidity. *Circulation* **78** (Suppl. I): I-179–I-184.
131. Christakis GT, Ivanov J, Weisel RD *et al.* (1989) The changing pattern of coronary artery bypass surgery. *Circulation* **80** (Suppl. I): 151–161.
132. Montague NT, Kouchoukos NT, Wilson TAS *et al.* (1985) Morbidity and mortality of coronary bypass grafting in patients 70 years of age and older. *Ann Thorac Surg* **39**: 552–557.
133. Roberts AJ, Woodhall DD, Conti CR *et al.* (1985) Mortality, morbidity, and cost-accounting related to coronary artery bypass graft surgery in the elderly. *Ann Thorac Surg* **39**: 426–432.
134. Varnauskas E and the European Coronary Surgery Study Group (1988) Twelve year follow up of survival in the randomised European Coronary Surgery Study. *N Engl J Med* **319**: 332–337.
135. Passamani E, Davis KB, Gillespie MJ, Killip T (1985) A randomised trial of coronary artery bypass surgery. *N Engl J Med* **312**: 1665–1671.
136. Robinson K, Conroy RM, Mulcahy R (1988) Risk factors and in hospital course of first myocardial infarction in the elderly. *Clin Cardiol* **11**: 519–523.
137. Kennedy RD, Caird FI (1972) The application of the Minnesota code to population studies of the electrocardiogram. *Gerontol Clin* **14**: 5–16.

138. Kitchin AH, Lowther CP, Milne JS (1973) Prevalence of clinical and electrocardiographic evidence of ischaemic heart disease in the older population. *Br Heart J* **35**: 946–953.
139. Rajala S, Kaltiala K, Haavisto M, Mattila K (1984) Prevalence of ECG findings in very old people. *Eur Heart J* **5**: 168–174.
140. Tinker GN (1981) Clinical presentation of myocardial infarction in the elderly. *Age Ageing* **10**: 237–240.
141. Williams BO, Begg TB, Semple T, McGuiness JB (1976) The elderly in a coronary unit. *Br Med J* **2**: 451–453.
142. Pathy MS (1967) Clinical presentation of myocardial infarction in the elderly. *Br Heart J* **29**: 190–199.
143. Wroblewski M, Mikulowski P, Steen B (1986) Symptoms of myocardial infarction in old age. *Age Ageing* **15**: 99–104.
144. Rodstein M (1956) The characteristics of non fatal myocardial infarction in the aged. *Arch Intern Med* **98**: 84–90.
145. Day JJ, Bayer AJ, Pathy MSJ (1987) Acute myocardial infarction: diagnostic difficulties and outcome in advanced old age. *Age Ageing* **16**: 239–243.
146. Black DA (1987) Mental state and presentation of myocardial infarction in the elderly. *Age Ageing* **16**: 125–127.
147. Day JJ, Bayer AJ, Chadha JS, Pathy MSJ (1988) Myocardial infarction in old people: the influence of diabetes mellitus. *J Am Geriatr Soc* **36**: 791–794.
148. Bayer AJ, Chadha JS, Farag RR, Pathy MSJ (1986) Changing presentation of myocardial infarction with increasing old age. *J Am Geriatr Soc* **34**: 263–266.
149. Solomon CG, Lee TH, Cook EF *et al.* (1989) Comparison of clinical presentation of acute myocardial infarction in patients older than 65 years of age to younger patients: the Multicentre Chest pain study experience. *Am J Cardiol* **63**: 772–776.
150. Swain DG, Nightingale PG, Gama R, Buckley BM (1990) Cardiac enzyme changes in elderly fallers. *Age Ageing* **19**: 207–211.
151. GISSI (1986) Effectiveness of intravenous thrombolytic treatment in acute myocardial infarction. *Lancet* **i**: 397–402.
152. AIMS Trial Study Group (1990) Long term effects of intravenous anistreplase in acute myocardial infarction: final report of the AIMS study. *Lancet* **335**: 427–431.
153. ISIS-2 (1988) Randomised trial of intravenous streptokinase, oral aspirin, both or neither among 17187 cases of suspected acute myocardial infarction. *Lancet* **ii**: 349–360.
154. Wilcox RG, Olsson CG, Skene AM *et al.* (1988) Trial of tissue plasminogen activator for mortality reduction in acute myocardial infarction. Anglo-Scandinavian Study of Early Thrombolysis (ASSET). *Lancet* **ii**: 525–530.
155. Rich MW, Bosner MS, Chung MK *et al.* (1991) Is age an independent predictor of mortality in patients with acute myocardial infarction? (Abstract). *J Am Coll Cardiol* **17** (2): 329A.
156. Coodley EI, Zebari D (1985) Characteristics of myocardial infarction in the elderly. In *Clinical Heart Disease in the Elderly Patient*, Coodley EL (ed.). PSG, Littleton, MA, pp. 334–344.
157. McDonald JB, Baillie J, Williams BO, Ballantyne D (1983) Coronary care in the elderly. *Age Ageing* **12**: 17–20.
158. Chaturvedi NC, Shivalingappa G, Shanks B *et al.* (1972) Myocardial infarction in the elderly. *Lancet* **i**: 280–228.
159. Sagie A, Rotenberg Z, Weinberger I *et al.* (1987) Acute transmural myocardial infarction in elderly patients hospitalized in the Coronary Care Unit versus the General Medical Ward. *J Am Geriatr Soc* **35**: 915.
160. Dudley NJ, Burns E (1991) Age related policies in coronary care units in the United

Kingdom (Abstract). *Age Ageing* **20** (Suppl. 1): 29.

161. Boon NA (1991) New deal for old hearts. *Br Med J* **303**: 70.

162. Pfeffer MA, Moye LA, Braunwald E *et al.* (1991) Selection bias in the use of thrombolytic therapy in acute myocardial infarction. *JAMA* **266**: 528–532.

163. Maggionia AP, Franzosi MG, Farina ML *et al.* (1991) Cerebrovascular events after myocardial infarction: analysis of the GISSI trial. *Br Med J* **302**: 1428–1431.

164. Behar S, Tanne D, Abinader E *et al.* (1991) Cerebrovascular accident complicating acute myocardial infarction: incidence, clinical significance, and short and long-term mortality rates. *Am J Med* **91**: 45–50.

165. Saunamaki KL (1984) Early post-myocardial infarction exercise testing in subjects 70 years or more of age: functional and prognostic evaluation. *Eur Heart J* **5** (Suppl. E): 93–96.

166. Deckers JW, Fioretti P, Brower RW *et al.* (1984) Ineligibility for predischarge exercise testing after myocardial infarction in the elderly: implications for prognosis. *Eur Heart J* **5** (Suppl. E): 97–100.

167. Turi ZG, Stone PH, Muller *et al.* (1986) Implications for acute intervention related to time of hospital arrival in acute myocardial infarction. *Am J Cardiol* **58**: 203–209.

168. Chaitman BR, Thompson B, Wittry MD *et al.* (1989) The use of tissue type plasminogen activator for acute myocardial infarction in the elderly. *J Am Coll Cardiol* **14**: 1159–1165.

169. Califf RM, Topol EJ, George BS *et al.* (1988) Haemorrhagic complications associated with the use of intravenous tissue plasminogen type activator in treatment of acute myocardial infarction. *Am J Med* **85**: 353–359.

170. Baillie SP, Furniss SS (1991) Thrombolysis for elderly patients—which way from here? *Age Ageing* **20**: 1–2.

171. Sherry S, Marder VJ (1991) Mistaken guidelines for thrombolytic therapy of acute myocardial infarction in the elderly. *J Am Coll Cardiol* **17**: 1237–1238.

172. SWIFT Trial Study Group (1991) SWIFT trial of delayed elective intervention v. conservative treatment after thrombolysis with anistreplase in acute myocardial infarction. *Br Med J* **302**: 555–560.

173. Gurwitz JH, Goldberg RJ, Gore JM (1991) Coronary thrombolysis for the elderly? *JAMA* **265**: 1720–1723.

174. ISIS I Collaborative group (1988) Mechanisms for the early mortality reduction produced by beta blockade started early in acute myocardial infarction. *Lancet* **i**: 921–923.

175. Dellborg M, Held P, Swedberg K, Vedin A (1985) Rupture of the myocardium: occurrence and risk factors. *Br Heart J* **54**: 11–16.

176. Bates RJ, Beutler S, Resnekov L, Anagnostopoulos CE (1977) Cardiac rupture: challenge in diagnosis and management. *Am J Cardiol* **40**: 429–437.

177. Gunderson T, Abrahmsen AM, Kjeksus J *et al.* (1982) Timolol related reduction in mortality and reinfarction in patients aged 65–75 years surviving acute myocardial infarction. *Circulation* **66**: 1179–1184.

178. Hjalmarson A, Elmfeld TD, Herlitz J *et al.* (1981) Effect on mortality of metoprolol in acute myocardial infarction. *Lancet* **ii**: 823–827.

179. Hawkins CM, Richardson DW, Vokonas PS (1983) Effect of propranolol in reducing mortality in old myocardial infarction patients: the beta blocker heart attack trial experience. *Circulation* **67**: (Suppl. 1): 1-94–1-97.

180. Lee TC, Laramee LA, Rutherford BD *et al.* (1990) Emergency percutaneous transluminal coronary angioplasty for acute myocardial infarction in patients 70 years of age and older. *Am J Cardiol* **66**: 663–667.

181. Holland KJ, O'Neill WW, Bates ER *et al.* (1989) Emergency percutaneous transluminal coronary angioplasty during acute myocardial infarction for patients

more than 70 years of age. *Am J Cardiol* **63**: 399–403.

182. Sleight P (1990) Do we need to intervene after thrombolysis in acute myocardial infarction? *Circulation* **81**: 1707–1709.
183. Gulati RS, Folsom A, Luepker RV *et al.* (1983) Cardiopulmonary resuscitation of old people. *Lancet* **ii**: 267–297.
184. Bedell SE, Delbanco TL, Cook EF, Epstein FH (1983) Survival after cardiopulmonary resuscitation in the hospital. *N Engl J Med* **309**: 569–576.
185. Tresch DD, Thakur RK, Hoffman RG *et al.* (1990) Comparison of outcome of paramedic witnessed cardiac arrest in patients younger and older than 70 years. *Am J Cardiol* **65**: 453–457.
186. Peach H, Pathy J (1979) Disability in the elderly after myocardial infarction. *J R Coll Physicians Lond* **13**: 154–157.
187. Pathy MS, Peach H (1981) Change in disability status as a predictor of long-term survival after myocardial infarction in the elderly. *Age Ageing* **10**: 174–178.
188. Williams MA, Maresh CM, Esterbrooks DJ *et al.* (1985) Early exercise training in patients aged older than age 65 years compared with that in younger patients after acute myocardial infarction or coronary artery bypass grafting. *Am J Cardiol* **55**: 263–266.
189. Registrar General for Scotland: Annual Report (1989) No. 135. Table C1.7, p. 46.
190. Elder AT, Fox KAA (1992) Thrombolytic treatment for elderly people. *Br J Med* **305**: 845–846.

18 Valve Disease in the Elderly

JEAN R. McEWAN AND CELIA M. OAKLEY

Hammersmith Hospital and The Royal Postgraduate Medical School, London, UK

Valve disorders rarely arise *de novo* in old age. They usually follow rheumatic endocarditis in earlier life or result from age-related degeneration, wear and tear (Figure 1). The decline in rheumatic heart disease and the increased longevity of the population have changed the prevalence and character of valvular heart disease. Mitral stenosis, which is almost always rheumatic in origin, is seen less frequently. Rheumatic aortic stenosis is also less prevalent. Stenosis caused by degenerative changes in congenitally bicuspid or previously normal tricuspid valves are now the usual cause of aortic valve disease and the ageing miral valve may become regurgitant. In 1989 37% of valve surgery in the UK was in patients over the age of 65 years (1) (Table 1). The improvement in outcome from cardiac surgery means that elderly people with valve disease should be assessed carefully and their possible need for surgery not neglectecd.

Elderly people present many different facets from younger people. Their disability may stem from causes other than the valve disease itself, such as the effects of atrial fibrillation, atriomegaly and lung disease. In addition, occult malignancy and deterioration in other vital systems, particularly renal, must be sought. The old person may blame the known valve disease for increasing disability which is really due to age and infirmity, and conversely may accept disability as caused by old age when it is the direct result of valve disease.

AORTIC STENOSIS

The frequency of aortic stenosis rises with increasing age. It is found in 5.5% of those aged over 75 years coming to post-mortem (2). It is more common in men than women (ratio 4:1) in surgically treated cases (3), although in populations over the age of 80, where women tend to predominate, the ratio is nearer 2:1 (4).

Pathology

Rheumatic aortic stenosis is caused by thickening of the free edge of the value cusps and fusion of the commissures (5). It is rarely seen without some

Geriatric Cardiology. Principles and Practice.   Edited by A. Martin and A. J. Camm
© 1994 John Wiley & Sons Ltd

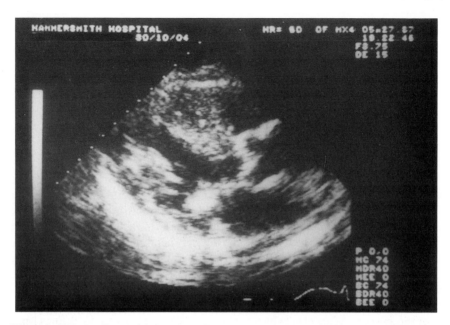

Figure 1. Echocardiographic imaging of the heart gives, like looking at a face, a good idea of a patient's age. Here is shown the long-axis view of the left ventricle of an 80-year-old woman. It shows annular mitral calcification, thickening of the aortic root and valve and bending of the long axis of the ventricle with protrusion of the septum into the outflow tract just below the aortic valve

Table 1. UK Heart Valve Registry (Department of Health): Number of heat valve procedures (% of total value operations)

	> 65	> 70	> 75 years
1986	30%	13%	3.7%
1989	37%	18%	7.4%

involvement of the mitral valve: combined mitral and aortic involvement occurs in at least a third of cases of rheumatic heart disease. In addition, since the development of rheumatic mitral stenosis is more rapid than that of aortic stenosis, a large number of patients who had only mild aortic stenosis when investigated and operated on for their mitral stenosis subsequently develop severe aortic stenosis requiring aortic valve replacement (6).

Estimates of the prevalence of congenitally bicuspid aortic valves lie between 0.4% and 2% of the population (7). The bicuspid valve usually has two asymmetric cusps with a central raphe replacing the third commissure and an eccentric valve orifice. Bicuspid valves are intrinsically mildly stenotic because they cannot open fully even in the absence of commissural fusion. They are more

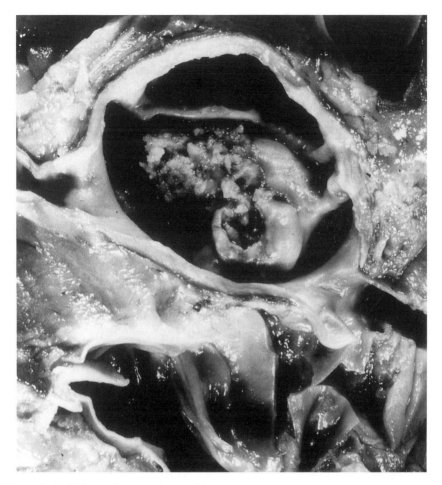

Figure 2. Calcific aortic stenosis found at autopsy in an 88-year-old man. The valve is grossly disorganized, with a greatly restricted eccentric orifice which was reduced to about 0.5 cm². The coronary arteries were large and free from significant atheroma

liable to endocarditis and to general wear and tear because of this. About half of them eventually calcify with stenosis or mixed stenosis and incompetence. A bicuspid valve is now the commonest cause of aortic stenosis, being found in over 40% of cases (4). Symptoms tend to develop from late middle life onwards.

Calcific stenosis of an originally normal aortic valve is becoming more common with increasing longevity of the population and is seen particularly in patients over the age of 70 (4). Calcific stenosis of both bicuspid and degenerated senile valves is characterized by thickened disorganized leaflets, but open commissures (Figure 2). The cusps have restricted movement and require good ventricular function to maintain adequate valve-opening force.

Symptoms

A normal aortic valve has an orifice of 3–4 cm². Symptoms begin to develop when the orifice is between 1 and 1.5 cm². Aortic stenosis presents with syncope, angina pectoris or heart failure. Syncope is probably due to abnormal barosensitivity stimulated by a rise in left ventricular pressure and the depressor reflex. Those episodes which have been closely observed have consisted of an abrupt fall in arterial pressure which if prolonged is followed by ventricular arrhythmia (8). The angina pectoris has several origins. Myocardial hypertrophy, prolonged systole, high left ventricular pressure, reduced coronary flow time on exercise and the Venturi phenomenon which impairs flow into the coronaries all contribute (9,10). When heart failure supervenes the outlook for the patient becomes much poorer. Symptoms increase greatly when the myocardium starts to fail.

Coronary artery disease is seen frequently in conjunction with aortic stenosis in elderly patients and may be the cause of angina pectoris in patients with otherwise asymptomatic aortic stenosis.

Signs

In aortic stenosis the apex beat may or may not be displaced laterally but will be forceful. The carotid and brachial pulses are slow rising with an anachronic notch, but with increasing age this may be masked by the sclerosis of the vascular tree. The jugular venous pressure is normal in the absence of congestive cardiac failure. The aortic component of the second heart sound may be absent or soft and delayed because of the prolonged ejection time and the reduced valve mobility. A thrill accompanying the midsystolic murmur suggests the stenosis is at least of moderate severity but its detection is largely dependent on the patient's body build. The murmur is loudest at the base of the heart and typically radiates into the neck.

Aortic sclerosis is the term applied when there is an aortic ejection systolic murmur, normal heart sounds and no transvalvular gradient. The origin of the murmur is usually a calcified aortic valve but this label is dangerous because underlying and often rapidly progressive stenosis may be neglected under this comforting term. Aortic stenosis is frequently underestimated or missed altogether in the elderly. Not only may the arterial pulses feel normal but the cardiac impulse is often impalpable, the murmur is soft and maximal at the apex and there is no thrill. This is particularly likely in men with barrel or big chests. No systolic murmur should be dismissed as of little significance in the elderly, particularly if there is angina or heart failure.

Investigation

The chest X-ray may show cardiac enlargement or may be normal. Calcium deposits in the valve are often seen, particularly in the lateral view. The

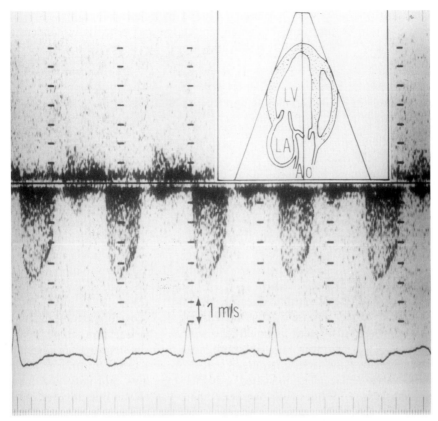

Figure 3. Continuous wave Doppler measurement of the peak flow velocity across the aortic valve was almost 5 m/s, giving a peak instantaneous gradient of 100 mmHg

electrocardiogram (ECG) will show left ventricular hypertrophy and repolarization changes. The echocardiogram will confirm the thickened disorganized valve with restricted movement, and Doppler studies allow objective assessment of the severity of the stenosis (Figure 3). The relationship of transvalvular gradient assessed by Doppler with that measured at cardiac catheterization is generally good (11) but, if cardiac output is poor, it must be remembered that a low gradient will still be of clinical significance. With increasing skills of echocardiography direct measurement of the aortic valve gradient is less important and the major purpose of the catheter is to examine the coronaries. Infrequently, in some older people the echo window may be poor and limit the application of echo Doppler, and in these patients catheterization still remains mandatory. At cardiac catheterization the stenotic valve may be crossed retrogradely, or the left ventricle may be entered via the trans-septal route and aortic and left ventricular pressures measured simultaneously. Exercise testing of patients with angina and an aortic outflow murmur should be deferred until significant aortic stenosis has been excluded by echocardiography. Exercise testing is unnecessary (and both uninterpretable and potentially dangerous) when the ECG is abnormal. It is safe and informative when the resting ECG is normal.

Treatment

The risk of sudden death during exercise makes surgery the favoured option in young patients who remain asymptomatic in the face of severe aortic stenosis. In the elderly, the risks of surgery are higher (see below) and 'prophylactic' aortic valve replacement is unjustified in the absence of symptoms, but careful follow-up is important. The development of shortness of breath, angina or syncope indicates a need to replace the valve. When heart failure supervenes, the risks of surgery are much higher but even then relief of the obstruction to outflow almost always improves both function and symptoms (12,13). Valvuloplasty has proved disappointing (see below), as the increase in orifice is rarely sufficient to relieve heart failure and is short lived. The only indication for valvuloplasty now is as a bridge to valve replacement and possibly in patients with a very short-term prognosis due to extracardiac disease.

Coronary artery disease is often the reason for the development of angina in patients whose aortic stenosis would otherwise have been asymptomatic. That is why angina as a symptom has a better prognosis in aortic stenosis than dyspnoea or syncope. In some series a requirement for coronary artery grafting as well as aortic valve replacement indicated a higher operative mortality and lower survival rate (14,15) but in our own series there was a lower operative mortality rate when the aortic valve replacement was for angina, despite associated coronary grafting, since the aortic valve replacement was carried out *before* the left ventricle failed.

The requirement for coronary artery bypass grafting must be reviewed in each patient. Grafting of coronary stenoses is important despite adding to the total duration of the procedure, firstly in ensuring that ischaemia does not limit the patient's ability to come off bypass and secondly if the patient's physical abilities improve after the valve surgery.

AORTIC REGURGITATION

Isolated aortic regurgitation is uncommon in the elderly. It may result from abnormal cusps or from disorders of the aortic wall.

Aortic regurgitation may be combined with stenosis in rheumatic heart disease or degenerative aortic valve disease. In either case stenosis of the aortic valve or involvement of the mitral valve in the rheumatic process usually overshadows the incompetence.

Aortic regurgitation may be caused by dilatation of the aortic root in long-standing hypertension (16). Chronic aortitis due to rheumatoid arthritis, Reiter's disease (17) or ankylosing spondylitis (18) may present in late life as aortic regurgitation, while syphilis, although rare, is still seen occasionally in elderly people and requires full treatment with penicillin (19). The inflammatory processes led to aortic root dilatation and weakening of the commissural support. Congenital 'collagen' abnormalities such as Marfan's syndrome and Ehlers–Danlos become symptomatic earlier in life, but a Marfan-type aortic root aneurysm or silent chronic dissection of the ascending thoracic aorta may present in old age. The most common causes of acute aortic regurgitation are endocarditis and aortic dissection.

Pathophysiology

With chronic aortic regurgitation the left ventricle dilates and hypertrophies. Even when severe the effective forward stroke volume remains normal, although this may mean a total left ventricular output of up to 25 l/min with a regurgitant flow of up to 20 l/min. The end-diastolic volume increases but end-systolic volume is initially maintained. With increasing regurgitation end-systolic volume rises but end-diastolic pressure remains normal. Eventually end-diastolic pressure rises, systolic function declines further and only then does exercise tolerance fall. Adaptation of the left ventricle to a large stroke volume and the ability to increment minute output by tachycardia (since an increased heart rate which shortens diastole decreases regurgitation (20,21) allow the patient to remain asymptomatic for years, even in the face of severe regurgitation.

As with other valvular heart disease, the best results of surgery are seen in patients with preserved preoperative left ventricular function. In the ideal situation valve replacement would be undertaken just before left ventricular function deteriorates but prediction of that point is very difficult (22). Recent observations of myocardial biochemistry using phosphorus nuclear magnetic resonance spectroscopy have revealed alterations in the metabolic profile of failing myocardium (23), and studies are currently under way to see whether such observations predate any clinical, echo or radiographic evidence of ventricular failure. Surgery is rarely needed for the elderly person, even with severe aortic regurgitation, who is asymptomatic. Symptoms are absent in chronic aortic regurgitation until the left ventricle starts to fail, and the indication for aortic valve replacement is recognition of deteriorating left ventricular ejection fraction by radionuclide or other means and particularly a failure to increase ejection fraction on exercise.

In severe acute aortic regurgitation, the adaptive processes have not come into play, so the heart may not be particularly enlarged but end-diastolic pressure will have risen quickly. The pulse pressure does not widen as much as in chronic aortic regurgitation. The mitral valve may close in mid-diastole because of the rapid rise in ventricular pressure.

Symptoms

Chronic aortic regurgitation has a long asymptomatic period followed by exertional dyspnoea, orthopnoea and paroxysmal nocturnal dyspnoea. Angina is less frequently seen than in aortic stenosis, and syncope is rare. Left ventricular dilatation leads to complaints of palpitation, particularly if ectopic activity develops. With acute aortic regurgitation the patient may develop circulatory failure with low output.

Signs

The pulse pressure is increased with increased systolic and a low diastolic pressure. In the elderly this must be distinguished from isolated systolic hypertension due to hardening of the peripheral arteries. The pulse is jerky (Corrigan's pulse) and may be bisferiens. This may be readily appreciated during the measurement of the blood pressure when a double knocking sound is heard when the systolic pressure is first reached. The Korotkoff sounds can often be heard right down to zero although diastolic pressure is usually no lower than 30 mmHg. As heart failure develops, the rising left ventricular end-diastolic pressure and peripheral vasoconstriction may result in a rise in arterial diastolic pressure.

The apex is displaced laterally and inferiorly and is hyperdynamic. A high-pitched decrescendo early diastolic murmur begins immediately after A2 and may obscure P2. On auscultation S1 is quiet and A2 is soft, with delayed closure of the aortic valve causing S2 to be split paradoxically. Alternatively, A2 may be absent, making S2 single. An S3 gallop is heard as the left ventricular end-systolic volume rises. The murmur is best heard using the diaphragm of the stethoscope in the left fourth intercostal space, with the patient sitting up, leaning forward in expiration. The murmur may change during the time course of the disease. Mild aortic regurgitation sounds like expired breath: in moderate and severe regurgitation the murmur is longer and lower. With the onset of left ventricular decompensation the murmur shortens again. The Austin Flint murmur is a low-pitched mid-diastolic rumble thought to be due to the regurgitant jet causing vibration and part closure of the anterior leaflet of the mitral valve. Acute aortic regurgitation has less obvious signs of the valve incompetence. There is usually a prominent summated gallop and only a short early diastolic murmur.

Investigations

The ECG typically shows left ventricular hypertrophy and strain pattern. Cardiomegaly on the chest X-ray is due to left ventricular enlargement. At angiography a rapid injection of dye into the aortic root (35 ml/s) demonstrates the regurgitation into the left ventricular cavity. Echocardiography shows that the left ventricular muscle is thickened, with increased end-diastolic and end-systolic volumes. The aortic root dimension can also be determined and abnormalities of the valve leaflets detected. With colour flow Doppler mosaic colours in the left ventricle illustrate the course of the regurgitant jet. The anterior leaflet of the mitral valve flutters in diastole and this is best seen using M-mode echocardiography. The Doppler studies and diastolic arterial pressure can allow estimation of the left ventricular end-diastolic pressure.

Management

Acute aortic regurgitation requires prompt surgical intervention, with interim use of afterload-reducing vasodilator therapy. Chronic aortic regurgitation, even if severe, is associated with a good outlook, with 75% of patients surviving 5 years and 50% 10 years after diagnosis (24). The onset of symptoms heralds rapid deterioration, heart failure being associated with death within 2 years. Patients who have no symptoms require no specific treatment but should be seen at 6-monthly intervals and some measurement of left ventricular size and function made, e.g. by echocardiography. Vasodilators, digitalis and diuretics may be given to elderly patients with mild (NYHA III or less) symptoms, but evidence of left ventricular dysfunction detected on echo requires that the elderly patient be considered for surgery.

MITRAL STENOSIS

Mitral stenosis does not arise *de novo* in old age. Rather, it is the result of inflammatory or degenerative processes begun earlier in life. Rheumatic heart disease is the commonest cause of mitral stenosis. Scarring from lupus endocarditis can also result in mitral stenosis. Amyloid infiltration of the valve leaflets and calcification of the mitral valve annulus are uncommon causes of mitral stenosis which is, at most, mild (25,26). With the virtual disappearance of acute rheumatic fever in the UK, almost all the rheumatic heart disease in the indigenous population is now seen in middle or old age. Symptoms often arise initially in the fourth or fifth decade and persist over many years, with a gradual deterioration in exercise tolerance which is hardly noticed by either patient or physician. The mitral stenosis may even go undetected until discovered by echocardiography carried out as part of a 'routine' screen for dyspnoea suspected to be cardiac in origin (27). It may be 20–25 years after the initial rheumatic fever before any symptoms develop but only 5 years from the onset of the symptoms of rheumatic mitral stenosis until class III symptoms develop. The older patients therefore tend to fall into two categories: those who have previously undergone conservative mitral valve surgery, and those with mild rheumatic heart disease which has only become symptomatic in late life.

Rheumatic heart disease is more common in females than males (two-thirds women). Pure mitral stenosis is found in 25% of patients, with 40% having mixed mitral valve disease.

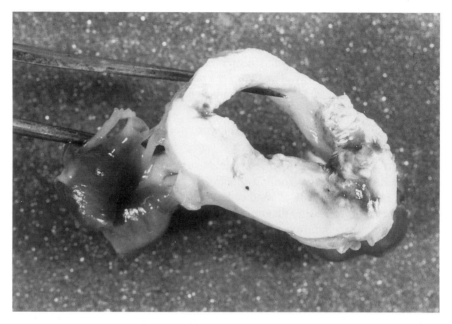

Figure 4. A typical example of mitral stenosis in older age is seen in this surgical specimen from a woman of 72 years. The valve is heavily calcified, the leaflets thickened and rigid, the chordae fused and shortened so that the papillary muscles seemed inserted almost directly into the leaflets. The patent had had a previous mitral valvotomy many years earlier. The commissures had not undergone re-fusion but re-stenosis with regurgitation had developed due to increasing immobilization of the leaflets, resulting in a funnel-shaped orifice which was actually smaller at chordal level below the valve than at the leaflet orifice

Pathology and pathophysiology

The valve leaflets are thickened and the commissures are fused. The chordae thicken, fuse and shorten and the whole apparatus becomes immobile and calcified (Figure 4).

The normal mitral valve orifice has an area of 4 cm². When it has decreased to 2 cm² the stenosis is mild and manifested mainly by an increase in the left atrial pressure on exertion. When the area is 1.5 cm² the cardiac output is reduced at rest, and when less than 1 cm² severe or critical mitral stenosis exists with pulmonary hypertension and a raised pulmonary vascular resistance. The mean transvalvular gradient then is about 20 mmHg, which means that a left atrial pressure of about 25 mmHg is necessary even to maintain cardiac output at rest. The increased pulmonary venous and pulmonary capillary pressures lead to dyspnoea on exertion. Increased heart rate on exercise or because of pyrexia or in uncontrolled atrial fibrillation decreases diastole and raises the left atrial pressure still further. The pressure gradient is proportional to the transvalvular flow squared, so doubling the flow rate quadruples the gradient. In severe mitral stenosis atrial contraction augments the cardiac output of those patients who remain in sinus rhythm, and the onset of atrial fibrillation can precipitate severe symptoms until the heart rate is controlled. Initially, atrial fibrillation lowers the cardiac output but once the heart rate is controlled left atrial pressure tends to be *lower* than in sinus rhythm. That is why atrial fibrillation is so well tolerated in mitral stenosis.

In pure mitral stenosis, the left ventricular end-diastolic pressure is normal, but when left ventricular function is impaired by long-standing ischaemic heart disease or hypertension (which are common in the elderly), or where mitral regurgitation coexists, the left atrial pressure needs to be even higher to maintain flow. In severe mitral stenosis the cardiac output may be low at rest because of pulmonary hypertension and as a consequence of administration of diuretics. Tiredness and exhaustion are the predominant symptoms in these circumstances.

Symptoms

Assessment of the significance of dyspnoea in an elderly person may be difficult because of coexisting respiratory disease, particularly chronic bronchitis. On the other hand, diminished mobility because of arthritis may mean that symptoms due to the mitral stenosis are not noted. Haemoptysis due to pulmonary venous hypertension is an uncommon symptom in the elderly. Some patients may complain of chest pain which may be difficult to distinguish from ischaemic heart disease. Previously undiagnosed rheumatic heart disease is an important cause of embolic stroke. Old people with no previous surgery on the mitral valve may be seen on account of dyspnoea and fatigue despite only modest compromise of the mitral valve orifice. They are invariably in atrial fibrillation with marked atrial dilatation and often some tricuspid regurgitation.

Signs

A low cardiac output is thought to be the reason for the purple patches across the cheeks and nose, caused by venous telangiectasia and known as mitral facies. The jugular venous pressure may be normal. A prominent 'a' wave may be seen when a patient with elevated pulmonary vascular resistance is still in sinus rhythm. Most patients are in atrial fibrillation with less severe mitral valve obstruction and lesser degrees of pulmonary hypertension but larger hearts on X-ray due to biatrial dilatation.

Palpation of the apex reveals a palpable S1 (tapping apex) and an apical diastolic thrill may rarely be felt. A right ventricular heave indicates right ventricular hypertrophy due to pulmonary hypertension, but an ill-sustained parasternal impulse may be caused by the left atrial v wave. If the mitral valve is still flexible the S1 is loud, but if calcified S1 will be soft. P2 may be loud. An opening snap indicates that some part of the valve is still flexible, and the closer it is to A2 then the higher is the left atrial pressure. The longer the low rumbling diastolic murmur, the higher the transvalvular gradient, but the murmur is frequently of too low intensity to hear throughout its length. Atrial contraction results in its loudness increasing (presystolic accentuation). Exercising the patient and the left lateral position both accentuate the murmur, which is loudest in expiration. A similar (but often more variable) murmur is found in left atrial myxoma.

In old people with symptoms the mitral orifice is only rarely tightly stenosed (0.6–1.0 cm²), more often moderately narrowed (1.0–1.5 cm²) and the signs may be modified by narrowed rib spaces (women), bulky lungs (men) or obesity.

Investigation

The ECG typically shows the patient to have atrial fibrillation, but if in sinus rhythm a large P wave (> 0.12 seconds) illustrates the left atrial enlargement. The classical chest X-ray shows left atrial enlargement with prominence of the appendage and valve calcification.

Two-dimensional echocardiography shows that the left atrium is enlarged, the thickened valve leaflets have reduced excursion and the anterior leaflet domes in diastole. On M-mode the reduced movement, leaflet thickening and slowed or flat diastolic closure are seen. The transvalvular gradient can be measured by Doppler from the pressure half-time and the pulmonary artery pressure estimated when tricuspid regurgitation is present.

All patients over the age of 40 need to be catheterized to assess the coronary arteries although echo imaging plus Doppler has reduced the requirement for catheterization otherwise. Multiple valve lesions and coexisting pulmonary disease may still merit confirmatory left and right heart studies.

MITRAL REGURGITATION

Mitral valve competence requires coordinated function of the mitral valve leaflets, chordae tendineae and annulus, papillary muscles and left ventricular muscle. Rheumatic heart disease, myxomatous degeneration and ischaemia may involve leaflets, chordae and papillary muscle. Dilatation of the mitral valve annulus occurs in any disease where the left ventricle is enlarged and dysfunctional, e.g. dilated cardiomyopathy or after ischaemic damage. Following infarction the papillary muscles can rupture, fibrose or their function may be impaired during reversible ischaemia. Calcification of the annulus spreading into the valve leaflets may impair both muscle leaflet contraction and mobility, and allow regurgitation. This is a particular problem in the elderly but is also seen in younger patients with disorders of calcium metabolism as in renal failure. Mitral regurgitation also occurs in hypertrophic cardiomyopathy.

Acute mitral regurgitation

Acute mitral regurgitation may occur if endocarditis destroys the leaflets or chordae and following infarction if there is sudden rupture of the head of a papillary muscle (rupture of a whole papillary muscle is rare and nearly immediately fatal). The apical systolic murmur is harsh and there may be a thrill. A third heart sound gallop results from increased left ventricular filling. The chest X-ray shows pulmonary oedema but often a near-normal-sized heart. The ECG may show only left ventricular volume overload, ST depression and T wave inversion from non-Q wave infarction or changes of major posterobasal infarction. A Swan–Ganz catheter pressure tracing is no longer necessary but if done it shows an elevated pulmonary capillary wedge pressure with regurgitant v waves. Echo and oxygen sampling differentiate acute regurgitation from ventricular septal rupture. The prognosis of severe acute mitral regurgitation is so bad that even elderly patients should be stabilized with intra-aortic balloon counter-pulsation after emergency pharmacological offloading, catheterized to check the coronary arteries and then valve replacement and revascularization carried out. Coronary angiography may be dispensed with in endocarditis, and left ventricular contrast injection should be avoided if the patient is hypotensive because of the risk of precipitating renal failure.

Pathophysiology

The left ventricle is relatively protected from the effects of chronic overload in mitral regurgitation by the fact that it can decompress into the left atrium. The tension developed by the ventricular myocardium is reduced at any given end-diastolic or systolic pressure and the velocity of myocardial fibre shortening is increased. The ventricle is able thereby to increase its total stroke and maintain forward output so that symptoms may be delayed for years. Eventually the left ventricular function deteriorates, its end-systolic volume increases, the shape becomes more globular, the mitral annulus is stretched and regurgitation increases further. Symptoms may develop only after ventricular impairment has already occurred. When surgery renders the valve competent the offloading into the left atrium is lost. The effect is analogous to giving the ventricle aortic stenosis and it is common for ventricular function to deteriorate sharply. The end-diastolic volume hardly changes and ejection fraction falls despite vigorous postoperative offloading and use of intravenous inotropes.

Symptoms

The main complaint is of chronic fatigue, tiredness and gradually decreasing exercise tolerance, and symptoms become troublesome only when the ventricle begins to fail. Presentation may be in congestive failure with oedema. In comparison with mitral stenosis, sudden deterioration such as when atrial fibrillation develops is uncommon.

Signs

The pulse volume is normal and has a sharp upstroke. The apex beat is hyperdynamic and displaced laterally and a third heart sound may be palpable.

On auscultation a holosystolic blowing murmur obscures S1 and extends beyond A2. It is loudest at the apex. Radiation depends on jet direction, either to the axilla or if the posterior leaflet prolapses then towards the aortic area. The second heart sound is widely split, P2 may be loud and a third sound gallop is usual.

Investigations

The ECG shows left atrial enlargement or atrial fibrillation. Sinus rhythm is often maintained in non-rheumatic disease. Left ventricular hypertrophy and strain pattern may occur. The chest X-ray shows left ventricular dilatation dwarfing left atrial enlargement. Calcification of the mitral valve annulus is best seen in the lateral or right anterior oblique view.

Echocardiography shows the large left atrium and the anatomy of the mitral valve's apparatus. Mitral prolapse (Figure 5), annular calcification or left ventricular hypertrophy can be visualized. The left ventricular size and function can also be seen. Doppler studies show the jet, the severity of the regurgitation being judged by the width of the jet as it emerges rather than the distance that it travels. However, assessment of severity by Doppler is full of pitfalls. Velocity is greater when the regurgitant orifice is smaller, and underestimation is a risk when the jet hits the atrial wall rather than being central as in rheumatic disease. It may even be missed altogether. Volume loading of the left ventricle should be recognized on imaging when reflex is severe. Transoesophageal echocardiography is a much more reliable way of visualizing the regurgitant jet.

The natural history of mitral regurgitation is often indolent for many years, so critical timing of invasive investigations and surgical intervention is imperative when the patient is elderly. Symptoms may be initially controlled by digoxin, diuretics and vasodilators but their onset indicates decompensation. While asymptomatic mitral regurgitation has a 5-year survival of $>80\%$, when symptoms develop this falls to 45%. Surgical treatment improves survival in patients with symptomatic mitral regurgitation, and both symptoms and left ventricular dilatation are an indication that the patient should be considered for surgery. Surgical outcome is related to left ventricular function and can be correlated with end-systolic volume (28). A volume of $>90\,\text{ml/m}^2$ of body surface area (BSA) has a poor surgical outcome, while one of $<30\,\text{ml/m}^2$ BSA heralds a good result. Age *per se* is no barrier to valve replacement, but when ejection fraction is less than 50% the risk of surgery is very high at any age.

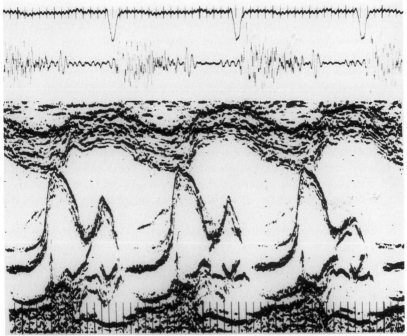

Figure 5. The directed M-mode beam is useful for accurate measurement of ventricular wall thickness and cavity size as well as in combination with phonocardiogram (shown here below the ECG) or mechanogram to display physiology—or in books without colour illustrations to show colour Doppler! Here we see increased excursion of both mitral leaflets with systolic prolapse of the posterior leaflet. The left ventricular walls show vigorous contraction and the cavity is slightly dilated in this patient with moderately severe mitral regurgitation

MANAGEMENT OF MITRAL VALVE DISEASE

Medical

Most elderly people can be improved by good control of the ventricular response to atrial fibrillation with digoxin. Anticoagulation is recommended for all patients with mitral stenosis and is mandatory in patients with atrial fibrillation. Loop diuretics are preferable to thiazides in the elderly but the dose should be the lowest possible needed to remove visible radiological evidence of pulmonary congestion. Angiotensin-converting enzyme (ACE) inhibitors coupled with controlled-release nitrates are often dramatically beneficial in mitral regurgitation.

Surgical

Closed mitral valvotomy is rarely useful for the elderly patient with mitral stenosis but an open commissurotomy may be effective if the valve is suitable.

The choice between mitral valve repair and replacement for mitral regurgitation depends largely on the ability of the surgeon. Controlled studies claim a more favourable outcome for mitral valve repair but report results from experienced surgeons in whose hands mitral valve repair does not substantially prolong bypass time (29). Preservation of the subvalvular apparatus (chordae, papillary muscles, etc.) improve results even with valve replacement.

It should be possible to determine whether the valve will be suitable for repair preoperatively. If the surgeon can be confident that he will not need to replace the valve, and left ventricular function is still good, valve repair will carry a lower risk than replacement with a better long-term prognosis for left ventricular function, and reduced embolic and infection risks (30,31). These considerations justify earlier operation or for choosing the surgical option rather than medical management in a patient for whom valve replacement might carry prohibitive risk.

The management of valve disease in elderly patients is summarized in Table 2.

GENERAL ASPECTS OF VALVE REPLACEMENT SURGERY IN ELDERLY PATIENTS

There was a sustained increase in total numbers of cardiac surgical operations in the UK during the 1980s (Professor K. M. Taylor, personal communication). Increased coronary artery bypass grafting accounts for most of this, heart valve surgery numbers having remained relatively constant. However, the proportion of patients undergoing valve replacement who are over the age of 65 has

Table 2. Summary of management of valve disease in elderly patients

Disease	Symptomatic	Asymptomatic
Aortic stenosis	Referral for surgery	Regular follow-up
Acute aortic regurgitation	Referral for surgery	—
Chronic aortic regurgitation	Referral for surgery, early	Regular follow-up
Mitral stenosis	Referral for surgery if uncontrolled medically	Regular follow-up, digoxin, diuretics
Acute mitral regurgitation	Stabilize using vasodilators and intra-aortic balloon counterpulsation, check coronaries then refer for emergency valve replacement and revascularization	—
Chronic mitral regurgitation	Diuretics and vasodilators (converting enzyme inhibitors) unless symptoms unacceptable with left ventricular function remaining reasonable	Regular follow-up, diuretics, offloading

Prophylactic use of antibiotics should be remembered for all non-aseptic interventional procedures (e.g. not for cardiac catheterization but for urinary catheterization, signoidoscopy, etc.) in elderly patients with valve disease.

increased (Table 1) and in the 1990s about 20% of valve surgery in Britain will be in patients over the age of 70. This will mean about 1000 valve operations per year in the UK in this group.

Operative mortality is greater in elderly than in younger people and also greater following valve surgery than coronary artery bypass grafting. Valve surgery mortality ranges from 6% for elective aortic valve replacement for isolated aortic stenosis (32,33) in a population aged >65 years to 25% in a population aged >80 years. Cerebral vascular accidents and renal failure are more common in elderly patients after cardiac surgery with total perioperative morbidity >35% in those aged over 80. Factors influencing operative mortality include the presence of coronary disease and poor left ventricular function (14,34). Associated tricuspid disease also has an adverse effect on survival (35). Nevertheless, reports of long-term survival after successful surgery are favourable, survival after aortic valve replacement being normalized after the first year (36). Survival at 7–8 years is 65–80%, which is lower than in younger patients where survival is 80–95%. Older patients with known coronary disease also have a reduced survival rate (15). As with all age groups there are marked differences in the results of elective surgery in the elderly when compared with those of emergency surgery, when the operative mortality can be >30% (37). Early consideration for elective surgery is to be recommended for aortic stenosis.

Limited life expectancy in the elderly population makes the use of a bioprosthesis justifiable, particularly in the aortic area, and in the mid-1980s those were the most popular valves. For older patients bioprostheses have the specific advantage that no long-term anticoagulation is required. Valve replacement merits a mehanical prosthesis if the patient's non-cardiac prognosis is likely to be 10 years, as bioprostheses have a limited life and degenerate more quickly in the mitral than aortic area. Atrial fibrillation indicates a need for anticoagulants, so viliating any advantages of a bioprosthesis.

Reoperation is infrequently undertaken in the elderly population but has a substantially higher mortality of up to 35%.

Careful selection of patients most likely to benefit from cardiac surgery should reduce perioperative mortality and morbidity, particularly that associated with cerebrovascular accidents, renal failure, myocardial infarction or peripheral vascular disease. More information is needed on the effect of anaesthesia and cardiopulmonary bypass on cerebral, renal and myocardial and respiratory function of elderly people.

Anticoagulation

The risks of thromboembolism in patients with mechanical prosthetic valves is about 4% per year in general. In Britain the recommended level of anticoagulation for such patients is for an international normalized ratio (INR) of between 3 and 5. The main problem with anticoagulation is the risk of serious haemorrhage, particularly in the elderly. A recent study comparing two different intensities of anticoagulation in patients with prosthetic heart valves suggested that a similar frequency of thromboembolism was seen in patients where anticoagulation averaged an INR of 2.65 in comparison to one of nine but, unsurprisingly, that bleeding complications were much lower in the patients on the lower anticoagulation regimen (38). The INR should be kept as close as possible to 3.0 and not allowed to creep above 3.5.

Balloon aortic valvuloplasty

The introduction of balloon aortic vavuloplasty gave hope of useful palliation of symptomatic severe aortic stenosis in patients in whom aortic valve replacement was considered to have too high a risk. This group includes very elderly patients as well as patients with poor left ventricular function and those with other medical conditions themselves life shortening or which make the risk of conventional anaesthesia and cardiopulmonary bypass unacceptable. The technique usually involves passing a large balloon catheter retrogradely across the aortic valve, through cuffed sheath inserted into the femoral artery or directly into the brachial artery, but an alternative access is venous with the valve crossed antegradely via a trans-septal route.

Early reports indicated moderate haemodynamic improvements following a successful procedure but a high incidence of procedure complications and an associated high mortality. Unfortunately follow-up studies reported a high rate of very rapid restenosis which approached 50% the first year after the procedure (39–41) and over 80% by 2 years (42). Recent reports from the Mansfield Scientific Balloon Aortic Valvuloplasty Registry have provided comprehensive information on patients treated over 10 months in 1987, i.e. relatively early experience with the technique. Careful review of this large series of patients has allowed clear evaluation of the application of balloon aortic valvuloplasty. Early mortality was 7.5% in 492 patients undergoing the procedure, 4.9% of the patients dying in the first 24 hours following the valvuloplasty (43). It must be noted, however, that the criteria for inclusion in the study included a patient being unacceptable for surgery, i.e. sick and old.

Multivariate analysis identified that a procedure-related complication (in over 20% and including vascular injury in 11% and myocardial perforation in 2% (44)), a lower initial left ventricular systolic pressure, a smaller final aortic valve area and a lower baseline cardiac output were all associated with increased mortality (45). The complication rate decreased substantially with increasing operator experience. The patients in this series had a 64% survival rate at 1 year (46) and an event-free survival rate (absence of death, repeat valvuloplasty or valve replacement) of 43%. Efficacy of valve dilatation was prognostic of patients' survival and of symptomatic relief. An initially low cardiac output with a low valve gradient was an indicator of high in-hospital mortality (11.9%) (45) and the actuarial probability of survival at 12 months was only 46% for such patients. On the other hand, age stratification showed that results are similar in old (> 80 years) and in younger (< 70, 70–79 years) patients despite the fact that the initial disease tends to be more severe in the older patients (47). Recurrence of symptoms is almost always associated with restenosis of the valve, although restenosis is also seen in more than half of patients who remain asymptomatic.

As with surgery, the results are best in those who have preserved myocardial function despite severe aortic stenosis. Thus, benefit is most likely where surgery is contraindicated because the patient has other severe disease, e.g. chronic respiratory problems. Patients who have a limited life expectancy because of malignancy could also gain. Patients with poor myocardial function will also do badly with valvuloplasty.

Sadly, balloon aortic annuloplasty has not lived up to initial optimistic expectation. At best it may be a bridge to aortic valve replacement in patients whose left ventricular function improves after the procedure. In such patients aortic valve replacement should not be delayed but carried out as soon as possible because of the certainty of rapid restenosis.

Balloon mitral commissurotomy

This is a much safer and more successful procedure than balloon aortic valvotomy. Although the best results are obtained in the young with valves which are free from superimposed degenerative changes, balloon mitral commissurotomy can offer good symptomatic relief in older patients with rheumatic mitral stenosis. The best results again are obtained in patients whose valves would have been suitable for open mitral valvotomy. In such patients the valve area may be doubled from 1.0 to a maximum of 2.0 cm²v with a < 5% chance of causing regurgitation severe enough to need surgery. Unacceptably high risk is encountered in patients with valve area < 0.6 cm², or severe pulmonary hypertension (pulmonary vascular resistance (PVR) > 6 mmHg/l/min) or low cardiac output (< 2 l/m²). The use of the Inoue balloon has reduced the time taken compared with the double balloon technique (48). Intraoperative trans-oesophageal echocardiography greatly aids the operator (49). The usual technique is with venous access and trans-septal approach. A small left-to-right shunt may remain afterwards.

The long-term results are still unknown. Restenosis can be anticipated but seems to be considerably slower than after balloon aortic valvuloplasty. The technique may be selected for patients deemed to be at higher risk from open heart surgery due to non-cardiac causes, particularly pulmonary disease.

Acknowledgement

With thanks to Professor K. M. Taylor for his permission to reprint data from the UK Heart Valve Registry, Department of Health.

REFERENCES

1. Taylor KM (1991) Heart valve surgery in the United Kingdom: present practice and future trends. *Br Heart J* **66**: 335–336.
2. Pomerance A (1965) Pathology of the heart with and without cardiac failure in the aged. *Br Heart J* **27**: 697–710.
3. Baker C, Sommerville J (1964) Results of surgical treatment of aortic stenosis. *Br Med J* **i**: 197–205.
4. Pomerance A (1972) Pathogenesis of aortic stenosis and its relation to age. *Br Heart J* **34**: 569–574.
5. Pomerance A (1965) Isolated aortic stenosis. In *Pathology of the Heart*, Pomerance A, Davies MJ (eds.) Blackwell Scientific, Oxford, pp. 327–342.
6. Seltzer A (1987) Changing aspects of the natural history of valvular aortic stenosis. *N Engl J Med* **317**: 91–98.
7. Roberts WC (1970) The congenitally bicuspid aortic valve: a study of 85 autopsy cases. *Am J Cardiol* **26**: 72–83.
8. Schwartz LS, Goldfisher J, Spragg GJ, Schwartz SP (1969) Syncope and sudden death in aortic stenosis. *Am J Cardiol* **23**: 647–658.
9. Lombard JT, Seltzer A (1987) Valvular aortic stenosis: clinical and haemodynamic profile of patients. *Ann Intern Med* **106**: 292–298.
10. Marcus ML, Doty DB, Hiratzkal LF *et al.* (1982) Decreased coronary reserve: a mechanism for angina pectoris in patients with aortic stenosis and normal coronary arteries. *N Engl J Med* **305**: 1362–1366.
11. Currie PJ, Hagler DJ, Seward JB *et al.* (1986) Instantaneous pressure gradient: a simultaneous Doppler and dual catheter correlation study. *J Am Coll Cardiol* **7**: 800–806.
12. Croke RP, Pifarra R, Sullivan H *et al.* (1977) Reversal of advanced left ventricular dysfunction following aortic valve replacement for aortic stenosis. *Ann Thorac Surg* **24**: 38–43.
13. Smith N, McAnulty JH, Rahimtoola SH (1978) Severe aortic stenosis with impaired left ventricular function and clinical heart failure: results of valve replacement. *Circulation* **58**: 255–264.
14. Fremes SE, Goldman BS, Ivanor J *et al.* (1989) Valvular surgery in the elderly. *Circulation* **80**: 177–190.
15. Bessone LN, Purpello DF, Hiro SP *et al.* (1988) Surgical management of aortic valve disease in the elderly: a longitudinal analysis. *Ann Thorac Surg* **46**: 264–269.
16. Waller BF, Zoltick JM, Rosen JH *et al.* (1982) Severe aortic stenosis from systemic hypertension (without aortic dissection) requiring aortic valve replacement. *Am J Cardiol* **49**: 473–477.
17. Paulus HE, Pearson CM, Pitts W Jr (1972) Aortic insufficiency in five patients with Reiter's syndrome: a detailed clinical and pathological study. *Am J Med* **53**: 464–472.
18. Roberts WC, Hollingsworth JF, Bulkley BH *et al.* (1974) Combined mitral and aortic regurgitation in ankylosing spondylitis: angiographic and anatomic features. *Am J Med* **56**: 237–243.
19. Prewitt TA (1970) Syphilytic aortic insufficiency: its increased incidence in the elderly. *JAMA* **211**: 637–639.
20. Kawanishi DT, McKay CP, Chandraratna AN (1985) Ejection fraction response to supine exercise in asymptomatic aortic regurgitation: relation to simultaneous haemodynamic measurements. *J Am Coll Cardiol* **5**: 847–855.
21. Laniado S, Yellen EL, Yoran C *et al.* (1982) Physiologic mechanisms in aortic insufficiency. (1) The effect of changing heart rate on flow dynamics. (2) Determinants for Austin Flint murmur. *Circulation* **66**: 226–235.

22. Zile MR (1991) Chronic aortic and mitral regurgitation: choosing the optimal time for surgical correction. *Clin Cardiol* **9**: 239–253.

23. Conway MA, Aliss J, Ouwerkerk KR *et al.* (1991) Detection of low phosphocreatinine to ATP ratio in failing hypertrophied human myocardium by ³¹P magnetic resonance spectroscopy. *Lancet* **338**: 973–976.

24. Rapaport E (1975) Natural history of aortic and mitral valve disease. *Am Cardiol* **35**: 221–257.

25. D'Cruz I, Panetta S, Cohen H, Glick G (1979) Submitral calcification or sclerosis in elderly patients: M-mode and two-dimensional echocardiography in 'mitral annulus calcification'. *Am J Cardiol* **44**: 31–38.

26. Hammer WJ, Roberts WC, de Leon AC (1978) 'Mitral stenosis' secondary to combined 'massive' mitral annular calcific deposits and small hypertrophied left ventricles: haemodynamic documentation of four patients. *Am J Med* **64**: 371–376.

27. Sherrid M, Goyle A, Delia E *et al.* (1991) Unsuspected mitral stenosis. *Am J Med* **90**: 189–192.

28. Borow K, Green LH, Mann T *et al.* (1980) End-systolic volume as a predictor of postoperative left ventricular performance and volume overload from valvular regurgitation. *Am J Med* **68**: 655–663.

29. Carpentier A (1984) Mitral reconstruction in predominant mitral incompetence. In *Recent Progress in Mitral Valve Disease*, Duran C, Anngle WW, Johnson AD, Oury JH (eds). Butterworths, London, pp. 265–276.

30. Scott ML, Stowe SL, Nunnally LC *et al.* (1989) Mitral valve reconstruction in the elderly population. *Ann Thorac Surg* **48**: 213–217.

31. Orszulak TA, Schaff HV, Danielson GK *et al.* (1985) Mitral regurgitation due to ruptured chordae tendineae: early and late results of valve repair. *J Thorac Cardiovasc Surg* **89**: 491–498.

32. Haraphongse M, Na Ayudhya RK, Haennel RG *et al.* (1990) Longterm follow-up after isolated aortic valve replacement. *Am J Cardiol* **6**: 236–240.

33. Galloway AC, Colvin SB, Crossi EA *et al.* (1990) Ten year experience with aortic valve replacement in 482 patients 70 years of age or older: operative risk and longterm results. *Ann Thorac Surg* **49**: 84–91.

34. Kriklin JK, Naffel DC, Blackstone EH *et al.* (1989) Risk factors for mortality after primary combined valvular and coronary artery surgery. *Circulation* **79**: 1185–1190.

35. Christakis GT, Weisel RD, David TE *et al.* (1988) Predictors of operative survival after valve replacement. *Circulation* **78**: I-25–I-34.

36. Lindblom D, Lindblom U, Invert T (1989) Heart valve replacement in septogenerians. *Scand J Thorac Cardiovasc Surg* **23**: 29–33.

37. Grondin CM, Thornton JC, Engle JC *et al.* (1989) Cardiac surgery in septogenerians: is there a difference in mortality morbidity? *J Thorac Cardiovasc Surg* **98**: 908–914.

38. Saour JN, Sieck JO, Mauro LAR, Gallus AS (1990) Trial of different intensities of anticoagulation in patients with prosthetic heart valves. *N Engl J Med* **322**: 428–432.

39. Block PC, Palacios IF (1988) Clinical and haemodynamic follow-up after percutaneous aortic valvuloplasty in the elderly. *Am J Cardiol* **62**: 760–763.

40. Letac B, Cribier A, Koning R, Belefleur J (1988) Results of percutaneous transluminal valvuloplasty in 218 adults with valvular aortic stenosis. *Am J Cardiol* **62**: 598–605.

41. Desnoyers MR, Isner JM, Pandian NG *et al.* (1988) Clinical and non-invasive haemodynamic results after aortic balloon valvuloplasty for aortic stenosis. *Am J Cardiol* **62**: 1078–1084.

42. Kuntz RE, Tosteson ANA, Berman AD *et al.* (1991) Predictors of even free survival after balloon aortic valvuloplasty. *N Engl J Med* **325**: 17–23.

43. Holmes DR, Nishimura RA, Reeder GS (1991) In-hospital mortality after balloon

aortic valvuloplasty: frequency and associated factors. *J Am Coll Cardiol* **17**: 189–192.

44. McKay RJ (1991) The Mansfield Scientific Aortic Valvuloplasty Registry: overview of acute haemodynamic results and procedural complications. *J Am Coll Cardiol* **17**: 485–491.

45. Nishimura RA, Holmes DR, Michela MA (1991) Follow-up of patients with low output, low gradient haemodynamics after percutaneous balloon aortic valvulo-plasty: the Mansfield Scientific Aortic Valvuloplasty Registry. *J Am Coll Cardiol* **17**: 828–833.

46. O'Neill WW (1991) Predictors of long-term survival after percutaneous aortic valvuloplasty: report of the Mansfield Scientific Balloon Aortic Valvuloplasty Registry. *J Am Coll Cardiol* **17**: 193–198.

47. Reeder GS, Nishimura RA, Holmes DR (1991) Patient age and results of balloon aortic valvuloplasty: the Mansfield Scientific Registry Experience. *J Am Coll Cardiol* **17**: 909–913.

48. Ribiero PA, Fawzy ME, Arafat MA *et al.* (1991) Comparison of mitral valve area result of balloon mitral valvotomy using Inoue and double balloon technique. *Am J Cardiol* **68**: 687–688.

49. Ramondo A, Chirillo F, Dan M *et al.* (1991) Value and limitation of trans-oeseophageal echocardiographic monitoring during percutaneous balloon mitral valvotomy. *Int J Cardiol* **31**: 223–233.

19 Muscle Disease

P. J. KEELING AND WILLIAM J. McKENNA
St George's Hospital Medical School, London, UK

The term cardiomyopathy has been used over the years to refer to any condition in which the primary disturbance is due to disease of the heart muscle. It is now recognized that there are a wide variety of conditions that predominantly affect heart muscle and include those in which there is no known cause. In this account, the term cardiomyopathy will be used in the latter sense, i.e. to mean an idiopathic heart muscle disorder which may be divided into three principal types: hypertrophic cardiomyopathy, dilated cardiomyopathy and restrictive cardiomyopathy. In addition other miscellaneous forms of cardiomyopathy are known which do not fall into any of the three above groups, but often have features of one, or more than one type of cardiomyopathy.

The diagnosis of cardiomyopathy is made by exclusion and, despite the introduction of including cardiac catheterization and endomyocardial biopsy, remains problematic, particularly at the extremes of age. In the elderly population additional cardiac diseases are common and extensive invasive cardiac investigation often cannot be justified in an elderly patient with a limited life expectancy. To add to these problems a number of physiological changes occur within the heart as a result of the normal ageing process (1–3); these include minor electrocardiographic changes, an increase in cardiothoracic ratio, ventricular hypertrophy and abnormalities in diastolic relaxation. For these reasons cardiomyopathy is probably considerably underdiagnosed or erroneously diagnosed in the elderly, and much of the information about cardiomyopathy in the elderly is incomplete and relies on the extrapolation of our knowledge of cardiomyopthy in the younger age group. Over recent years there have been considerable advances in our understanding of the cardiomyopathies and in the near future this should enable us to improve our clinical management of patients of all ages (4).

HYPERTROPHIC CARDIOMYOPATHY

Background

Early reports of hypertrophic cardiomyopathy (HCM) described young and middle-aged patients with a high incidence of sudden death (5–7). The first

Geriatric Cardiology. Principles and Practice. Edited by A. Martin and A. J. Camm
© 1994 John Wiley & Sons Ltd

detailed characterization of a patient with HCM was in 1958 by the pathologist Donald Teare (8), who described asymmetrical septal hypertrophy in the hearts of young siblings who had died suddenly. In the early 1960s Goodwin *et al.* (9,10), Braunwald *et al.* (11) and Wigle *et al.* (12) characterized the clinical aspects of HCM. The introduction of mode echocardiography in the 1970s stimulated great interest in the condition, and asymmetrical septal hypertrophy became recognized as a cardinal feature of the condition (13). Since the advent of cross-sectional echocardiography, however, a wider spectrum of HCM has become apparent (14,15). Left ventricular hypertrophy may be symmetrical, asymmetrical predominantly involving areas of the septum, or localized in the distal or right ventricles. In the past HCM was considered to be a rare disease with a poor prognosis, but with the increased sensitivity of our screening tests more HCM has become recognized and the true incidence is uncertain. Recent blood pressure and echocardiographic evaluation of a large cohort from the Framingham study suggests that unexplained left ventricular hypertrophy is much more common than has been previously recognized and that abnormal patterns of hypertrophy are present in approximately 2% of normotensive elderly patients (16). It is probable that HCM is more common but carries a less ominous prognosis than previous information would have led us to believe. In the elderly population HCM is not uncommon and carries a relatively favourable prognosis. Whether this arises from elderly HCM being a 'naturally selected' benign form of the condition or from their disease developing at a later stage in life is not known.

Diagnosis

HCM is defined as an idiopathic heart muscle disorder characterized by unexplained left ventricular hypertrophy (17,18). The diagnostic difficulties in elderly HCM are numerous and include previous unrecognized hypertension, physiological age-related ventricular hypertrophy and mild concomitant aortic valve disease. The recent discovery of genetic markers for HCM promises much in the identification of the condition in all age groups and will undoubtedly clarify the situation considerably.

The striking clinical and pathological features of HCM have been defined almost exclusively in the young and only recently has elderly HCM received much attention (19,20). The clinical features of HCM in the elderly population are summarized in Table 1. Clinical recognition of HCM in the elderly may be difficult for a number of reasons. Arterial pulses tend to be of higher volume and more rapidly rising because of inelastic arteries, so that the character of the arterial pulses may not be helpful; systolic murmurs due to sclerosis/stenosis of the aortic valve or to mitral regurgitation/mitral leaflet prolapse can give rise to late systolic murmurs very similar to those common in HCM. In addition elderly people with HCM may have no murmurs attributable to the condition because of accompanying ventricular dilation which diminishes outflow tract obstruction.

Table 1. Relation of age and clinical features at diagnosis

	Age at diagnosis (years)				
	≤14 n = 27	15–30 n = 67	31–45 n = 69	46–60 n = 64	≥60 n = 121
Syncope	9 (33%)	10 (15%)	8 (12%)	4 (7%)	28 (23%)
Exertional chest pain	5 (19%)	17 (25%)	20 (29%)	24 (38%)	70 (58%)
Dyspnoea					
class II	12 (44%)	21 (31%)	22 (32%)	22 (34%)	68 (56%)
classes III–IV	0	3 (5%)	5 (7%)	6 (9%)	

Furthermore if atrial fibrillation develops, as is common in elderly HCM, another clinical sign—the palpable atrial beat—disappears. The chest X-ray provides no particular help, usually showing a somewhat enlarged heart, some atrial distension and pulmonary venous congestion. In such patients the electrocardiogram (ECG) and echocardiography become very important.

Although the ECG may be normal in children with HCM, it is very rare for the ECG to be normal in old age. When sinus rhythm is present the ECG may show marked changes of left or biatrial hypertrophy but these signs are lost in atrial fibrillation. Evidence of a marked left ventricular disorder is nearly always present in the elderly with HCM whether or not they are in heart failure. Left anterior hemiblock is common (20%) but left or right bundle branch block is rare. The QRS is often widened and if there is left anterior hemiblock midseptal V leads show qS waves suggestive of previous infarction. Atrioventricular block has been described in HCM but is unusual and probably the result of chance rather than as one of the complications of HCM. Other patients may show a non-specific picture of left ventricular disorder with absent Q waves in leads I, AVL, V5 and V6, a slightly broadened QRS and minor repolarization changes in left ventricular leads.

The diagnosis of HCM relies upon the demonstration of unexplained left ventricular hypertrophy and is thus heavily dependent on echocardiography. When performing echocardiography in the elderly subject it is often technically difficult to obtain high-quality echocardiograms. Furthermore many of the characteristic echocardiographic features of HCM (systolic anterior motion of the mitral valve and midsystolic closure of the aortic valve) disappear with increasing age. Reliance solely upon abnormalities of left ventricular wall thickness for a diagnosis of HCM is dangerous (spurious increase in septal thickness by incorporating tricuspid papillary muscle, off-axis scans, etc). However, the major limitation of the M-mode technique in HCM is that it visualizes only a single slice through the upper (and perhaps mid) anterior septum and posterior wall. The mid and distal portion of the left ventricle as well as the entire posterior septum and free wall are not visualized.

Cross-sectional or two-dimensional echocardiography is currently the best available means to detect and to assess the distribution of left ventricular hypertrophy. Reliable measurements of myocardial wall thickness can be made in the anterior and posterior septum and in the left ventricular free and posterior wall in both the upper and the lower left ventricle. The diagnosis of HCM is made by the demonstration of an unexplained increase in myocardial thickness greater than two standard deviations from the mean of the normal population, i.e. >1.5 cm. Occasionally hypertensive heart disease can present as normotensive left ventricular hypertrophy because of the associated left ventricular systolic dysfunction. In this situation the left ventricle is invariably dilated and there may be evidence of renal or ocular involvement, or a family history suggestive of HCM may be found in family members. Another diagnostic difficulty is posed by the patient who presents with mild elevation in blood pressure but with moderate or severe left ventricular hypertrophy in the absence of other target organ manifestations of severe systemic hypertension. In this case, the importance of making the diagnosis of HCM relates strictly to prognosis and to the possibility of other family members being affected. If family studies are negative we would not diagnose HCM in such a patient but would attempt to identify additional factors which may be of prognostic importance, such as arrhythmias.

It has always been assumed that HCM in old age did not differ from HCM at any other age, but as other forms of heart disease becomes increasingly common with advancing age other diagnoses tended to be preferred. In a recent report (21) on 44 elderly patients in whom a clinical diagnosis of obstructive HCM was made on the basis of severe left ventricular hypertrophy, small left ventricular end-diastolic dimensions, supernormal ejection fractions and outflow tract obstruction on Doppler echocardiography (mean peak gradient 50 ± 28 mmHg). Further investigation, however, showed that 39% had a history of hypertension, a great predominance of females, uniform concentric left ventricular hypertrophy and marked diastolic dysfunction from which it was concluded that these patients were either not truly cases of HCM or represented a distinct form of the condition from that recognized in young adults.

Other studies, however, have provided conflicting results, and one such report (22) describes a subgroup of 52 elderly patients (mean age 69 years, range 60–84, 45 female) with obstructive HCM in whom certain clinical and morphological features differed importantly from those of many other patients with this disease. The majority (50/52, 96%) of the patients were asymptomatic or mildly symptomatic for most of their lives until their sixth or seventh decade, when they presented with progressive, intractable heart failure which was resistant to drug therapy and often required surgery. Echocardiographic examination showed a relatively small heart with modest ventricular septal hypertrophy but with marked distortion of the left ventricular outflow tract and anterior displacement of the mitral valve within the left ventricular cavity. Large deposits of calcium were seen posterior to the mitral valve within the mitral annulus and significantly contributed to the outflow tract narrowing, and has been confirmed by other workers (23). Marked systolic anterior motion of the mitral valve was common and was often severe (total 62%, subtotal 38%). The mechanism by which this occurred in most elderly patients differed from that observed more typically in younger patients with HCM in that anterior excursion of the mitral valve leaflets was relatively restricted and systolic apposition between the mitral valve and septum resulted largely from posterior excursion of the septum.

Arrhythmias

Arrhythmias are common in HCM (24,25) and are of similar incidence in the middle-aged and the elderly (Table 2). More than one-quarter of patients will have ventricular tachycardia of three beats or more during 48-hour ambulatory electrocardiographic monitoring. Such episodes are invariably asymptomatic and are a marker of patients at risk of sudden death. In our experience conventional class I antiarrhythmic agents (quinidine, disopyramide, mexiletine) and symptomatic therapy with β-blockers or verapamil are poorly tolerated and often unsuccessful in achieving sustained abolition of ventricular arrhythmia in patients with HCM (25). We have found that amiodarone is particularly useful in the treatment of symptomatic ventricular tachycardia. In addition, for the past 10 years we have used prophylactic low-dose amiodarone (median daily dose 200 mg) in patients with HCM and episodes of non-sustained ventricular tachycardia, and have noted a decrease in mortality over this time period (7% versus < 1% annual mortality).

Supraventricular arrhythmias are also common (24,25) and have an increased prevalence in the middle aged and elderly (Table 1). Approximately 10% of patients are in established atrial fibrillation and a further 30% have paroxysmal atrial fibrillation or supraventricular arrhythmias during electrocardiographic monitoring. Although atrioventricular nodal blocking drugs, (digoxin, β-blockers, verapamil) may control the ventricular response during supraventricular tachycardia they do not significantly reduce their incidence. In contrast amiodarone will suppress paroxysmal supraventricular tachycardia and restore sinus rhythm in approximately one-third of patients with chronic atrial fibrillation and may obviate the need for anticoagulation (26). Many of the unwanted effects of amiodarone therapy are related to dose and duration of

Table 2. The incidence of arrhythmia in relation to age in 177 patients with hypertrophic cardiomyopathy

	Age (years)				
	$\leqslant 15$ $n = 20$	$16-30$ $n = 50$	$31-45$ $n = 32$	$46-60$ $n = 52$	> 60 $n = 23$
Atrial fibrillation	0	0	2 (6%)	4 (8%)	2 (9%)
Supraventricular tachycardia	1 (5%)	8 (16%)	12 (40%)	17 (35%)	8 (38%)
Ventricular tachycardia	0	8 (16%)	10 (31%)	14 (27%)	6 (26%)

therapy; they do not appear to have a higher incidence in the elderly (27). One possible exception is hypothyroidism, which is seen in 1–2% of elderly patients receiving amiodarone and may represent an increased incidence of hypothyroidism in those patients on amiodarone compared to age-matched controls.

Natural history

Adverse risk factors have been well characterized in young/middle-aged adults (28). Stepwise discriminant analysis has revealed that a young age at diagnosis, 'malignant family history', presence of syncopal attacks and non-sustained ventricular tachycardia are all associated with a significant adverse risk of sudden death. The prognosis of patients diagnosed as having HCM at advanced age has not been well defined. It had always been assumed that elderly HCM simply represented the end spectrum of adult HCM, which by natural selection represented a benign form of the condition. One recent study (29) details the follow-up of 95 patients diagnosed as having HCM at age greater than or equal to 65 years. Seventy-five per cent of patients were symptomatic, as defined by the presence of chest pain, dyspnoea or syncope, and the mean ventricular septal thickness was 20 mm. The median duration of follow-up study was 4.2 years. The survival rate at 1 and 5 years was 95% and 76%, respectively, which was not significantly different from that in an age- and gender-matched control group, and symptomatic progression was not observed. These results suggest that following the diagnosis of HCM in the sixth or seventh decade the prognosis of patients is generally favourable.

Investigations and treatment

Left ventricular angiography and invasive haemodynamic measurements are not necessary for the diagnosis or the characterization of young or elderly patients with HCM. All patients should, however, undergo cross-sectional echocardiography and 48-hour electrocardiographic monitoring at the time of diagnosis. This allows the extent and pattern of left ventricular hypertrophy to be determined and provides a baseline for subsequent comparisons. All cases of newly diagnosed HCM should be assessed for familial disease, which is present in 50% of cases, by screening the first-degree relatives for the conditions. This can reliably be performed in an adult by a clinical examination, 12-lead ECG and two-dimensional echocardiogram. Difficulties are encountered, however, in the child/adolescent (in whom complete ventricular growth has not been completed), the athlete (who may have marked ventricular hypertrophy) or patients with concomitant disease (as previously discussed). In cases where doubt remains about the diagnosis, we recommend referral to a centre specializing in screening for HCM.

Treatment of HCM is largely symptomatic. The aetiology and treatment of dyspnoea and chest pain in HCM are uncertain, and troublesome chest pain in particular may require cardiac catheterization in order to exclude occlusive coronary artery disease. If stenotic coronary artery lesions are associated with severe refractory symptoms, coronary artery bypass grafting is indicated. Propanolol is the treatment of choice for dyspnoea and exertional or atypical chest pain. If the predominant haemodynamic abnormality is impaired relaxation or filling, combined use of propranolol and nifedipine (30) or verapamil alone may be effective (31,32). True left ventricular outflow tract obstruction may also be helped by the use of these medications, although surgical myectomy may occasionally be needed in refractory cases (33,34). Approximately 10–15% of patients with HCM have impaired systolic function. Treatment of these patients is more difficult as they are prone to cardiac failure following the administration of negative inotropic agents, and these drugs must be administered cautiously. Rarely patients may develop severe mitral regurgitation and may benefit from a mitral valve replacement with a low-profile prosthesis. It remains to be determined if prophylactic amiodarone is of benefit in the elderly with HCM.

The follow-up of patients with HCM should be directed at the prevention of complications, particularly endocarditis, embolic events and sudden death. Antibiotic prophylaxis is recommended in all patients with turbulent blood flow (left ventricular outflow tract gradient or mitral regurgitation) when undergoing invasive dental or other procedures. Patients in established atrial fibrillation and those patients with a high incidence of supraventricular arrhythmias are prone to the development of emboli and should be anticoagulated. We aim to follow up patients with HCM on at least an annual basis and perform clinical evaluation, echocardiography and 24-hour electrocardiographic monitoring in these patients at each visit.

Conclusion

Recent advances in clinical and molecular genetics have provided us with important information concerning the pathogenesis and familial nature of HCM. The molecular basis of familial HCM has now been defined and is determined by defects in the cardiac β-heavy chain myosin gene (35–37). Further analysis of both the familial and sporadic forms of HCM are currently under way and may provide us with a genetic marker for the disease and allow us to (a) reliably diagnose the condition in patients and family members, (b) accurately determine incidence, prevalence and natural history of HCM, and (c) enable accurate genetic counselling to family members of a patient with HCM.

DILATED CARDIOMYOPATHY

Background

Idiopathic dilated cardiomyopathy (DCM) has been defined as an idiopathic heart muscle disease characterized by a dilated and hypocontractile left and/or right ventricle (38). It occurs throughout the world although its true incidence is not known. An autopsy study from Sweden has suggested that it occurs as frequently as 10 per 100 000 and would suggest up to 5500 new cases a year in the UK alone (39). Diagnosis relies on the exclusion of specific cardiac disease and thus these estimates are likely to represent a considerable underestimate, and the true incidence may be much higher. Dilated cardiomyopathy has a long preclinical phase and usually presents at a late stage as severe biventricular heart failure with an associated poor long-term prognosis. In the elderly population treatment is largely symptomatic and it is only relatively recently that the widespread use of vasodilators has offered an improved prognosis, cardiac transplantation rarely being a realistic therapeutic option (40). Over the last few years considerable progress has been made in assessing the pathogenic mechanisms involved in DCM and determining individual risk, and promises great clinical benefits in the near future (41).

Aetiology

Aetiology and pathogenesis remain speculative and controversial. They are, however, important as they are likely to influence not only the natural history of the disease but also its specific treatment. Dilated cardiomyopathy may be a heterogeneous condition in which different mechanisms may be operating in different patients to produce a wide spectrum of clinical disease. Several distinct aetiological factors have been implicated in the pathogenesis of DCM and include Coxsackie B virus infection, autoimmune and inherited disease (42). Each alone may be capable of inducing chronic myocardial dysfunction; however, they are not mutually exclusive, and a viral infection may trigger the induction of an autoimmune disease in a genetically predisposed individual (43).

Viral infection

Enteroviruses, and particularly Coxsackie B viruses, are believed to be important in the pathogenesis of myocarditis and DCM (44). Although there is considerable support for an aetiological role of Coxsackie virus in murine myocarditis and DCM (45), direct evidence in man is lacking (46). The principal supporting evidence linking enteroviral infection to DCM is derived from serological studies (47,48) and the recent application of recombinant DNA technology to the detection of enteroviral genome within myocardial tissue from patients with DCM (49,50).

Autoimmunity

There has been much recent interest in the possibility that DCM, at least in a subset of patients, is an organ-specific autoimmune disease. Supporting evidence includes the demonstration of an association with a specific HLA phenotype

(DR4) (51), the inappropriate expression of major histocompatability complex class II antigens on endocardium and cardiac endothelium in patients with DCM (52), and the demonstration of an organ-specific cardiac antibody against α- and β-heavy chain myosin in 26% of patients with DCM (53). Further work is in progress to define this antibody response, which promises to provide us with an important serological marker for this condition.

Genetic factors

Until recently the only evidence that genetic factors were important in DCM came from anecdotal reports of familial DCM, which have suggested widespread degrees of familial aggregation ranging from 2% to 50%. Recently there have been two large prospective studies from Italy (42) and USA (54) which have shown that DCM is familial in at least 20% of cases, inheritence being most consistent with an autosomal dominant condition. The prevalence of familial DCM in the UK is at present unknown.

Alcoholic cardiomyopathy

Chronic excessive consumption of alcohol has been associated with DCM for many years, although the mechanism of its cardiac toxicity remains unclear (55). Alcoholism is a common problem in the elderly but there have been no specific studies on alcoholic cardiomyopathy in the elderly. Despite considerable effort to identify a reliable technique for assessing the importance of alcohol in the pathogenesis of DCM (56,57) the diagnosis of alcoholic DCM can only be inferred from a history of 'excessive alcohol consumption' over many years (e.g. > 6–8 units per day for 5–10 years) and a raised MCV and γGT. Abstinence from alcohol is now accepted as a prerequisite for recovery (58) and full recovery can be achieved in conjunction with conventional medical therapy.

Diagnosis

The diagnosis of DCM is based on World Health Organization criteria (59) with the demonstration of a dilated and poorly contracting left and/or right ventricle in the absence of coronary heart disease, valvular or pericardial disorders, and specific heart muscle diseases. What constitutes a 'dilated' and 'poorly contract-ing' ventricle is poorly defined and contributes to the difficulties in diagnosis and the interpretation of the literature. It is believed that there is a long preclinical phase in which the patient remains largely asymptomatic and that DCM commonly presents at a late stage with heart failure associated with a severe ventricular dysfunction. A minority of patients present with an associated symptom (e.g. chest pain), or a complication of DCM (e.g. arrhythmia, thromboembolism, heart block or sudden death) and may present at an earlier stage in the natural history of the condition when ventricular function is better preserved. The clinical characteristics of our series of 119 patients with DCM, of which 11 (9.2%) were above the age of 60 years at the time of diagnosis, are shown in Table 3.

There are no specific physical findings in DCM and the signs are those of low-output biventricular failure. The ECG is almost invariably abnormal in DCM but has no specific features and may show ST/T changes, ventricular hypertrophy, pathological Q waves, bundle branch block, atrial fibrillation or degrees of conduction disturbance (60,61). Echocardiography confirms left ventricular dilatation (an end-diastolic dimension of >55 mm or >112% of the predicted normal, using age and body surface area as variables (62)) and impaired systolic contraction (shortening fraction of <25%) are generally accepted, although different centres use different criteria. Left ventricular wall thickness is usually normal, although ventricular mass is often increased and correlates with voltage hypertrophy on the ECG (63). Echocardiographic assessment of the right ventricle is technically more difficult and assessment less reliable.

Radionuclide imaging may show biventricular dilatation and impaired contractility. Thallium-201 scintography provides a non-invasive method of identifying cardiac ischaemia, but has proven unhelpful in DCM because of the widespread presence of both fixed and reversible defects in this condition (64). The role of exercise testing in heart failure has been the subject of much debate. Exercise duration suffers from problems in reproducibility in patients with moderate to severe failure, and cardiopulmonary exercise testing with the monitoring of respiratory gases exchange is now an essential part of the assessment of chronic heart failure. Measurements made during cardiopulmonary exercise testing have been shown to be reliable parameters for evaluation of the severity of heart failure and are sensitive enough to detect the efficacy of therapeutic intervention for heart failure (65).

Cardiac catheterization allows angiographic and haemodynamic confirmation of left ventricular dysfunction and demonstrates an absence of coronary disease. Difficulties are, however, encountered when severe left ventricular dysfunction is documented in associated with minor degrees of coronary artery disease (e.g. <50% coronary stenoses), particularly when the left anterior descending coronary artery is spared. The role of endomyocardial biopsy in DCM remains controversial. Although an endomyocardial biopsy may be useful in excluding specific heart muscle disease (66), the histopathological findings are non-specific and include myocyte damage, myofibre loss and patchy interstitial fibrosis (67). In specialized centres, however, endomyocardial biopsy provides tissue for study, which will allow a better understanding of disease pathogenesis and ultimately lead to improved clinical management of these patients.

Natural history

The condition often presents at a late stage and is associated with a poor long-term prognosis with an annual mortality of between 10% and 20% (68).

Table 3. Clinical characteristics of patients with DCM above and below 60 years of age

	Age >60 years	Age <60 years
Number	11 (9%)	108 (91%)
Age (range, years)	12.3–59.9	60–73.9
NYHA class	I–4, II–3, III–2, IV–2	I–43, II–20, III–30, IV–15
Duration Sx	77 (70)	32 (43)**
Alcohol	4 (36%)	63 (77%)
AF	3 (27%)	21 (19%)
LBBB	LBBB–4 (36%)	LBBB–30 (28%)
Voltage LVH	3 (27%)	20 (14%)
LVWT (mm)	8.8 (3.5)	10.3 (2.9)
LVEDD (mm)	73.3 (14.6)	67.4 (10.7)
FS (%)	12.8 (7.2)	13.9 (7.7)
LVEDP (mmHg)	19.1 (7.2)	18.4 (8.1)
LVEF (%)	22.1 (10.1)	26.7 (10.5)
Peak mets	4.2 (1.7)	5.9 (3.1)
Outcome		
Duration (mean; range, years)	22.1 (3–63)	21 (1–136)
Transplant	1	20
Pacemaker	1	7
Death	0	13

$p < 0.05$; *$p < 0.01$. All results are expressed as mean (s.d.).
Abbreviations: LVWT (mm), left ventricular wall thickness; LVEDD (mm), left ventricular end-diastolic dimension; LBBB, left bundle branch block; AF, atrial fibrillation; Voltage LVH, left ventricular hypertrophy (S2 + R5 > 40 mm); FS (%), fractional shortening; LVEDP (mmHg), left ventricular end-diastolic pressure; LVEF (%), left ventricular ejection fraction; Peak mets, metabolic equivalents achieved at peak exercise; Sx, symptoms.

Accumulated data suggest that older patients have a worse prognosis but this is not our experience (see Table 3). Most deaths are related to intractable heart failure but sudden deaths account for about one-quarter of cases (69). The mechanism of sudden death in DCM is controversial (70) and has been assumed to be tachyarrhythmic; however, recently the importance of bradyarrhythmias has been emphasized (71) and bradycardic death has been documented on the Holter monitor (72). Our attention has also been drawn to the frequent occurrence of pulmonary and systemic emboli in this condition (73,74). Autopsy studies have demonstrated an annual incidence of between 3.5% and 5.5% and shown that these emboli are largely unsuspected during life and a relatively frequent cause of death in these patients. Many studies have attempted to identify patients at risk of sudden death or progressive heart failure in DCM (75–80). However, risk stratification for DCM has been disappointing largely because of our lack of understanding of the mechanisms involved. The most generally accepted and clinically useful predictors of sudden death in DCM are NYHA functional class, low ejection fraction, sustained ventricular tachycardia, impaired exercise capacity and increased neurohumoral responses. In our own experience patients with progressive heart failure are best identified and monitored by serial assessments over time.

Treatment

Treatment in DCM is largely symptomatic and involves the appropriate treatment of heart failure, arrhythmias and thromboembolism, and apart from vasodilator therapy and cardiac transplantation treatment has made little difference to survival. The introduction of vasodilator therapy, particularly with angiotensin-converting enzyme inhibitors (ACE inhibitors), has been shown not only to improve symptoms but also to reduce the progression of the disease and improve survival (81,82). However, there are a number of practical difficulties with the current use of ACE inhibitors in patients with chronic heart failure; although the patients were elderly (average age 70 years) in the Consensus Study only those with severe heart failure (NYHA class IV) were included; no study to date has demonstrated a reduction in the occurrence of sudden death and it is not known whether there is any benefit in using ACE inhibitors in combination with other vasodilators. It is our practice to introduce ACE inhibitor therapy at an early stage in patients with DCM and this can often be performed on an outpatient basis, even in the elderly patient, using a small nocturnal test dose of a short-acting agent (e.g. captopril 6.25 mg). Cardiac transplantation is usually not applicable in the elderly patient because of the limitations imposed by the scarcity of donor organs and the age limits which are commonly used at most cardiac transplantation centres.

The role of long-term anticoagulation has been advocated in patients with DCM (73); however, the evidence for this is controversial. Patients in atrial fibrillation and those who have previously suffered from thromboembolism probably benefit from anticoagulation (83,84). The timing and duration of therapy, and the optimal level of anticoagulation, are unknown and warrant further evaluation (85). Treatment of arrhythmias in DCM has been disappointing in that it is often unsuccessful and made little impact of survival (86,87). The one possible exception is treatment with low-dose amiodarone (plasma levels of < 1.0 mg/l), which has been shown to be effective in the treatment of paroxysmal atrial fibrillation and ventricular tachycardia and in which a reduction in sudden deaths has been reported in some studies (88) but not in others (89). Patients with DCM, particularly those who have a resting tachycardia, can show a clinical improvement after the introduction of β-blocker therapy. Unfortunately this can worsen the situation and provoke cardiac failure in some patients (90), and until we can identify the appropriate patients for treatment we do not advise their useage except under closely monitored conditions.

Conclusion

For many years DCM went unrecognized but recently there has been a great deal of interest, particularly in disease pathogenesis and risk stratification. Novel techniques such as signal averaging (91,92), molecular hybridization (50,93) and medical genetics in conjunction with the new application of existing technologies (52,53,94,95) promise great benefits in our understanding of the condition that should enable us rapidly to improve the clinical management of such patients.

RESTRICTIVE CARDIOMYOPATHY

Restrictive cardiomyopathy represents a heart muscle characterized by rapid early diastolic filling ('restrictive physiology') with preserved systolic contraction in the absence of specific heart muscle diseases and significant ventricular hypertrophy or dilatation. The restrictive cardiomyopathies are usually classified by the presence of peripheral blood eosinophilia and by the endomyocardial histology into Loeffler's eosinophilic endomyocardial disease and endomyocardial fibrosis, respectively. Restrictive cardiomyopathy is rare in the UK, and particularly so in the elderly age group, although hereditary forms of restrictive cardiomyopathy do occur and are being increasingly recognized. In the elderly age group restrictive heart muscle disease is usually associated with specific heart muscle disease which shows restrictive physiology, particularly infiltrative diseases, such as cardiac amyloidosis or sarcoidosis, or are induced by therapeutic doses of external radiation.

Cardiac amyloidosis

Cardiac amyloidosis was first observed by Vichow in 1957 and since then many cases have been documented. The condition is caused by the pathological deposition of an extracellular protein in the form of a β-pleated sheet (a form not normally found in man) in the walls of small blood vessels, where it interferes with tissue oxygenation and causes pressure atrophy. Many different proteins have been reported to be involved in amyloidosis but can be broadly classified into immunogobulin amyloid fibril (AL) and amyloid fibril proteins (AA). The former, previously called primary amyloidosis, is associated with immunological diseases such as myelomatosis, while the latter, previously known as secondary amyloidosis, is associated with inflammatory diseases such as connective tissue disorders. In addition several heredofamilial forms of the condition have been described that can predominantly affect the heart. Why different types of amyloid protein predominantly affect the heart is not understood but the heart can be involved in any form of amyloidosis. Protein is deposited within the subendocardium, the conducting tissue and between the myocardial fibres, and the pattern of this involvement dictates the cardiac disease produced, which includes cardiac failure, conduction disease and arrhythmias. Cardiac amyloidosis commonly produces low-voltage complexes, poor R wave progression and conduction block on the ECG. Conventional echocardiography usually reveals a small non-compliant left ventricle, biatrial enlargement, symmetrical ventricular hypertrophy with exaggerated systolic wall thickening and an unusual speckled granular appearance (96,97). Although echocardiographic tissue characterization (98) promises to be of use, the diagnosis relies on tissue being examined histopathologically using special stains (99).

Senile cardiac amyloidosis is probably the commonest cardiomyopathy seen in the elderly and occurs in up to half the hearts of elderly patients at autopsy. In these cases amyloid protein is found almost exclusively within the atria and not in the ventricle or other organs and seems to be of little clinical importance. A specific form of senile cardiac amyloidosis, distinct from AL, is now recognized in which the ventricle (and other organs) are involved and is associated with significant cardiac disease (100). In a large study (101) of 45–99-year-olds ($n = 1625$) this form of senile cardiac amyloidosis was found in 22.4% of autopsies. In these patients congestive heart failure is common, as is conduction block and atrial fibrillation, and the condition is largely unsuspected antemortem (102). The application of newly developed immunohistochemical techniques have shown that in these patients cardiac involvement occurs at a relatively young age and is associated with a longer survival than patients with primary systemic amyloidosis (103). Systemic amyloidosis has been considered a theoretical contraindication for heart transplantation because of the concern that amyloidosis is a systemic disease that could potentially recur in the allograft (104). Recently heart transplantation has been performed in patients with cardiac amyloidosis with a good long-term outcome (105). The results of further research in this area are awaited and will surely be greatly helped by the establishment of a new murine model for accelerated senescence—the senescence accelerated mouse (SAM)—which shows a high incidence of senile amyloidosis with cardiac involvement (106).

Cardiac sarcoidosis

Although the diagnosis of myocardial sarcoidosis is difficult to establish clinically, the heart may be involved at autopsy in up to a third of cases of sarcoidosis and may only become apparent many years after the initial diagnosis of systemic sarcoidosis (107). The hallmark of the condition is the histopathological replacement of large areas of myocardium and conducting tissue with non-caseating granulomas and fibrosis. Cardiac sarcoidosis may remain occult, or may present with arrhythmia, conduction block or clinically as DCM (108). The incidence of sudden death in cardiac sarcoidosis is high (up to 60%) (109). Electrocardiographic and echocardiographic features are non-specific and diagnosis relies on tissue histology. There are remarkable reports of rapid and maintained responses to immunosuppression in the literature (110) and it is important that if systemic sarcoidosis is present or even suspected several biopsies should be performed to overcome the sampling errors, which are considerable, particularly from the right ventricle. In addition conduction block should be treated at an early stage by the insertion of a permanent pacemaking device.

REFERENCES

1. Decourt LV, deAssis RV, Pileggi F (1988) Structural changes in the aged heart. *Arq Bras Cardiol* **51**: 7–22.
2. Kitzman DW, Scholz DG, Hagen PT *et al.* (1988) Age-related changes in normal human hearts during the first 10 decades of life. Part II (maturity): A quantitative anatomic study of 765 specimens from subjects 20 to 99 years old. *Mayo Clin Proc* **63**: 137–146.
3. Waller BF. The old-age heart: normal aging changes which can produce or mimic cardiac disease. *Clin Cardiol* **11**: 513–517.
4. Abelmann WH, Lorell BH (1989) The challenge of cardiomyopathy. *J Am Coll Cardiol* **13**: 1219–1239.
5. Frank S, Braunwald E (1968) Idiopathic hypertrophic subaortic stenosis: clinical analysis of 126 patients with emphasis on the natural history. *Circulation* **37**: 759–788.
6. Hardarson T, de La Calzada CS, Curiel R, Coodwin JF (1973) Prognosis and mortality of hypertrophic obstructive cardiomyopathy. *Lancet* **ii**: 1462–1467.
7. McKenna WJ, Goodwin JF (1981) The natural history of hypertrophic cardiomyopathy In *Current Problems in Cardiology*, Vol. VI, Harvey P (ed.). Year Book Medical Publishers, Chicago, pp. 5–26.
8. Teare D (1958) Asymmetrical hypertrophy in the heart in young adults. *Br Heart J* **20**: 1–8.
9. Goodwin IF, Hollman A, Cleland WP, Teare ND (1960) Obstructive cardiomyopathy simulating aortic stenosis. *Br Heart J* **22**: 403–414.
10. Cohen I, Effat H, Goodwin JF *et al.* (1964) Hypertrophic obstructive cardiomyopathy. *Br Heart J* **26**: 16–32.
11. Braunwald E, Morrow AS, Cornell WP *et al.* (1960) Idiopathic hypertrophic subaortic stenosis: clinical, hemodynamic and angiographic manifestations. *Am J Med* **29**: 924–945.
12. Wigle ED, Heinbecker RO, Gunton RW (1962) Idiopathic ventricular septal hypertrophy causing muscular subaortic stenosis. *Circulation* **26**: 325–340.
13. Henry WL, Clark CF, Epstein SF (1973) Asymmetric septal hypertrophy: echocardiographic identification of the pathognomonic anatomic abnormality of IHSS. *Circulation* **47**: 225–233.
14. Maron BJ, Gottdiener JS, Bonow RO, Epstein SE (1981) Hypertrophic cardiomyopathy with unusual locations of left ventricular hypertrophy undetectable by M-mode echocardiography. *Circulation* **63**: 409–418.
15. Maron BJ, Gottdiener JS, Epstein SE (1981) Patterns and significance of distribution of left ventricular hypertrophy in hypertrophic cardiomyopathy. *Am J Cardiol* **48**: 418–428.
16. Maron BJ, Bonow RO, Seshagiri TNR *et al.* (1982) Hypertrophic cardiomyopathy with ventricular septal hypertrophy localized to the apical region of the left ventricle (apical hypertrophic cardiomyopathy). *Am J Cardiol* **49**: 1838–1848.
17. Maron BJ, Epstein SE (1980) Hypertrophic cardiomyopathy. Recent observations regarding the specificity of three hallmarks of the disease: asymmetric septal hypertrophy, septal disorganization and systolic anterior motion of the anterior mitral leaflet. *Am J Cardiol* **45**: 141–153.
18. Goodwin JF (1974) Prospects and predictions for the cardiomyopathies. *Circulation* **50**: 210–219.
19. Pelliccia F, Cianfrocca C, Romeo F, Reale A (1991) Natural history of hypertrophic cardiomyopathy in the elderly. *Cardiology* **78**: 329–333.
20. Lever HM, Karam RF, Currie PJ, Healy BP (1989) Hypertrophic cardiomyopathy

in the elderly: distinctions from the young based on cardiac shape. *Circulation* **79**: 580–589.

21. Agatson AS, Polakoff R, Hippogoankar R *et al.* (1989) The significance of increased left ventricular outflow tract velocities in the elderly measured by continuous wave Doppler. *Am Heart J* **117**: 1320–1326.
22. Lewis JF, Maron BJ (1989) Elderly patients with hypertrophic cardiomyopathy: a subset with distinctive left ventricular morphology and progressive clinical course late in life. *J Am Coll Cardiol* **13**: 36–45.
23. Aronow WS, Kronzon I (1988) Prevalence of hypertrophic cardiomyopathy and its association with mitral annular calcium in elderly patients. *Chest* **94**: 1295–1296.
24. Savage DD, Seides SF, Maron BJ *et al.* (1979) Prevalence of arrhythmia during 24 hour electrocardiographic monitoring and exercise testing in patients with obstructive and non-obstructive hypertrophic cardiomyopathy. *Circulation* **59**: 866–875.
25. McKenna WJ, England D, Dioi YL *et al.* (1981) Arrhythmia in hypertrophic cardiomyopathy. I. Influence on prognosis. *Br Heart J* **46**: 168–172.
26. McKenna WJ, Harris L, Rowland E *et al.* (1984) Amiodarone for long term management in hypertrophic cardiomyopathy. *Am J Cardiol* **54**: 802–810.
27. Harris L, McKenna WJ, Rowland E *et al.* (1983) Side effects of longterm amiodarone therapy. *Circulation* **67**: 45–51.
28. McKenna WJ, Deanfield JE, Faruqui A *et al.* (1981) Prognosis in hypertrophic cardiomyopathy: role of age and clinical electrocardiographic and haemodynamic features. *Am J Cardiol* **47**: 532–538.
29. Fay WP, Taliercio CP, Ilstrup DM *et al.* (1990) Natural history of hypertrophic cardiomyopathy in the elderly. *J Am Coll Cardiol* **16**: 821–826.
30. Landmark K, Sire S, Thaulow E *et al.* (1982) Haemodynamic effects of nifedipine and propranolol in patients with hypertropitic obstructive cardiomyopathy. *Br Heart J* **48**: 19–26.
31. Bonow RO, Rosing DR, Bacharach SL *et al.* (1981) Effects of verapamil on left ventricular systolic function and diastolic filling in patients with hypertrophic cardiomyopathy. *Circulation* **64**: 787–796.
32. Hanrath P, Mathey DG, Kremer P *et al.* (1980) Effect of verapamil on left ventricular isovolumic relaxation time and regional left ventricular filling in hypertrophic cardiomyopathy. *Am J Cardiol* **45**: 1258–1264.
33. Koch JP, Maron BJ, Epstein SE, Morrow AG (1980) Results of operation for obstructive hypertrophic cardiomyopathy in the elderly. *Am J Cardiol* **46**: 963–966.
34. Beahrs MM, Tajik AJ, Seward JB *et al.* (1983) Hypertrophic obstructive cardiomyopathy: ten- to 21-year follow-up after partial septal myectomy. *Am J Cardiol* **51**: 1160–1166.
35. Tanigawa G, Jarcho JA, Kass S *et al.* (1990) A molecular basis for familial hypertrophic cardiomyopathy: an alpha/beta cardiac myosin heavy chain hybrid gene. *Cell* **62**: 991–998.
36. Geisterfer LA, Kass S, Tanigawa G *et al.* (1990) A molecular basis for familial hypertrophic cardiomyopathy: a beta cardiac myosin heavy chain gene missense mutation. *Cell* **62**: 999–1006.
37. Jarcho JA, McKenna WT, Pare P *et al.* (1989) Mapping a gene for familial hypertrophic cardiomyopathy to chromosome 14ql. *N Engl J Med* **321**: 1372–1378.
38. Goodwin JF, Oakley CM (1972) The cardiomyopathies. *Br Heart J* **34**: 545–552.
39. Torp A (1978) Incidence of congestive cardiomyopathy. *Postgrad Med J* **54**: 435–439.
40. Goodwin JF (1989) Clinical decisions in the management of the cardiomyopathies. *Drugs* **38**: 988–999.
41. Caforio ALP, Stewart J, McKenna WJ (1990) Idiopathic dilated cardiomyopathy.

Br J Med **300**: 890–891.

42. Mestroni L, Miani D, Di LA *et al.* (1990) Clinical and pathologic study of familial dilated cardiomyopathy. *Am J Cardiol* **65**: 1449–1453.

43. Neu N, Craig SW, Rose NR *et al.* (1987) Coxsackievirus induced myocarditis in mice: cardiac myosin autoantibodies do not cross-react with the virus. *Clin Exp Immunol* **69**: 566–574.

44. Burch GE, De Pasquale, NP (1964) *Viral Myocarditis. Cardiomyopathies.* Churchill, London, Ch. 5, pp. 99–115.

45. Wilson FM, Mirander QR, Chason JL *et al.* (1969) Residual pathologic changes following murine coxsackie virus A and B myocarditis. *Am J Pathol* **55**: 253–265.

46. Woodruff JF (1980) Viral myocarditis: a review. *Am J Pathol* **101**: 425–484.

47. Cambridge G, MacArthur CG, Waterson AP *et al.* (1979) Antibodies to Coxsackie B viruses in congestive cardiomyopathy. *Br Heart J* **41**: 692–696.

48. Muir P, Nicholson F, Tilzey AJ *et al.* (1989) Chronic relapsing pericarditis and dilated cardiomyopathy: serological evidence of persistent enterovirus infection. *Lancet* **i**: 804–807.

49. Archard L, Bowles N, Olsen E, Richardson P (1987) Detection of persistent coxsackie b virus RNA in dilated cardiomyopathy and myocarditis. *Eur Heart J* **8** (Suppl. J): 437–440.

50. Tracy S, Wiegand V, McManus B *et al.* (1990) Molecular approaches to enteroviral diagnosis in idiopathic cardiomyopathy and myocarditis. *J Am Coll Cardiol* **15**: 1688–1694.

51. Anderson JL, Carlquist JF, Lutz JR *et al.* (1984) HLA A B C and DR typing in idiopathic dilated cardiomyopathy: a search for immune response factors. *Am J Cardiol* **53**: 1326–1330.

52. Caforio AL, Stewart JT, Bonifacio E *et al.* (1990) Inappropriate major histocompatibilty complex expression on cardiac tissue in dilated cardiomyopathy: relevance for autoimmunity? *J Autoimmun* **3**: 187–200.

53. Caforio AL, Botazzo GF, McKenna WJ *et al.* (1990) Class II major histocompatibility complex antigens on cardiac endothelium: an early biopsy marker of rejection in the transplanted human heart. *Transplant Proc* **22**: 1830–1833.

54. Michels VV, Moll PP, Miller FA *et al.* (1992) The frequency of familial dilated cardiomyopathy in a series of patients with idiopathic dilated cardiomyopathy. *N Engl J Med* **326**: 77–82.

55. Dancy M, Maxwell JD (1986) Alcohol and dilated cardiomyopathy. *Alcohol Alcohol* **21**: 185–198.

56. Ferriere M, Rouy S, Rouy JM *et al.* (1983) [Histological aspects of congestive cardiomyopathy caused by alcohol: comparison with so-called primary cardiomyopathies]. *Ann Cardiol Angeiol Paris* **32**: 225–232.

57. Richardson PJ, Wodak AD, Atkinson L *et al.* (1986) Relation between alcohol intake, myocardial enzyme activity, and myocardial function in dilated cardiomyopathy: evidence for the concept of alcohol induced heart muscle disease. *Br Heart J* **56**: 165–170.

58. Juilliere Y, Gillet C, Danchin N *et al.* (1990) Abstention from alcohol in dilated cardiomyopathy: complete regression of the clinical disease but persistence of myocardial perfusion defects on exercise thallium-201 tomography. *Eur J Nucl Med* **17**: 279–281.

59. Bradenberg RO, Chazov E, Cherian G *et al.* (1981) Report of the WHO/ISFC task force on definition and classification of the cardiomyopathies. *Circulation* **64** (437A): 1397–1399.

60. Soria R, Desnos M, Benoit P *et al.* (1987) Dilated cardiomyopathy: electrocardiographic forms. *Arch Mal Coeur* **80**: 581–588.

61. Wilensky RL, Yudelman P, Cohen AI et al. (1988) Serial electrocardiographic changes in idiopathic dilated cardiomyopathy confirmed at necropsy. Am J Cardiol 62: 276–283.

62. Henry WL, Gardin JM, Ware JH (1980) Echocardiographic measurements in normal subjects from infancy to old age. Circulation 62: 1054–1061.

63. Brohet C, Ntahorubuze H, Vanoverschelde JL et al. (1990) Electrovectorcardiographic diagnosis of left ventricular hypertrophy in complete left bundle-branch block. Ann Cardiol Angeiol Paris 39: 207–212.

64. Takata J, Doi Y, Chikamori T (1989) [Prognostic significance of large perfusion defects on thallium-201 myocardial scintigraphy in dilated cardiomyopathy]. J Cardiol 19: 1081–1088.

65. Itoh H, Koike A, Taniguchi K, Marumo F (1989) Severity and pathophysiology of heart failure on the basis of anaerobic threshold (AT) and related parameters. Jpn Circ J 53: 146–154.

66. Unverferth DV, Baker PB (1986) Value of endomyocardial biopsy. Am J Med 80: 22–32.

67. Davies MJ (1984) The cardiomyopathies: a review of terminology, pathology and pathogenesis. Histopathology 8: 363–393.

68. Dolara A (1989) [Natural history of dilated cardiomyopathy (editorial)]. G Ital Cardiol 19: 121–122.

69. Juilliere Y, Danchin N, Briancon S et al. (1988) Dilated cardiomyopathy: long-term follow-up and predictors of survival. Int J Cardiol 21: 269–277.

70. Packer M (1985) Sudden unexpected death in patients with congestive heart failure: a second frontier. Circulation 72: 681–685.

71. Bayes DLA, Coumel P, Leclercq JF (1989) Ambulatory sudden cardiac death: mechanisms of production of fatal arrhythmia on the basis of data from 157 cases. Am Heart J 117: 151–159.

72. Radhakrishnan S, Kaul U, Bahl VK et al. (1988) Sudden bradyarrhythmic death in dilated cardiomyopathy: a case report. PACE 11: 1369–1372.

73. Fuster V, Gersh BJ, Giuliani ER et al. (1981) The natural history of idiopathic dilated cardiomyopathy. Am J Cardiol 47: 525–531.

74. Roberts WC, Siegel RJ, McManus BM (1987) Idiopathic dilated cardiomyopathy: analysis of 152 necropsy patients. Am J Cardiol 60: 1340–1355.

75. Hagege A, Desnos M, Fernandez F et al. (1988) Prognostic factors in dilated cardiomyopathies. Arch Mal Coeur 81: 1473–1479.

76. Komajda M, Jais JP, Goldfarb B et al. (1990) Analysis of predictive factors of mortality in dilated cardiomyopathy: a cooperative study by the Cardiomyopathy Working Group. Arch Mal Coeur 83: 899–906.

77. Oakley C (1978) Diagnosis and natural history of congested (dilated) cardiomyopathies. Postgrad Med J 54: 440–450.

78. Razzolini R, Boffa GM, Stritoni P et al. (1989) Natural history of dilated cardiomyopathy. G Ital Cardiol 19: 114–120.

79. Romeo F, Pelliccia F, Cianfrocca C et al. (1989) Determinants of end-stage idiopathic dilated cardiomyopathy: a multivariate analysis of 104 patients. Clin Cardiol 12: 387–392.

80. Zanchetta M, Pedon L, Carlon R et al. (1990) Dilated cardiomyopathy: multivariate discriminant analysis of main hemodynamic-angiographic indices. G Ital Cardiol 20: 15–19.

81. Consensus Trial Study Group (1987) Effects of enalapril on mortality in severe congestive heart failure: results of the Cooperative North Scandinavian Enalapril Survival Study (Consensus). N Engl J Med 316: 1429–1435.

82. Cohn JN, Archibald DG, Ziesche S et al. (1986) Effect of vasodilator therapy on

mortality in chronic congestive heart failure: results of a Veterans Administration Cooperative Study. *N Engl J Med* **314**: 1547–1552.

83. The Boston Area Anticoagulation Trial for Atrial Fibrillation Investigators (1990) The effect of low-dose warfarin on the risk of stroke in patients with nonrheumatic atrial fibrillation. *N Engl J Med* **323**: 1505–1511.

84. Chesebro JH, Fuster V, Halperin JL (1990) Atril fibrillation: risk marker for stroke. *N Engl J Med* **22**: 1556–1558.

85. Falk RH (1990) A plea for a clinical trial of anticoagulation in dilated cardiomyopathy. *Am J Cardiol* **65**: 914–915.

86. Oakley C (1991) Genesis of arrhythmias in the failing heart and therapeutic implications. *Am J Cardiol* **67**: 26–28.

87. Poll DS, Marchlinski FE, Buxton AE *et al.* (1984) Sustained ventricular tachycardia in patients with idiopathic dilated cardiomyopathy: electrophysiologic testing and lack of response to antiarrhythmic drug therapy. *Circulation* **70**: 451–456.

88. Neri R, Mestroni L, Salvi A *et al.* (1987) Ventricular arrhythmias in dilated cardiomyopathy: efficacy of amiodarone. *Am Heart J* **113**: 707–715.

89. Keogh AM, Baron DW, Hickie JB (1990) Prognostic guides in patients with idiopathic or ischemic dilated cardiomyopathy assessed for cardiac transplantation. *Am J Cardiol* **65**: 903–908.

90. Fisher ML, Plotnick GD, Peters RW, Carliner NH (1986) Beta-blockers in congestive cardiomyopathy: conceptual advance or contraindication? *Am J Med* **80**: 59–66.

91. Iannucci G, Villani M, Alessandri N *et al.* (1990) Late potentials in idiopathic dilated cardiomyopathy. *G Ital Cardiol* **20**: 549–554.

92. Fauchier JP, Cosnay P, Moquet B *et al.* (1988) Late ventricular potentials and spontaneous and induced ventricular arrhythmias in dilated or hypertrophic cardiomyopathies: a prospective study about 83 patients. *PACE* **11**: 1974–1983.

93. Keeling, PJ, Jeffery S, Caforio ALP *et al.* (1992) Similar prevalence of enteroviral genome within the myocardium from patients with idiopathic dilated cardiomyopathy and control by the polymerase chain reaction. *Br Heart J* **68**: 554–559.

94. Sleight P (1988) Importance of cardiovascular reflexes in disease. *Am J Med* **83**(3A): 92–96.

95. Farrell TG, Paul V, Cripps TR *et al.* (1991) Baroreflex sensitivity and electrophysiological correlates in patients after acute myocardial infarction. *Circulation* **83**: 945–952.

96. Klein HH (1991) [Significance of electro- and echocardiogram for the diagnosis of cardial amyloidosis]. *Dtsch Med Wochenschr* **116**: 13–17.

97. Nishikawa H, Nishiyama S, Nishimura S *et al.* (1988) Echocardiographic findings in nine patients with cardiac amyloidosis: their correlation with necropsy findings. *J Cardiol* **18**: 121–133.

98. Chandrasekaran K, Aylward PE, Fleagle SR *et al.* (1989) Feasibility of identifying amyloid and hypertrophic cardiomyopathy with the use of computerized quantitative texture analysis of clinical echocardiographic data. *J Am Coll Cardiol* **13**: 832–840.

99. Pellikka PA, Holmes DJ, Edwards WD *et al.* (1988) Endomyocardial biopsy in 30 patients with primary amyloidosis and suspected cardiac involvement. *Arch Intern Med* **148**: 662–666.

100. Westermark P, Johansson B, Natvig JB (1979) Senile cardiac amyloidosis: evidence of two different amyloid substances in the ageing heart. *Scand J Immunol* **10**: 303–308.

101. Serov VV, Zykova LD, Vinogradova OM, Sekamova SM (1988) [Senile cardiac amyloidosis]. *Arkh Patol* **50**(8): 3–12.

102. Johansson B, Westermark P (1991) Senile systemic amyloidosis: a clinico-pathological study of twelve patients with massive amyloid infiltration. *Int J Cardiol* **32**: 83–92.
103. Gertz MA, Kyle RA, Edwards WD (1989) Recognition of congestive heart failure due to senile cardiac amyloidosis. *Biomed Pharmacother* **43**: 101–106.
104. Valantine HA, Billingham ME (1989) Recurrence of amyloid in a cardiac allograft four months after transplantation. *J Heart Transplant* **8**: 337–341.
105. Conner R, Hosenpud JD, Norman DJ *et al.* (1988) Heart transplantation for cardiac amyloidosis: successful one-year outcome despite recurrence of the disease. *J Heart Transplant* **7**: 165–167.
106. Ogawa H (1988) Senile cardiac amyloidosis in senescence accelerated mouse (SAM) *Jpn Circ J* **52**: 1377–1383.
107. Swanton RH (1988) Sarcoidosis of the heart. *Eur Heart J* Suppl 9: 169–174.
108. Flora GS, Sharma OP (1989) Myocardial sarcoidosis: a review. *Sarcoidosis* **6**: 97–106.
109. Fleming HA (1974) Sarcoid heart disease. *Br Heart J* **36**: 54–68.
110. Lorell B, Alderman EL, Mason JW (1978) Cardiac sarcoidosis: diagnosis with endomyocardial biopsy and treatment with corticosteroids. *Am J Cardiol* **42**: 143–146.

20 Cardiac Arrhythmias in the Elderly

FRANCIS D. MURGATROYD, YAVER BASHIR AND A. JOHN CAMM

St George's Hospital Medical School, London, UK

Cardiac arrhythmias occurring in the elderly create several substantial challenges. Firstly, their incidence, both as a manifestation of cardiopulmonary disease and in apparently healthy individuals, rises steeply with age. Secondly, the diversity and vagueness of presentations caused by arrhythmias, overlapping considerably with those of other common pathologies (in particular cerebrovascular and pulmonary), create considerable difficulties of differential diagnosis. Impairment of ventricular function and reflex responses to hypotension, and coexisting vascular disease, cause arrhythmias which may be well tolerated in some patients and give rise to haemodynamic collapse in others. Drug therapy may be complicated by unpredictable pharmacokinetics and the increased frequency of certain side-effects. Finally, the option for interventional treatments, such as catheter ablation and sophisticated pacemakers, may be overlooked, either because of the unfounded fear of distressing procedures, or the reduced priority often given to elderly patients when economic stringencies apply.

In general, the principles of managing cardiac arrhythmias do not differ with the age of the patient. However, certain arrhythmias are of particular importance because of their frequency and connotations. In this chapter, the nature, symptomatology and diagnosis of tachycardias will be discussed in general, before individual arrhythmias are discussed in terms of their cause, diagnosis and management. The bradycardias, including the sick sinus syndrome, will be dealt with elsewhere.

Mechanisms of arrhythmias

Cardiac arrhythmias are thought to arise from one of two mechanisms. *Increased automaticity* is an accentuation of the inherent ability of many cardiac tissues to generate an independent rhythm. A variety of pathological states (including ischaemia) may excite a focus of tissue to discharge at a rate exceeding that of the sinus node, and thus dominate the cardiac rhythm. This is thought to be the mechanism of many atrial tachycardias (Figure 1a). However, the majority of

Geriatric Cardiology. Principles and Practice. Edited by A. Martin and A. J. Camm
© 1994 John Wiley & Sons Ltd

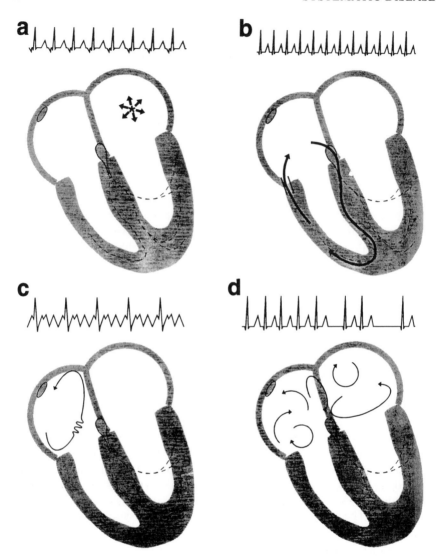

Figure 1. (a) *Atrial tachycardia* is usually caused by an ectopic atrial focus (in this case, in the left atrium). Unless this is close to the sinus node, the P wave is of abnormal morphology or axis. (b) *Atrioventricular re-entrant tachycardia* is caused by a re-entrant circuit with a fixed anatomic substrate. In the orthodromic form, excitation passes from atrium to ventricle via the atrioventricular node and returns via an accessory pathway: a narrow-complex tachycardia results. In the antidromic form, this circuit is reversed: this is one cause of broad-complex tachycardia. (c) *Atrial flutter* is caused by a single re-entrant circuit, almost always within the right atrium. This circuit passes round the venae cavae, and usually involves an area of slow conduction in the low right atrium. (c) *Atrial fibrillation* is caused by multiple re-entrant wavelets within the atria. These continually bombard the atrioventricular node, giving rise to an irregular ventricular rhythm

arrhythmias are thought to arise from *re-entry*. In its classical form, this consists of a wave of excitation repeatedly circulating around a fixed anatomical obstacle, such as a zone of infarction. The time taken for one circulation depends on the size of the circuit and the conduction velocity, and it must exceed the refractory period of any part of the circuit, so that the wavefront continually encounters excitable tissue; otherwise it will be extinguished. Much of the evidence for the nature of arrhythmias comes from the demonstration of an 'excitable gap' during which, for example, a correctly timed extrastimulus may reset or interrupt the circuit. The clearest example of classical re-entry is seen in the Wolff–Parkinson–White syndrome (Figure 1b). Re-entry may also occur around a zone of functional block, maintained in a constantly refractory state by the circulation itself, or around a combination of fixed and functional obstacles: this is the likely mechanism of atrial flutter (Figure 1c). Finally it is thought that fibrillation consists of multiple irregular wavelets propagating within the myocardium, constantly coalescing, dividing and invading adjacent excitable tissue (Figure 1d).

Presentation and diagnosis

Arrhythmias may cause symptoms due to awareness of the heart beat itself, reduced blood flow, or inadequate cardiac pump function. Arrhythmias tend to be less well tolerated in elderly patients, especially those with coexisting cardiovascular disease. With increasing age, a patient is less likely to complain of palpitations, and more likely to present with one of a variety of manifestations of heart failure and organ hypoperfusion, ranging from impaired mental function, dizziness and syncope (and resulting falls and trauma), to renal failure and thromboembolism. An arrhythmia must therefore fall within the differential diagnosis of many presentations. It should also be suspected as the cause of acute or paroxysmal deterioration of a pre-existing condition, or indeed of its first presentation. Furthermore, idiopathic arrhythmia is relatively infrequent in the elderly: atrial fibrillation in particular occurs as a complication of many metabolic disorders and virtually any form of cardiac disease. Conversely, other arrhythmias have close associations with specific diagnoses. The clinician should not be satisfied with diagnosing and treating the arrhythmia alone, but should satisfy himself that treatable underlying pathologies have been excluded.

The diagnosis of an arrhythmia and its response to therapy always requires electrocardiographic documentation (Table 1). Ambulatory monitoring has historically been the principal tool for recording paroxysmal arrhythmias, but is rarely applicable for periods of more than 24–48 hours. Increasing use is therefore being made of patient-activated electrocardiographic devices, the more sophisticated of which have 'loop' memory facilities (enabling the electrocardiogram (ECG) prior to a symptomatic event to be recorded), and the ability to transmit by telephone. The more sophisticated pacemakers have elementary Holter facilities, which often yield useful information about coexistent tachy-

Table 1. Electrocardiographic techniques used in the diagnosis of arrhythmias

Passive techniques	
Resting electrocardiography	12-lead surface ECG
	Oesophageal electrogram
Ambulatory monitoring	Telemetry (in hospital)
	Holter monitoring
	Holter/statistical features in implanted pacemakers
Event monitoring	Transtelephonic devices
	'Memory loop' recorders
Provocative techniques	
Exercise testing	Treadmill
	Bicycle ergometer
Drug bolus injection	Adenosine
	Isoprenaline
	Ajmaline
	Atropine
Autonomic manoeuvres	Valsalva manoeuvre
	Diving reflex
Electrophysiological study	Programmed electrical stimulation

cardias. In addition to these passive recording techniques, a number of methods can be used to provoke arrhythmias and give information about underlying cardiac disease.

ATRIAL ARRHYTHMIAS

Atrial premature beats

Atrial premature beats (APBs) occur with great frequency in the elderly. Couplets or short runs of APBs are an almost universal finding on 24-hour tapes, and their frequency is increased in those with cardiac disease and with advancing age. Frequent APBs can give rise to a pulse that is difficult to distinguish from atrial fibrillation. APBs *per se* do not require treatment, but they may give rise to symptoms (usually an APB itself is not felt, as it has a low stroke volume; it is more common for patients to complain of 'missed' beats), or initiate tachycardia. The natural 'firing' rate of ectopic foci is relatively slow, so APBs tend to be more common at times of relative sinus bradycardia, or in the presence of sinus node disease. Conversely, atrial ectopic activity which increases with exercise may reflect myocardial ischaemia or a raised atrial pressure and should alert the physician to the possibility of organic heart disease, as should frequent and multifocal APBs.

Atrial tachycardia

This is a regular tachycardia with a P wave morphology different from that associated with sinus rhythm, and a P–R interval which may vary with rate.

Varying degrees of atrioventricular (AV) block may also be seen. Commonly, but not always, the tachycardia starts abruptly, and it frequently accelerates following initiation. A benign, slow, short-lived variety of atrial tachycardia (AT) has been noted in Holter recordings from 28% of healthy adults over 65 and may virtually be considered a normal finding in this group (1). AT itself is not affected by physiological manoeuvres that increase vagal tone, but such manoeuvres may reduce the ventricular rate by causing AV block. Electrophysiological studies have demonstrated that the majority of cases of AT are automatic, i.e. caused by a single rapidly firing focus, but a small proportion are caused by a re-entrant circuit within the atrium: re-entrant AT can usually be initiated and terminated by single atrial premature beats. The two mechanisms are difficult to distinguish from surface ECG recordings alone.

Two types of AT are of particular diagnostic and therapeutic significance: 'multifocal' AT and 'AT with block'.

Multifocal atrial tachycardia

This is most commonly seen in acutely ill elderly patients, particularly those with decompensated chronic obstructive pulmonary disease. The rate is usually less than 140 beats/min, and multiple atrial foci can usually be distinguished from their differing P wave morphologies. The competition between the foci causes an irregular P–P, and therefore R–R, interval. The P waves may not be readily apparent on a bedside monitor and, unless a 12-lead ECG is carefully examined, the rhythm may be confused with atrial fibrillation. This may lead to therapy with digoxin, which is ineffective for the arrhythmia. Multifocal AT is one of the many arrhythmias associated with digoxin toxicity, and it has also been seen with toxic levels of theophylline and tricyclic antidepressants. Chronic multifocal AT may degenerate into atrial fibrillation. Management should initially be directed at identifying and correcting an underlying cause: the administration of oxygen alone may cause reversion to sinus rhythm. Multifocal AT is associated with a poor prognosis, chiefly because of the severity of the underlying illness rather than the arrhythmia, but the tachycardia itself may cause haemodynamic decompensation.

Atrial tachycardia with block

Wenckebach second-degree AV block generally accompanies AT when the atrial rate exceeds 150 beats/min, but can occur in association with an ageing AV node at much lower rates. It is usually seen in patients with organic heart disease but, most importantly, the majority of cases are caused by digoxin toxicity (2): this must be assumed to be the cause, until proven otherwise, in a patient known to be on digoxin. The serum potassium level should be maintained at the upper end of the normal range, and digoxin should be withdrawn. Additional treatment with antiarrhythmic drugs may not be necessary, and indeed may further complicate the arrhythmia, but phenytoin, which does not slow AV conduction, is

Type 1   **Type 2**

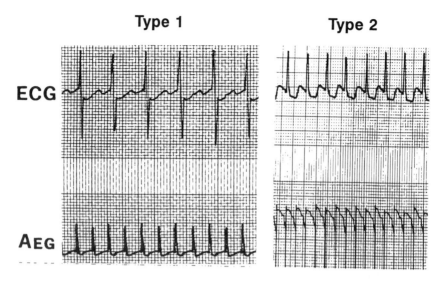

Figure 2. Atrial flutter. ECG = surface electrocardiogram; AEG = atrial electrogram.
Reproduced from Wells *et al.* (4) with permission

traditionally recommended, and digoxin-specific antibody fragment, which
causes rapid inactivation of circulating digoxin, is useful when a dangerous
arrhythmia is due to digoxin toxicity (3).

Atrial flutter

Paroxysmal episodes of atrial flutter (AFl) may occur without evidence of
cardiac abnormality, but persistent AFl usually accompanies organic heart
disease or metabolic abnormalities. The regular atrial activity in AFl is caused by
a re-entrant circuit, and the rate and regularity of the ventricular response
depend on the characteristics of AV conduction for the individual. The majority
of cases of AFl have the classical (type I) pattern (Figure 2) with an atrial rate
between 250 and 350 beats/min, and usually remarkably close to 300 beats/min.
Type II AFl, with an atrial rate between 350 and 450 beats/min, is much rarer (4).
Characteristic flutter waves, usually best demonstrated in the inferior limb leads
and V1, are not always seen even on a full 12-lead ECG, and AFl should be
suspected whenever there is evidence of regular atrial activity at this rate.
Furthermore, regular 2:1 AV conduction makes atrial activity difficult to
distinguish, causing AFl to be frequently misdiagnosed and treated as AV or AV
nodal re-entrant tachycardia. In this situation, vagal manoeuvres, such as carotid
sinus massage, or the administration of adenosine (0.05–0.25 mg/kg by rapid
intravenous bolus), are useful for diagnostic purposes: the transient AV block
produced by these measures makes the atrial arrhythmia easily visible (while

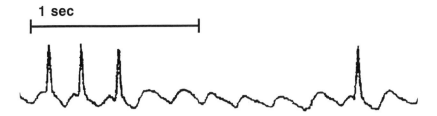

Figure 3. Use of adenosine in the diagnosis of atrial flutter. An intravenous bolus of adenosine causes transient atrioventricular block, during which flutter waves, previously difficult to discern because of a rapid ventricular response, are revealed

leaving it unaffected) in AFl (Figure 3), and usually terminates re-entrant tachycardias involving the AV node.

AFl differs in many important respects from atrial fibrillation (AF). Recurrent, brief episodes are less common than with AF: AFl tends to be more persistent, lasting for weeks or months. However, chronic AFl eventually tends to degenerate into AF. Attempted 'pharmacological' cardioversion is usually unsuccessful (5), but sinus rhythm may be restored by synchronized DC shock, usually with relatively low energies, or, as this is a re-entrant tachycardia, by rapid atrial pacing (6). The latter can be performed non-invasively using a transoesophageal electrode: this can be useful in those for whom anaesthesia is undesirable, or cardioversion dangerous (e.g. digoxin toxicity) (7). Because the atrial activity is organized, and the atria are therefore mechanically active, AFl does not seem to carry the same risk of thromboembolism as atrial fibrillation (8). Therapy is therefore usually limited to rate control, or attempted prevention of symptomatic paroxysmal episodes, along the same lines as in AF. If anything, these goals are harder to achieve in AFl than in AF.

Atrial fibrillation

Prevalence and aetiology (Figure 4)

The prevalence of chronic AF has a slight male predominance and increases steeply with age, rising sharply over the age of 55, so that more than half of patients with AF are over 70. In the Framingham study, cardiovascular causes such as rheumatic heart disease, cardiac failure and hypertension were found to increase the risk of AF three- to fivefold, and diabetes was also found to be a major risk factor (9,10).

Mortality (Figure 5)

AF is associated with an increased mortality in both men and women: this is entirely attributable to an excess in cardiovascular deaths (9). Mortality rises

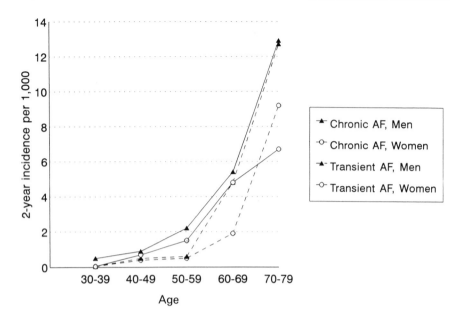

Figure 4. The incidence of atrial fibrillation. Data from the Framingham study (9)

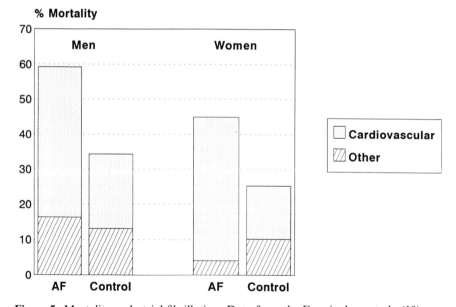

Figure 5. Mortality and atrial fibrillation. Data from the Framingham study (10)

steeply with age and the degree of heart failure present at the time of diagnosis. There is little difference in mortality between groups with different structural cardiac diseases (rheumatic, hypertensive, coronary), but those in whom the arrhythmia is associated with thyrotoxicosis and those with 'lone' AF have an appreciably lower mortality (11). The degree to which AF itself contributes to mortality is less clear. Where structural cardiac disease is present, comparison with control patients with similar severity of disease, but still in sinus rhythm, does show increased mortality in the AF group. However, conflicting results have emerged from follow-up studies of patients with 'lone' AF, some indicating a benign prognosis, others showing a significant increase in mortality, particularly with sustained (as opposed to paroxysmal) AF. Much of the difference between studies probably arises from the different study populations: hospital-based studies invariably demonstrate higher risk than those arising from life insurance examinations. The higher mortality seen in the Framingham series may reflect the fact that they were older, and not as rigorously investigated (echocardiography not being routine at the time): it is likely that many patients did not have truly 'lone' AF. It is becoming increasingly clear (see later) that the chief contribution of AF to mortality is the increased risk of stroke and other manifestations of thromboembolic disease. Other than this, it has not been demonstrated that AF is a risk factor in itself, rather than simply a marker of disease severity.

Autonomic factors and atrial fibrillation

Measures of cardiovascular autonomic function, such as the baroreflex and tilt tests, uniformly demonstrate depressed responses in the elderly, especially in the presence of other disease, such as hypertension and diabetes (12). This finding may go some way to explain the increased incidence of AF in the elderly, in the light of the recent description of groups of patients in whom the onset of paroxysmal AF is associated with extremes in the vagal/sympathetic balance of heart rate control. Patients with the 'vagotonic' pattern of attacks typically experience symptoms at times of low heart rate (e.g. at night and postprandially) (13). Increased vagal tone may cause electrophysiological changes in the atria which render them vulnerable to AF initiated by an APB occurring during or following a long R–R interval. Conversely, the 'adrenergic' form of paroxysmal AF causes symptoms principally on exertion, and typically starts with frequent APBs becoming AT, which degenerates into AF (14). These patterns are increasingly recognized in patients referred to specialist centres with refractory arrhythmia, but their prevalence within the general population of patients with paroxysmal AF, and the importance of autonomic factors in the initiation of sustained AF, are unknown.

Treatment of atrial flutter and fibrillation

Control of ventricular rate

Most patients in AF show little haemodynamic or symptomatic compromise if their heart rate is adequately controlled. Where therapy is needed to control ventricular rate, digoxin remains the mainstay of treatment, and carries the considerable advantage of not being negatively inotropic. The main disadvantage of digoxin is its narrow therapeutic ratio, requiring caution in its prescription and monitoring of drug levels. While it is unusual for digoxin (of appropriate dosage, in combination with a normal serum potassium) not to control the resting ventricular rate adequately, the rate often rises sharply on exertion, and this should be suspected in patients in AF with a disproportionate level of exertional dyspnoea (15). The addition of a β-blocker or a calcium antagonist usually improves the rate control, but this advantage is offset by their negative inotropy (16): where this is a problem, careful dose optimization or the use of diltiazem instead of verapamil may help (17).

Anticoagulation

In rheumatic AF, the risk of systemic embolism is 17 times that in controls in sinus rhythm: the benefit of anticoagulation is so clear that a controlled trial is unlikely. The role of anticoagulation in non-rheumatic AF (NRAF) has been more debatable, but the Framingham study demonstrated a fivefold increase in the incidence of stroke in this group taken as a whole (10). The Copenhagen AFASAK trial, in all forms of NRAF, showed a reduction in stroke incidence from 5.5% to 2.0% per annum with warfarin (international normalized ratio (INR) = 2.8–4.2), but this was offset by a 3% withdrawal rate due to bleeding. No significant benefit was seen with aspirin 75 mg per day (18). The Boston Area Anticoagulation Trial for Atrial Fibrillation (BAATAF) employed a low-dose warfarin regimen (INR 1.5–2.7) and demonstrated a reduction in the incidence of stroke from 3% to 0.4% (19). The Stroke Prevention in Atrial Fibrillation (SPAF) trial also demonstrated significant benefit from warfarin (INR = 2.0–3.5) (20). However, the SPAF investigators considered advanced years to be a contraindication to anticoagulant therapy, and consequently half of the population examined was excluded from randomization: most patients in the study were under 76 years. The Canadian Atrial Fibrillation Anticoagulation trial also examined the use of warfarin in non-rheumatic AF: although discontinued prematurely because of the results of the other studies, its results were consistent with a benefit from warfarin (INR = 2–3) (21).

Of these trials, only BAATAF was able to show a significant reduction in mortality. Nevertheless, the case for anticoagulant therapy to prevent embolic complications in patients with NRAF, taken as a group, is now established. The role of aspirin is less clear, but it is perhaps significant that the patients in AFASAK (in whom aspirin 75 mg per day was not shown to be beneficial) were significantly older, and had a higher incidence of other coexisting disease, than those in SPAF (in whom aspirin 325 mg per day significantly reduced the incidence of thromboembolism). It therefore seems that aspirin is likely to be a less effective prophylactic therapy in older patients than warfarin. The SPAF-2 study is directly comparing the two treatments in patients in whom neither is considered contraindicated.

Subgroup analysis in these studies has demonstrated, as has long been suspected, that the risk of thromboembolic complications in 'lone' AF, particularly in its paroxysmal form, is far lower than that in patients with AF and associated hypertensive or congestive heart disease. However, none of the studies had sufficient individual power to detect or exclude a benefit from antithrombotic therapy in patients with 'lone' AF.

It is now clear that all patients with chronic AF and structural heart disease should be formally anticoagulated unless this is absolutely contraindicated. There is also a strong case for anticoagulating older patients with 'lone' AF, at least with a 'low-dose' warfarin regimen. Despite its value in reducing the incidence of stroke and (myocardial) ischaemic events in patients with cerebrovascular disease, aspirin must be considered a poor second to warfarin in the elderly patient with AF: this presumably reflects the different pathological processes involved.

Maintenance of sinus rhythm

While the control of heart rate in sustained AF is not difficult in most patients, the prevention of recurrence of AF following cardioversion or in those with paroxysmal episodes remains controversial. Digoxin remains widely prescribed in both groups of patients, but until recently there was no evidence that it has any effect in preventing recurrence of AF, or even reducing the heart rate during arrhythmic episodes. A recently completed randomized controlled trial of digoxin in the prevention of paroxysmal AF showed that digoxin does cause a modest reduction in the frequency of symptomatic episodes (22). It remains unclear whether this is due to a true suppression of AF, or simply a lessening of symptoms due to a reduction in the ventricular rate.

The only drugs widely agreed to be effective in the prevention of AF are amiodarone and the class Ic drugs flecainide and propafenone; there is also growing evidence that sotalol is useful (23–25). However, these drugs can only be recommended with caution in the elderly in view of their potential for side-effects (particularly amiodarone and sotalol) and proarrhythmia in patients with structural heart disease (particularly the class I drugs). More established drugs, particularly quinidine and disopyramide, should probably be tried first: unfortunately, their usefulness is often limited by anticholinergic side-effects, and even quinidine may be proarrhythmic. In those with clear-cut exercise-induced arrhythmia, a β-blocker is often usful.

JUNCTIONAL ARRHYTHMIAS

The presence of two electrical communications between atrium and ventricle, either an accessory pathway (as in the Wolff–Parkinson–White syndrome), or dual AV nodal pathways, provides the substrate for re-entrant circuits at the AV

Table 2. Diagnostic approaches in broad complex tachycardia

---

1. Clinical features
2. 12-lead surface ECG:
3. Atrial ECG:
   —Transvenous
   —Transoesophageal
4. Adenosine during tachycardia
5. Intracardiac electrophysiological study
6. Other (e.g. echocardiography)

---

junction. Where these give rise to narrow-complex tachycardias, the differential diagnosis is with atrial tachycardia and flutter. The ECG during sinus rhythm may show, or be made to show (Table 1) evidence of pre-excitation, and careful examination of the timing, morphology, and axis of P waves during tachycardia aids diagnosis. If junctional tachycardias do not excite the ventricles via a healthy His–Purkinje system, a broad-complex tachycardia (Table 2) may result, which may be difficult to distinguish from ventricular tachycardia (VT): although various electrocardiographic features can be used to differentiate the two, if any doubt exists a presumptive diagnosis of VT should be made as the spontaneous occurrence of new junctional tachycardias in the elderly is far lower than that of new VT (see below) in a group of patients with a high prevalence of structural heart disease.

Two major advances have dramatically changed the management of junctional tachycardias in the last decade. Firstly, the recognition that adenosine is at least as effective as any other intravenous drug for the termination of these arrhythmias, and is considerably safer, has made adenosine the treatment of choice in the acute situation (26). If the diagnosis in incorrect or in doubt, the very short half-life of adenosine means that little if any harm is caused, and useful diagnostic information is often gained (27). Secondly, since the advent of steerable catheters and radiofrequency energy sources, the ablation of accessory atrioventricular or dual atrioventricular nodal pathways can be performed under local anaesthesia in specialist centres with a high degree of safety and efficacy (28). It can now be argued that every patient who has junctional arrhythmias of sufficient frequency, severity, or risk, is a candidate for catheter ablation rather than drug therapy, and this is particularly the case in older patients, in whom antiarrhythmic drugs are generally less safe and less well tolerated.

VENTRICULAR ARRHYTHMIAS

Both symptomatic and asymptomatic ventricular arrhythmias are commonplace among the elderly: ambulatory ECG monitoring discloses high-grade ventricular ectopic activity in 35–50% of healthy subjects over the age of 65 years (29). This is largely a reflection of the prevalence of coronary artery disease, hypertension and other structural heart disorders in older populations, but age-related alterations in cardiac morphology and physiology such as increased left ventricular wall thickness, myocardial fibrosis and declining arterial baroreflex sensitivity also favour the development of arrhythmias. The arrhythmogenic effects of commonly prescribed drugs such as digoxin, theophyllines and dopaminergic agents may also play a role in the aetiology of the arrhythmia, and diuretic-induced electrolyte imbalance may be a particularly important factor.

The commonest ventricular arrhythmia encountered in clinical practice is monomorphic ventricular tachycardia, which usually occurs against a background of prior myocardial infarction, and this arrhythmia has a re-entrant mechanism. Other causes include hypertension, aortic stenosis, cardiomyopathy and drug toxicity. The clinical management of ventricular arrhythmias in the elderly is essentially no different from that of other patients although, partly due to resource limitations, a more conservative approach is often adopted with regard to non-pharmacological strategies such as ablation therapy and implantable antitachycardia/defibrillator devices.

Clinical presentation and diagnosis

The clinical presentation of ventricular tachycardia (VT) depends on the degree of haemodynamic disturbance produced by arrhythmia. This ranges from palpitations in stable cases through to dizziness, syncope and ultimately complete circulatory collapse with sudden cardiac death. The factors determining the haemodynamic stability of an episode of VT are not clearly understood, and the spectrum of severity cannot be explained simply on the basis of tachycardia rate and left ventricular function: it is likely that impaired vasomotor regulation during tachycardia is a major factor (12).

Ventricular tachycardia gives rise to a classic surface ECG appearance of broad complex tachycardia (Figure 6). The differential diagnosis includes supraventricular tachycardia with rate-related aberrant conduction or pre-existing bundle branch block, and pre-excited arrhythmias in patients with accessory AV pathways. Unfortunately, awareness of these alternative possibilities seems to have resulted in a widespread tendency to misdiagnose cases of VT as supraventricular arrhythmias with pre-excited or aberrant conduction (30). Serious errors of management may occur, particularly administrative of intravenous verapamil, with the associated risk of hypotension or even cardiac arrest. This has prompted the development of numerous diagnostic schemes to guide emergency management of broad complex tachycardia. Many of these algorithms, such as the one suggested by Dancy and Ward (Figure 7) (31), are based on electrocardiographic criteria. A 12-lead ECG recording of tachycardia must be obtained if the patient's haemodynamic state permits. Electrocardiographic features of ventriculoatrial dissociation (independent P waves, capture or fusion beats) are diagnostic of VT (Figure 6) but are only present in 25–30% of cases. QRS duration >140 ms (right bundle branch block shape) or >160 ms

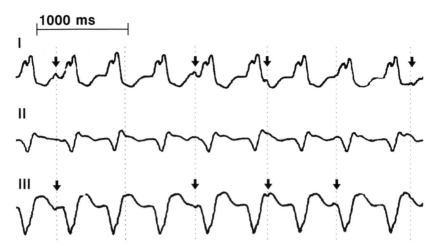

Figure 6. Ventricular tachycardia. Atrioventricular dissociation is demonstrated by the presence of independent P waves (arrowed)

(left bundle branch block shape) and marked left axis deviation favour the diagnosis of VT, as do the findings of particular tachycardia morphologies or ventricular concordance. In addition, specific QRS configurations in the precordial leads may provide some information (32). A recent approach has been proposed which employs four diagnostic criteria in a stepwise fashion and achieves 98.7% sensitivity and 96.5% specificity in the detection of VT (33).

Although more than 90% of cases of VT can be correctly diagnosed on the basis of electrocardiographic criteria, these can be difficult to memorize and apply in the acute setting. Recently, there has been greater emphasis on the diagnostic value of simple clinical criteria. Evidence of structural heart disease, in particular previous myocardial infarction or heart failure, is a very strong pointer to VT: indeed, in surveys of broad complex tachycardia, a history of myocardial infarction consistently emerges as the most powerful predictor of VT in multivariate analysis, ahead of all the ECG criteria mentioned above (34,35). On the other hand, it is still not generally appreciated that a stable haemodynamic state is of little value in differentiating VT from supraventricular tachycardia.

An important new development for the emergency management of broad complex tachycardia is the use of adenosine, an endogenous purine nucleoside with an extremely short half-life (10–30 seconds) and potent negative dromotropic effects. Intravenous adenosine can be given in incremental bolus doses to produce transient AV block without any risk of precipitating haemodynamic collapse. Adenosine terminates junctional tachycardias and slows the ventricular response to atrial flutter/tachycardia but has no effect on VT. Although occasional false positives and negatives do occur (for example, adenosine terminates certain rare forms of exercise-induced VT and can transiently accelerate pre-excited arrhythmias), recent studies have shown that adenosine is

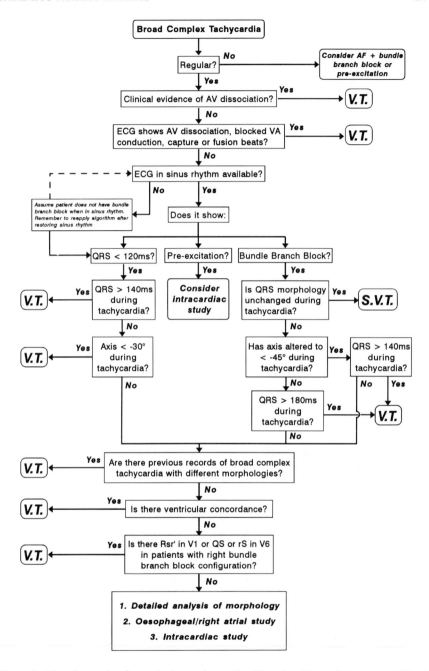

Figure 7. The diagnosis of ventricular tachycardia. The algorithm of Dancy and Ward (31). V.T. = ventricular tachycardia; S.V.T = supraventricular tachycardia

an extremely accurate, simple and, above all, safe diagnostic tool in broad complex tachycardia and should be made available in all casualty departments and coronary care units (36). It should be emphasized, however, that adenosine has no therapeutic effect in most cases of VT.

By application of clinical and ECG criteria and use of intravenous adenosine, the correct diagnosis of broad complex tachycardia (usually VT) can be reached in over 95% of cases. Occasionally, recording of the atrial electrogram by an oesophageal or right atrial electrode may be necessary to clarify the diagnosis (37).

Management: emergency treatment

Arrhythmia termination and suppression of recurrent episodes are the goals of acute management. Clearly, immediate DC cardioversion is required if the patient presents in a state of haemodynamic collapse, but otherwise bolus intravenous administration of antiarrhythmic drugs is usually the first approach despite a low (less than 50%) success rate. Lignocaine, although relatively ineffective (15–30%), remains the drug of first choice because of its short half-life and low side-effect profile: a higher efficacy is achieved with a second class I drug (disopyramide, procainamide, flecainide), but at the expense of a higher incidence of adverse effects (38). If this also fails, DC cardioversion should be performed either under neuroleptic sedation or general anaesthesia as soon as possible—at all costs, the practice of serial antiarrhythmic drug administration should be avoided, since this usually results in a downward spiral of progressive haemodynamic deterioration and/or serious proarrhythmic effects.

Following restoration of sinus rhythm, maintenance oral or intravenous antiarrhythmic therapy should be commenced (see below). Early or frequent breakthrough of VT presents a difficult management problem, particularly if repeated DC cardioversion is required. In this common situation, emergency transvenous overdrive pacing is much underused as a method for terminating VT episodes and preventing their re-emergence (39). Most coronary care units keep external pacing generators with a ' × 3' function specifically for this purpose. Pacing termination is often perceived as invasive and dangerous, but it is considerably safer and more comfortable for patients than repeated cardioversions under general anaesthesia or frequent changes in antiarrhythmic therapy.

The vast majority of patients with recurrent VT can be brought under control acutely by a combination of these measures. Failure usually occurs because insufficient time has been allowed for the effectiveness of amiodarone to build up or because overuse of multiple antiarrhythmic drugs has resulted in arrhythmia aggravation.

Management: long-term drug therapy

Maintenance antiarrhythmic therapy is almost always required for VT, except for those cases arising in the acute phase of myocardial infarction or with some remediable cause such as an electrolyte imbalance. The choice of drug is largely empirical, although there is an increasing tendency to early use of amiodarone, particularly if there are signs of heart failure or evidence of severe left ventricular dysfunction (40,41). The major drawback of amiodarone in the acute setting is its slow onset of action: even with high-dose intravenous or oral loading, antiarrhythmic efficacy may not be attained for 7–10 days or even longer, during which time breakthrough episodes of VT can occur and require treatment. In some cases, VT episodes may be so frequent that a second antiarrhythmic agent is required to cover the period of amiodarone loading: bretylium infusion is often effective, exhibiting broadly similar class III activity to amiodarone, although hypotension may be a problem. It is also important to optimize the patient's haemodynamic and metabolic state: electrolyte imbalance must be corrected (particularly potassium and magnesium depletion), cardiac decompensation treated with diuretics and vasodilators and any proarrhythmic drugs withdrawn.

Empirical selection of long-term antiarrhythmic therapy is associated with a high recurrence rate (including sudden deaths) and, accordingly, there is now more emphasis on assessment of therapeutic efficacy. The two most widely used techniques are Holter monitoring and programmed electrical stimulation. Holter monitoring has the important advantages of being inexpensive, non-invasive and widely available outside cardiac centres. Studies have shown that abolition of spontaneously occurring non-sustained VT runs and/or suppression of high-grade ventricular ectopic activity on treatment indicate long-term antiarrhythmic efficacy. Unfortunately, these arrhythmic markers are only consistently present in 30–50% of patients in the drug-free state, and ambulatory monitoring cannot at present be used to guide therapy in the remainder. However, recent advances in Holter technology may considerably extend the repertoire and scope of the technique: two important developments are high-resolution signal-averaged electrocardiography for detection of low-amplitude 'late potentials' (probably representing the substrate for re-entrant VT) and analysis of cardiac autonomic tone from heart rate variability and possibly diurnal QT fluctuation (42,43). Further work is required to ascertain whether these parameters can be used to improve antiarrhythmic drug testing.

Programmed electrical stimulation (PES) involves insertion of a transvenous ventricular pacing electrode and stepwise application of progressively more aggressive combinations of pacing and extrastimuli in an attempt to provoke VT resembling the clinical arrhythmia (44). This is possible in approximately 90% of patients with recurrent VT occurring against a background of past myocardial infarction, but VT is not so easily provoked when cardiomyopathy is the cause. The stimulation protocol is repeated after administration of an antiarrhythmic drug: if the inducibility of the tachycardia is significantly reduced, long-term prescription of that drug is planned (45). PES is generally considered the best method for selecting antiarrhythmic therapy in VT, although some have questioned the validity of this approach and further work is needed to clarify the significance of partial responses, and preliminary findings from the ESVEM study suggest that PES may be inferior to Holter-based selection of antiarrhythmic drug therapy (46). PES also currently plays a crucial role in the selection of 'drug-refractory' patients for non-pharmacological therapies. The technique is invasive but has an excellent safety record (47).

In general, there has been a trend away from the use of class I agents, including newer class Ic drugs such as flecainide, towards class III agents, particularly amiodarone. Apart from lesser therapeutic efficacy, there is concern about the negative inotropic and proarrhythmic effects of class I drugs in patients with impaired LV function, particularly in the aftermath of the Cardiac Arrhythmia Suppression Trial (CAST), which reported higher sudden death rates in flecainide and encainide-treated postinfarction patients with complex (albeit asymptomatic) ventricular arrhythmias (48). The major problem with long-term amiodarone therapy is the high incidence of extracardiac toxicity, including photosensitivity, thyroid dysfunction and the less common but more serious complications of hepatic injury or pulmonary fibrosis (49). Good results have also been reported with sotalol, a β-blocker with additional class III activity, in recurrent VT (41), but this may not be tolerated if there is severe left ventricular dysfunction. Several new 'pure' class III agents are under development and show great promise. It may soon be possible to achieve the same therapeutic efficacy as amiodarone without the side-effects and with a more suitable pharmacokinetic profile. For the moment, amiodarone will continue to be the most widely utilized drug in recurrent VT. Refractory cases may respond to a combination of amiodarone with a class I agent or low-dose β-blockade to offset the facilitatory role of increased sympathetic tone in arrhythmogenesis. Recent work suggests that adjuvant treatment with xamoterol (a β-receptor partial agonist) may be particularly effective in this situation, and surprisingly well tolerated even in patients with fairly severe LV dysfunction, although xamoterol alone is contraindicated in patients with severe heart failure (50,51).

Finally, in the aftermath of CAST, it is clear that there is no indication for treatment of asymptomatic ventricular arrhythmias detected by Holter monitoring. This is particularly important in elderly patients, given the prevalence of asymptomatic high-grade ventricular ectopy and the increasing use of ambulatory monitoring to investigate blackouts or dizzy spells. CAST was primarily concerned with the use of class I agents, and several studies are currently being undertaken to establish whether amiodarone can reduce the incidence of sudden death in high-risk postinfarction patients.

ANTIARRHYTHMIC DRUG THERAPY IN THE ELDERLY: GENERAL CONSIDERATIONS

Drug dosing and plasma concentrations

The altered and variable pharmacokinetics of the elderly patient complicates all prescribing: this is particularly the case with antiarrhythmic drugs, because of their low therapeutic ratio. In general, drug absorption is not significantly altered in the elderly, but the bioavailability of drugs with an extensive first-pass metabolism (notably propranolol and flecainide) may be considerably increased. The volume of distribution of water-soluble drugs is reduced, as is that of drugs extensively bound to skeletal muscle (such as digoxin), and that of fat-soluble drugs is variable. Elimination, however, is the most important pharmacokinetic variable affecting dosing in the elderly. The age-related fall in glomerular filtration rate affects all drugs when the principal route of excretion is renal, and this is further reduced in the presence of lowered cardiac output. The elimination of those drugs which are predominantly metabolized in the liver is more variably affected by age: this presumably reflects the multiplicity of enzymatic pathways involved.

Digoxin is particularly sensitive to many of these factors, with a fixed daily dose giving wide inter-individual variation in plasma concentration. Although dosing nomograms exist which allow for altered distribution and elimination, they should not be considered a substitute for therapeutic monitoring (52). There is a well-documented therapeutic range for digoxin prescribed to control the ventricular rate in chronic AF (with very little effect at levels below 1.0 mg/ml, and toxicity unlikely below 2.0 mg/ml), and monitoring of plasma drug concentration is essential. For other antiarrhythmic drugs, the concept of a therapeutic range is not as useful. Treatment should be individualized by starting each patient on the minimum dose, and gradually increasing this until either efficacy or limiting side-effects are obtained: this implies the necessity for clear endpoints, such as symptom frequency or presence of arrhythmia on Holter recordings. Although assays for several antiarrhythmic drugs are readily available (in particular the class I drugs quinidine, procainamide, lignocaine and flecainide, and amiodarone and its des-ethyl ester), these are generally used, when treatment is ineffective, to document adequate dosing before changing the drug; and additionally in situations of suspected toxicity.

Side-effects

The other major consideration in prescribing antiarrhythmic drugs in the elderly is the frequency of side-effects, due to the increasing prevalence of coexisting disease, both cardiac and non-cardiac.

Virtually all antiarrhythmic drugs, but particularly digoxin and β-blockers (and to a lesser extent verapamil), may cause sinus bradycardia or pauses: this is a particularly common finding on 24-hour tapes in patients being treated for AF, but is not necessarily dangerous unless accompanied by symptoms. The same agents may, through their action on the ageing AV node, give rise to more sudden and dangerous bradycardia by causing complete heart block. These bradycardic effects often make it impossible to treat tachycardias adequately without additionally implanting a pacemaker, and this is particularly the case in the sick sinus syndrome. The overwhelming proportion of elderly patients with arrhythmias which require treatment have significant organic heart disease (in particular, ischaemic, hypertensive and valvular): this further limits the safe use of antiarrhythmic drugs. Apart from digoxin (and, perhaps, oral amiodarone), all have a significant negative inotropic effect which may precipitate heart failure in patients with impaired ventricular function or aortic stenosis. Furthermore, the CAST study and other observational reports have highlighted the increased risk of proarrhythmia in the presence of structural heart disease (48,53).

Finally, the extracardiac side-effects of antiarrhythmic drugs may limit their usefulness, and these are all more frequent and less well tolerated in older patients. For example, lipid-soluble β-blockers (such as atenolol), which cross the blood–brain barrier, may disturb sleep patterns, and toxic doses of lignocaine and mexiletine cause impaired consciousness and seizures. The calcium antagonists may cause postural hypotension and syncope through vasodilatation, but the most frequent side-effect of verapamil in elderly patients is probably constipation. Poor peripheral circulation may be revealed or exacerbated by β-blockers (the more cardioselective agents such as bisoprolol may be better tolerated) and they are contraindicated in those with obstructive airways disease. The anticholinergic properties of quinidine and disopyramide, which are but a nuisance in most patients under 60 years, may provoke glaucoma or acute urinary retention in older individuals predisposed to these conditions. To an extent, this side-effect can be reduced by the concomitant prescription of cholinesterase inhibitors such as neostigmine, but careful dosing is required to avoid swings in 'cholinergic status', and in general these combinations are best avoided in all but the most compliant patients.

NON-PHARMACOLOGICAL TREATMENTS FOR CARDIAC ARRHYTHMIAS

Certain specialized centres can now offer a variety of new approaches to the therapy of atrial arrhythmias refractory to conventional treatment. Atrial foci can be ablated electrically with a transvenous catheter or with a cryoprobe at surgery, and surgical incisions can be made in the atria to interrupt the re-entrant circuits involved in both AFl and, more recently, AF (54). Consistent success can be obtained by abandoning the control of the atrial arrhythmia altogether and causing complete heart block by destroying the AV node or His bundle: the ventricles are then driven by an artificial pacemaker (55). This can be achieved by many methods, but catheter-based techniques using radio-frequency energy can be performed under local anaesthesia with low complication rates and minimal distress to the patient (56). The technique of His bundle ablation is now well established and, though invasive, offers the promise of considerable symptomatic improvement without the use of drugs: it can be appropriate even in frail patients.

Patients with drug-refractory VT may be treated by ablation (surgical or transcatheter), implantable antitachycardia devices or cardiac transplantation, although clearly the latter is less appropriate in the elderly. Arrhythmias with a re-entrant basis are often terminable by pacing/extrastimulus techniques, but for many years the role of antitachycardia pacing in VT was restricted due to the risk of accelerating haemodynamically stable tachycardias and causing sudden death. The recent development of implantable devices with the capability for automatic recognition and defibrillation of life-threatening ventricular arrhythmias has transformed the situation. Newer systems incorporating both antitachycardia pacing and back-up defibrillation offer flexible and highly efficacious therapy for many patients with refractory VT (57). To date, most of these devices have been implanted via thoracotomy, but newer transvenous systems require a much simpler implantation procedure with reduced morbidity and mortality. Unfortunately, it seems likely that access to this excellent new modality of antiarrhythmic therapy will be severely restricted for elderly patients because of resource limitations rather than on any clinical grounds. In such circumstances, there is still a limited but useful role for magnet-activated (by physician) antitachycardia pacemakers without defibrillator back-up in a subset of patients with recurrent episodes of haemodynamically stable VT (58). Although these patients have to attend hospital before activating their devices (in case of acceleration), they may still be saved the need for repeated admission and DC cardioversion.

If VT is drug-refractory and occurs frequently or becomes incessant, ablative therapy is the only option. Arrhythmia surgery involves mapping to identify the tachycardia focus or circuit and destruction of the re-entrant substrate by endocardial stripping or cryotherapy (59). Although successful in experienced hands, the mortality and morbidity are substantial. Such open-heart operations are seldom appropriate in elderly patients, even as a last resort. Transcatheter ablation may have far greater applicability, but has been considerably less successful than when applied to the treatment of junctional tachycardias (60). To a great extent, this is because the substrate is less discrete and localized, and because of haemodynamic instability during VT, but improvements in technique and the development of better power sources may improve this situation in the near future.

REFERENCES

1. Fleg JL, Kennedy HL (1982) Cardiac arrhythmias in a healthy elderly population: detection by 24-hour ambulatory electrocardiography. *Chest* **81**: 302–307.
2. Bigger JT Jr (1985) Digitalis toxicity. *J Clin Pharmacol* **25**: 514–521.
3. Wenger TL, Butler VP Jr, Haber E *et al.* (1985) Treatment of 63 severely digitalis-toxic patients with digoxin specific antibody fragments. *J Am Coll Cardiol* **5**: 118A–123A.
4. Wells JLJ, MacLean WA, James TN, Waldo AL (1979) Characterization of atrial flutter: studies in man after open heart surgery using fixed atrial electrodes. *Circulation* **60**: 665–673.
5. Nathan AW, Camm AJ, Bexton RS, Hellestrand KJ (1987) Intravenous flecainide acetate for the clinical management of paroxysmal tachycardias. *Clin Cardiol* **10**:

317–322.

6. Waldo AL, Maclean WAH, Karp RB *et al.* (1977) Entrainment and interruption of atrial flutter with atrial pacing: studies in man following open heart surgery. *Circulation* **56**: 737.

7. Crawford W, Plumb VJ, Epstein AE, Kay GN (1989) Prospective evaluation of transesophageal pacing for the interruption of atrial flutter. *Am J Med* **86**: 663–667.

8. Arnold AZ, Mick MJ, Mazurek RP *et al.* (1992) Role of prophylactic anticoagulation for direct current cardioversion in patients with atrial fibrillation or atrial flutter. *J Am Coll Cardiol* **19**: 851–855.

9. Kannel WB, Abbott RD, Savage DD, McNamara PM (1982) Epidemiologic features of atrial fibrillation: the Framingham study. *N Engl J Med* **306**: 1018–1022.

10. Wolf PA, Dawber TR, Thomas HE, Kannel WB (1978) Epidemiologic assessment of chronic atrial fibrillation and risk of stroke: the Framingham study. *Neurology* **28**: 973–977.

11. Kopecky SL, Gersh BJ, McGoon MD *et al.* (1987) The natural history of lone atrial fibrillation: a population base study over three decades. *N Engl J Med* **317**: 669–674.

12. Gribbin B, Pickering TG, Sleight P, Peto R (1971) Effect of age and high blood pressure on baroreflex sensitivity in man. *Circ Res* **29**: 424–431.

13. Coumel P, Attuel P, Lavallée JP *et al.* (1978) Syndrome d'arythmie auriculaire d'origine vagale. *Arch Mal Coeur* **71**: 645–656.

14. Coumel P, Escoubet B, Attuel P (1984) Beta-blocking therapy in atrial and ventricular tachyarrhythmias: experience with nadolol. *Am Heart J* **108**: 1098–1108.

15. Falk RH, Leavitt JI (1991) Dogoxin for atrial fibrillation: a drug whose time has gone? *Ann Intern Med* **114**: 573–575.

16. DiBianco R, Morganroth J, Freitag JA *et al.* (1984) Effects of nadolol on the spontaneous and exercise-provoked heart rate of patients with chronic atrial fibrillation receiving stable dosages of digoxin. *Am Heart J* **108**: 1121–1127.

17. Salerno DM, Dias VC, Kleiger RE *et al.* (1989) Efficacy and safety of intravenous diltiazem for treatment of atrial fibrillation and atrial flutter: the Diltiazem–Atrial Fibrillation/Flutter Study Group. *Am J Cardiol* **63**: 1046–1051.

18. Petersen P, Boysen G, Godtfredsen J *et al.* (1989) Placebo-controlled, randomised trial of warfarin and aspirin for prevention of thromboembolic complications in chronic atrial fibrillation: the Copenhagen AFASAK study. *Lancet* **i**: 175–179.

19. The effect of low-dose warfarin on the risk of stroke in patients with nonrheumatic atrial fibrillation: the Boston Area Anticoagulation Trial for Atrial Fibrillation Investigators. *N Engl J Med* **323**: 1505–1511.

20. Stroke Prevention in Atrial Fibrillation Study (1991) Final results. *Circulation* **84**: 527–539.

21. Connolly SJ, Laupacis A, Gent M *et al.* (1991) Canadian Atrial Fibrillation Anticoagulation (CAFA) Study. *J Am Coll Cardiol* **18**: 349–355.

22. Murgatroyd FD, O'Nunain S, Gibson SM *et al.* (1993) The results of CRAFT-1: a multi-center, double-blind, placebo-controlled crossover study of digoxin in symptomatic paroxysmal atrial fibrillation (Abstract). *J Am Coll Cardiol* **21**: 478A.

23. Anderson JL, Gilbert EM, Alpert BL *et al.* (1989) Prevention of symptomatic recurrences of paroxysmal atrial fibrillation in patients initially tolerating antiarrhythmic therapy: a multicenter, double-blind, crossover study of flecainide and placebo with transtelephonic monitoring. Flecainide Supraventricular Tachycardia Study Group. *Circulation* **80**: 1557–1570.

24. Connolly SJ, Hoffert DL (1989) Usefulness of propafenone for recurrent paroxysmal atrial fibrillation. *Am J Cardiol* **63**: 817–819.

25. Antman EM, Beamer AD, Cantillon C *et al.* (1990) Therapy of refractory symptomatic atrial fibrillation and atrial flutter: a staged care approach with new

antiarrhythmic drugs. *J Am Coll Cardiol* **15**: 698–707.

26. DiMarco JP, Miles W, Akhtar M *et al.* (1990) Adenosine for paroxysmal supraventricular tachycardia: dose ranging and comparison with verapamil. Assessment in placebo-controlled, multicenter trials. The Adenosine for PSVT Study Group. *Ann Intern Med* **113**: 104–110.

27. Rankin AC, Oldroyd KG, Chong E *et al.* (1989) Value and limitations of adenosine in the diagnosis and treatment of narrow and broad complex tachycardias. *Br Heart J* **62**: 195–203.

28. Jackman WM, Wang XZ, Friday KJ *et al.* (1991) Catheter ablation of accessory atrioventricular pathways (Wolff–Parkinson–White syndrome) by radiofrequency current. *N Engl J Med* **324**: 1605–1611.

29. Fleg JL (1988) Ventricular arrhythmias in the elderly: prevalence, mechanisms, and therapeutic implications. *Geriatrics* **43**: 23–29.

30. Dancy M, Camm AJ, Ward D (1985) Misdiagnosis of chronic recurrent ventricular tachycardia. *Lancet* **ii**: 320–323.

31. Dancy M, Ward D (1985) Diagnosis of ventricular tachycardia: a clinical algorithm. *Br Med J* **291**: 1036–1038.

32. Kindwall KE, Brown J, Josephson ME (1988) Electrocardiographic criteria for ventricular tachycardia in wide complex left bundle branch block morphology tachycardias. *Am J Cardiol* **61**: 1279–1283.

33. Brugada P, Brugada J, Mont L *et al.* (1991) A new approach to the differential diagnosis of a regular tachycardia with a wide QRS complex. *Circulation* **83**: 1649–1659.

34. Tchou P, Young P, Mahmud R *et al.* (1988) Useful clinical criteria for the diagnosis of ventricular tachycardia. *Am J Med* **84**: 53–56.

35. Akhtar M, Shenasa M, Jazayeri M *et al.* (1988) Wide QRS complex tachycardia: reappraisal of a common clinical problem. *Ann Intern Med* **109**: 905–912.

36. Griffith MJ, Linker NJ, Ward DE, Camm AJ (1988) Adenosine in the diagnosis of broad complex tachycardia. *Lancet* **i**: 672–675.

37. Levine JH, Kadish AH (1990) Transesophageal pacing and recording. In *Cardiac Electrophysiology from Cell to Bedside*, Zipes DP, Jalife J (eds). Saunders, Philadelphia, pp. 858–863.

38. Griffith MJ, Linker NJ, Garratt C *et al.* (1990) Relative efficacy and safety of intravenous drugs for termination of sustained ventricular tachycardia. *Lancet* **336**: 670–673.

39. Fisher JD (1990) Antitachycardia pacing in the acute care setting. In *Electrical Therapy for Cardiac Arrhythmias*, Saksena S, Goldschlager N (eds). Saunders, Philadelphia, pp. 411–423.

40. Herre JM, Sauve MJ, Malone P *et al.* (1989) Long-term results of amiodarone therapy in patients with recurrent sustained ventricular tachycardia or ventricular fibrillation. *J Am Coll Cardiol* **13**: 442–449.

41. Multicentre randomized trial of sotalol vs amiodarone for chronic malignant ventricular tachyarrhythmias: Amiodarone vs Sotalol Study Group. *Eur Heart J* **10**: 685–694.

42. Gomes JA, Winters SL, Martinson M *et al.* (1989) The prognostic significance of quantitative signal-averaged variables relative to clinical variables, site of myocardial infarction, ejection fraction and ventricular premature beats: a prospective study. *J Am Coll Cardiol* **13**: 377–384.

43. Kleiger RE, Miller JP, Bigger JTJ, Moss AJ (1987) Decreased heart rate variability and its association with increased mortality after acute myocardial infarction. *Am J Cardiol* **59**: 256–262.

44. Wellens HJ, Brugada P, Stevenson WG (1985) Programmed electrical stimulation of

the heart in patients with life-threatening ventricular arrhythmias: what is the significance of induced arrhythmias and what is the correct stimulation protocol? *Circulation* **72**: 1–7.

45. Kuchar DL, Garan H, Ruskin JN (1988) Electrophysiologic evaluation of antiarrhythmic therapy for ventricular tachyarrhythmias. *Am J Cardiol* **62**: 39H–45H.

46. The EVSEM Investigators (1993) Determinants of predicted efficacy of antiarrhythmic drugs in the electrophysiologic study versus electrocardiographic monitoring trial. *Circulation* **87**: 323–329.

47. Horowitz LN (1986) Safety of electrophysiologic studies. *Circulation* **73**: II-28–II-31.

48. The Cardiac Arrhythmia Suppression Trial (CAST) Investigators (1989) Preliminary report: effect of encainide and flecainide on mortality in a randomized trial of arrhythmia suppression after myocardial infarction. *N Engl J Med* **321**: 406–412.

49. Frobel TR, Miller PE, Mostow ND, Rakita L (1989) A general overview of amiodarone toxicity: its prevention, detection, and management. *Prog Cardiovasc Dis* **31**: 393–426.

50. Paul V, Griffith M, Ward DE, Camm AJ (1989) Adjuvant xamoterol or metoprolol in patients with malignant ventricular arrhythmia resistant to amiodarone. *Lancet* **ii**: 302–305.

51. The Xamoterol in Severe Heart Failure Study Group (1990) Xamoterol in severe heart failure. *Lancet* **336**: 1–6.

52. Jelliffe RW, Brooker G (1974) A nomogram for digoxin therapy. *Am J Med* **57**: 63–68.

53. Murgatroyd FD, Camm AJ (1992) Pro-arrhythmic effects of anti-arrhythmic drugs. In *Recent advances in Cardiology 11*, Rowlands DJ (ed.). Churchill Livingstone, Edinburgh, pp. 145–176.

54. Cox JL, Boineau JP, Schuessler RB *et al.* (1991) Operations for atrial fibrillation. *Clin Cardiol* **14**: 827–834.

55. Scheinman MM, Morady F, Hess DS, Gonzalez R (1982) Catheter induced ablation of the atrioventricular junction to control refractory supraventricular arrhythmias. *JAMA* **248**: 851–855.

56. Borggrefe M, Hindricks G, Haverkamp W *et al.* (1990) Radiofrequency ablation. In *Cardiac Electrophysiology: From Cell to Bedside* Zipes DP, Jalife J (eds). Saunders, Philadelphia, pp. 997–1004.

57. Bardy GH, Troutman C, Poole JE *et al.* (1992) Clinical experience with a tiered-therapy, multiprogrammable antiarrhythmia device. *Circulation* **85**: 1689–1698.

58. Fisher JD, Johnston DR, Furman S *et al.* (1987) Long-term efficacy of antitachycardia pacing for supraventricular and ventricular tachycardias. *Am J Cardiol* **60**: 1311–1316.

59. Manolis AS, Rastegar H, Payne D *et al.* (1989) Surgical therapy for drug-refractory ventricular tachycardia: results with mapping-guided subendocardial resection. *J Am Coll Cardiol* **14**: 199–208.

60. Evans GTJ, Scheinman MM, Zipes DP *et al.* (1988) The Percutaneous Cardiac Mapping and Ablation Registry: final summary of results. *PACE* **11**: 1621–1626.

21 Metabolic and Endocrine Disease in the Elderly

CAROL A. SEYMOUR[a] **AND JOHN RECKLESS**[b]
[a]*St George's Hospital Medical School, London, UK*
[b] *Royal United Hospital, Bath, UK*

Definition of the elderly is important since illness in old age is characterized by vague, often atypical presenting features which because of the slowness in onset may be missed or incorrectly attributed to the ageing process. This is particularly so for metabolic/endocrine disorders which affect the cardiovascular system. Thus hypothyroidism may be associated with bradycardia, and diabetes mellitus with a wide range of complications affecting the cardiovascular and peripheral vascular systems. Although most clinicians and lay persons can instinctively diagnose human ageing by its appearance, precise definition of the 'elderly' and understanding of the underlying mechanisms are often less clear.

There are many theories to explain biological ageing; disease itself can 'age' an individual, hence the statement 'man is as old as his arteries'. A more usually accepted definition is that of a series of accumulated changes occurring in a biological system with time. However, if pathophysiological processes, such as atheroma, can be accelerated or exacerbated by disease, ageing is both a physiological and a pathological process. Metabolic diseases are a particularly good example; age may alter or obscure the typical presentation of common diseases such as thyrotoxicosis or diabetes, which may be based in part on a decreased body metabolic rate. It is well established that in animals diet/calorie restriction can extend life-span by up to 40%, even though the relationship between calorie restriction, metabolic rate and longevity remains controversial. There is no one theory of ageing, and the ultimate test for any proposed mechanism might be that interference should slow the process. This may only be true with acquired ageing processes such as atheroma, where it is possible to reduce or reverse accelerated atheroma in at-risk patients due to hypercholesterolaemia, by reducing cholesterol levels with treatment.

In this chapter, the effect of ageing on metabolism, particularly of the common conditions affecting the heart and large arteries, will be reviewed, such as hyperlipoproteinaemia, glucose intolerance, diabetes and thyroid disease. Discussion of the rarer endocrine problems and inborn errors of metabolism (e.g. homocystinuria) which rarely present in the elderly will not be included.

Geriatric Cardiology. Principles and Practice.   Edited by A. Martin and A.J. Camm
© 1994 John Wiley & Sons Ltd

LIPIDS AND CARDIOVASCULAR DISEASE IN THE ELDERLY

Introduction

There is considerable evidence that levels of plasma lipids (predominantly cholesterol) correlate with an increased risk of coronary heart disease (CHD) (1). Further, interventional studies such as the Lipid Research Clinics Coronary Primary Prevention and Helsinki Heart Trials have suggested that drug-induced lowering of cholesterol also reduces mortality from CHD (2,3). Dyslipidaemia is thus a modifiable risk factor for CHD at least in young and middle-age adults (3). Cardiovascular disease is also a major cause of death and disability in the elderly, but there has been a paucity of evidence for specific risk factors for CHD in this group of patients, since atherosclerosis is considered a natural ageing process. It can thus be expected to be more advanced in the elderly. The significance of the circulating lipid and lipoprotein levels in older individuals is therefore more controversial than in younger age groups (<60 years) (4). Some reports suggest that screening and treatment of lipid disorders in the elderly are unwarranted (5).

Epidemiology of coronary heart disease in the elderly

More recently there have been a number of studies specifically seeking to determine the answers to these problems in older patients. Circulating cholesterol is known to rise with age, as shown by the Framingham (6), Lipid Research Clinics (2), Minnesota Heart Health Program and the Honolulu Heart Study and others (7).

However, of all age groups both men and women over 60 years have a higher prevalence of elevated serum cholesterol level but only a few studies have addressed the issue as to whether there is a greater total CHD risk attributable to cholesterol or dyslipidaemic condition in the elderly (8,9). This suggests that total cholesterol is not as reliable a predictor of CHD in the elderly as it is in the younger patient (9).

Recently the Bronx Study (10) looked prospectively at elderly volunteers (mean age at entry to the study was 79 years) to assess risk factors for CHD, dementia and cerebrovascular disease. Low high-density lipoprotein (HDL) cholesterol (HDL-C) was found to be a powerful predictor for men, whilst elevated low-density lipoprotein (LDL) cholesterol (LDL-C) was important in myocardial infarction in women. The combination of reduced HDL-C and increased LDL-C were important risk factors for cardiovascular and cerebrovascular disease for both elderly men and women (10).

Ettinger *et al.* (11) investigated the significance of lipoprotein lipid concentrations in 2106 men and 2732 women with an average age of 65 years. This is, to date, the *only* study which suggests that plasma cholesterol levels were in general lower than previously reported. In this study, the LDL-C was markedly reduced in men, and increased triacylglycerol (TG) concentrations were associated in women with obesity, central fat distribution, glucose intolerance and oestrogen preparations, and in men with the use of β-blockers. Negatively associated factors included age, renal disease, use of alcohol and socio-economic status. In addition the total cholesterol: HDL-C ratio (which should take into account the cholesterol content of atherogenic apolipoprotein B (apoB) and protective effect of HDL-C particles) were all lower than reported in previous studies (11,12). One possible explanation is that health care programmes could have had a beneficial effect as well as improved nutrition, general health and life-style behaviour of these individuals. In addition, in the 79–85-year old, it is likely that those with markedly atherogenic profiles may have died already. However, even in this encouraging study of the elderly, 39% were in the borderline high-risk category (total cholesterol 5.17–6.12 mmol/l), 24% were in the high-risk group (>6.2 mmol/l), 40% had borderline high LDL-C and 46% had high LDL-C levels, suggesting that it is important to screen the older age groups particularly when CHD is severe and interventional therapy (angioplasty and coronary artery bypass graft (CABG) surgery) is being considered.

Normal lipids and lipoprotein metabolism

Lipoproteins are macromolecular complexes of lipids and protein and are synthesized mainly by the liver and intestine and catabolized by hepatic and extrahepatic tissues. They are comprised of cholesterol, TG, phospholipid and apolipoproteins (see Table 1). Their main function is to transport dietary and other endogenously synthesized lipids from one organ to another for use in biosynthesis and repair. Components of these particles have important physio-logical and pathological consequences at all ages. Increased plasma concentra-tions of various lipoprotein particles and their components are strongly associated with the development of macrovascular disease leading to morbidity and mortality from myocardial ischaemia, from cerebrovascular and peripheral vascular disease. Mortality statistics in the industrialized world show that deaths attributable to vascular disease account for half of all deaths (13); with a higher percentage occurring in men (31%) and lower in women (24%), with most deaths in the age range 65–74 years, and over the age of 75 years (14). Factors (such as

Table 1. Biochemical characteristics of the major lipoprotein particles in human plasma

Particle	Cholesterol	Triglyceride	Major apolipoproteins
Chylomicron	+	+ + + + +	apo-B_{48}, apo-E, apo-C
VLDL	+	+ + + + +	apo-B_{100}, apo-E, apo-C
IDL	+ + +	+ + +	apo-B_{100}, apo-E
LDL	+ + + + +	+	apo-B_{100}
HDL	+ + + + +	+	apo-A

+ indicates proportion of cholesterol or triglyceride contained in a lipoprotein particle insulin and non-esterified fatty acids (NEFA)) affecting synthesis and secretion of lipoprotein particles (e.g. very low-density lipoprotein, VLDL) by the liver are important because they have the potential to alter properties of these particles and in turn affect vascular disease, both in normal subjects and patients with diabetes mellitus.

Lipoprotein metabolism

A dynamic relationship exists between the transport of TG as a source of energy and transport of cholesterol, which is used as a constituent of cell membranes, and a precursor of steroid hormones and bile acids. The pathway and metabolism of absorbed lipids from dietary triglycerides are shown in Figure 1. Cholesterol ester, absorbed as free cholesterol, is resynthesized in the intestinal epithelium. TG and cholesterol esters are secreted to lymph bound to apolipo-proteins apo-A_1 and B_{48}. VLDL are mainly products of endogenous synthesis in the liver and are markedly suppressed by postprandial chylomicrons. TG are synthesized in the liver or come from the plasma compartment having been recycled as NEFA after TG hydrolysis in adipose tissue. Intrahepatic TG is complexed with apo-B_{100} and secreted to the plasma compartment as VLDL with cholesterol, phospholipid and apolipoproteins C and E on the surface.

A number of lytic enzymes (lipases, lecithin cholesterol acyltransferase (LCAT)) are involved in cholesterol and TG metabolism (shown in Figure 1). Chylomicrons and VLDL, substrates of lipoprotein lipase, are influenced by hormones such as insulin and can be inhibited from binding to capillary sites by heparin. Postlipolytic lipoproteins (remnant particles) are small and dense with lower TG content, and are acted on by LCAT esterifying free cholesterol and partly hydrolysed lipid on the surface of the particle.

Triacylglycerol

Progress has been made in the last 30 years in identifying risk factors for the development of CHD. In the 1980s physicians began endorsing the cessation of smoking as a preventive measure of both IHD and lung cancer. In the 1970s, the US National High Blood Pressure Program had a campaign against hyperten-sion and set guidelines for proper diagnosis and management, and more recently the same has occurred in the UK with respect to elderly people (15). In the 1980s, more emphasis was laid on guidelines for management and diagnosis of hypercholesterolaemia, most recently culminating in the European Atheros-clerosis Society's (EAS's) new clinical guidelines for prevention of CHD (16). The identification and attention to specific management of these risk factors in the Western world and the USA have very likely contributed to the decreased annual rate of cardiovascular mortality—approximately 25% from 1968 to 1987. However, cardiovascular mortality is still a predominant cause of death in many industrialized nations and most recently attention has become focused on

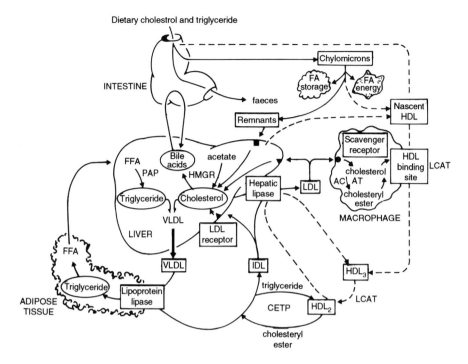

Figure 1. Lipoprotein metabolism. ACAT, acyl CoA:cholesterol acyltransferase; LCAT, lecithin:cholesterol acyltransferase; HMGR, HMG CoA reductase: PAP, phosphatidic acid phosphatase; CETP, cholesteryl ester transfer protein; FA, fatty acids; FFA, free fatty acids. Reproduced by kind permission of James Shepherd

hypertriglyceridaemia as a cardiovascular risk factor. Previous studies have suggested that hypertriglyceridaemia may be a separate and independent risk factor for CHD, as subjects with angiographically proven CHD have increased plasma TG concentrations when compared with controls (17).

Plasma TG measurements are the sum of TG contained within the various lipoprotein particles, and all particles contain TG in varying amounts. Following absorption from the intestine, dietary fat is packaged in large TG-rich particles (chylomicrons) containing surface apolipoproteins A_1, A_{IV} and B_{48}, and after secretion to chyle acquires apo-C_2 and apo-E from HDL. Chylomicron particles are lysed by circulating lipoprotein lipase (see Figure 1) and the remnant particle is cleared by the liver, which then synthesizes, assembles and secretes the lipoprotein particle VLDL. These may vary in size; large particles are converted to remnant particles, cleared and do not add to the LDL pool. Small VLDL particles are rapidly converted to LDL and are main contributors to the LDL pool (18). Circulation times of the VLDL remnants are determined by apo-E content and activity of the apo-B/E receptor, which has a central role in lipid metabolism (19). Receptor activity on the hepatocyte is finely regulated by intracellular cholesterol concentration within the cell and controlled through the rate-limiting enzyme, hydroxymethylglutaryl coenzyme A (HMGCoA) reductase. A low-affinity component for LDL and VLDL remnant removal is present in cells but is easily exceeded in adults, leading to increased plasma concentrations. These remnants can be modified and taken up by scavenger macrophage cells and lead to increasing cholesterol accumulation since macrophages do not down-regulate receptors. To a certain extent apo-B/E receptors on the hepatocyte divert lipoprotein overload to the scavenger cell pathway and promote atheroma (20). It has also been shown that stimulated macrophages from hypertriglyceridaemic subjects release increased amounts of superoxide compared with control macrophages.

Plasma TG is related to HDL concentrations, and patients with low HDL may have exaggerated postprandial lipaemia (21). Plasma TG also contributes to the increased risk of CHD by increased activity of cholesterol ester transfer protein, promoting exchange of TG to HDL. The latter promote transfer of cholesterol ester delivery to macrophages, as TG-rich HDL is a good substrate for hepatic lipase, leading to an overall increase in macrophage cholesterol ester and decreased HDL.

Reverse cholesterol transport

HDL particles are disc-shaped precursors derived from cholesterol esters. Action of LCAT esterifies cholesterol and converts HDL to a mature spherical-shaped particle which has two subfractions: HDL_2 and HDL_3. HDL_2 concentration varies between individuals, with age and with postprandial hyperlipaemia, and is higher in individuals with high lipoprotein lipase activity who may be at less risk from CHD, whilst those with low lipase activity have a higher HDL_3 with consequent increased CHD risk (22). Reverse cholesterol transport refers to binding of free tissue cholesterol from peripheral tissues to apo-A_1 and conversion of cholesterol ester within the HDL molecule, catalysed by LCAT.

Lipid metabolism and hormone/drugs

Lipid metabolism may be affected by hormones (cf. insulin secretion—see sections on diabetes, thyroid and sex hormones) (23) as well as by nutrients, including alcohol.

A variety of drugs may affect circulating cholesterol and TG, but commonest are oestrogens and antihypertensive agents, particularly thiazides and β-blocking agents.

Secondary causes of hyperlipidaemia

Interaction with other risk factors for CHD can occur, such as obesity (body mass index (BMI) >30) glucose intolerance and central fat distribution.

Table 2. Causes of secondary dyslipidaemia

Obesity
Diabetes mellitus
Alcohol abuse
Drugs: thiazides, β-blockers, cimetidine, immunosuppressives
Hypothyroidism
Chronic renal disease (renal failure/nephrotic syndrome)
Chronic cholestasis (e.g. primary biliary cirrhosis)
Myeloma

Previous studies have shown that these factors all have a positive correlation with increased VLDL and a negative correlation with HDL-C. In women, these are also correlated with higher LDL-C particularly after the menopause. In both sexes there is an increase in glucose intolerance with age (24,25), which may also account for body fat composition and distribution. These are all modifiable risk factors for CHD in the elderly.

Concurrent use of medications for coexisting medical conditions is more common in the elderly than in younger or middle-aged populations. Table 2 outlines disorders of other systems and drugs which may affect cholesterol and TG patterns. Varying changes in cholesterol and TG occur in renal disease at all ages (26), which may be separate risk factors from the renal disease or the accompanying hypertension. In one study serum creatinine, which decreases with age, correlated best with TG and LDL-C in women and negatively with serum HDL-C, suggesting that renal function *per se* may be an important modifier of lipoprotein levels in the elderly.

Other diseases (e.g. renal disease, systemic lupus erythematosus and myeloma) may also affect circulating lipid levels and predispose to an increased risk of ischaemic heart disease at any age (see Table 2).

Lipid disorders

It is useful to classify lipid disorders (see Table 3) in order to assign a treatment category. This is as helpful for the elderly as for younger age groups. However, primary genetic forms are very unlikely to occur in the elderly, except possibly heterozygotes interacting with age and other diseases or drugs. Polygenic causes of hyperlipidaemia are most likely to predispose to heart disease in the elderly.

The clinical significance of LDL is not as clear in old age as in the younger age groups (10,11). Recent reports indicate that males and females over 60 have a higher prevalence of serum cholesterol, and that high total cholesterol and LDL are good predictors of risk of CHD in patients > 60, but the predictive power may not be as accurate as in the younger age group because of the rising prevalence of competing diseases, atheroma and other risk factors.

Recent intervention studies suggest that screening of elderly subjects is viable and may reduce the risk of disabling CHD and cerebrovascular disease (27,28).

Table 3. The major primary dyslipoproteinaemias[a]

Hypercholesterolaemia
  Polygenic hypercholesterolaemia (IIa or IIb)
  Familial hypercholesterolaemia (IIa)
  Familial combined hyperlipidaemia (IIb)

Hypertriglyceridaemia
  Familial hypertriglyceridaemia (V or IV)
  Familial combined hyperlipidaemia (IV)
  Familial hyperchylomicronaemia (I)

Mixed hyperlipidaemia
  Familial combined hyperlipidaemia (IIb)
  Familial dysbetalipoproteinaemia (III)
  (remnant hyperlipidaemia)

---

[a]Corresponding Frederickson/WHO classification coding is
indicated in parentheses.

Lipid-lowering therapy in the elderly

The benefits of hyperlipidaemic therapy must outweigh possible side-effects in patients of any age but particularly in the elderly. The specific therapy for lowering LDL or TG should be used with care in the elderly since the benefits of a reduced cholesterol level, and efficacy/benefit for prolonging life or preventing further CHD in the elderly still needs to be evaluated by clinical trials. Side-effects may be commoner than in other age groups because of coexisting disease or therapy. Drug therapy for abnormal circulating lipoproteins must therefore be determined specifically for each patient, and education of each individual and assessment of compliance are the objectives of a good physician.

Diet

Lipid lowering in any patient must start with assessment and adjustment of dietary intake, in combination with the appropriate alteration in life-style for the age of the subject. This applies as much to the elderly as to any other patient. Attention should be paid to weight, exercise, alcohol and hypertension. Exercise advice should be modified since there may be less mobility in the elderly than in younger patients. The principle of dietary control of cholesterol is to restrict saturated fats and increase polyunsaturated and monounsaturated fats so as to reduce the flux through the chylomicron remnants and up-regulate apo-B/E receptors. This increases LDL clearance, reduces LDL concentration and down-regulates HMG CoA reductase. This can often be achieved through restriction of calorie intake and dietary changes.

For predominant hypertriglyceridaemia it is more appropriate to control weight with a low-carbohydrate, low-fat diet and reduce alcohol, and in the elderly there may be no need for any more specific therapy. However, it is important that diet must provide an elderly patient with adequate nutrition (e.g. calcium), since recent studies suggest that many elderly patients both in and out of hospital are malnourished (29). The balance must be determined by the physician considering each patient's needs. In some patients, it may be better to leave a higher saturated fat in the diet than is ideal, in order to avoid over-treating to reduce calories and producing risks of osteomalacia and bone problems (see 'Hormone replacement therapy', p. 449).

Pharmacological therapy

Available treatment has a wide repertoire and has been well reviewed (9,30).

Cholesterol-lowering therapy

With better understanding of lipids as risk factors for ischaemic heart disease, it is now becoming possible to define some therapy for specific defects in patients. In the elderly subject, however, these may be less clearly defined and the generic approach may be justified. It is clear that patients of any age undergoing interventional therapy for CHD (CABG surgery or angioplasty) should have their lipid status investigated and treated as appropriate with medication as well as diet just as for patients of younger age range, although possibly with reduced drug doses.

Bile acids sequestrants (Colestipol, Cholestyramine)

These are considered by some to be the drugs of first choice in the elderly since they are not absorbed, but act in the intestine, interfering with the absorption and reabsorption of cholesterol and bile acids, eventually leading to uptake of LDL-C and up-regulating LDL-C receptors. Cholestyramine may reduce the total cholesterol by 11–25% (2). This information comes from studies carried out in middle-aged men and these resins may not be so efficient in the > 65-year-old. Lower doses (4–5 g twice daily) should be used in the first instance in the elderly patient and only increased if the patient tolerates the drug but does not show a good cholesterol-lowering response. Such low-dose regimens can be expected to reduce cholesterol by up to 0.65–1.15 mmol/l, whilst high doses (8–10 g/twice daily) can reduce cholesterol by up to 30% l/l (2,31). Possible side-effects have been summarized in Table 4. Constipation may prevent use of these drugs in some elderly subjects. In addition, compliance may be more difficult to achieve in the elderly, who may be taking other medications. Thus the theory of not taking other medications within an hour before taking resins or 4 hours after taking them may be impractical.

Table 4. Drug treatment of hypercholesterolaemia

Drug	Effect	Potency	Comments
Bile acid sequestrants Colestipol Cholestyramine	LDL reduction	+ + + +	Most effective when taken before food. Side-effects of dyspepsia and flatulence less problematic if introduced slowly. *Good features*: safety well established; systemic side-effects rare. *Adverse effects*: may block absorption of other drugs; may cause reciprocal increase in VLDL
Fibrate drugs Bezafibrate Gemfibrozil Fenofibrate Ciprofibrate	LDL reduction	+ + +	Best taken after food. *Good features*: generally safe and well tolerated; HDL-C increased. *Adverse effects*: occasional dyspepsia, reversible myositis, impotence, lens opacities. Reduce dose in renal failure
Nicotinic acid drugs Nicotinic acid Acipimox Nicofuranose	LDL reduction	+ + +	Best taken after food to avoid major problems of pruritus and flushing seen with parent compound; derivatives less troublesome. Aspirin premedication may control symptoms. *Good features*: generally safe; HDL-C increased. *Adverse features*: occasional dyspepsia, urticaria, gout and changes in liver enzymes
HMG CoA reductase inhibitors Simvastatin Pravastatin	LDL reduction	+ + + + +	Best taken in evening. Rare incidence of myopathy increased considerably when combined with cyclosporin, fibrates and possibly nicotinic acid drugs. *Good features*: effective and convenient. *Adverse features*: occasional dyspepsia, rash, headache and changes in liver enzymes, reversible myositis, sleep disturbance; full safety profile not yet establibshed. Potentiates action of warfarin

HMG CoA reductase inhibitors

The statins are known to be effective in treating both pure and combined hypercholesterolaemia and should be used to treat hypercholesterolaemia only if severe in elderly patients, although some patients will have been taking this medication since a younger age and should continue to do so. All reviews confirm the efficiency of this class of drug which reduces LDL-C (by reducing synthesis) and VLDL-C by promoting clearance from circulation. An increase in HDL has been reported, but the significance of this in the elderly patient is uncertain. To date there is no reported primary or secondary trial of statins in the elderly. All information comes from studies of middle-aged patients (30,32) where LDL is reduced by 25–40%.

There are a number of drug side-effects which may be more important in elderly patients than in younger age groups. Symptoms such as myalgia/myositis with increased serum creatine kinase and much rarer myopathy syndrome may occur with associated muscle weakness, myoglobinuria and rarely renal failure (33). This is more common in females than males and must be looked for carefully in elderly patients with incipient renal failure. These side-effects are dose-related and reversible on discontinuing treatment. Other side-effects include sleep disturbance, which may be important in the elderly, exacerbation of predisposed depression and non-accidental death (34). Statins should therefore be reserved for use in elderly patients with severe hypercholesterolaemia undergoing therapy for CHD, with careful monitoring and in low dose.

Triglyceride-lowering therapy

Fibric acid derivatives

These are effective in treating hypertriglyceridaemia and combined hypertriglyceridaemia. They can also be used in combined hypercholesterolaemic conditions because they moderately reduce LDL-C and increase HDL concentration (35). Fibrates are particularly useful when increased circulating TG are risk factors for pancreatitis. VLDL are very atherogenic in some individuals, particularly the elderly, where they interact with other risk factors (e.g. diabetes). Thus there may be less indication for drug treatment of TG in the elderly except where VLDL levels are markedly elevated. The European Atherosclerosis Guidelines have suggested treatment levels but these may be adhered to less rigidly in the elderly subject (16). Actions and side-effects of fibrates are summarized in Table 5.

Gemfibrozil was used in the Helsinki Heart Study (3), with reduction of CHD and deaths from non-fatal myocardial infarction, but associated with a number of unexplained side-effects and causing a reduction in HDL. It is usually given in a dose of up to 600 mg twice daily and may reduce LDL-C by 0.5–0.8 mmol/l. Possible side-effects are outlined in Table 4 but, as for the fibrates, gallstones are the most important side-effect since surgery (even with minimally invasive

Table 5. Drug treatment of hypertriglyceridaemia

Drug	Effect	Potency	Comments
Fibrate drugs Bezafibrate Gemfibrozil Ciprofibrate Fenofibrate	VLDL reduction	+++	See general notes in Appendix 1. Tends to correct low HDL commonly associated with hypertriglyceridaemia
Nicotinic acid drugs Nicotinic acid Acipimox Nicofuranose	VLDL reduction	+++	See general notes in Appendix 1. Tends to correct low HDL commonly associated with hypertriglyceridaemia
Omega-3-fatty acids Maxepa	VLDL reduction	+++++	Good features: may lessen risk of thrombosis. *Adverse features:* long-term safety not established; reciprocal LDL increase with standard dosage; relatively expensive

endoscopy) has an increased risk in the elderly. Cataracts are also a potentially important side-effect of all fibrates and need to be looked for in all patients given this therapy. This is therefore not the drug of choice in elderly patients.

Nicotinic acid

Nicotinic acid reduces hepatic synthesis of TG and LDL-C and raises HDL-C and therefore is effective in treating combined hypercholesterolaemia and combined hypertriglyceridaemia. Data are available for secondary prevention of coronary heart disease by nicotinic acid (36), from the Coronary Drug Project, where it reduced second heart attacks in patients with CHD and in long-term follow-up prolonged life-span (37). Since this drug increases HDL, the strongest lipid predictor for CHD in the elderly, it would seem to be the drug of choice for mixed hyperlipidaemia in this group.

Low doses (100 mg per day) should be used initially and given with the evening meal, and increased slowly to a maximum of 3 g per day with careful monitoring of liver tests and lipoprotein profile over 4–6 weeks. Existing studies suggest that reduction of cholesterol could be of the order of 0.5–0.8 mmol/l (90) and with high doses 0.8–1.05 mmol/l. There is a high frequency of side-effects (see Table 5) but flushing may be the most important in elderly patients (which may be averted in some patients by prior use of low-dose aspirin). Dryness of eyes and mouth, indigestion and constipation are also likely to be more prominent in the elderly, and nicotinic acid may induce diabetes. Careful monitoring of liver tests and symptoms is needed if this drug is used in the elderly since hepatotoxicity has been reported. Review of the literature suggests that two-thirds of elderly patients tolerate nicotinic acid well (9).

Combination therapy

There is no doubt that combined use of agents such as statins and resins are effective in reducing and ameliorating lipoprotein profiles. This has been used in younger patients to control familial hypercholesterolaemia and familial combined hypercholesterolaemia. In general this will not be as necessary in elderly patients unless there is a failure to respond to simple therapy particularly in patients who have had interventional therapy for their cardiac state, or when the patient has commenced combination therapy at a younger age. Side-effects may be more prominent with combination therapy and need to be monitored closely in all patients.

Other therapy may need to be considered for control of non-lipid risk factors, such as aspirin for reducing the likelihood of thrombosis, and agents such as vitamins E and C that may reduce oxidized LDL and peroxidation, which may otherwise exacerbate atheroma.

Hormone replacement therapy

After the menopause the risk of CHD increases markedly in females and approaches the incidence in males, but interestingly does not overtake it (38). Serum cholesterol increases up to the seventh decade and so approaches that for males, where serum cholesterol appears to plateau at the fifth decade. Approximately 30% of women (age 55–64) may have serum cholesterol levels > 7.8 mmol/l.

Since cardiovascular disease is rare in women before the menopause, oestrogen is believed to be protective in women. Clinical trials suggest that the taking of unopposed oestrogen by postmenopausal women has a beneficial effect on serum lipids and reduced both total and cardiovascular mortality (39). Since addition of progestins to reduce the possibility of endometrial carcinoma, in non-hysterectomized women, it has been suggested that combined oestrogen–progestin regimens do not show benefits of cardiovascular disease protection (40).

Whom to treat and whether to treat

There is now overwhelming evidence that increased circulating cholesterol in the elderly contributes to the high prevalence of CHD, even taking into account that atherosclerosis is a natural ageing process. Postmenopausal females are equally at risk as men in the same age group and treatment should be reserved for those who have already been taking lipid-lowering therapy from younger ages and for those who have undergone interventional therapy for CHD. EAS guidelines suggest low thresholds for treatment in the elderly, but the basis of any therapeutic regimen should also be diet, which should be used in the first 6 months before addition of any therapy. There are clearly elderly patients who are at increased risk of CHD who should be treated but these diminish as age increases.

However, physicians should also have courage enough to decide when not to treat the elderly as well as when to treat. Side-effects must be taken into account and, for the healthy elderly patient or patient with significant disease in other systems, this may result in using diet alone particularly if the LDL-C is only just outside the normal range. Thus drug treatment for cholesterol lowering must be predominantly for secondary and is rarely used for primary prevention. With LDL-C > 5 mmol/l it may be necessary to take into account the presence of other disease and drug interactions before commencing therapy as recommended by the EAS guidelines for younger people.

Conclusion

Treatment of hyperlipidaemia in patients over 65 has been a controversial issue, but there is increasing evidence that the relationship of lipid risk and the response to lipid lowering in the elderly is the same as for those between 35 and 55. Treatment should be used in elderly patients who have had interventional therapy for CHD and should be continued in patients who have had lipid-lowering therapy from younger age because of personal and familial risks. However, the dose should be reduced in the elderly.

The question of cost-effectiveness of lowering cholesterol in the older age group is as yet unanswered. Females outnumber males in the older individuals with high cholesterol levels and yet are thought to have a lower risk of CHD even after the menopause. If all elderly individuals were to be prescribed hypo-lipidaemic therapy this would result in a significant rise in the nation's health care costs.

The role of other factors such as oxidized LDL, lipoprotein (a) and thrombogenesis is still unanswered in the elderly. Low-dose aspirin is effective at all ages and also good prophylaxis in the prevention of stroke and cerebrovascular disease.

Finally, the question of hypocholesterolaemia needs to be addressed. The significance of hypocholesterolaemia from epidemiological studies is still uncertain. Elderly Scandinavian subjects treated in a 10-year study with an initial cholesterol level of > 7.0 mmol/l showed that low cholesterol levels predicted an excess risk of cancer and were associated with haemorrhagic stroke (41). Until this matter is clarified by prospective epidemiological studies in the elderly, it is uncertain whether aggressive therapy for lowering lipids in the elderly is always justified because it might produce unfavourable risk factor profiles.

IMPAIRED GLUCOSE TOLERANCE AND DIABETES MELLITUS IN THE ELDERLY

Introduction

Following the introduction of insulin in 1922 death rates in younger diabetics fell (42), but subsequently macrovascular disease increasingly contributed to mortality (43–45). CHD causes considerable morbidity and is the commonest cause of death in diabetic subjects, and in addition peripheral and cerebrovascular disease is considerably increased (43,46,47). In the USA 33% of all individuals will die of atherosclerosis, but 75% of diabetics (48) will do so, with over 50% dying of CHD.

Microvascular disease in diabetes, and arterial medial sclerosis and calcification, may coexist with macrovascular disease, which is similar in diabetics and non-diabetics (44). Macrovascular disease is not confined to a particular type of diabetes (50), while duration of diabetes and its control are only partly related to CHD occurrence.

Increased CHD risk occurs with impaired glucose tolerance (IGT) as well as in overt diabetes (47), shown both in prospective studies of those with IGT and non-insulin-dependent diabetes mellitus (NIDDM) (51–53), and in those with insulin-dependent diabetes mellitus (IDDM) from 10 to 15 years after diabetes onset (54).

Prevalence of diabetes mellitus in the elderly

Prevalence of known diabetes mellitus in all age groups in the UK is 1.0–1.3% (55), approximately 30% of whom are taking insulin (not all with IDDM). In California (56), by WHO criteria 14.7% of 997 men and 11.3% of 1243 women aged 50–89 years have diabetes. Prevalence was lower when based on fasting hyperglycaemia (5% and 2.2%) or on diabetes history (5.7% and 3.1%) for males and females respectively). Prevalence increased systematically with age ($p < 0.001$) and was more common in men up to the age of 80 years, above which 19.7% of men and 22.6% of women had diabetes (only 0.3% of this elderly population having IDDM) (56). In the 65–74-year-old population in the NHANES II study (57), diabetes prevalence was higher than in the California study (56) in men (19.1% versus 11.9%) and women (17.0% versus 12.9%), as it also was in Mexican Americans (58) and Hispanics (59). Rural Italians aged > 60 years (60) had a prevalence of 12.6% (males) and 18.1% (females), while rates in Western Australia (61) were lower in those aged 65–74 years (6.5% and 8.6%), but rose (18.9% and 11.8%, respectively) in those aged > 75 years. Similar rates are seen in Japan (62), where prevalence of diabetes in the age range 45 to > 75 years was about 12%, and of IGT was about 16%.

The prevalence of IGT increases less steeply with age (1.5-fold per decade) (63–64) than does NIDDM prevalence (56,63–65). The true increase in NIDDM and IGT risk with age is likely to be higher, because prevalence studies underestimate risk more at older than at younger ages due to selective survival (66).

Diabetes in the elderly, associated factors and cardiovascular risk

Glucose tolerance deteriorates with ageing (67), fasting and 2-hour glucose increasing by 0.06 and 0.05 mmol/l, respectively, each decade after age 50 years (67,68). NIDDM and IGT risk prevalences doubled when BMI was >27 (men) or >25 kg/m (women), and tripled with central adiposity and family history (65.4%:24.1% (men); 52.8%:19.6% (women)) in 1300 subjects aged 65–74 years (69), but these three factors explained only 10% of the variance in 2-hour glucose values.

Finnish elderly subjects ($n = 1431$; 65–74 years) with NIDDM or IGT were more obese, had higher waist:hip ratio, and were more hypertensive than normal individuals, as well as having higher triglycerides and apolipoprotein B, and lower HDL-C and apo-A$_1$ (70). These hyperglycaemic men had 1.5-fold more angina pectoris and ECG changes than normoglycaemic men, and the women also had more frequent ischaemic ECGs, suggesting that asymptomatic hyper-glycaemia in the elderly is not benign (71). That elderly males in this study (71) had more CHD than females is in contrast to general findings in NIDDM (72,73). Previous cross-sectional (74) and prospective (75,76) studies in diabetes compared to controls have shown middle-aged diabetic women to have a greater relative risk than men.

Coronary heart disease mortality in diabetes

Assessment of relative CHD risk in diabetes is imprecise due to selection bias in population comparisons, high CHD prevalence and incidence in general or non-diabetic populations, as well as variations in rigour of diabetes diagnosis. This is particularly so in the elderly, where asymptomatic and undiagnosed diabetes is frequent. Even where diabetes has been diagnosed, death certification is unreliable, severely under-reporting diabetes (43–45,77,78). Ochi et al. (78) found the rate of reporting diabetes as cause of death to be 8.5 (per 100 000 patient-years), but 31.5 for diabetes as a contributory or underlying cause, and 82.7 if all deaths in diabetics were counted. In a follow-up of 5971 known British Diabetic Association members, diabetes was omitted in one-third of 2134 death certificates (77).

In Birmingham (UK), diabetics (largely NIDDM) aged over 40 years showed a 1.59-fold excess of circulatory disease deaths in 2278 males, and a 1.81-fold excess in 3727 females. The latter showed increasing mortality with longer diabetes duration. The risk increased with concurrent hypertension in both genders (79).

In Oslo (46), 3832 diabetics, newly identified in 1925–1955 and traced to 1965, showed all-cause mortality ratios of 2.92 for males and 2.82 for females, and of

3.87 and 3.62, respectively, for CHD mortality. Males in Oslo reaching age 70 or more had a mortality ratio of 2.4 compared to the general population, while the ratio was 4.3 for those failing to reach 70 years. (Female ratios were 2.8 and 8.6, respectively.) Thus relative risk and CHD risk attributable to diabetes were less in older individuals. However, both CHD rates and diabetes prevalence increase with age, so that CHD events become increasingly common. A retrospective study in Warsaw (80) of 5261 diabetics aged 30–68 years at diagnosis showed ratios for overall mortality of 1.31- and 1.27-fold for males and females, for cerebrovascular disease of 2.95- and 1.47-fold, and for CHD of 1.95- and 1.75-fold, respectively. Data from the Steno Memorial Hospital, Denmark, looked at long-term survival of diabetics diagnosed prior to 1933 at or below age 30 years (81). Forty per cent were alive, and all-cause mortality was two to six times higher in the (by now) elderly population compared to controls, in a ratio of 50% to 10%. Diabetics diagnosed before age 10 years had a worse prognosis than those diagnosed at age 21–30 years. Diabetic females survived longer than men, not entirely accounted for by the better prognosis of women in general, and despite a tendency to have an increased risk ratio compared to men in many studies of diabetes.

Of a cohort of 2560 East German diabetics diagnosed in 1966, 1054 had died by 1976—63% from cardiovascular causes (82). Ratios of excess mortality, largely from CHD, which ranged from 2.0 to 1.1, decreased with age. This decline in relative mortality with advancing age has been shown elsewhere (44–46,79).

Extensive long-term follow-up data from the Joslin Clinic in Boston, USA, from before insulin therapy into the 1970s (44,45), showed changes in mortality causes. Mortality ratios by age and gender are shown in Table 6 (83). Age of onset of diabetes had different relationships to microvascular and macrovascular disease. Microvascular problems were increased in younger patients. Macrovascular disease was increased at diabetes onset above age 20 years (Table 7) (45,84) accounting for 70% of all deaths, with over 50% from CHD. Frequency of CHD death increased with diabetes duration for those with onset at <40 years, but in

Table 6. Mortality of Joslin Clinic diabetics, and general population. Mortality of diabetics originally seen 1950–1958 and followed to 1 January 1961 (58)

Age at onset (years)	Males		Females	
	Deaths per 1000	Ratio	Deaths per 1000	Ratio
<24	3.2[a]	3.1	0.8[a]	2.0
25–34	10.3[a]	7.4	15.3	13.9
35–44	16.1	4.4	10.4[a]	4.5
45–54	21.5	2.1	18.2	3.1
55–64	44.9	1.8	35.7	2.4
64–74	84.8	1.6	85.5	2.4

[a]Based on less than 20 deaths.

Table 7. Vascular mortality (as percentage of total deaths) in 9214 Joslin Clinic diabetics dying between 1956 and 1958 (2,252)

| | Age at onset (years) | | | | | | | |
| | Males | | | | Females | | | |
Cause of death	<20	20–39	40–59	60+	<20	20–39	40–59	60+
Cardiovascular–renal	80	79	75	73	75	76	78	76
Macrovascular	32	62	71	70	32	62	73	73
Cardiac	26	53	57	52	25	53	56	51
Cerebral	5	7	11	13	6	7	14	18
Other vascular	1	2	3	5	1	2	3	4
Microvascular	48	17	4	2	43	14	6	3
Nephopathy	41	13	2	0	38	7	3	1
Other renal	6	5	2	2	6	7	3	2

older patients there was no evidence of increasing risk with prolonged diabetes duration despite increased CHD rates in the elderly.

Expectation of life can be estimated from Joslin Clinic data for diabetic compared to non-diabetic populations. As these data reflect diabetes care and experience in the 1950s to 1960s, it may be that relative prognosis in diabetes will have improved. None the less, Figure 2 demonstrates a 30% reduction in life expectancy at any age of diabetes onset, including the elderly (45,84).

A further problem related to the increasing prevalence of diabetes in the elderly is that the prevalence of undiagnosed diabetes and of IGT also increase. It is estimated that the onset of IDDM was at least 4–7 years, and perhaps 9–12 years, before clinical diagnosis (85), so that initial presentation is with microvascular or macrovascular complications of diabetes rather than with diabetes itself. Preclinical diabetes has equal prevalence to clinical diabetes. This raises many public health issues (86), since addition of diabetes may increase the CHD risk to an individual. Thus greater attention needs to be given not only to diabetes control but also to other CHD risk factors (dietary and pharmacological treatment, life-style and behavioural changes).

Age-related glucose intolerance

Development of IGT with age was found in 1920 in people over 60 years (87). While no or little deterioration in fasting blood glucose (0.0–0.1 mmol/l per decade) occurs with ageing (88), the blood glucose 1–2 hours after a glucose load rises by 0.33–0.71 mmol/l per decade, women being 0.5 mmol/l higher than men (88). Age-related deterioration in glucose intolerance is distinct from NIDDM and obesity (88), with impairment of insulin secretion and especially insulin action. The latter results in delayed postprandial hepatic glucose output and

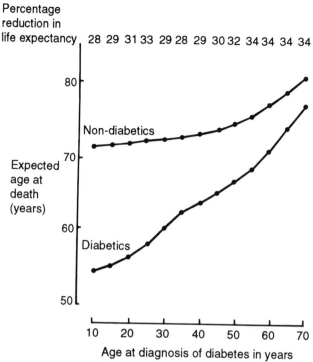

Figure 2. Expectation of life in diabetics and non-diabetics. For different attained ages the expected ages at death are shown for diabetics and for the general population. The relative reduction in life expectancy is shown as a percentage. Thus at any age a person developing diabetes has a life expectancy one-third less than a non-diabetic of a similar age. Values for older ages are likely to be fairly accurate, but for younger ages less so. Diabetic data exclude deaths within 1 week of first observation or hospital discharge. Data from Marks and Krall (45)

peripheral glucose disposal. The principal postreceptor defect is decreased glucose transport secondary to a reduced number of membrane glucose transporters. Jackson (88) suggests that in most elderly subjects delayed initial insulin secretion, changes in body composition (reduced muscle mass, obesity), decreased physical activity, changes in diet and raised free fatty acid levels probably play no significant role in predisposing to age-related glucose intolerance.

Pathological mechanisms linking diabetes and atherosclerosis

Atheroma and diabetes

Cerebrovascular disease, peripheral vascular disease and CHD, common in the elderly, are more common in those with diabetes. Atheroma may be an ageing process but age of occurrence of clinical events will reflect predisposing risk factors, such as cigarette smoking, hypertension and lipoprotein abnormalities. High levels of insulin (89) and fibrinogen (90) have also been implicated. However, even allowing for these, diabetes remains a risk factor *per se*. While attributable risk for CHD, from hypercholesterolaemia for example, becomes somewhat less strong with advancing age, many of these risk factors become more common with advancing age (91), so that the contribution of any one factor to atherosclerotic event risk will increase. In the elderly, average cholesterol and triglyceride levels may be a little lower, but may reflect other changes (e.g. weight), or may reflect differential mortality and selective culling of high-risk individuals from the population (92).

Atherosclerosis risk may also be linked to age-related changes in the arterial wall, affecting fibroblasts, endothelial cells and smooth muscle cells (89). Cell proliferation and injury repair may be impaired, ability to catabolize LDL may be reduced, and platelet changes may favour a hypercoagulable state.

Macrovascular disease is similar in non-diabetic, IDDM and NIDDM populations (49,50), and is not directly related to levels of glycaemia achieved or the treatment used to achieve diabetic control (49,50). The common risk factors (hypercholesterolaemia, hypertension and cigarette smoking) have the same relationship to CHD in diabetic and non-diabetic populations (93), and do not explain the increased risk (94). Prevalences of diabetes and atherosclerosis increase with age, but diabetes predisposes to accelerated premature atheroma (50) which may progress more rapidly after first clinical appearance. As in the non-diabetic population, the excess atheroma risk diminishes but does not disappear in elderly diabetic subjects (92). HDL levels, inversely related to cardiovascular disease, fall slightly with advancing age (95); they are low in NIDDM or in insulin-treated NIDDM but higher in IDDM with satisfactory control (96). It is clear that other changes may affect lipoproteins and their metabolism, and account for some of the increased CHD risk in diabetes, which cannot be explained by other known CHD risk factors (see pp. 456 below and 10).

Diabetes, hypertension and atheroma

Hypertension prevalence increases as glucose intolerance deteriorates from normal, through IGT and undiagnosed diabetes, to diagnosed diabetes (97), augmenting the diabetes morbidity from stroke, cerebral haemorrhage and CHD. Advancing age increases blood pressure in diabetes (98), contributing to CHD morbidity and mortality. Systolic hypertension has been underrated as a CHD and stroke risk factor (49), yet can be safely treated in the elderly (99), although evidence that this intervention will reduce vascular disease is not yet available.

Lipids, diabetes and atheroma

A similar association occurs between lipoprotein abnormalities and CHD in diabetes and control populations. Diabetics with CHD tend to have higher

Table 8. Disturbances in lipoprotein metabolism in diabetes

Alteration in metabolisms	Lipoprotein effects
↓ Lipoprotein lipase (LPL)	↑ Chylomicron and VLDL remnants[a]
	↑ Triglycerides
	↓ HDL
	Altered composition
↓ Hepatic lipase (HL)	↑ Remnant particles[a]
	↓ HDL
↓ Lecithin cholesterol acyltransferase (LCAT)	Altered composition
↓ Cholesteryl ester transfer protein (CETP)	Altered composition
↓ LDL receptor activity	↑ LDL
↑ VLDL synthesis/secretion	↑ Triglycerides
↑ Lipoprotein glycosylation	↑ LDL?
	↑ Scavenger pathway removal
↑ Oxidation of LDL	↑ LDL
	↑ Macrophage uptake

Adapted from Roelfsema and Frolich (151).
[a]If severe.

plasma TG levels, lower HDL cholesterol, and normal or slightly higher LDL cholesterol, than do diabetics without CHD (100). Hypertriglyceridaemia of diabetes is linked to glycaemic control, but even when controlled some patients with NIDDM have persistent moderate TG increases with lower HDL cholesterol levels (101). This atherogenic profile only partly explains excess CHD risk (72,73,93).

Various disturbances in lipid metabolism have been reported in diabetes (Table 8) (102). Increased hepatic TG synthesis and secretion of VLDL-TG and VLDL-apo B (103) have been noted in NIDDM patients with moderate hypertriglyceridaemia. Clearance of chylomicrons, VLDL and remnant particles may be impaired in elderly NIDDM patients, as the enzyme lipoprotein lipase (LPL) is insulin-dependent, leading to remnant particle accumulation and hypertriglyceridaemia (104). Classical diabetic lipaemia occurs because of decreased clearance of TG-rich lipoproteins. This results in impaired provision of their surface components to HDL, and lower HDL concentrations (105), while VLDL particles themselves are larger and more triglyceride-rich (106). Remnants may accumulate with impaired activity of hepatic lipase, an insulin-sensitive enzyme (107).

VLDL remnants, removed by the liver or metabolized to LDL, also provide cholesterol to peripheral tissues. Insulin deficiency/resistance may reduce LDL clearance by impairing LDL receptor binding and uptake (108). Non-enzymatic glycation of proteins occurs at higher rates in diabetic subjects, especially if poorly controlled. Thus apo-B, the structural protein of VLDL and LDL, is glycated (86,109), and glycated LDL is less readily recognized by the LDL receptor (109). In elderly NIDDM subjects, glycation of arterial subintimal glycosoaminoglycans and collagen may trap LDL, predisposing to oxidation and increased removal by the arterial wall macrophages (20), potentially enhancing atherogenesis (110).

Qualitative lipoprotein changes in diabetes and atheroma

Qualitative changes in lipoprotein structure and composition may affect CHD risk. Thus small, dense LDL particles are more atherogenic, with higher CHD risk (111–113). Such LDL particles (pattern B LDL subclass) may be determined by elevated serum TG levels (114,115). In hypertriglyceridaemic individuals the concentration of LDL-C may be reduced and, paradoxically, may rise as plasma TG responds to treatment (115,166). Such changes are frequent in hypertrig-lyceridaemic diabetic subjects (101,117,118).

James and Pometta (117) showed that improved metabolic control of diabetic subjects reduced the concentration of pattern B LDL particles, correcting density distribution towards a normal LDL pattern A. Alteration towards a more normal, less atherogenic, LDL is associated with restoration of LDL-C:TG ratio, with reduction in serum VLDL-TG and higher HDL-C levels (115,117–119). This may reflect reduced plasma residence time of VLDL, reduced transfer of lipids between TG-rich and cholesterol-rich lipoproteins, reduced CETP activity, and more normal transfer of surface VLDL components to HDL during catabolism. Increased secretion and size of VLDL particles occurring in NIDDM improve with glycaemic control (120).

These alterations in VLDL, LDL and HDL composition have been identified as an atherogenic lipoprotein phenotype and proposed as a genetic marker for premature CHD (111–113). Treatment of hypertriglyceridaemia, with or without concomitant diabetes, by weight loss, diet or fibrate drugs as described previously (114–116, 121) tends to improve the profile. With increasing prevalence of diabetes and CHD with age, these findings have particular relevance in the elderly NIDDM patients. In younger, non-diabetic, mainly male populations, two-thirds of anticipated benefit is evident often within 2 years of initiation of hypolipidaemia treatment. Currently, little evidence of effects of therapy is available from primary intervention studies of diabetic, female or elderly populations. Some data, from the Helsinki Heart Study (3,122), have implications for diabetes since 135 of the 4081 men (40–55 years old at entry) studied for 5 years had NIDDM. These had lower HDL cholesterol, higher TG, higher BMI and more hypertension ($p < 0.001$) than control subjects. Incidence of myocardial infarct and cardiac death was twice as high in the diabetics (7.4%:3.3%), while CHD incidence in the gemfibrozil group was 3.4%, compared to 10.5% in the placebo-treated group. In multivariate analyses, diabetes, age, smoking, low HDL-C and high LDL-C were independently related to CHD incidence (3,122). Careful, sensible extrapolation of currently available data suggests that attention to CHD risk factors is appropriate particularly to high-risk NIDDM elderly populations.

Glycaemic control, hyperlipidaemia and CHD

The relationship between glycaemic control and diabetic complications is not clear (123), and indeed glycaemia may not necessarily be the correct measure of diabetic metabolic control. A quarter of individuals with diabetes do not develop complications, and this is independent of diabetic control (51). It may be that there is a genetic predisposition to complications, as evidenced by studies of HLA status, capillary basement change, familial clustering of complications (124) and predisposition to hypertension. However, clinical trials provide some evidence that early retinopathy, microalbuminuria and nerve conduction may improve with near normoglycaemia, as do the lipoprotein abnormalities (125). Such improvements do have a potential cost to the patient in terms of treatment requirements, interference with daily living and risks of and from hypoglycaemia (123,126).

Most but not all studies (127) have failed to show that CHD should increase with diabetes duration (133), suggesting that glycaemia and diabetes mellitus directly cause CHD. Relative risk ratios for CHD are increased in those with diabetes, both known or newly diagnosed, and with IGT (128), but not especially in the elderly. Blood glucose levels in the upper 5% of the general population distribution are associated with excess CHD risk (75,127,129,130).

The recently reported Diabetes Control and Complications Trial (DCCT) showed highly significant reductions in microvascular complications in an intensively treated group, compared to a conventionally treated group of young insulin-dependent diabetic patients. The macrovascular disease event rate was also 42% lower, albeit non-significantly reduced because of the lower overall event rate in this young population (176).

Insulin resistance, diabetes and coronary heart disease

Insulin resistance is an important association between CHD risk and glucose intolerance in the elderly, linked also with hyperlipidaemia (especially high plasma TG and low HDL-C), hypertension, gout, hyperuricaemia and central obesity (127,131). In two groups of obese diabetic patients closely matched for age, glucose intolerance and indices of obesity, the group with hypertriglyceridaemia had an increased TG content of abdominal adipocytes (fat cell size) and raised fasting plasma insulin (132), which correlated best with adipocyte TG, suggesting a link between insulin resistance and central adiposity (132). Insulin may promote atherosclerosis directly, and in some epidemiological studies (128,129,138) hyperinsulinaemia was predictive for subsequent CHD in men, but not in women (133). The relationship of fasting insulin to CHD has also been found in NIDDM patients (100,134), but in the Bedford study development of CHD was higher in people with IGT and lower plasma insulin (75), which may reflect depletion of pancreatic islet β cell function with longer duration of glucose intolerance, or may be confounded by secretion of split proinsulin in NIDDM (135)—aspects which are important to consider in the elderly.

If insulin resistance and resulting hyperinsulinaemia appear before NIDDM and CHD, any relationship of duration of NIDDM with CHD risk will weaken. The relative protection of non-diabetic females from CHD may relate to increased insulin sensitivity compared to men, protection being lost when IGT or NIDDM develops (136), particularly in the elderly patient with NIDDM.

Treatment aspects in the elderly

Initial management of the elderly person with IGT and NIDDM is of life-style and environmental factors, since hyperinsulinaemia is associated with atherogenic risk factors in prediabetic patients, and increases CHD risk. Weight loss and exercise improve insulin sensitivity and reduce both diabetes and CHD (137). In many individuals hypertriglyceridaemia and associated lipoprotein abnormalities respond to control of glucose metabolism and to weight loss, obesity exacerbating any genetic predisposition to hyperlipidaemia. Excess alcohol intake may contribute to hyperlipidaemia, as may other secondary causes such as hypothyroidism, or concurrent drug treatments (e.g. β-blockers or thiazides for hypertension). In such individuals, hypertension treatment with agents not negatively affecting lipid metabolism (e.g. angiotensin-converting enzyme inhibitors, calcium channel antagonists or α-blockers) may be preferable, although large long-term intervention studies to show morbidity and mortality benefit have not been undertaken in elderly diabetic subjects.

Where diet and life-style measures in the elderly NIDDM patients are insufficient, diabetic control should be improved with oral hypoglycaemic agents, and in a proportion with insulin therapy. A small number of IGT/NIDDM subjects with markedly abnormal hypertriglyceridaemia may require insulin therapy because of severity of hypertriglyceridaemia and the pancreatitis risk, rather than for poor glycaemic control.

Where NIDDM subjects have continued hyperlipidaemia after diet, especially where HDL levels are low, where there are other CHD risk factors, where there is a poor family history for CHD or where the individual already has CHD, the lipaemia should be treated (see pp. 445–9) appropriately.

ACROMEGALY

Introduction

Acromegaly is due to growth hormone overproduction usually of pituitary origin, with morbidity and mortality related to local effects of the tumour and systemic effects of the excess hormone production. While acromegaly is mainly a disorder of middle age, it affects the patient over decades. The long-term vascular morbidity is usually late in the natural history of the disease and will often present in the elderly. The prevalence of acromegaly is about 50 per million, while the yearly incidence is around 304 per million (138).

Secretion of growth hormone in the elderly

With ageing the anterior pituitary gland undergoes patchy fibrosis, focal necrosis, vascular alterations, iron deposition, microadenoma formation and moderate size reduction (139). The reduction in protein synthesis and decrease in lean body mass usually seen with ageing suggest that secretion and/or action of growth hormone may be reduced in the elderly. In normal males over age 60 years growth hormone treatment can increase lean body mass (140). Basal and 24-hour integrated growth hormone levels are higher in females than males, and decrease with age (139,141). Mean pulse amplitude, duration and fraction of growth hormone secreted in pulses during 24 hours, but not the pulse frequency, decrease with age (141). Compatible with an age-related decrease in basal secretion, but not the action of growth hormone, are reductions in basal somatomedin secretion but unchanged sensitivity of somatomedin C (insulin-like growth factor 1) secretion in response to growth hormone (141).

Cardiovascular morbidity and mortality of acromegaly

The gradual onset of symptoms and signs in most individuals developing acromegaly results in a mean duration of disease estimated at 8.7 years in 885 patients from various series diagnosed at a mean age of 42 years (142). Epidemiological studies have shown increased mortality, partially ameliorated with therapy, although frequently this will have been only partly effective (138,142–144). Wright's study (144), with 54 deaths in 194 patients, showed twice the expected death rates, primarily from cardiovascular and cerebrovascular disease, with death rates higher in those with hypertension or diabetes. Alexander (138) showed 4.8-fold increased mortality in 70 men (significantly increased from malignancy, respiratory, cardiovascular and cerebrovascular diseases) and 2.4-fold in 94 women (significantly increased from cerebrovascular disease). Bengtsson (143) similarly showed significant increases in vascular and malignant disease.

One-third of acromegalic patients may present with cardiac disease (142,145,146). Echocardiography may demonstrate concentric left ventricular wall or asymmetrical septal hypertrophy and decreased ventricular ejection fraction, even without previous history of hypertension or other cause, but without a clear relationship to disease duration or severity of growth hormone elevation (142,145). Some improvement in muscle hypertrophy and dysfunction may follow effective acromegaly treatment (145). Symptomatic cardiac disease occurs in about a sixth of patients (142,145–147). Most cardiac disease in acromegaly appears to be associated with CHD or hypertension, although cardiomyopathy may occur with myocardial interstitial fibrosis and interstitial mononuclear infiltrate (145,147). Congestive cardiac failure may relate to CHD, hypertension or a cardiomyopathy, and may be easier to control following effective treatment of the acromegaly (146), due in part to a reduction in sodium retention seen in active acromegaly (148).

Hypertension is three- to fourfold more common in acromegaly (142,147,149), partly ameliorated by pituitary ablative treatment (149). Hypertension in acromegaly is associated with low renin and aldosterone, and sodium retention. Carbohydrate intolerance is present in up to half and diabetes mellitus in a fifth of acromegalics (142,144,147), the latter being associated with increased mortality (161). Effective treatment may result in resolution of diabetes in two-thirds of patients (147), and even treatment with octreotide, which can directly impair insulin secretion, can improve glucose tolerance as growth hormone is lowered (150). In acromegaly, fasting plasma insulin and insulin response to intravenous glucose are elevated, and the insulin resistance associated with growth hormone seems to be due to a postinsulin receptor defect (142). As in some other secondary causes of diabetes mellitus, the progression to IGT and NIDDM is associated with lower insulin levels than those with normal glucose intolerance, indicating that a progressive pancreatic islet β cell failure precedes the glucose intolerance. In a small number of acromegalic patients with NIDDM in whom growth hormone levels were normalized, abnormalities of insulin secretion persisted even though glucose tolerance returned to normal (151).

Acromegaly, coronary heart disease and the elderly

The cardiovascular and cerebrovascular disease associated with acromegaly may occur at initial presentation, but are linked to duration of untreated or inadequately treated acromegaly. Macrovascular disease, common in the elderly, is even more common in the elderly acromegalic, and at least partly attributable to the associated increased rates of hypertension and diabetes mellitus. Active and effective treatment of acromegalic patients at an early stage is indicated only to diagnose the subsequent possibility of hypopituitarism, but also to reduce the late vascular complications and accelerated mortality.

THYROID GLAND

Introduction

Although involutional changes and reduction in sensitivity of many organs occur with age, the thyroid gland is particularly important and has practical effects on the cardiovascular and peripheral vascular systems. Alteration in thyroid function may often be missed in the ageing individual until the later stages of the disease. Although not part of the ageing process, hypothyroidism is common in elderly patients, particularly females (152). Diagnosis may be more difficult to make than in a younger person because of the insidious onset and the presence of a 'subclinical' form.

Hypothalamic–pituitary function

With age, both animals and man have an associated reduction in hypothalamic concentration of neurotransmitters such as catecholamines, γ-aminobutyric acid and acetylcholine. Age is also associated with a decline in sensitivity of the hypothalamus to the concentration of hormones and metabolites. Thus high glucose concentrations are needed to inhibit and high corticoid activity is needed to suppress in the elderly.

One in 10 men over the age of 60 have high thyrotrophin (TSH) levels (153). These are normally associated with clinical hypothyroidism or biochemically low circulating thyroxine (T_4) levels, and vary with the health of the individual. In healthy elderly patients, standard thyrotrophin-releasing hormone (TRH) doses release normal TSH concentrations as for any other age, and TSH sensitivity of the pituitary does not change with age. However, in a recent study of subjects aged >60 years (154), high TSH levels were more common in women (11.6%) than in men (2.9%), and antithyroid antibodies were found in 60% of those with an increased TSH, only 5.8% of whom had subnormal TSH levels.

Thyroid gland

The size of the thyroid gland is unchanged overall with age but may reduce in weight on becoming fibrotic. Histological abnormalities include reduction in follicle size and in colloid content, and an increasing proportion of connective tissue with glandular epithelial atrophy.

Thyroid hormones and ageing

A number of physiological alterations occur with age. These include a reduction in basal metabolic rate (BMR) (an early measure of thyroid status), which is usually due to reduction in lean body mass. Thyroid radioactive iodine uptake and the absolute thyroid iodine uptake index both decrease progressively from age 50 to 90 (155). In association with this, production rates of both T_4 and triiodothyronine (T_3) are reduced by about 25–33%. Changes in the latter are due to a reduced availability of T_4 in peripheral tissues for deiodination. Reduction in T_3 production with age is not as well recognized but may be associated with illness and some age-related reduction in deiodination of T_4 and production of reverse T_3. Resin T_3 uptake (marker of serum thyroid hormone binding) and serum thyroid binding globulin (TBG) do not change with age.

Thyrotrophin

Basal serum TSH concentrations vary with age as compared with younger individuals, and are associated with a small increase, more usually seen in women. Sawin *et al.* (156) showed that 7.1% of females and 2.7% of elderly males had TSH levels of >10 iu/l. Fourteen per cent of all patients have TSH of >5 iu/l, but when those with positive antibodies were eliminated there was no increase in TSH with age alone. Sensitivity of the pituitary gland to changes in thyroid hormone concentrations, assessed by the TSH response to TRH, is reduced in elderly subjects; only 50% showed an augmented TSH response to TRH (157) more marked in men than women. This has led to the suggestion that normal serum TSH levels may not always be a reliable index of the euthyroid state in the elderly.

Thus alterations in thyroid physiology with age are primarily a reduced degradation of T_4 with maintenance of normal serum thyroid hormone concentration. Reduction in measured levels of thyroid hormones (T_4, T_3) alone should not be regarded as hypothyroidism.

Thyroid disease

Hypothyroidism

This is often missed in the elderly because the symptoms and signs of thyroid disease are masked. Thus all individuals showing gradual and recent deterioration, both mentally and physically, should be screened for hypothyroidism, but only when they have recovered from other acute illness. This is important since biochemical tests for thyroid function may be affected by acute illness. Since pituitary hypothyroidism is uncommon in the elderly, only primary hypothyroidism will be considered in this section.

Hypothyroidism has been well reviewed (158) and is more common in females than males, with an overall prevalence in the community of about 2% (157), but recent large surveys in the UK, Europe and the USA suggest a prevalence as high as 3.9%, with two-thirds remaining undiagnosed before admission to hospital or clinic.

Aetiology

The commonest cause of hypothyroidism is autoimmune thyroiditis. Postmortem studies show lymphocyte infiltration in 25% of the female thyroid gland. There is a wide range of antibodies which react positively to thyroglobulin or microsomes (159) and which are commoner in women. These autoimmune conditions vary from Hashimoto's disease to primary atrophy.

It is also apparent that variable T_3 changes occur with reduction in function in healthy patients with variable degradation, but the response of T_3 to TRH is normal. Reverse T_3 is unchanged in the elderly. Population studies (160) show that serum TSH is increased most often in those over 65 years old, where females predominate over males (10.7%:5.9%, respectively) whereas in younger age groups (e.g. less than 55) the gender ratio is more marked (10%:1.9%). Even when hypothyroidism has been diagnosed there is often a high frequency of failure to treat (152). In the Framingham study, thyroid hormone replacement was only found in 10% of women, of whom 19% were being treated inappropriately. However, 37% of these were definitely hypothyroid, with an elevated TSH greater than 10 iu/l despite thyroid therapy (155).

Hypothyroidism may occur following treatment for Graves' disease; overt hypothyroidism developed in 6–20% of patients who were initially euthyroid following thionamide (carbimazole or propylthiouracil) therapy—fewer than occurred with radiotherapy, radioiodine or surgery. The prevalence of anti-thyroid antibodies in those developing late hypothyroidism treated with drugs suggests that coexisting autoimmune thyroiditis may be the cause of the hypothyroidism. It is known that markers of autoimmune thyroiditis increase with age, especially in females. Patients may develop hypothyroidism secondary to thyroidectomy if subsequently unmonitored or secondary to radioactive iodine (^{131}I) therapy (161). The incidence is lower with partial thyroidectomy than with ^{131}I treatment, but 10 years post surgery up to 40% may be hypothyroid.

Natural history

Hypothyroidism progresses slowly from normal through mild to overt disease. Information comes from patients treated with ^{131}I for thyrotoxicosis, assessed on the basis of a reduced free T_4 index, increased basal TSH with normal free T_3 index, or abnormally enhanced TSH response to the TRH stimulation with normal basal TSH and free T_4 index. Mean corrected T_4 levels, unlike mean free T_4 index, were lower in treated patients with normal TSH response to TRH, or in control subjects. Thus normal T_4 levels in patients with a high basal TSH or with increased response of TSH to TRH suggest hypothyroidism. Similarly the frequency of antibodies is greater in the female than is the frequency of serum TSH increase. A number of studies evaluated presence of antibody as a means of detection or identifying those at risk of hypothyroidism (one-third of elderly patients with raised TSH levels do not have antithyroid antibodies, and only 5.7% of subjects per year become frankly hypothyroid) (160).

Clinical features

Clinical features of hypothyroidism in the elderly are summarized in Table 9. Hypothyroidism may have an insidious onset over many years. Initial features such as alopecia, dry skin, cold weather intolerance, constipation and mental changes could overlap with changes that could be also attributed to age. In one survey, no increased TSH levels in patients with clinical abnormalities were noted.

Chest pain may be present in 25% and dyspnoea may be present in more than 50% of patients (161). Enlargement of the heart also may occur due to

Table 9. Clinical features associated with hypothyroidism in the elderly

System	Clinical/laboratory feature
Cardiovascular	Bradycardia Heart failure Cardiomyopathy
Central nervous	Syncope, fits Deafness, dizziness Vertigo, tinnitus Carpal tunnel syndrome Slow reflexes Apathy Depression Myxoedema 'madness'
Haematological	Macrocytic anaemia
Metabolic	↑ Cholesterol ↑ Triglyceride

pericardial effusion or cardiomyopathy. In secondary hypothyroidism, which is rare, other features of hypopituitarism may be present (e.g. hypoadrenalism, hypogonadism and hypopigmentation).

Subclinical hypothyroidism
This term refers to subjects who are clinically normal, with a normal T_4 and T_3, often raised basal TSH levels and an increased TSH response to TRH. Epidemiological studies of thyroid disease in an English community found no association of subclinical hypothyroidism with lipid abnormalities and cardiovascular disease (162). Other studies looking for patients treated for subclinical hypothyroidism and seeking to detect improvement in cardiovascular disease and lipids noted some changes (163), which included the syndrome of premyxoedema of Fowler, where hypercholesterolaemia can be used as a diagnostic indicator of the syndrome. Two studies from Edinburgh showed that left ventricular ejection function on exercise assessed by radionuclide ventriculography was improved (158,163). In addition, changes in the cardiac output with treatment suggested that there is a true reduction in myocardial contractile activity, and both at rest and with exercise stroke volume was reduced in subclinical hypothyroidism (164).

Other systems may be affected; thus dementia and paranoia, with functional psychoses which occur with clinical hypothyroidism, may also occur in subclinical hypothyroidism, but the condition may only be confirmed by a TRH test. Overall there is only weak evidence for a causal relationship or association between subclinical hypothyroidism and neurotic depression.

Diagnosis

Although hypothyroidism may be diagnosed by clinical features which include a slow reaction phase of the ankle jerks, this can now be assessed more accurately by photomotography, when the ankle jerk is present. A recent study, however, suggests that there is no really effective scoring system for detecting hypothyroidism in the elderly (152). Two recent reports have defined the role of hypothyroidism in cardiovascular findings (158,165). The presence of hypothyroid cardiomyopathy was shown to be reversible by treatment and could be detected by echocardiography (165). A related diastolic hypertension was present in 1.2% of the referred population of patients. In the clinically apparently euthyroid patient, biochemical tests are essential for confirming the diagnosis of hypothyroidism.

It is important to remember in hospitalizing sick individuals that total T_4 and free T_4 index alter because of tissue catabolism and release of inhibitors of the thyroid hormone binding to thyroid-binding globulin. Similarly in recovery from acute illness, marked reduction of T_4 levels with an increase in TSH above the normal range can occur (166). It is therefore advisable to test elderly patients when they have recovered from acute illness. In this respect it is also important to note that treatment has an effect on the severely ill patient and thyroid function since dopamine and high glucocorticoid levels may be associated with reduction in TSH to normal in overt primary hypothyroidism. Thus a high index of suspicion is needed when testing for hypothyroidism in the elderly, particularly in hospitalized and sick patients. T_4 and TSH levels should ideally be assessed during or after the recovery phase from the original illness if possible.

Laboratory diagnosis

The laboratory diagnosis for hypothyroidism is straightforward, with a reduction in serum T_4, normal T_3 and increased TSH (> 10 iu/ml), often with the presence of antithyroid antibodies (to thyroglobulin and thyroid microsomes). Hypothyroidism is also suggested by correction of T_4 by T_3 uptake to obtain a reduced free T_4 index, and an increase in basal TSH which is detected by TRH stimulation.

In the absence of a hypopituitary condition (which is rare in the elderly) TSH is the most sensitive way to detect hypothyroidism, and this has been further improved by the development of a very sensitive assay (167). Increased circulating levels of creatine kinase and aspartate transaminase (AST) may persist with significant hypothyroidism—an important association which may incorrectly be attributed to myocardial ischaemia or infarction.

Some patients with mild or subclinical hypothyroidism may only be detected by carrying out a TRH stimulation test which, however, should be reserved only for those who do not have clear clinical features of hypothyroidism and where only a small increase in TSH is associated with a low or low normal T_4 level.

Any criteria for laboratory diagnosis of hypothyroidism must be carefully interpreted in sick patients since changes in total T_4 and free T_4 index may not be

Table 10. Drug-induced changes in thyroid hormones in the elderly

Drug	T_4 change	T_3 change
Carbamazepine	↓	↓
Diazepam	↓	—
Heparin	↓	—
Iodide	↓	↓
Phenothiazine	↓	—
Phenytoin	—	↓
Propranolol	↓	—
Salicylates	↓	↓
Stanazolol	↓	—
Sulphonylurea	↓	—
Oestrogen	↑	—
Thiazine	—	↑

Adapted from Wenzel (168).

diagnostic in the euthyroid sick patient. In addition changes in circulating glucocorticoids or therapy such as dopamine infusions can reduce TSH levels to within the normal range and must therefore be taken into account when assessing whether a seriously ill patient has hypothyroidism. Suspected subclinical hypothyroidism in the sick patient can be confirmed by TSH levels which remain elevated on recovery from the illness, and often associated with a persistent rise in antithyroid antibodies. More usually TSH normalizes on recovery and the antibodies are negative. In a recent study (152) only 50% of the increased TSH levels (>20 iu/l) in sick patients was due to thyroid disease.

Thus appropriate laboratory tests are needed to confirm clinical and to detect subclinical hypothyroidism in the elderly. Where possible, T_4 and TSH levels should be measured in the recovery phase rather than during the initial or acute admission. Table 10 shows drugs which alter T_4 and T_3 levels in the elderly (168).

Treatment
A number of studies suggest that lower T_4 replacement is needed in the elderly (158,169). Most studies agree that doses should be 20–30% lower than those used in younger patients, to a final dose of 50–100 µg per day, particularly in the frail elderly patient. In the healthy >65-year-old, 100 µg per day may be too little. A new ultra-sensitive radioimmunoassay of TSH (167) has enabled a better monitoring of the efficacy of therapy in elderly patients. However, it is important in the elderly not to induce replacement hyperthyroidism, which can be present even with normal T_4 and T_3 levels, and which may be associated with osteoporosis and increased bone loss. This can be assessed by a TRH test, where the response is flat with an increase in the mean nocturnal heart rate, reduced TSH levels and associated red blood cell ouabain-binding capacity which is significantly more than in controls but not as low as in the untreated patients with

hyperthyroidism (170). In addition the systolic time interval may be increased in the presence of subclinical hyperthyroidism.

It has been suggested that lean body mass is a predictor of the absolute thyroid requirement, and in addition lower doses may be needed where other illness coexists. Thus therapy needs to be tailored to the individual and higher initial doses can be given in the elderly if there is no concurrent ischaemic heart disease. When ischaemic heart disease is present, doses need to be introduced more slowly because of the risk of tachycardia, increased myocardial oxygen demand and exacerbation of angina. If, as is more likely in the elderly, marked coronary artery disease is present, low-dose L-thyroxine medication should commence with 12.5–25 μg per day and then be titrated slowly over 4–6 weeks to the final dose (50–100 μg per day). Close follow-up of symptoms referable to the cardiovascular system, such as tachycardia, and monitoring of the T_4 and TSH levels are essential. Patients with the mildest form of subclinical hypothyroidism detected with TRH stimulation tests may need only the lower replacement dose of T_4, and management is still controversial (169), although subjective and objective improvement in cardiac parameters may occur. Following surgery or radioiodine therapy replacement could be faster, starting at 50 μg per day and increased within the subsequent 2–4 weeks. Regular monitoring of thyroid function should be by measurement of TSH levels.

In the presence of marked ischaemic heart disease, it may not be possible to achieve biochemically normal T_4 and TSH levels without exacerbating the symptoms of angina; thus doses of other cardiac medications may need to be increased. Particular care is needed in the elderly to be aware of drug interactions.

If treatment of secondary hypothyroidism is undertaken, then hydrocortisone therapy must be initiated before starting therapy with L-thyroxine in order to avoid an adrenal crisis.

Side-effects of therapy

Apart from subclinical hyperthyroidism there are few side-effects of T_4 therapy, but arrhythmias, heart failure and myocardial infarction are important side-effects in the elderly patient with atherosclerotic heart disease with angina.

Hyperthyroidism

Incidence

Prevalence of hyperthyroidism is 5–12 times as common in the female than the male (171), and increases with age. The prevalence of females over 60 years old with thyrotoxicosis was 1.9% (158); in one series 10% were over the age of 75.

Aetiology

Graves' disease is still the most common cause of hyperthyroidism, but unlike the young patient, where diffuse toxic goitre is common, in the elderly toxic multinodular goitre or autonomously functioning goitres are common. In one study (81 patients) 70% of patients over 60 had toxic goitre (172) and in a series of 349 patients with autonomous functioning thyroid glands 55% were over 60 (173).

A similar proportion of patients have hyperthyroidism due to low thyroid uptake of ^{131}I, which would include iodine-induced hyperthyroidism, amiodarone-induced and lithium-induced thyrotoxicosis and subacute thyroiditis forms such as de Quervain's, and where excess T_4 has been given.

Clinical features

Whilst these may be typical and the same as in younger patients, they may also be as shown in Table 3. Symptoms affecting the cardiovascular system are common, such as tiredness, palpitations, angina, shortness of breath and heart failure. Cardiomegaly is often associated with atrial fibrillation. Mental and emotional symptoms are also common. Increased appetite, diarrhoea, heat intolerance, lid lag, stare and exophthalmos are all rare in the elderly as compared to younger age groups. Tremor is difficult to assess. It is important to note that apathetic hyperthyroidism in the elderly may present with depression, absence of hyperkinetic activity and slowed mental activity (see Table 11) but is also more likely to present with cardiac problems.

Pathogenesis

There is evidence of autoimmunity in Graves' disease with IgG antibodies capable of activating the TSH receptor on thyroid follicular cells. This can be detected either as a stimulating thyroid antibody or inhibiting thyroid receptor-binding antibody. Up to 80% may present in Graves' disease but heterogeneous

Table 11. Clinical features associated with hyperthyroidism in the elderly

System	Clinical features
Cardiovascular	Tachycardia Arrhythmia—atrial fibrillation Heart failure
Central nervous	Apathy, lethargy Anxiety Depression
Muscular	Asthenia Proximal muscle weakness
Gastrointestinal	Anorexia Weight loss Constipation

antibodies and a high prevalence of other antibodies (microsomal) may be present.

The incidence of toxic nodular goitre has been reviewed (174); it may occur in long-standing goitres which have become autonomous escaping from TSH control. Initially these may be detectable only by failure to suppress TSH or abolish the TSH response to intravenous TRH. Nodules may be palpable or detectable by thyroid scan showing a nodular pattern due to a combination of fibrosis with scarring and necrosis. Only a few nodules may be overactive, presumably due to stimulation by immunoglobulin. Solitary toxic nodular goitre is rare in the elderly.

Iodine-induced hyperthyroidism can (including that induced by seaweed from health food shops) occur in both normal glands and in previous multinodular goitre given iodine.

Increasing use of amiodarone in the elderly with dysrhythmias may cause hyperthyroidism. Amiodarone contains 40% by weight of atomic iodine, with about 3 mg per day liberated per 100 mg of amiodarone. This drug is also a potent inhibitor of 5-monodeiodinase, converting T_4 to T_3 and also deiodinating T_3. This leads to an increase in circulating T_4 over T_3 and in reverse T_3, whilst TSH levels remain normal. In some areas of iodine deficiency, the drug causes hyperthyroidism and vice versa when dietary iodine saturation is high. Reversal of the hyperthyroid state by discontinuing the drug is not so simple, since tissues accumulate the drug and its half-life is many months (175). Thus thyroid function tests should be checked before giving amiodarone baseline.

Investigations

Measurements of both T_4 and T_3 is necessary for diagnosis of hyperthyroidism. T_3 is usually disproportionately increased in relation to T_4 because of preferential secretion from the thyroid. The most sensitive screening test is T_4, which is increased in 86% of elderly subjects, and free T_3, which is increased in 89%. T_3 toxicosis is common with an autonomous functioning thyroid nodule may be missed because there is a reduction in T_3 when the patients are sick or treated with propanolol, or iodinated contrast material is used. Thus interpretation of T_4 and T_3 levels need more careful evaluation in the elderly than in younger age groups.

Twenty-four-hour uptake of ^{131}I may not be helpful but could be used to exclude thyroiditis. TSH may be low and this may not be typical in elderly patients. There may be a need, where the TSH level is normal, for a TRH test to exclude thyrotoxicosis. This could be misleading if the patient is taking steroids or dopamine. Patients with sublinical T_3 toxicosis (i.e. low TSH and obtunded TSH response to TRH) account for about 10% of all patients with lone atrial fibrillation (176).

An increased ratio of T_4 to T_3 occurs with iodine overload, amiodarone, thyroiditis or exogenous T_4 administration. In these cases suppressed TSH or a flat TRH test may confirm the diagnosis.

Treatment

Initially treatment may start with control of the cardiovascular symptoms, e.g. β-blockade or digoxin for angina, heart failure and atrial fibrillation. Doses should be tailored in the elderly patient because of renal and hepatic impairment which are more common than in young patients.

β-Blockers (such as propranolol) can be used to control anxiety, tachycardia and atrial fibrillation, and to reduce tremor in the elderly as in younger patients. Particular β-blockers (nadolol, metoprolol and sotalol) also partially inhibit peripheral conversion of T_4 to T_3 and increase reverse T_3 but are more expensive than propranolol. Contraindications are the same as in non-thyroid and younger patients, but it is particularly important in the elderly to note shortness of breath and congestive cardiac failure. However, while cardiac failure is a real problem, there are occasions when β-blockade is effective without failure because the benefits of reducing catechol stimulation outweigh the negative inotropic effects. β-blockade could be used while awaiting treatment with radioiodine and also can be used with digoxin to control atrial arrhythmias.

In the elderly thyrotoxic patient with known heart disease (and also with other medical conditions), radioactive iodine is the treatment of choice where there is comparatively little risk of genetic abnormality and teratogenicity is small.

Antithyroid drugs

Carbimazole (CBZ), methimazole and propylthiouracil (PTU) are widely used in the $>$40-year-olds, as in the younger patient. These drugs are concentrated in thyroid tissue, and inhibit T_4 synthesis by an effect on iodination of tyrosine residues and coupling of iodotyrosines. They may also suppress thyroid antibody synthesis. PTU also inhibits peripheral T_4 to T_3 conversion. In elderly patients it is used to render patients euthyroid whilst awaiting ablation therapy either by surgery or radioiodine. Remission is common with Graves' disease, but unusual with multinodular goitre and therefore PTU is contraindicated for use in such patients.

CBZ is given once daily (30–45 mg), and PTU is given in a dose of 300–450 mg per day because of its shorter half-life. Either drug is taken for about 4–6 weeks until a euthyroid state is ensured. The doses are then reduced to about a third as maintenance. Side-effects of rashes and pruritus (5% of patients) and more rarely agranulocytosis may occur, and are dose-related. The latter can be as high as one in 500.

Radioiodine

This is the treatment of choice in elderly patients with thyrotoxicosis, Graves' disease and for many with toxic nodular goitres. It is easy to give, and in the elderly there is no increased risk of long-term malignancy. Hypothyroidism may arise subsequently in both young and elderly patients, and thyroid function must be monitored regularly after initial treatment. It has been suggested that large ablative doses of ^{131}I should be used, followed by early T$_4$ replacement; in one study this had the added advantage of reversing atrial fibrillation to sinus rhythm. The more accepted treatment is low-dose ^{131}I estimated on gland size, which appears to reduce the incidence of hypothyroidism by 10 years. However, antithyroid drugs may be needed in the early stages to render the patient euthyroid. High-dose ^{131}I may be preferable in the elderly, but since replacement therapy is necessary the compliance of elderly patients needs to be taken into consideration when planning this therapy.

Patients with toxic nodular goitre have a lower uptake than those with Graves' disease, and in these patients further doses of ^{131}I may be needed. There is a risk of radiation thyroiditis in the first 2 weeks after ^{131}I therapy, when thyroid hormones are released into the circulation and a thyroid storm may occur. This could be hazardous in the elderly patient, particularly in the presence of cardiovascular disease.

Surgery
Surgery is recommended for those with large toxic multinodular goitres causing local pressure effects, some of which may need pretreatment with ^{131}I. Use of antithyroid drugs (e.g. Lugol's iodine) may need to be given to render the patient euthyroid before surgery, and propranolol may also be used in the elderly as in younger patients.

Treatment of thyroid storm
This is a rare life-threatening condition where exacerbation of the thyrotoxic state occurs with tachycardia, hyperpyrexia, confusion, heart failure and cardiovascular collapse. This may be precipitated by infection, surgery or in a patient with unsuspected hyperthyroidism or within 24 hours of a partial thyroidectomy or treatment with ^{131}I therapy. Management involves intravenous fluids with electrolytes and appropriate sedation, treatment of infection and Lugol's iodine three times a day to prevent the release of preformed thyroid hormone. Carbimazole (60 mg daily) may be given orally to block the thyroid hormone release, and intravenous hydrocortisone should be given 6-hourly to reduce potential allergic effects. Propranolol may be useful in controlling cardiovascular arrhythmias (e.g. 80 mg 6-hourly) but a careful watch for heart failure is necessary. Digoxin and diuretics should be used in conjunction with these drugs in a patient with a history of previous heart failure.

Treatment of iodine-induced hyperthyroidism
The best example of this, particularly in the elderly, is amiodarone therapy since with other iodide-induced therapies the treatment of choice is withdrawal of the treatment. Amiodarone, however, has a long half-life. Carbimazole (45 mg daily) should be used to decrease the preformed thyroid hormone synthesis but does not stop its release. When the patient is euthyroid, T$_3$ therapy is added and the patient may also respond to prednisolone 50–100 mg daily.

Follow-up of treated thyrotoxicosis

All patients with treated thyrotoxicosis should be followed up, initially no later than 3 months after ^{131}I, and reviewed at 6-monthly intervals and annually thereafter. Regular measurement of TSH will detect those at risk of progression to overt hyperthyroidism. Thyroid carcinoma may develop in nodules but is not especially relevant to the elderly patient with cardiovascular disease.

Acknowledgement

The authors are grateful to Professor Pyörälä and Dr Mykkänen for help, and permission to quote from Dr Mykkänen's thesis submitted to the University of Kuopio, Kuopio, Finland.

REFERENCES

1. Stamler J, Wentworth D, Neaton JD (1986) The MRFIT Research Group: is the relationship between serum cholesterol and risk of premature death from coronary heart disease continuous or graded? *JAMA* **256**: 2823–2828.
2. Lipid Research Clinics Program (1984) Coronary primary prevention trial results. i. Reduction incidence of coronary heart disease. ii. The relationship of reduction in incidence of coronary heart disease to cholesterol lowering. *JAMA* **251**: 351–374.
3. Frick MH, Elo O, Haapa K *et al.* (1987) Helsinki Heart Study: primary prevention trial with gemfibrozil in middle aged men with dyslipidaemia. *N Engl J Med* **317**: 1237–1245.
4. Brody JA, Brock DB, Williams TR (1987) Trends in the health of elderly population. *Annu Rev Public Health* **8**: 211–234.
5. Garber AM, Littenberg B, So HC *et al.* (1991) Costs and health consequences of cholesterol screening for asymptomatic older Americans. *Arch Intern Med* **151**: 1089–1095.
6. Kannel WB, Wolf PA, Garrison J (1992) Framingham Study: an epidemiological investigation of cardiovascular disease. Section 36. Framingham Heart Study 30 year Followup. National Heart, Lung and Blood Institute publication No. NIH 88-2970.
7. Wallace RB, Colsher PL (1992) Blood lipid distributions in older persons: prevalence and correlates of hyperlipidaemia. *Ann Epidemiol* **2**: 15–21.
8. Frishman WH, Ooi WL, Derman DP *et al.* (1992) Serum lipids and lipoproteins in advanced age: intra-individual changes. *Ann Epidemiol* **2**: 43–50.
9. Denke MA, Grundy SM (1990) Hypercholesterolaemia in elderly persons: resolving the treatment dilemma. *Ann Intern Med* **112**: 780–792.
10. Zimetbaum P, Frishman WH, Ooi WL *et al.* (1992) Plasma lipids and lipoproteins and the incidence of cardiovascular disease in the very elderly: the Bronx Study. *Arterioscl Thrombos* **12**: 416–423.
11. Ettinger WH, Wall PW, Kuller LH *et al.* (1992) Lipoprotein lipids in old people. *Circulation* **86**: 858–869.
12. Bagdade JD, Albers JJ (1992) Hypercholesterolaemia predicts early death for coronary heart disease in elderly men but not women. *Ann Epidemiol* **2**: 77–83.
13. Consensus Conference (1985) Lowering blood cholesterol to prevent heart disease. *J Ann Med Soc* **253**: 2080–2086.
14. Data from Office of Population Censuses and Survey Monitor (1988).

15. MRC Working Party Group (1992) MRC trial of treatment of hypertension in older age groups. *Br Med J* **304**: 405–412.

16. Prevention of coronary heart disease (1992) Scientific background and new clinical guidelines. Recommendations of European Atherosclerosis Society prepared by the International Task Force for Prevention of Coronary Heart Disease. *Nutr Metab Cardiovasc Dis* **2**: 113–156.

17. Barbir M, Wile D, Trayner I *et al.* (1988) High prevalence of hypertriglyceridaemia and apolipoprotein abnormalities in coronary artery disease. *Br Heart J* **60**: 397–403.

18. Shepherd J, Krauss RM (1991) Pathophysiology of triglyceride-rich particles. *Ann J Cardiol* **68**: 5A–7A.

19. Brown MS, Kovanen PT, Goldstein JL (1981) Regulation of plasma cholesterol by lipoprotein receptors. *Science* **212**: 628–635.

20. Parthasarathy S, Quinn MT, Schwenke DC *et al.* (1989) Oxidative modification of beta-very low density lipoprotein, potential role in monocyte recruitment and foam cell formation. *Arterioscl* **9**: 398–404.

21. Berr F, Kern JR (1987) Evidence of saturated hepatic chylomicron remnant uptake after a lipid meal. *J Hepatol* **5**: S10.

22. Gotto AM, Patsch J, Yamomoto A (1991) Postprandial hyperlipidaemia. *Ann J Cardiol* **68**: 11A–12A.

23. Series JJ, Biggart EM, O'Reilly D St J *et al.* (1988) Thyroid dysfunction and hypercholesterolaemia in the general population of Glasgow, Scotland. *Clin Chim Acta* **172**: 217–222.

24. Haffner SM, Stern MP, Hazuda HP *et al.* (1990) Cardiovascular risk factors in confirmed prediabetic individuals. *JAMA* **263**: 2893–2898.

25. Savage PJ, Wall PT, Tracy RP, Ettinger WH (1991) Association of abnormal glucose tolerance with coronary heart disease in older men and women: the Cardiovascular Health Study. *Circulation* **84**: II-2176.

26. Appel G (1991) Lipid abnormalities in renal disease. *Kidney Inf* **39**: 169–183.

27. Miller JP (1992) Significance of hyperlipidaemia in the elderly. *Prog Cardiol* **5**: 93–102.

28. Miller JP (1992) Screening for hyperlipidaemia and its treatment in women and the elderly. *Postgrad Med J* **68**: 876–877.

29. Thomas AJ, Bunker VW, Hinks LJ, Sodha N, Mullee MA, Clayton BE (1988) Energy, protein, zinc and copper status of twenty one elderly inpatients: analysed dietary intake and biochemical indices. *Br J Nutr* **S9**: 181–191.

30. Thompson GR (1989) Drug treatment of hyperlipidaemia. In *A Handbook of Hyperlipidaemia*, Thompson GR (ed.), Ch. 12. Current Science; London, pp. 179–194.

31. Beil V, Crouse JR, Einarsson K, Grundy SM (1982) Effects of interruption of the enterohepatic circulation of bile acids on the transport of very low density lipoprotein triglycerides. *Metabolism* **31**: 438–444.

32. Illingworth DR, Bacon SP, Larsen KK (1988) Long term experience with HMG CoA reductase inhibitors in therapy of hypercholesterolaemia. *Atherosclerosis Rev* **18**: 161–187.

33. Heidemann H, Bock KD, Kruzfelder E (1981) Rhabdomyolysis and bezafibrate therapy in renal insufficiency. *Klin Wochenschr* **59**: 413–414.

34. Pekkanen J, Nissinen A, Punsar S, Karvonen MJ (1989) Serum cholesterol and risk of accidental or violent death in a 25 year follow-up: the Finnish cohorts of the 7 countries study. *Arch Intern Med* **149**: 1589–1591.

35. Illingworth DR (1990) Treatment of hyperlipidaemia. *Br Med Bull* **46**: 1025–1058.

36. Coronary Drug Project Research Group (1985) Clofibrate and niacin in coronary

heart disease. *JAMA* **231**: 360–381.

37. Canner PL, Berge KG, Wenger NK *et al.* (1986) 15 year mortality in coronary drug project patients: long term benefit with niacin. *J Am Coll Cardiol* **8**: 1245–1255.

38. Bush TL (1990) The epidemiology of cardiovascular disease in post-menopausal women. *Ann NY Acad Sci* **592** 263–271.

39. Sullivan JM, Zwaag RV, Hughes JP *et al.* (1990) Estrogen replacement and coronary disease. *Arch Intern Med* **150**: 2557–2562.

40. Seed M (1992) Oral contraception, hormone replacement therapy and hyper-lipidaemia. *Postgrad Med J* **68**: 877–878.

41. Agner E, Hansen PF (1983) Fasting serum cholesterol and triglycerides in a 10 year prospective study in old age. *Acta Med Scand* **214**: 33–41.

42. Stocks P (1944) Diabetes mortality in 1861–1942 and some of the factors affecting it. *J Hygiene* **43**: 242–247.

43. West KM (1978) *Epidemiology of Diabetes and its Vascular Lesions.* Elsevier, New York, pp. 172–176, 357–360, 389–402.

44. Krowleski AS, Warram JH, Christlieb AR (1985) Onset, course, complications and prognosis in diabetes mellitus. In *Joslin's Diabetes Mellitus* 12th edn, Marble A, Krall LP, Bradley RF *et al.* (eds). Lea & Febiger, Philadelphia, pp. 251–277.

45. Marks HH, Krall LP (1971) Onset, course, prognosis and mortality in diabetes mellitus. *Joslin's Diabetes Mellitus*, 11th edn, Marble A, White P, Bradley RF, Krall LP (eds), Lea & Febiger, Philadelphia, pp. 209–254.

46. Westlund K (1969) *Mortality of Diabetes.* Life Insurance Companies' Institute for Medical Statistics at the Oslo City Hospitals. Report No. 13.

47. Bradley RF (1971) Cardiovascular disease. In *Joslin's Diabetes Mellitus*, 11th edn, Marble A, White P, Bradley RF, Krall LP (eds). Lea & Febiger, Philadelphia, pp. 417–477.

48. Steiner G (1981) Diabetes and atherosclerosis: an overview. *Diabetes* **30** (Suppl. 2): 1–7.

49. Strandness DE, Priest RE, Gibbons GE (1964) Combined clinical and pathologic study of diabetic and nondiabetic peripheral arterial disease. *Diabetes* **13**: 366–372.

50. Stout RW (1981) Blood glucose and atherosclerosis. *Arteriosclerosis* **1**: 227–234.

51. Pirart J (1978) Diabetes mellitus and its degenerative complications: a prospective study of 4400 patients observed between 1947 and 1973. *Diabetes Care* **1**: 166–188, 252–263.

52. Fuller JH, McCartney P, Jarrett R *et al.* (1979) Hyperglycaemia and coronary heart disease: the Whitehall study. *J Chronic Dis* **32**: 721–728.

53. Kannel WB, McGee DL (1979) Diabetes and cardiovascular disease: the Framing-ham study. *JAMA* **241**: 2035–2038.

54. Crall FV, Roberts WC (1978) The extramural and intramural coronary arteries in juvenile diabetes mellitus: analysis of nine necropsy patients aged 19–38 years with onset of diabetes before age 15 years. *Am J Med* **64**: 221–230.

55. Higgs ER, Kelleher A, Simpson HCR, Reckless JPD (1992) Screening programme for microvascular complications and hypertension in a community diabetic population. *Diabetic Med* **9**: 550–556.

56. Wingard DL, Sinsheimer P, Barrett-Connor EL, McPhillips JB (1990) Community-based study of prevalence of NIDDM in older adults. *Diabetes Care* **13** (Suppl. 2): 3–8.

57. Barrett-Connor E (1980) The prevalence of diabetes mellitus in an adult community as determined by history or fasting hyperglycaemia. *Am J Epidemiol* **111**: 705–712.

58. Hanis CL, Ferrell RE, Barton SA *et al.* (1983) Diabetes among Mexican Americans in Starr County, Texas. *Am J Epidemiol* **118**: 659–672.

59. Stern MP (1985) Diabetes in Hispanic Americans. In *Diabetes in America.* US

Government Printing Office, Washington DC, NIH Publication No. 85-1468.
60. Verrillo A, de Teresa A, La Rocca S, Giarrussso PC (1985) Prevalence of diabetes mellitus and impaired glucose tolerance in rural area of Italy. *Diabetes Res* **2**: 301–306.
61. Glatthaar C, Welborn TA, Stenhouse NS, Garcia-Webb P (1985) Diabetes and impaired glucose tolerance: a prevalence estimate based on the Busselton 1981 survey. *Med Aust* **143**: 436–440.
62. Sekikawa A, Tominaga M, Takahashi K *et al.* (1993) Prevalence of diabetes and impaired glucose tolerance in Funagata area, Japan. *Diabetes Care* **16**: 570–574.
63. Harris MI, Hadden WC, Knowler WC, Bennett PH (1987) Prevalence of diabetes and impaired glucose tolerance and plasma glucose levels in US population aged 20–74 years. *Diabetes* **36**: 523–534.
64. McPhillips JB, Barrett-Connor E, Wingard DL (1990) Cardiovascular disease risk factors prior to the diagnosis of impaired glucose tolerance and non-insulin dependent diabetes mellitus in a community of older diabetics. *Am J Epidemiol* **131**: 443–453.
65. Laakso M, Reuanen A, Klaukka T (1991) Changes in the prevalence and incidence of diabetes mellitus in Finnish adults, 1970–1987. *Am J Epidemiol* **133**: 850–857.
66. Mykkänen L (1993) Non-insulin dependent diabetes mellitus and impaired glucose tolerance in the elderly: prevalence and association with cardiovascular risk factors and atherosclerotic vascular disease. MD thesis, in preparation (personal communication).
67. Davidson MB (1979) The effect of aging on carbohydrate metabolism: a review of the English literature and a practical approach to the diagnosis of diabetes mellitus in the elderly. *Metabolism* **28**: 688–705.
68. Keen H, Ng Tang Fui S (1982) The definition and classification of diabetes mellitus. *Clin Endocrinol Metab* **11**: 279–305.
69. Mykkanen L, Laakso M, Uusitupa M, Pyorala K (1990) Prevalence of diabetes and impaired glucose tolerance in elderly subjects and their association with obesity and family history of diabetes. *Diabetes Care* **13**: 1099–1105.
70. Mykkanen L, Laakso M, Pentilla I, Pyorala K (1991) Asymptomatic hyperglycaemia and cardiovascular risk factors in the elderly. *Atherosclerosis* **88**: 153–161.
71. Mykkanen L, Laakso M, Pyorala K (1992) Asymptomatic hyperglycaemia and atherosclerotic vascular disease in the elderly. *Diabetes Care* **15**: 1020–1030.
72. Pyorala K, Laakso M (1983) Macrovascular disease in diabetes mellitus. In *Diabetes in Epidemiological Perspective*, Mann JI, Pyorala K, Teuscher A (eds). Churchill Livingstone, Edinburgh, pp. 183–247.
73. Pyorala K, Laakso M, Uusitupa M (1987) Diabetes and atherosclerosis: an epidemiologic view. *Diabetes Metab Rev* **3**: 463–524.
74. Keen H, Rose G, Pyke DA *et al.* (1965) Blood sugar and arterial disease. *Lancet* **ii**: 505–508.
75. Jarrett RJ, McCartney P, Keen H (1982) The Bedford Survey: ten year mortality rates in newly diagnosed diabetics, borderline diabetics and normoglycaemic control and risk indices for coronary heart disease in borderline diabetics. *Diabetologia* **22**: 79–84.
76. Pan W-H, Cedres LB, Liu K *et al.* (1986) Relationship of clinical diabetes and asymptomatic hyperglycaemia to risk of coronary heart disease mortality in men and women. *Am J Epidemiol* **123**: 504–516.
77. Fuller JH, Elford J, Goldblatt P *et al.* (1983) Diabetes mortality: new light on an underestimated public health problem. *Diabetologia* **24**: 336–341.
78. Ochi JW, Melton LJ, Palumbo PJ *et al.* (1985) A population-based study of diabetes mortality. *Diabetes Care* **8**: 224–229.

79. Hayward RE, Lucena BC (1965) An investigation into the mortality of diabetics. *J Inst Actuaries* **91**: 286–315.
80. Krowleski AS, Czyzyk A, Janeczko D *et al.* (1977) Mortality from cardiovascular diseases among diabetics. *Diabetalogia* **13**: 345–350.
81. Deckert T, Poulsen JE, Larsen M (1978) Prognosis of diabetics with diabetes onset before the age of thirty-one: survival, causes of death, and complications. *Diabetologia* **14**: 363–370.
82. Panzram G, Zabel-Langhennig R (1981) Prognosis of diabetes mellitus in a geographically defined population. *Diabetologia* **20**: 587–591.
83. Entmacher PS, Root HF, Marks HH (1964) Longevity of diabetic patients in recent years. *Diabetes* **13**: 373–377.
84. Reckless JPD (1987) The epidemiology of heart disease in diabetes mellitus. In *Diabetes and the Heart* Taylor KG (ed.). Castle House, Tunbridge Wells, pp. 1–18.
85. Harris MI, Klein R, Welborn TA, Knuiman MW (1992) Onset of NIDDM occurs at least 4–7 years before clinical diagnosis. *Diabetes Care* **15**: 815–819.
86. Harris MI (1993) Undiagnosed NIDDM: clinical and public health issues. *Diabetes Care* **16**: 642–652.
87. Spence JW (1992–21) Some observations on sugar tolerance with special reference to variations found at different ages. *Q J Med* **14**: 314–326.
88. Jackson RA (1990) Mechanisms of age-related glucose intolerance. *Diabetes Care* **13** (Suppl. 2): 9–19.
89. Stout RW (1990) Diabetes, atherosclerosis and aging. *Diabetes Care* **13** (Suppl. 2): 20–23.
90. Kannel WB, Wolf PA, Castelli WP, D'Agostino RB (1987) Fibrinogen and risk of cardiovascular disease: the Framingham study. *JAMA* **258**: 1183–1186.
91. Kreisberg RA (1987) Aging, glucose metabolism, and diabetes: current concepts. *Geriatrics* **42**: 67–72.
92. Bierman EL (1978) Atherosclerosis and aging. *Fed Proc* **37**: 2832–2836.
93. Garcia MJ, McNamara PM, Gordon T, Kannel WB (1974) Morbidity and mortality in diabetics in the Framingham population: sixteen year follow-up study. *Diabetes* **23**: 105–111.
94. Stamler J, Wentworth D, Neaton J *et al.* (1984) Diabetes and risk of coronary, cardiovascular, and all causes mortality: findings for 356,000 men screened by the multiple risk factor intervention trial (MRFIT). *Circulation* **70** (Suppl. II): 161.
95. Green MS, Heiss G, Rifkind BM *et al.* (1985) The ratio of plasma high density lipoprotein cholesterol to total and low density lipoprotein cholesterol: age related changes and race and sex differences in selected North American populations. The Lipid Research Clinics' Program Prevalence Study. *Circulation* **72**: 93–104.
96. Reckless JPD, Betteridge DJ, Wu P *et al.* (1978) High density and low density lipoproteins and prevalence of vascular disease and diabetes mellitus. *Br Med J* i: 883–886.
97. Harris MI (1980) National Diabetes Data Group: National Health and Nutrition Examination Survey, 1967–1980. US Government Printing Office, Washington, DC.
98. Kannel WB, Dawber TR, McGee DL (1980) Perspectives on systolic hypertension: the Framingham Study. *Circulation* **61**: 1179–1182.
99. Hulley SB, Furberg CD, Garland B *et al.* (1985) Systolic hypertension in the elderly program (SHEP): antihypertensive efficacy of chlorthalidone. *Am J Cardiol* **56**: 913–920.
100. Ronnemaa T, Laakso M, Kallio V *et al.* (1989) Serum lipids, lipoproteins, and apolipoproteins and the excessive occurrence of coronary heart disease in non-insulin dependent diabetic patients. *Am J Epidemiol* **130**: 632–645.

101. Taskinen M-R (1990) Hyperlipidaemia in diabetes. *Clin Endocrinol Metab* **4**: 743–745.
102. Orchard TJ (1990) Dyslipoproteinaemia and diabetes. *Endocrinol Metab Clin North Am* **19**: 361–380.
103. Kissebah AH, Alfarsi S, Evans DJ, Adams PW (1983) Plasma low density lipoprotein transport kinetics in non-insulin dependent diabetes mellitus. *J Clin Invest* **71**: 655–667.
104. Pfeiffer MA, Brunzell JD, Best JD *et al.* (1983) The response of plasma triglyceride, cholesterol, and lipoprotein lipase to treatment in non-insulin dependent diabetic subjects without familial hypertriglyceridaemia. *Diabetes* **32**: 525–531.
105. Eisenberg S (1984) High density lipoprotein metabolism. *J Lipid Res* **25**: 1017–1058.
106. Howard BV (1987) Lipoprotein metabolism in diabetes mellitus. *J Lipid Res* **28**: 613–628.
107. Harno KE, Nikkila EA, Kuusi T (1993) Plasma HDL-cholesterol and postheparin plasma hepatic endothelial lipase activity: relationship to obesity and non-insulin dependent diabetes.
108. Hiramatsu K, Bierman EL, Chait A (1985) Metabolism of low density lipoproteins from patients with diabetic hypertriglyceridaemia by cultured human skin fibroblasts. *Diabetes* **34**: 8–14.
109. Steinbrecher UP, Witztum JL (1984) Glucosylation of low density lipoproteins to an extent comparable to that seen in diabetes slows their catabolism. *Diabetes* **33**: 130–134.
110. Brownlee M (1992) Glycation products and the pathogenesis of diabetic complications. *Diabetes Care* **15**: 1835–1843.
111. Austin MA, Breslow JL, Hennekens CH *et al.* (1988) Low density lipoprotein subclass patterns and risk of myocardial infarction. *JAMA* **260**: 1917–1921.
112. Austin MA, Krauss RM (1986) Genetic control of low density lipoprotein subclasses. *Lancet* **ii**: 592–595.
113. Austin MA, King MC, Vranizan KM, Krauss RM (1990) Atherogenic lipoprotein phenotype: a proposed genetic marker for coronary heart disease risk. *Circulation* **82**: 495–506.
114. Eisenberg S, Gavish D, Oscry Y *et al.* (1984) Abnormalities in very low, low, and high density lipoproteins in hypertriglyceridaemia: reversal towards normal with bezafibrate treatment. *J Clin Invest* **74**: 470–482.
115. Lahdenpera S, Tillt-Kiesi M, Vuorinen-Markkola H *et al.* (1993) Effects of gemfibrozil on low density lipoprotein particle size, density distribution, and composition in patients with type II diabetes. *Diabetes Care* **16**: 584–592.
116. Shen D-C, Fuh MMT, Shieh S-H *et al.* (1991) Effects of gemfibrozil treatment in sulfonylurea-treated patients with non-insulin dependent diabetes mellitus. *J Clin Endocrinol Metab* **73**: 503–510.
117. James RW, Pometta D (1991) The distribution profiles of very low density and low density lipoproteins in poorly-controlled male type II (non-insulin dependent) diabetic patients. *Diabetologia* **34**: 246–252.
118. Barakat HA, Carpenter JW, McLendon VD *et al.* (1990) Influence of obesity, impaired glucose tolerance, and NIDDM on LDL structure and composition: possible link between hyperinsulinaemia and atherosclerosis. *Diabetes* **39**: 1527–1533.
119. Bagdade JD, Buchanan WE, Kuusi T, Taskinen M-R (1990) Persistent abnormalities in lipoprotein composition in non-insulin dependent diabetes after intensive insulin therapy. *Arteriosclerosis* **10**: 232–239.
120. Taskinen M-R, Packard CJ, Shepherd J (1990) Effect of insulin therapy on metabolic fate of apolipoprotein-containing lipoproteins in NIDDM. *Diabetes* **39**:

1017–1027.

121. Shepherd J, Griffin B, Caslake MJ *et al.* (1991) The influence of fibrates on lipoprotein metabolism. In *Atherosclerosis Reviews*, Vol. 22, Gotto AM, Paoletti R (eds). Raven Press, New York, pp. 163–169.

122. Koskinen P, Manttari M, Manninen V *et al.* (1992) Coronary heart disease in NIDMM in the Helsinki Heart Study. *Diabetes Care* **15**: 820–825.

123. Strowig S, Raskin P (1992) Glycaemic control and diabetic complications. *Diabetes Care* **15**: 1126–1140.

124. Seaquist ER, Goetz FC, Rich S, Barbosa J (1989) Familial clustering of diabetic kidney disease: evidence for genetic susceptibility to diabetic nephropathy. *N Engl J Med* **32**: 1161–1165.

125. Pietro AO, Dunn FL, Grundy SM, Raskin P (1983) The effect of continuous subcutaneous insulin infusion on very low density lipoprotein triglyceride metabolism in type I diabetes mellitus. *Diabetes* **32**: 75–81.

126. DCCT Research Group (1991) Epidemiology of severe hypoglycaemia in the Diabetes Control and Complications Trial. *Am J Med* **90**: 450–459.

127. Donahue RP, Orchard TJ (1992) Diabetes mellitus and macrovascular complications. *Diabetes Care* **15**: 1141–1155.

128. Eschwege E, Richard JL, Thibult N *et al.* (1985) Coronary heart disease mortality in relation with diabetes, blood glucose, and plasma insulin levels: the Paris Prospective Study, ten years later. *Hormone Metab Res* **15** (Suppl.): 41–46.

129. Welborn TA, Wearne K (1979) Coronary heart disease incidence and cardiovascular mortality in Busselton with reference to glucose and insulin concentrations. *Diabetes Care* **2**: 154–160.

130. Wilson PWF, Cupples A, Kannel WB (1991) Is hyperglycaemia associated with cardiovascular disease? The Framingham Study. *Am Heart J* **121**: 586–590.

131. Donahue RP, Skyler JS, Schneiderman N, Prineas RJ (1990) Hyperinsulinaemia and elevated blood pressure: cause, confounder or coincidence? *Am J Epidemiol* **132**: 827–836.

132. Reckless JPD, Clifton-Bligh P, Galton DJ (1975) The triglyceride content of adipocytes and plasma of patients with diabetes mellitus. *Hormone Metab Res* **7**: 407–410.

133. Pyorala K (1979) Relationship of glucose tolerance and plasma insulin to the incidence of coronary heart disease: results from two population studies in Finland. *Diabetes Care* **2**: 131–141.

134. Ronnemace T, Laakso M, Pyorala K, Puukka P (1991) High fasting insulin is an indicator of coronary heart disease in non-insulin dependent diabetic patients and non-diabetic subjects. *Atherosclerosis* **11**: 80–90.

135. Temple R, Clark PMS, Hales CN (1992) Measurement of insulin secretion in type 2 diabetes: problems and pitfalls. *Diabetic Med* **9**: 503–512.

136. Modan M, Or J, Karasik A *et al.* (1991) Hyperinsulinaemia, sex and risk of atherosclerotic cardiovascular disease. *Circulation* **84**: 1165–1175.

137. Helmrich S, Ragland D, Leung RW, Paffenbarger RS (1991) Physical activity and reduced occurrence of non-insulin dependent diabetes mellitus. *N Engl J Med* **325**: 147–153.

138. Alexander L, Appleton D, Hall R *et al.* (1980) Epidemiology of acromegaly in the Newcastle region. *Clin Endocrinol* **12**: 71–79.

139. Blackman MR (1987) Pituitary hormones and aging. *Endocrinol Metab Clin North Am* **16**: 981–994.

140. Rudman D, Feller AG, Nagraz HS *et al.* (1990) Effects of human growth hormone in men over 60 years old. *N Engl J Med* **323**: 1–6.

141. Ho KY, Evans WS, Blizzard RM *et al.* (1987) Effects of sex and age on the 24-hour

profile of growth hormone secretion in man: importance of endogenous estradiol concentrations. *J Clin Endocrinol Metab* **64**: 51–58.

142. Molitch ME (1992) Clinical manifestations of acromegaly. *Endocrinol Metab Clin North Am* **21**: 597–614.

143. Bengtsson B-A, Eden S, Ernest I *et al.* (1988) Epidemiology and long term survival in acromegaly. *Acta Med Scand* **223**: 327–335.

144. Wright AD, Hill DM, Lowy C *et al.* (1970) Mortality in acromegaly. *Q J Med* **39**: 1–16.

145. Hayward RP, Emanuel RW, Nabarro JDN (1987) Acromegalic heart disease: influence of treatment of the acromegaly on the heart. *Q J Med* **62** (NS): 41–58.

146. McGuffin WL, Sherman BM, Roth J *et al.* (1974) Acromegaly and cardiovascular disorders: a prospective study. *Ann Intern Med* **81**: 11–18.

147. Nabarro JDN (1987) Acromegaly. *Clin Endocrinol* **26**: 481–512.

148. McLellan AR, Connell JMC, Beastall GH *et al.* (1988) Growth hormone, body composition and somatomedin C after treatment of acromegaly. *Q J Med* **69** (NS): 997–1008.

149. Souadjian JV, Schirger A (1967) Hypertension in acromegaly. *Am J Med Sci* **254**: 629–633.

150. James RA, Moller N, Chatterjee S *et al.* (1991) Carbohydrate tolerance and serum lipids in acromegaly before and during treatment with high dose octreotide. *Diabetic Med* **8**: 517–523.

151. Roelfsema F, Frolich M (1985) Glucose tolerance and plasma immunoreactive levels in acromegalics before and after selective trans-sphenoidal surgery. *Clin Endocrinol* **22**: 531–537.

152. Parle JV, Franklyn JA, Cross KW *et al.* (1991) Prevalence and follow up of abnormal thyrotrophin (TSH) concentrations in the elderly in the United Kingdom. *Clin Endocrinol* **34**: 77–83.

153. Sawin CT, Geller A, Hershman JM *et al.* (1989) The Ageing Thyroid. The use of thyroid hormone in older persons. *JAMA* **261**: 2635–2655.

154. Parle JV, Franklyn JA, Cross KW *et al.* (1991) Assessment of a screening process to detect patients age 60 years and over at high risk of hypothyroidism. *Br J Gen Pract* **41**: 417–420.

155. Hansen JM, Skovsted L, Siersback-Nielsen K (1975) Age dependent changes in iodine metabolism and thyroid function. *Acta Endocrinol* **79**: 60–65.

156. Sawin CT, Chopra D, Azizi F (1979) The ageing thyroid-increased prevalence of elevated serum thyrotrophin levels in the elderly. *JAMA* **242**: 247–250.

157. Tunbridge WMG, Evered DC, Hall R *et al.* (1977) The spectrum of thyroid disease in a community: the Wickham Survey. *Clin Endocrinol* **7**: 481–493.

158. Griffin JE (1990) Review: hypothyroidism in the elderly. *Am J Med Sci* **299**: 334–345.

159. Doniach D, Bottazzo GF, Russell RCG (1979) Goitrous auto-immune thyroiditis (Hashimoto's disease). *Clin Endocrinol Metab* **8**: 63–80.

160. Tunbridge WMG, Brewis M, French JM *et al.* (1981) Natural history of autoimmune thyroiditis. *Br Med J* **282**: 258–262.

161. Hurley JR (1983) Thyroid disease in the elderly. *Med Clin North Am* **67**: 497–515.

162. Tunbridge WMG, Evered DC, Hall R *et al.* (1977) Lipid profiles and cardiovascular disease in the Wickham area with reference to thyroid failure. *Clin Endocrinol* **7**: 495–508.

163. Forfar JC, Wathen CG, Todd WTA *et al.* (1983) Left ventricular performance in subclinical hypothyroidism. *Q J Med* **57**: 857–865.

164. Bell GM, Todd WTA, Forfar JC *et al.* (1985) End organ responses to thyroxine therapy in subclinical hypothyroidism. *Clin Endocrinol* **22**: 83–89.

165. Shenoy MM, Goldman JM (1987) Hypothyroid cardiomyopathy: echo-cardio-

graphic documentation reversibility. *Ann J Med Sci* **294**: 1–9.

166. Wong ET, Bradley SG, Schulz AL (1989) Elevation of thyroid stimulating hormone during acute nonthyroidal illness. *Arch Intern Med* **141**: 873–875.

167. Cobb WE, Lamberton RP, Jackson IMD (1984) Use of a rapid sensitive immunoradiometric assay for thyrotrophin to distinguish normal from hyperthyroid subjects. *Clin Chem* **30**: 1558–1560.

168. Wenzel KW (1981) Pharmacological interference with in vitro tests of thyroid function. *Metabolism* **30**: 717–732.

169. Kabadi UM (1987) Variability of L-thyroxine dose replacement in elderly patients with primary hypothyroidism. *J Fam Pract* **24**: 473–477.

170. Wilcox AH, Levin GE (1986) Erythrocyte ouabain-binding capacity in hypothyroid patients receiving thyroxine. *J Endocrinol* **108**: 185.

171. MacLennan WJ, Peden NR (1988) Hyperthyroidism. In *Metabolic and Endocrine Problems in the Elderly*. MacLennan WJ and Peden NR (eds), Springer-Verlag, Berlin, pp. 44–61.

172. Davis PJ, Davis FB (1974) Hyperthyroidism in patients over 60. *Medicine (Baltimore)* **53**: 161–181.

173. Hamburger JL (1980) Evolution of toxicity in solitary non-toxic autonomously functioning thyroid nodules. *J Clin Endocrinol Metab* **50**: 1089–1093.

174. Studer H, Peter HJ, Gerber H (1985) Toxic nodular goitre. *Clin Endocrinol Metab* **14**: 351–372.

175. Holt DW, Incker GT, Jackson PR (1983) Amiodarone pharmacokinetics. *Am Heart J* **106**: 840–847.

176. The Diabetes Control and Complications Trial Research Group (1993) The effect of intensive treatment of diabetes on the development and progression of long-term complications in insulin-dependent diabetes mellitus. *New Engl J Med* **329**: 977–986.

Appendix 1. Serum cholesterol according to age and risk profile

Age	Target cholesterol (mmol/l) without risk factor[a]
20–30	< 6.5
31–40	< 7.0
41–50	< 7.5
51–60	< 8.0
61–70[b]	< 8.0

[a]Add 0.5 mmol/l for premenopausal women.
[b]As total cholesterol (and LDL fraction) rises with age, it may not be necessary to measure total cholesterol in patients over 70 years unless cardiovascular therapy or interventional procedures are envisaged.

Part V

SYNDROMES

22 Faints and Falls: Pathophysiology and Clinical Evaluation of Syncope in the Elderly

DAVID G. BENDITT, KEITH LURIE, YOICHI KOBAYASHI AND STEPHEN REMOLE
University of Minnesota Medical School, Minneapolis, Minnesota, USA

Faints and falls in the elderly are frequent causes for medical consultation, and form an important source of morbidity in this age group. Although orthopaedic complications, such as hip fractures, are of particular concern (1–3), other injuries may be equally disabling and signal the end of an independent lifestyle for many older patients. The origins of isolated faints or falls often remain obscure. Even the aetiology of recurrent episodes may prove elusive. In many cases it may be difficult to differentiate a simple accident contributed to by deteriorating vision, a less acute sense of balance, or diminished agility, from a syncopal episode associated with any of a wide range of clinical conditions (Table 1). In either case, the medical history, upon which considerable reliance is usually placed, may be unclear and/or incomplete especially for unwitnessed events. This review focuses primarily on the problem of syncope in older individuals, addressing its frequency, pathophysiology, potential causes, evaluation and current therapies.

EPIDEMIOLOGY OF SYNCOPAL EVENTS

The Framingham Study has provided the most thorough insight into the frequency with which syncope occurs among free-living individuals in the Western world. Findings were based upon a biennial survey of over 5200 subjects, ranging in age from 30 to 62 years (mean 46 years) at entry into the study in 1950, and indicated that at least one syncopal episode may be anticipated in 3% of men and 3.5% of women during their lifetime (4). The age at which the initial syncopal event occurred ranged widely; the mean age was 52 years (range 15–78 years) and 50 years (range 13–87 years), respectively, for men and women. Syncope recurrences were reported by 30% of men and 27% of women. In most cases the events occurred in the absence of evident cardiac or neurological disease, and therefore were considered to be 'isolated'.

Geriatric Cardiology. Principles and Practice. Edited by A. Martin and A. J. Camm
© 1994 John Wiley & Sons Ltd

Table 1. Syncope: clinical conditions, differential diagnosis

CARDIOVASCULAR DISORDERS

Cardiac/pulmonary disease
  Mechanical disturbances (obstruction to flow, inadequate flow)
  Cardiac valvular disease
  Myocardial infarction
  Obstructive cardiomyopathy
  Pericardial disease/tamponade
  Pulmonary embolus
  Primary pulmonary hypertension

  Rhythm disturbances
  Sinus node dysfunction (including bradycardia/tachycardia syndrome)
  Atrioventricular conduction system disease
  Paroxysmal supraventricular tachycardias
  Paroxysmal ventricular tachycardia (including Torsade de pointes)
  Implanted pacing system malfunction, pulse generator/lead failure, pacemaker-
    mediated tachycardia, 'pacemaker syndrome'

  Vascular disturbances
  Cerebrovascular (including disorders of the posterior circulation)
  Non-cerebral vessels (eg. subclavian steal, aortic aneurysm dissection)
  Autonomic neuropathies
  Drug or dehydration-induced orthostasis

Neurally mediated reflex syncope
  Emotional (vasovagal) faint
  Carotid sinus syncope
  Cough syncope and related disorders
  Gastrointestinal, pelvic or urological origin (swallowing, defaecation, post-
    micturition)
  Airway stimulation
  Glossopharyngeal neuralgia
  Drug-induced

NON-CARDIOVASCULAR DISORDERS

Central nervous system substrates
  Seizure disorders
  Subarachnoid hemorrhage
  Narcolepsy
  Hydrocephalus

Metabolic/endocrine disturbances
  Hypoglycaemia
  Volume depletion (dehydration, haemorrhage, Addison's disease, pheo-
    chromocytoma)
  Hypoxaemia
  Hyperventilation (hypocapnia)

Psychiatric disorders
  Panic attacks
  Hysteria

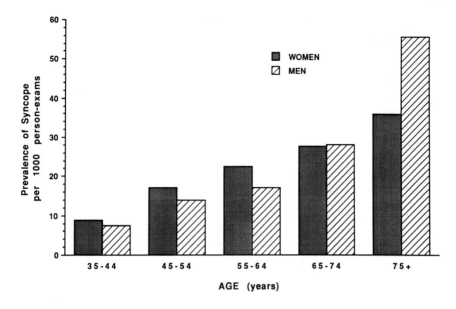

Figure 1. Graph modified from Savage *et al.* (4) illustrating the tendency for syncopal episodes to occur more frequently with increasing age. Results are similar in both women and men

Age-specific syncope prevalance rises with passing years (Figure 1), being particularly notable among individuals over age 65 (4). Further, Framingham data indicated that recurrent syncope was common, a finding additionally supported by the studies of Kapoor *et al.* (5–7). Consequently, given the potential for physical injury as well as the potential costs of disability and subsequent hospitalizations associated with recurrences of syncope, early identification of the cause and institution of appropriate therapy should be a medical priority (6,8,9).

Cardiac, vascular and neurological disease occur frequently in older individuals and are common possible contributors to syncopal events. Indeed, Kapoor *et al.* (6) indicated that in their experience 'mortality and incidence of sudden death were most likely determined by underlying cardiovascular diseases regardless of recurrences of syncope'. This view seems to be supported by findings in their original report (5) in which patients with syncope and associated cardiovascular disease were significantly older (72% greater than 55 years of age), and exhibited a higher frequency of congestive heart failure, ventricular arrhythmias, atrial fibrillation and left ventricular hypertrophy than did patients with syncope unassociated with cardiovascular disorders. On the other hand, in a selected group of elderly individuals with syncope admitted to a medical intensive care unit, subsequent 1-year mortality has been estimated to be 50% higher than that expected of an age-matched cohort (10). Clearly, the independent role syncope may play in determining subsequent mortality is a topic which warrants further study.

PATHOPHYSIOLOGY OF SYNCOPE IN THE ELDERLY

It has been estimated that maintenance of consciousness requires cerebral oxygen (O_2) delivery of at least 3.5 ml O_2 per 100 g tissue each minute (11,12). In the healthy young to middle-aged individual, cerebral blood flow averages 50–60 ml/min per 100 g tissue, and in the absence of severe hypoxemia O_2 requirements are easily achieved. Further, maintenance of this necessary level of blood flow is achieved over a relatively wide range of perfusion pressures due to the 'autoregulatory' features of the cerebrovascular bed (13). Additionally, in the healthy younger individual cerebral blood flow is also maintained by various compensatory and control mechanisms. Thus, diminished oxygen tension (pO_2) or elevated carbon dioxide tension (pCO_2) results in cerebral vasodilation, while the carotid baroreceptors provide protection for cerebral perfusion by altering heart rate and adjusting systemic vascular resistance to accommodate for hypotensive states. Finally, vascular volume is protected by normal renal function (usually unimpeded by drugs) in conjunction with hormonal influences, particularly those attributable to the renin–angiotensin–aldosterone system and vasopressin.

In the elderly patient, many of the compensatory and protective mechanisms associated with the more youthful cerebrovascular bed may become compromised. Ageing alone has been associated with diminution of cerebral blood flow by up to 25% between ages 20 and 70 years (14,15), while hypertension, a common accompaniment of the ageing process, is associated with a shift of the autoregulatory curve to higher pressures (Figure 2). Additionally, coexisting diseases may contribute to a less effective compensatory response. For example, diabetes alters the chemoresponsiveness of the cerebrovascular bed (16). Finally, the carotid baroreceptors become functionally less reliable with age. It has been pointed out that the carotid baroreceptors are less sensitive to either phenylephrine-induced blood pressure increases or negative pressure or drug-induced hypotension in the elderly (17). Thus, compensatory heart rate and vascular changes may be inadequate to adjust for even such relatively transient disturbances as postural change, cough, straining or dehydration, let alone more serious problems such as arrhythmias or haemorrhage. On the other hand, from time to time the carotid baroreceptors appear to be overactive in the older patient and may contribute to transient neurological disturbances (18–24). The latter circumstance, commonly termed 'carotid sinus syndrome', may occur randomly or may be contributed to by altered structure in the head and neck blood vessels such as may occur in patients who have undergone neck surgery and/or irradiation (Figure 3).

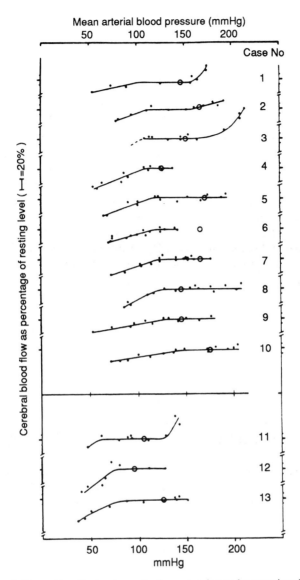

Figure 2. Graph illustrating the tendency for hypertension to be associated with a shift of the cerebrovascular autoregulatory curve to higher pressures. The ordinate depicts cerebral blood flow as a percentage of resting level in hypertensive patients (top) and normal blood pressure subjects (bottom). The unfilled circle indicates each patient's usual mean blood pressure. Reprinted with permission from Stransgaard S, Olesen J, Skinhoj E, Lassen NA. Autoregulation of brain circulation in severe arterial hypertension. *Brit Med J* 1973; 1:507–510

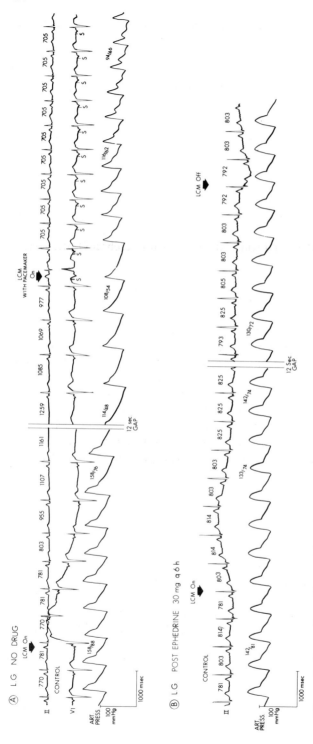

Figure 3. Recordings illustrating the cardioinhibitory and vasodepressor components in an elderly patient with carotid sinus hypersensitivity and suspected carotid sinus syndrome. (A) Recordings from top to bottom are ECG leads II and V1, and arterial pressure. Cardiac cycle length is indicated in milliseconds. The arrow at the top left indicates initiation of left-sided carotid sinus message (LCM). Subsequent bradycardia and marked drop in systemic pressure are noted. The nadir of the systemic pressure occurred approximately 14 s after onset of LCM. At the right, atrial pacing was initiated at a cycle length of 705 ms. Despite the maintenance of both rate and AV synchrony, substantial hypotension persisted. (B) ECG lead II and arterial pressure recordings from the same patient as in panel A. In this case left-sided carotid massage was conducted following treatment with oral ephedrine. Both the cardioinhibitory and vasodepressor components were eliminated. The left-hand arrow indicates onset of a vigorous period of carotid massage lasting more than 20 s. Carotid massage of this duration is not usually recommended, but was used in this case to further confirm the efficacy of ephedrine in this individual patient

Diminution of cerebral O_2 delivery below minimum requirements for 10 seconds or longer may be expected to be accompanied by loss of both consciousness and postural tone, while briefer periods may initiate a transient sensation of imminent loss of consciousness (25). Due to the physiological changes associated with ageing, and especially in the presence of concomitant medical conditions which may further reduce cardiac output, diminish cerebrovascular flow, and/or decrease the O_2-carrying capacity of blood, the brain's nutrient flow is far more tenuous in the older patient than is the case in youth. Lipsitz (26) provided a clearly illustration of the potential for multiple factors to tip the balance against adequate cerebral perfusion in the elderly patient. He notes that cerebral blood flow averages 50 ml/min per 100 g tissue in healthy individuals over 75 years of age, but is only in the 40 ml/min range in elderly hospitalized patients with hypertension or atherosclerotic disease. In the presence of lower baseline blood flow, concomitant anaemia and/or hypoxia may substantially diminish the usual wide safety factor for cerebral O_2 delivery.

CLINICAL CONDITIONS ASSOCIATED WITH SYNCOPE IN THE ELDERLY PATIENT

Clinical conditions contributing to syncope may be broadly classified as cardiovascular and non-cardiovascular in origin (Table 1). The former primarily includes syncope due to: (i) cardiac and pulmonary disease; (ii) vascular disease; and (iii) neurally mediated reflex disturbances. Non-cardiovascular aetiologies encompass: (i) structural central nervous system (CNS) substrates; (ii) metabolic and endocrine disturbances; and (iii) psychiatric disorders. It should be kept in mind, however, that there are important overlaps among the categories. Thus, syncope associated with aortic stenosis has well-known neural reflex contributions (27,28). The same may also be true for syncope thought to be primarily 'orthostatic' in origin.

Syncope of cardiovascular origin

Cardiac/pulmonary disease

Mechanical disturbances (obstruction/inadequate flow)
Syncope, occurring as a result of obstruction to left ventricular outflow (e.g. aortic stenosis, hypertrophic obstructive cardiomyopathy) is typically associated with physical exertion. The mechanism of the faint may be due in part to inadequate blood flow as a result of mechanical obstruction, but ventricular mechanoreceptor-mediated bradycardia and vasodilatation may be an equally important contributor (27,28). The latter mechanism appears to be triggered from mechanoreceptors in the ventricular walls, and utilizes neural reflex pathways discussed in more detail below. In the case of obstructive cardiomyopathy, an entity which has become of greater concern in the elderly

population (29), the spontaneous occurrence of atrial tachyarrhythmias may also be associated with diminution of forward flow and thereby contribute directly to a syncopal event.

Left ventricular inflow obstruction may also provoke syncope on exertion in patients with mitral stenosis, or at unpredictable times in patients with atrial myxoma. However, these conditions are relatively uncommon causes of syncope. More often, the older patient may suffer a syncopal episode in conjunction with acute myocardial ischaemia or infarction (30,31), due to either transient reduction of cardiac output, neural reflex mechanisms, cardiac arrhythmias, or a combination of these and other factors. According to Pathy (30), syncope was a presenting symptom of acute myocardial infarction in 7% of older patients (age > 65 years). Other acute medical conditions such as pulmonary embolism or pericardial tamponade also need to be considered. Right ventricular outflow obstruction and/or right-to-left shunting secondary to pulmonic stenosis or pulmonary hypertension may also cause syncope, but these are vanishingly rare in the elderly population.

Rhythm disturbances

Cardiac rhythm disturbances are among the most frequent and potentially hazardous causes of syncope and dizziness in all age groups. In the elderly patient, bradyarrhythmias due to sinus node dysfunction and/or conduction system disease are important considerations. However, ventricular tachyarrhythmias are at least as frequent, and may be of even greater prognostic importance. Additionally, supraventricular tachyarrhythmias may cause symptomatic hypotension, although relatively infrequently.

Sinus node dysfunction Disturbances of 'sinus node function' encompass a variety of sinotrial, atrial and at times atrioventricular (AV) electrophysiological abnormalities (32–36). Thus, electrocardiographic (ECG) manifestations of sinus node dysfunction (SND) may include severe sinus bradycardia, sinus pauses or sinus arrest, sinoatrial exit block, chronic atrial tachyarrhythmias, and alternating periods of atrial bradyarrhythmias and tachyarrhythmias. Additionally, increasing recognition of exertional symptoms due to abnormal heart rate responses during physical exercise or emotional stress (so-called 'chronotropic incompetence') provides another facet to sinoatrial disease (37–39).

Clinical manifestations of SND vary widely. Many individuals with ECG evidence of SND are essentially asymptomatic, while others exhibit a range of complaints as a result of persistent or intermittent diminution of blood flow to critical organ systems, particularly the brain. The latter may be the result of inappropriate bradycardia, paroxysmal tachycardias or repetitive embolic events. Thus syncope and dizziness may be manifestations of SND. However, inasmuch as these symptoms are transient events, it is usually difficult to substantiate a causal relationship between symptom occurrence and ECG findings. Further, the range of normal ECG findings and heart rate variations observed in health, and especially in the elderly population, complicate unequivocal identification of SND. Consequently, many elderly patients with symptomatic SND may go undiagnosed unless an extremely vigorous evaluation is undertaken.

Conduction system disease Cardiac conduction system disease is common in elderly patients, and accounts for approximately one-half of permanent pacemaker implantations in Western countries (40,41). In the USA alone, it has been estimated that 50 000 new cases of complete heart block occur annually, and that syncope is associated with 50% of these cases (42). In the older individual, structural disturbances of the cardiac conduction system may be the result of acute ischaemic syndromes, as well as the effects of long-standing atherosclerotic disease, cardiomyopathy, hypertension and valvular heart disease. However, not infrequently the aetiology cannot be specified and a chronic degenerative process is assumed. As a rule, the pathology of the conduction system in patients exhibiting the more chronic disease states tends towards widespread fibrosis, and exists in concert with regional or generalized myocardial disease. Thus, patients with conduction system disorders often exhibit the substrate for other arrhythmias (particularly ventricular tachyarrhythmias), and not infrequently it is these tachyarrhythmias rather than AV block which account for symptoms. Finally, it must always be borne in mind that concomitant drug treatment (e.g. cardiac glycosides, β-adrenergic blockers, calcium channel blockers and membrane-active antiarrhythmics) may contribute to symptomatic conduction system disturbances.

Electrophysiological testing for evaluation of conduction disturbances is discussed in more detail below. However, it is important to note that in the absence of a clear-cut association between spontaneous symptoms and bradycardia (e.g. during ambulatory ECG monitoring) the presence of ECG evidence of conduction system disease should not lead to the assumption that the cause of symptoms has been determined. As alluded to above, susceptibility to ventricular tachyarrhythmias is common in patients with conduction system disease. In fact, up to one-quarter of syncope patients with pre-existing bundle branch block have been shown to exhibit inducible sustained ventricular tachycardia (including macro-bundle re-entry) during programmed electrical stimulation of the heart (43,44). Furthermore, among 30 patients (ages 55–63 years) with chronic bifascicular block and syncope reported by Dhingra *et al.* (45), the ultimate cause of symptoms was determined to be ventricular tachycardia in nine (30%) and AV block in five (17%). A variety of aetiologies comprised the remaining diagnoses, with no cause being identified in nine (30%) cases. On the other hand, in one study evaluating results of electrophysiological testing in syncope patients with bundle branch block over 75 years of age (46), only 5% manifested ventricular tachycardia, while 68% were believed (but not proven) to have manifested susceptibility to bradyarrhythmias as evidenced by H–V interval prolongation (65–130 ms, mean 88 ms). Probably the H–V interval measurement was misleading in many of these cases, underscoring the importance of a thorough electrophysiological assessment during the diagnostic evaluation of these patients.

Supraventricular and ventricular tachyarrhythmias Abrupt onset of tachyarrhythmias may be accompanied by hypotension with consequent dizziness or syncope. The latter might be especially anticipated in the individual with coexisting cardiac or vascular disease, particularly if onset of arrhythmia occurs when the patient is in the upright posture.

As a rule, supraventricular tachyarrthythmias (SVT) are only infrequently implicated as causes of syncope among patients referred for electrophysiological assessment of syncope of unknown origin. In a survey of published studies incorporating patients of all ages, Camm and Lau (47) concluded that SVT accounted for only 8% of diagnoses. In the older patient group, in whom inducible atrial fibrillation and flutter are relatively common, this number is probably even lower. Indeed, Sugrue *et al.* (46) were unable to attribute symptoms to SVT in any of their elderly patients, although 10% exhibited atrial fibrillation or flutter in the laboratory.

Among the various causes of cardiac syncope, the ventricular tachycardias are the most frequent and serious. The overview provided by Camm and Lau (47) suggests a causal frequency of 20% among syncope patients of all ages. This percentage may be even higher among older patients in whom the prevalance of concomitant heart disease is high. On the other hand, ventricular arrhythmias occur commonly in older patients. Evidence of this is provided by Camm *et al.* (48), who noted that 30% of 106 asymptomatic individuals over 75 years of age had high-grade ventricular arrhythmias, with 6% exhibiting runs. These findings are additionally supported by Fleg and Kennedy (49), who reported occurrence of ventricular tachycardia in 4% of 98 patients aged 60–85 years. Consequently, the mere presence of ventricular tachycardia does not provide a definitive diagnostic endpoint in the older patient undergoing assessment for syncope. As is the case with other diagnoses, careful symptom correlation is crucial.

Programmed electrical stimulation of the heart during electrophysiological testing has proved highly effective for eliciting susceptibility to ventricular tachyarrhythmias in patients with structural heart disease. Although the specificity of such testing is uncertain in the elderly, the procedure has proved safe and as a consequence can contribute importantly to both the establishment of a diagnosis and assessment of therapy. However, certain forms of ventricular tachycardia may not be amenable to study in this fashion. For instance, conventional stimulation techniques are not typically able to identify susceptibility to 'torsades de pointe', while pause-dependent ventricular tachycardia (such as is often associated with proarrhythmic effects of certain antiarrhythmic drugs) (Figure 4) may only come to light if 'long–short' stimulation sequences are employed.

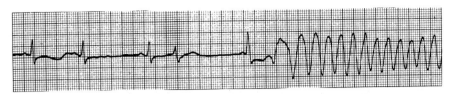

Figure 4. Electrocardiographic rhythm strip illustrating initiation of a pause-dependent ventricular tachycardia in an older patient. This individual was being treated with a type IC antiarrhythmic agent for control of paroxysmal primary atrial tachyarrhythmias. Recurrent syncopal spells became a new clinical problem, and were attributed to non-sustained polymorphus ventricular tachycardia

Orthostatic/autonomic vascular control disturbances

Symptomatic hypotension associated with movement to the upright posture may be the consequence of: (i) transient or chronic diminution of intravascular volume; and/or (ii) abnormal vasomotor compensatory mechanisms of various aetiologies. In either case presyncope or syncope can occur. In fact, such occurrences are believed to be quite common in elderly individuals, having been reported to be present in one-third to one-half of those over 75 years of age, with institutionalized patients tending to be even more susceptible (50,51).

Diminution of intravascular volume Actual or relative central vascular volume depletion with consequent abrupt onset of posturally related symptomatic hypotension is probably one of the most common causes of syncope and dizziness in elderly patients. Iatrogenic factors such as excessive diuresis or overly aggressive use of antihypertensive agents are common contributors. Environmental factors (e.g. excessive heat), diminished mobility and/or a reduced appetite may preclude the physically impaired older patient from achieving sufficient intake to maintain circulatory homeostasis. Additionally, complications associated with other medical conditions (e.g. haemorrhage, third space fluid loss, dehydration) may tip the balance. Less commonly, disease processes resulting in adrenal insufficiency, diabetes insipidus or hyperglycaemia, among others, may provoke the same result.

Abnormal vasomotor compensation Postural hypotension in the presence of an intact compensatory neural reflex response would be expected to produce tachycardia, diaphoresis and peripheral vasoconstriction, resulting in pallor and cool extremities. In some instances, however, even in the presence of a reasonably intact attempt by the autonomic nervous system to maintain the circulation, abrupt posturally induced central volume depletion may result in a clinical picture reminiscent of neurally mediated hypotension–bradycardia (comparable perhaps to that observed in the second stage of haemorrhage). Thus, absence of tachycardia in association with so-called orthostatic hypotension does not absolutely indicate the presence of an abnormal autonomic–vasomotor compensatory state. Nonetheless, both primary and secondary forms of autonomic nervous system insufficiency occur in elderly patients, and may be responsible for transient neurological symptoms.

Idiopathic orthostatic hypotension due to primary autonomic nervous system dysfunction may occur in the absence of other neurological disturbances, or in association with multiple system involvement (Shy–Drager syndrome). More commonly, however, the disturbance of the autonomic nervous system is secondary in nature—for example, neuropathies of alcohol or diabetic origin, spinal cord lesions, paraneoplastic syndromes, or even prolonged periods of physical inactivity such as occur during hospitalizations. Additionally, a wide range of commonly used vasoactive drugs or sedatives impair neural reflex compensation and increase susceptibility to symptomatic orthostasis.

Neurally mediated reflex syncope
Although neurally mediated reflex syndromes (Table 1) are believed to be the most common source of spontaneous syncope in all age groups, only a few of these syndromes occur frequently (e.g. 'emotional' or vasovagal faint) while most (e.g. carotid sinus syndrome, micturition syncope, cough syncope) are relatively rare. In the older patient, numerous ancillary factors including drug therapy, hypovolaemia, venous insufficiency and chronotropic incompetence may contribute to development of neurally mediated hypotension and bradycardia, and obscure the correct diagnosis. Additionally, the elderly are more likely to exhibit structural cardiac, vascular and neurological disorders than are younger patients. Such findings, although not directly responsible for symptoms, may complicate recognition of the actual aetiological diagnosis.

The 'emotional' or vasovagal faint and carotid sinus hypersensitivity have been the most thoroughly studied of the neurally mediated syncopal syndromes, and clinical and experimental findings in these conditions form the basis for current hypotheses regarding mechanisms of spontaneous hypotension and bradycardia. Essentially, the origin of the afferent signals in each of these conditions appears to be receptors which respond to mechanical stimuli, pain or, less commonly, temperature change. In the so-called vasovagal faint, the most common of the neurally mediated syncopal syndromes, mechanoreceptors (and probably other receptors as well, e.g. chemoreceptors, temperature receptors) located in any of a variety of organ systems appear to provide stimuli initiating a cascade of CNS responses (52–55). In many instances contributing factors such as pain and anxiety are important.

Both venous and arteriolar dilatation appear to be critical to development of symptomatic hypotension in patients with vasovagal episodes. The former directly impairs stroke volume and cardiac output, which drop substantially despite reduced resistance to ejection. The latter directly reduces systemic pressure, and in the presence of a reduced cardiac output probably diminishes the time during which the cerebrovascular bed remains in its autoregulatory range.

For purposes of convenience the neurally mediated syncopal syndromes will be subdivided into (i) the emotional faint, (ii) carotid sinus syndrome, (iii) drug-induced syncope, (iv) various forms of situational syncope and (v) head-up tilt and haemorrhage.

'Emotional' (vasovagal or vasodepressor) faint Numerous factors have been associated with triggering 'emotional' or vasovagal faints in susceptible individuals, including noxious smells or unpleasant sights, unanticipated pain, abrupt movement to or prolonged exposure to upright posture, heat, dehydration, physical exercise and venipuncture. As a rule, the temporal sequence of events documented in both spontaneous and tilt table-induced episodes reveal an initial period of moderate but progressive hypotension preceding onset of marked bradycardia (56,57).

Despite the importance of vascular phenomena in the pathophysiology of neurally mediated syncopal syndromes, it is usually the heart rate slowing (especially when extreme) which draws the greatest clinical attention (Figure 5). The latter, although not often documented during spontaneous fainting episodes, has been recorded in some instances. Based on such recordings, it appears likely that asystolic periods of 10–20 seconds (and perhaps longer) are common accompaniments of the emotional faint.

Carotid sinus syncope Carotid sinus stimulation can result in various degrees of sinus bradycardia or pauses, paroxysmal AV block, and vasodilatation with hypotension (Figure 3) (18–24,58). However, the frequency with which carotid sinus hypersensitivity is responsible for syncopal symptoms is uncertain. This difficulty is due in part to the fact that many individuals, especially the elderly, exhibit marked bradycardia with carotid sinus stimulation (carotid sinus hypersensitivity) (20,23), and in part as a result of the complexity of establishing a clear-cut association between spontaneous syncope and demonstrable carotid sinus hypersensitivity (21,22,59–61). Estimates suggest that only 5–20% of patients exhibiting carotid sinus hypersensitivity actually have syncope of carotid sinus origin (19,22,61). Clinically the diagnosis is suspected if the attack is triggered by or associated with turning or extending the neck, tight collars or ties, previous neck surgery or irradiation or in some cases physical exertion. Exclusion of extracranial vascular disease as a cause of syncope is a crucial and often confounding element of the diagnostic evaluation in these patients.

Drug-induced syncope Drug-related effects are among the most common factors triggering syncope in the elderly. Not only are older patients far more likely to be exposed to one or often several agents capable of causing syncope (e.g., nitrates, diuretics, angiotensin-converting enzyme (ACE) inhibitors and other antihypertensives), but their cardiac, vascular and renal compensatory mechanisms are more limited than is the case in younger individuals (62).

In general, drug-induced syncope has been considered primarily a volume

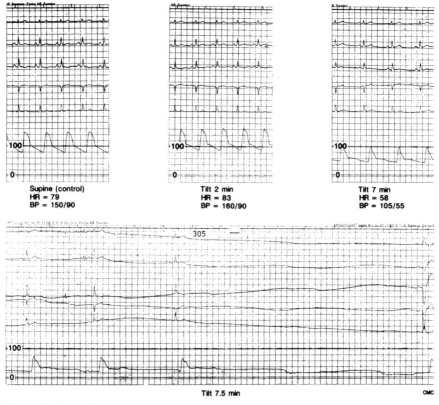

Figure 5. Recordings obtained in a patient undergoing head-up tilt testing for evaluation of susceptibility to neurally mediated syncope. In each of the top panels the timing with respect to the tilt study, heart rate and blood pressure is indicated. It is evident that by 7 min of head-up tilt the patient was exhibiting a marked drop in systemic arterial pressure with only modest bradycardia. In the lower panel (7.5 min of head-up tilt), marked bradycardia and a prolonged asystolic pause occurred. Resumption of the supine posture resulted in prompt recovery

depletion and/or an orthostatic problem. However, neurally mediated reflex hypotension–bradycardia may be an important contributing factor as well. The latter is probably particularly relevant in patients being treated with nitrates for ischaemic heart disease, since nitrates may effect marked venous dilatation with a consequent decrease in the volume of blood returning to the heart. Typically the resulting diminished cardiac output and systemic pressure elicit a compensatory carotid baroreceptor response with initial parasympathetic withdrawal and increasing sympathetic 'drive'. The result is tachycardia accompanied by an enhanced cardiac inotropic state. However, in older patients this compensatory response may be inadequate (perhaps related to diminished carotid baroreceptor sensitivity) and the resulting accentuation of central cardiopulmonary mechanoreceptor afferent activity may be unbalanced and trigger an episode of symptomatic neurally mediated hypotension–bradycardia (18,63–65).

'Situational' syncope A number of syncopal syndromes have been associated with increased intrathoracic pressure, (e.g. cough and sneeze syncope, syncope associated with playing certain musical instruments or lifting heavy objects, straining during bowel movement) (66–69). The basis for these forms of syncope is believed to be primarily related to a critical diminution of systemic venous return with consequent reduction of cardiac output and cerebral blood flow (67). However, other factors may facilitate the faint, especially in the elderly patient. For instance, compensatory attempts to overcome the impact of a diminished stroke volume (in part carotid baroreceptor mediated) may be inadequate. Furthermore, in cough or sneeze syncope a concussive effect may directly activate vascular mechanoreceptors, resulting in more prolonged periods of hypotension than would seem likely if diminished venous return were the sole cause.

Postmicturition syncope is typically thought to occur most frequently as an isolated event in young males, although older males and occasionally females may manifest the disorder (70). The syncopal episode tends to be closely associated with having arisen from sleep to empty the bladder, and occurs a few moments after bladder emptying has been completed. In general, marked bladder distension results in systemic vasoconstriction via a spinal cord reflex, (71,72). The latter is compensated for by baroreceptor diminution of sympathetic activity in an attempt to prevent hypertension in association with bladder distention (72–75). The mechanism of syncope in this setting has been attributed to an excessive or prolonged compensatory response.

Syncope may be associated with defaecation, and other forms of pelvic stimulation. Vagal afferents from the bowel wall transmit impulses from tension receptors, with the frequency of the signals being related to the rapidity of the distention or contraction (76). As a result, defaecation or even bowel instrumentation (e.g. sigmoidoscopy, colonoscopy) may initiate afferent neural signals which trigger symptomatic hypotensive/bradycardia episodes. Defaecation syncope is thought to be a more frequent problem in constipated individuals using laxatives, or in association with the evacuation of a large quantity of stool (77). Thus, elderly patients may tend to be at greater risk.

'Swallow' syncope is rare and usually associated with oesophageal or other pharyngeal abnormalities (3,78–81). Syncope tends to occur during or immediately after swallowing food, although oesophageal spasm may play a role in triggering the neural signals in some patients (81). Furthermore, severe bradycardia during passage of a gastroscope or feeding tube, and syncope associated with swallowing a very cold drink or vomiting, are probably related to 'swallow' syncope (75,82). In all these situations, afferent neural impulses arise in territories subserved by the glossopharyngeal or vagus nerves. In this regard, the glossopharyngeal nerve incorporates afferents from the carotid sinus and the posterior pharyngeal wall (3). Consequently the pain associated with glossopharyngeal neuralgia may trigger hypotension and bradycardia directly (83–85).

Airways stimulation (e.g. during endotracheal intubation) may initiate both marked bradycardia and a substantial vasopressor action and consequently is of particular relevance in the care of older patients. Abrupt exposure of the airways to cold (e.g. cold water) may elicit a similar outcome (75). Neurally mediated hypotension/bradycardia may also occur in association with or immediately following exercise in individuals without apparent structural heart disease, (54,86–91). In general this syndrome has been almost exclusively associated with younger otherwise healthy individuals. However, one report detailed occurrence of an 11-second asystolic pause with a prolonged syncopal event after completion of a maximal treadmill exercise test in a 52-year-old male (86). This patient had apparently experienced a similar event following treadmill exercise 4 years earlier. It is unlikely that many elderly patients are candidates for this form of syncope.

Head-up tilt and haemorrhage-induced hypotension/bradycardia Under normal conditions upright posture is associated with reduced venous return to the heart and a consequent diminution of stroke volume and cardiac output. Concomitant dehydration and/or inefficient dependent venoconstriction (such as may occur in elderly individuals exposed to prolonged bed rest or suffering from venous insufficiency and/or certain neuropathies) would exacerbate these haemodynamic stresses. The normal adaptive response is a combination of tachycardia and vasoconstriction. However, in the ill or older patient compensation may be inadequate, with the result being symptomatic hypotension. Additionally, in susceptible individuals the impact of central volume changes and the resulting compensatory increase in cardiac inotropic state may induce both hypotension and paradoxical bradycardia secondary to afferent signals generated by both carotid sinus baroreceptors and central cardiopulmonary mechanoreceptors (see discussion above). Abrupt haemorrhage may produce a similar scenario. In the latter case, the initial tachycardia associated with blood loss may transform into the so-called 'second' stage of haemorrhage in which marked bradycardia and vasodilatation develop (92–95).

Syncope of non-cardiovascular origin

In patients, especially the elderly, the historical description of transient neurological events may be sufficiently imprecise as to preclude differentiating recurrent syncope or presyncope from other complaints such as dizziness (including vertigo), episodic weakness, transient loss of attentiveness, and seizures. Thus, differential diagnostic considerations in such cases must include a variety of vascular, space-occupying, inflammatory and metabolic disturbances which affect CNS function either directly or indirectly. Only a brief overview of some of the more important conditions is offered here.

Central nervous system substrates

Vascular disease
Transient ischaemic attacks due to vertebrobasilar system insufficiency may cause syncope, although more commonly the presenting symptoms encompass ataxia, diploplia, dysarthria and vertigo. In general, when syncope is associated with a vertebrobasilar aetiology there are also identifiable transient or fixed focal neurological abnormalities. In those cases where a vertebrobasilar aetiology seems likely, the cause may be atherosclerotic narrowings or extrinsic mechanical compression of the vertebral arteries (e.g. cervical spondylosis, cervical osteoarthritis, cervical rib). Mechanical disturbances should receive particular consideration if attacks are associated with positional changes of the head, particularly extension or lateral rotation. The latter history, of course, is also compatible with carotid sinus syndrome (see above).

Subclavian 'steal' syndrome or severe carotid artery disease (e.g. atherosclerotic disease, Takayasu's disease) may be the cause of syncope in some patients. In the former, narrowing of the subclavian artery at its origin results in syncope or dizziness in conjunction with upper extremity exercise as blood is shunted from the brain to the exercising limb via the vertebral artery system. Usually a bruit can be detected over the affected subclavian artery, along with diminution of ipsilateral brachial artery pressure.

Seizures
The incidence of epilepsy increases after age 60 (96), and *de novo* seizure disturbances in elderly patients may result in apparent syncopal symptoms (97). As a rule, differentiation of seizure disorders from syncope may be suggested by the fact that seizures tend to be positionally independent whereas syncope is most commonly associated with upright posture. Additionally, seizures are often preceded by an aura, may be accompanied by convulsive activity and loss of bowel or urinary continence, and are typically followed by a confusional state. On the other hand, occurrence of apparent 'seizure-like' motor activity accompanying transient loss of consciousness should not be considered diagnostic of a primary seizure disturbance, since such activity may be observed in association with transient cerebrovascular hypotension of many aetiologies. However, in the latter cases the motor activity tends to be relatively brief and unassociated with either bladder or bowel incontinence. Conversely, absence of motor activity does not exclude seizures. Although akinetic seizures are more frequent in children, they may occur in the older patient. In such cases the presence of a postictal state may be helpful in suggesting the diagnosis. However, syncope of any aetiology in the older patient may be followed by a lengthy period of confusion mimicking a postictal state.

Metabolic/endocrine disturbances

In general, metabolic/endocrine disturbances are not frequent causes of syncope, but are more often responsible for confusional states or behavioral disturbances.

In the elderly, it is not uncommon for several disease processes to interact, resulting in abnormalities of cerebral nutrient or oxygen supply. Thus, hypoxaemia due to heart failure, pneumonia or pulmonary embolism may compound a chronic anaemia in an ill older patient. Hypoglycaemia or excessive hyperglycaemia could similarly contribute to an altered state of consciousness. Finally, concomitant drug therapy (e.g. diuretics, sedatives and hypnotics) through electrolyte disturbances or accumulation of metabolic products may result in transient neurological disturbances. Retrospectively, it may be difficult to differentiate such symptoms from syncope or presyncope by history alone. As a rule, though, unlike true syncope these conditions do not tend to resolve in the absence of active therapeutic intervention.

Psychiatric disorders

Apparent syncope may be the result of anxiety attacks or hysteria. The former may be associated with hyperventilation and hypocapnia, while the latter tends to be relatively dramatic, occurring in the presence of onlookers and being unassociated with alterations of heart rate, systemic pressure or skin colour. As a rule, the 'psychiatric' aetiologies for 'syncope' tend to be relatively uncommon in older patients. However, in the elderly patient the potential contributing effects of prescribed or over-the-counter drugs on mental state should be kept in mind. For example, sedatives, β-adrenergic blockers or drugs with anticholinergic properties (e.g. certain antidiarrhoeal agents, cold preparations and antiarrhythmics) may have substantial impact on cognitive function in the ill elderly patient. Alcohol also continues to be an important source of morbidity, while other 'recreational' agents may be somewhat less of a problem than is the case in younger individuals.

DIAGNOSTIC METHODS

In most published studies examining the problem of unexplained syncope, the usual diagnostic evaluation includes a detailed medical history and physical examination, haematological and biochemical assessment, 12-lead ECG, and ambulatory ECG recordings (24- or 48-hour, magnetic tape, continuous-loop event recorders). Signal-averaged ECG (SAECG) and exercise testing are also included in some reports. In addition, neurological consultation is often obtained, and usually entails an electroencephalogram (EEG) and either computed axial tomography (CAT) or magnetic resonance imaging (MRI) studies. Individuals in whom the diagnosis is still unclear tend to be referred for invasive cardiac electrophysiological studies (EPS) (44,47,98–107). Finally, head-up tilt testing has recently been introduced and appears to be a particularly useful diagnostic procedure for patients with cardiovascular disease in whom the basis for syncope remains unclear, or as a screening procedure in syncope patients without evident cardiovascular disease (52–55,57).

History and physical examination

A detailed medical history and a thorough physical examination are both crucial to the evaluation of syncopal episodes. Indeed, it has been suggested that these tools alone provide a 'working' diagnosis in more than 60% of cases (26). However, actual confirmation of a suspected diagnosis is far more difficult, and for the most part was not achieved in early studies of syncope patients (5,8). Current clinical practice may be similarly deficient in this regard. Assessment of a syncopal event requires detailed historical information. Apart from the patient's account of the event, witnesses should be sought. In particular, the patient's appearance, evidence of seizure activity, and documentation of the state of respiration and pulse may be queried. Additionally, observations regarding the patient's status prior to the episode may be of value (e.g. general state of health and hydration, rapid assumption of upright posture, abrupt turning of the head and neck). Family members or friends may provide knowledge of medications, alcohol intake or other factors which may have contributed to symptoms. The circumstances surrounding the syncopal episode, prodromal symptoms, the rapidity with which loss of consciousness occurred, its duration and the speed of recovery should be noted. Typically, non-sustained cardiac arrhythmias and transient AV block result in rapid onset and prompt resolution of symptoms. Neurally mediated syncopal syndromes often have prodromes which may include any of a variety of symptoms such as hearing loss, loss of peripheral vision, nausea and diaphoresis. Additionally the history may suggest the diagnosis if the episode was associated with a painful or emotionally upsetting experience, or accompanied abrupt head movement, coughing, micturition or defaecation. As a rule, neurally mediated hypotension-bradycardia resolves relatively rapidly once the patient is supine. However, a confusional state may persist for many minutes, especially in older patients. Thus, a clear history may not be obtainable, and the presence of the confusional state may in fact mistakenly suggest a postictal picture following a seizure disturbance.

Physical examination at the time of syncope would be helpful, but for obvious reasons is not often possible. Nonetheless, bystanders may provide a description of the patient and perhaps some documentation of the rate, regularity and strength of the peripheral pulse. Thus, marked pallor in conjunction with a slow feeble pulse may lead to suspicion of a neurally mediated reflex syncopal syndrome. Cyanosis and/or tachypnoea would on the other hand lead to a completely different set of considerations. Examination subsequent to the syncopal event should assess susceptibility to orthostatic hypotension, bearing in mind that healthy elderly individuals often exhibit a 20–40 mmHg drop of systolic pressure (26). Additionally, the status of the carotid vessels must be assessed, often with the aid of ultrasonic studies or other imaging techniques. Physical examination of the carotid upstroke may be misleadingly brisk in older patients with valvular heart disease (26). Consequently, the echocardiogram has become an essential tool in the initial assessment of the functional importance of suspected valve lesions, as well as for assessment of ventricular function and exclusion of pericardial disease and intracardiac tumours. The role of measures such as carotid sinus massage and Valsalva manoeuvre is less certain at this stage. Inasmuch as these tests are best conducted with the aid of both ECG monitoring and arterial pressure recordings, they are probably better reserved for inclusion as part of a complete battery of autonomic studies (including head-up tilt testing, see later).

Haematological and biochemical studies

Routine batteries of haematological and biochemical studies, while always carried out, only rarely pay dividends. Selective testing, based on the history and physical examination, is more prudent. Thus, in the older patient with a history suggestive of acute or chronic gastrointestinal bleeding, the presence of anaemia and/or occult blood in the stool may provide a remediable cause of syncope. In patients taking diuretics or who are being treated for hypertension or cardiac disease, electrolyte disturbances may be clinically relevant, especially if a cardiac arrhythmia is suspected. Similarly, assessment of blood glucose in the diabetic patient may provide a tentative diagnosis. On the whole, however, such studies must be interpreted carefully in light of the medical history surrounding symptomatic events.

Electrocardiographic recordings

ECG recordings (particularly long-term ambulatory recordings) may be of value by documenting underlying conduction system disease and/or arrhythmias, and on occasion by fortuitous capture of an arrhythmic basis for syncopal symptoms. The latter, although rare, could provide a definitive diagnosis and for the most part obviate further evaluation. However, even in such instances the question remains whether the dysrhythmia is due to underlying structural heart or conduction system disease, or the result of a functional disturbance such as one of the neurally mediated mechanisms discussed above.

In general the role of the 12-lead ECG in assessment of patients with recurrent syncope is limited to the initial search for evidence of underlying cardiac disease. However, such findings only rarely contribute directly to identification of a specific diagnosis. Thus, certain uncommon ECG findings such as ventricular pre-excitation or Q–T interval prolongation may directly suggest a mechanism for syncope, whereas common findings such as sinus bradycardia and bifascicular block are more often than not unrelated to the cause of symptoms. The lack of specificity of the 12-lead ECG is a particular problem in elderly patients, in whom baseline ECG abnormalities are more frequent than is the case in younger individuals.

The role of the SAECG in evaluation of patients with syncope is as yet ill defined. An abnormal SAECG in a patient with structural heart disease raises suspicion of the substrate for ventricular tachyarrhythmias. Unfortunately, a large percentage of elderly individuals may show such abnormalities due to a relatively high prevalence of heart disease. Further critical assessment of this technique is required.

Obtaining ECG documentation of symptomatic arrhythmia, if possible at all, usually requires repetitive or 'continuous' ECG recording techniques. In general, this approach is neither convenient nor particularly cost-effective. Further, it entails exposing the patient to the potential harm associated with recurrent symptoms. Overall, unless symptoms are very frequent, the conventional 24-hour or 48-hour ambulatory ECG ('Holter type') is not a very effective tool. This is probably even truer for evaluation of syncope than for assessment of symptomatic arrhythmias. A further problem with ambulatory ECG monitoring is that many 'abnormalities' of heart rhythm are present in the general population (e.g. sinus pauses, second-degree Mobitz type I AV block), and particularly in the elderly (48,108–112). Thus, detection of certain abnormalities, unless clearly associated with symptoms, cannot be considered unequivocally diagnostic. For instance, asymptomatic sinus pauses of > 2 seconds have been reported to occur in up to 11% of patients undergoing ambulatory ECG monitoring, and are even more common in trained athletes. In regard to longer pauses, both Ector et al. (113) and Hilgard et al. (114) noted that pauses of > 3 second were uncommon during ambulatory monitoring (2.4% and 0.8% of patients, respectively), but differed on their significance. Ector et al. (113) indicated that pauses of this duration were usually associated with symptoms, whereas Hilgard et al. (114) found the opposite, and further indicated that prognosis was unaltered by pacing. On the other hand, ambulatory ECG evidence for Mobitz type II AV block, sustained or non-sustained ventricular tachycardia, or torsades de pointe, carries stronger diagnostic weight, although doubts may persist even with these arrhythmias in the absence of concomitant symptoms.

Since syncopal symptoms tend to be infrequent, the most useful long-term portable ECG monitors are those of the 'event' recorder type (115). These systems can be employed in a 'continuous-loop' mode for patients whose symptoms preclude responding appropriately when the episode begins. However, important limitations remain. For instance, the need for daily replacement of, and the skin irritation associated with, long-term skin electrodes may discourage compliance. Furthermore, if the patient is unconscious for a prolonged period of time (1 minute or more), current devices will not be triggered in sufficient time to save from 'memory' the cardiac rhythm at the initiation of symptoms. The benefit of the recording will have been lost. Perhaps development of longer-term recorders (possibly implantable in some instances), capable of detecting both haemodynamic and ECG events, will circumvent some of these limitations.

Exercise testing is of limited utility in the evaluation of syncope. In rare instances it may permit detection of rate-dependent AV block, or exertionally related tachyarrhythmias (86). Additionally, certain forms of neurally mediated syncope associated with exertion may come to light (54,89,91). However, unless the history clearly implicates exertion, exercise testing is not particularly valuable, especially in evaluation of the older syncope patient.

Clinical cardiac electrophysiological studies

As noted above, careful evaluation of the medical history, physical examination and non-invasive laboratory findings may lead to a presumptive diagnosis in many patients. However, the term 'presumptive' needs to be emphasized, particularly in the elderly patient population where many possible 'causes' of syncope might be discovered. Consequently, additional supportive diagnostic information is often required, and invasive clinical electrophysiological studies (EPS) and/or autonomic function testing may be indicated.

Conventional EPS comprise specialized methods of intracardiac recording and electrical stimulation to assess the status of both the sinoatrial node and the cardiac conduction system, and evaluate susceptibility to inducible supraventricular and ventricular brady- and tachyarrhythmias. Comprehensive reviews of EPS techniques, their indications and limitations have been published elsewhere (36,116–118). Such testing may lead to the establishment of a potential basis for syncopal symptoms in a patient in whom non-invasive techniques have been entirely unsuccessful, or in whom doubt remains. In general, the EPS approach has proved most helpful for defining probable arrhythmic causes of syncope in those patients with underlying congenital or acquired structural heart disease. On the other hand, EPS has been less successful among patients without overt structural substrate for arrhythmia (98–100). The latter group is probably primarily comprised of individuals with various forms of neurally mediated syncope who are more likely to be identified by autonomic function testing (see below). Table 2 summarizes reported results of EPS diagnostic testing in patients with syncope of otherwise uncertain origin, with an emphasis on those studies in whom a substantial number of older patients were included.

Despite the apparent utility of EPS in the evaluation of syncope, it is important to keep in mind the possibility that elderly patients, especially those with coexisting heart disease, may manifest abnormal EPS findings which are not clinically relevant. Furthermore, EPS testing may fail to identify a subtle or fastidious abnormality (107), or discern the haemodynamic significance of a finding (119). In regard to the former problem, Fujimura et al. (107) reported EPS findings in 21 patients (mean age 63 ± 13 years) with documented symptomatic bradyarrhythmias (AV block, 13; sinus pauses, eight). Of the 13 patients with AV conduction system disturbances, EPS provided a corresponding abnormality in only two patients (sensitivity 15.4%), whereas unrelated abnormalities were quite frequent. In the subgroup of patients with sinus pauses, EPS correctly identified the problem in three of eight (sensitivity 37.5%), while a further three patients were found to have abnormalities unrelated to the

Table 2. Electrophysiological (EP) testing in syncope of unknown origin

Reference	Number of patients	Number with heart disease	Overall EP positive	EP-positive with heart disease	EP-positive without heart disease
(100)	30	18	16 (53%)	15 (83%)	1 (8%)
(105)	53	38	30 (57%)	27 (71%)	3 (20%)
(156)	150	75	112 (75%)	64 (85%)	48 (64%)
(120)	94	42	26 (28%)	16 (38%)	10 (20%)
Total	327	173	184 (56%)	122 (71%)	62 (36%)

Adapted from Camm and Lau (47).

documented spontaneous arrhythmia. Therefore, the specificity and sensitivity of EPS testing in syncope patients needs further assessment, and the presence of an abnormality needs to be interpreted cautiously.

Sinus node dysfunction

The sensitivity of EPS for detection of SND is variable, being reported to range from 35% to 100% for sinus node recovery time (SNRT) measurements alone, and from 15% to 75% for sinoatrial conduction time (SACT) alone, with an estimated combined sensitivity of 70% (36). Thus, the usually employed sinus node function tests may be expected to miss a substantial number of bona fide SND cases. On the other hand, the estimated combined specificity of these tests is in the range of 90% (36), suggesting that a positive test is probably important in the context of identifying the presence of SND. However, in the elderly, the identification of SND by EPS does not guarantee a causative role in patients' symptoms. Careful assessment of all clinically related data is essential before a conclusion can be drawn.

There is some reason to believe that the greater the abnormality detected during sinus node function testing, the greater the likelihood of both a bradycardic origin for symptoms and a positive response to cardiac pacing (35,120). However, this point is not well established, and in our view sinus node function abnormalities can be misleading. Specifically, available evidence suggests a relatively poor correspondence between identified EPS abnormalities of SND function and the documented type of symptomatic spontaneous arrhythmia in those cases where such a comparison has been possible. For instance, Strauss *et al.* (121) reported that abnormal SNRT prolongation was

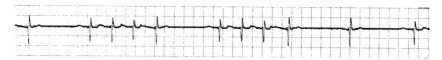

Figure 6. Rhythm strip illustrating occurrence of both intermittent atrial tachycardia and bradycardia in an elderly patient with recurrent dizzy spells and sick sinus syndrome. Subsequent evaluation revealed the dizzy spells to be closely correlated with prolonged episodes of sustained bradycardia. Cardiac pacing with a rate-adaptive dual-chamber pacemaker (DDDR mode) was utilized in conjunction with antiarrhythmic drug therapy. The patient has been asymptomatic since initiation of treatment

more frequent than SACT abnormalities, whether the spontaneous arrhythmia was a presumed disturbance of automaticity (i.e. sinus pause) or a disturbance of sinoatrial conduction (i.e., sinoatrial exit block). Furthermore, in patients with SND and prolonged SNRT, it is possible that spontaneous symptoms could result from either intermittent tachycardia or post-tachycardia pauses (Figure 6). Thus, despite the fact that EPS may be helpful in identifying the presence of SND, doubt may remain as to whether bradycardia or tachycardia is the source of symptoms.

The prognostic attributes of sinus node function testing remain incompletely explored. Gann *et al.* (122) followed the clinical course (mean 4.6 years) of 103 patients with sinus bradycardia in whom corrected SNRT (CSNRT) was measured on entry into the study. Thirty-five patients were asymptomatic initially. Of these 35 individuals, 11 had abnormal CSNRT and seven of these 11 patients (64%) required pacemaker therapy. On the other hand, of the 24/35 patients with normal CSNRT, a lesser number (7/35, 29%) eventually needed pacemakers. Among symptomatic patients (dizziness, syncope), 30/68 had abnormal CSNRT and 26 ultimately needed pacemakers (although one of these continued to have symptoms). Of the 38 patients with normal CSNRT, a smaller but still substantial number of patients (16/38) were eventually paced. Thus, we can conclude that abnormal sinus node function testing in patients with dizziness or syncope without other explanation has a high specificity and suggests that cardiac pacing will be beneficial. However, a normal CSNRT does not exclude this possibility. Additional similar studies are essential in order to confirm these observations.

Conduction system disease

EPS testing in patients with syncope is probably diagnostic if infra-Hisian block can be demonstrated, and no other abnormalities surface. However, more commonly only suggestive evidence of potentially symptomatic conduction system disease is obtained, with the clinical decision resting upon the duration of the H–V interval (i.e. the interval of time taken for a cardiac electrical impulse to traverse the His bundle and initiate ventricular excitation, typical normal values being 35–55 ms). There has been considerable controversy surrounding interpretation of this value. Nonetheless, the findings of Scheinman *et al.* (123) suggest that an H–V interval of >70 ms is of modest concern (approximately a 12% progression to high-grade AV block in 3 years), whereas an H–V interval of >100 ms is clearly worrisome (24% progression to complete heart block in 3-year follow-up).

Relying solely on H–V interval measurements to identify pacemaker candidates must be tempered by the fact that, among the studies which have examined the predictive value of the H–V interval, relatively few syncope patients have been studied and followed. Consequently, the implications of these reports in the subgroup of elderly syncope patients is not clear. Perhaps strict reliance on the 100 ms benchmark may result in certain patients with symptomatic conduction system disease being overlooked. Therefore, additional provocative measures are warranted, such as 'stressing' the conduction system by atrial pacing and/or infusion of an antiarrhythmic drug (e.g., procainamide) in order to unmask susceptibility to infra-Hisian block (124,125). In the case of atrial pacing, Dhingra *et al.* (124) found a strong correlation between pacing-induced infra-Hisian block and subsequent development of spontaneous high-grade AV block, suggesting that such an observation in a patient with syncope warrants pacemaker implantation. Alternatively, the important association between HV interval prolongation, heart disease and susceptibility to tachyarrhythmias should not be forgotten (43,44). Thus, tachycardia (especially ventricular tachyarrhythmias) rather than bradycardia may be the cause of syncope in many of these individuals, and must be excluded as much as possible prior to proceeding with prophylactic pacing.

Supraventricular tachyarrhythmias

As a rule, paroxysmal supraventricular tachycardias (PSVT) are relatively rare causes of syncope. However, a rapid heart rate of any aetiology in the elderly patient may be associated with marked hypotension, especially at the onset of the attack. The latter may be particularly likely if the patient is in the upright posture and/or has concomitant cardiac or vascular disease. Susceptibility to PSVT may often be demonstrated during EPS, and the mechanism elucidated. In the elderly patient, primary atrial tachycardias (e.g. paroxysmal atrial fibrillation or flutter) and re-entry within the AV node tend to be the more frequent aetiologies. Nonetheless, PSVT utilizing accessory connections of congenital origin are observed from time to time.

During EPS, the haemodynamic significance of induced PSVT may not be readily apparent unless continuous intra-arterial pressure recordings are obtained. Subjecting patients to upright posture (by use of a tilt table) during the arrhythmia can also be of crucial diagnostic value (119). Under such conditions, an increase in tachycardia rate and/or a marked fall in systemic pressure may provide conclusive support for the tachyarrhythmia being the source of dizziness or syncope.

Apart from the diagnostic value of EPS in patient with symptomatic PSVT, these studies are often useful for optimizing therapy. Given the potential risks associated with syncope in the elderly, there is little room for empirical treatment in this setting. EPS offers the opportunity to assess pharmacological management directly, and provides the information necessary to recognize when transcatheter or surgical ablative procedures may be appropriate.

Ventricular tachyarrhythmias

Induction of ventricular tachycardia (VT) during EPS evaluation of syncope has been interpreted to provide a presumptive diagnosis in approximately 20% of cases (47). In particular, EPS-induced sustained monomorphic VT is highly suggestive of a basis for syncope (104,105), with almost all reported cases responding to EPS-directed therapy with symptom remission. On the other hand, induction of only non-sustained or polymorphic VT or ventricular fibrillation is of doubtful significance (105). In the case of non-sustained VT, Morady *et al.* (105) noted failure to suppress symptoms in almost 40% of patients. It is essential to consider that elderly patients with a high prevalence of heart disease may readily manifest inducible VT, and consequently the clinical significance of this observation must be carefully viewed in light of the patient's medical history and ancillary findings.

The aggressiveness of the stimulation protocol is an important determinant of the specificity of EPS techniques when applied to the assessment of VT susceptibility. In fact, induction of 'non-clinical' ventricular tachyarrhythmias has been reported in up to 45% of patients in whom such an observation was entirely unexpected (126–130), suggesting the importance of not 'over-interpreting' the results. On the other hand, certain forms of VT, such as torsades de pointe, are well known to cause syncopal symptoms, yet are not usually amenable to EPS induction. Overall, in the case of the 'search' for a potential but previously undocumented VT in a syncope patient, most centres now restrict the level of provocation to a maximum of two extrastimuli from two ventricular sites in an attempt to preserve specificity of the test. Additionally, 'long–short' interval stimulation may be included in those cases where 'pause-dependent' VT is suspected. The role of catecholamine infusion is less certain, but may be beneficial if clinical circumstances strongly favour a tachyarrhythmia aetiology. Finally, in certain cases where a proarrhythmic event may be suspected, restudy on the probable 'offending' agent may be necessary.

Autonomic testing for neurally mediated syncopal syndromes

Head-up tilt testing in conjunction with other tests of autonomic neural control, such as carotid sinus massage, and Valsalva manoeuvre, are the most commonly employed techniques for evaluation of susceptibility to neurally mediated syncopal syndromes. Lower body negative pressure techniques, while of physiological importance, have not been adequately evaluated in the clinical setting. Assessment of observed intrinsic heart rate may also be used to evaluate the relative predominance of parasympathetic and sympathetic control on sinus node and AV node electrophysiological properties (36). Additionally, estimation of circulating blood volume and its distribution has been advocated in some studies, although its clinical utility has recently been questioned (131).

The physiological responses to upright posture during tilt table testing have been the subject of study for some time, particularly in aviation and aerospace environments. Only recently, however, has head-up tilt testing become a standard technique for assessing susceptibility to neurally mediated reflex syncopal syndromes (52,54,57,132–142). The rationale for upright tilt testing in this setting is evident from the discussion provided previously of the physiological effects of upright posture, and its role in eliciting neural reflex activity believed critical to initiating hypotension and bradycardia. Based on similarities between their clinical and neuroendocrine features, it seems reasonable to conclude that the hypotension/bradycardia induced by head-up tilt provides a model of spontaneous neurally mediated 'vasovagal' syndromes (52,57,139). However, the manner in which tilt testing is conducted in the clinical laboratory will markedly affect its sensitivity and specificity as a diagnostic tool in patients undergoing evaluation for syncope. Methodological considerations including tilt table design, tilt angle, duration of the procedure and other factors are currently the subject of active study, and their discussion is beyond the scope of this review.

Observations on the use of head-up tilt testing in evaluation of patients with unexplained syncope

The neural reflexes thought responsible for neurally mediated syncopal syndromes appear to be universally present in humans. Although evidence suggests that age may diminish sensitivity of these reflexes (9,143), these findings are disputed (144) and it is evident that reflex activity of this type does contribute to occurrence of spontaneous syncopal events in older patients (137,142). Furthermore, it is likely that upright tilt testing, like carotid sinus massage, will result in a 'positive' response in some asymptomatic individuals (i.e. false positive test). Fortunately, at least among younger otherwise healthy individuals, such 'false positive' tests occur only infrequently. For example, Fitzpatrick and Sutton (137,145) indicated that prolonged (45-minute) 60° upright tilt was accompanied by development of syncope in only 7% of 27 control subjects (mean time to syncope, 35 ± 5 minutes). Our own experience is comparable (146).

Recently, Vardas *et al.* (147) extended the tilt table experience in asymptomatic individuals by examining responses to 60° upright tilt (45 minutes duration) in patients with marked sinus bradycardia, but without a history of syncope. Among the 28 patients evaluated (19 males, nine females, age range 38–72 years), only two (7%) developed syncopal symptoms (time to syncope 15 and 20 minutes, respectively). Thus, even in patients with asymptomatic sinus bradycardia, head-up tilt testing appears to be relatively free of an excessive number of 'false positive' outcomes.

The response to upright tilt table testing in patients with suspected neurally mediated syncope is quite different from that observed in either asymptomatic control subjects or in syncope patients in whom conventional PES testing proved 'diagnostic' (i.e. induced tachyarrhythmias, conduction system disease). For example, Abi-Samra et al. (134) found tilt table testing effective for reproducing symptoms in 27/34 (79%) patients with previously unexplained syncope. Further, among 71 patients with recurrent syncope, Fitzpatrick and Sutton (136) found that 60° upright tilt reproduced symptoms in 53 (74%), of whom 40 exhibited both hypotension and bradycardia, while 13 manifested primarily vasodepression. A recent abstracted update from this same group has further confirmed this finding (137). In our laboratory, Almquist et al. (52) reported that 10-minute duration 80° upright tilt (using isoproterenol infusion as an adjunctive provocative measure when necessary) reproduced symptoms in nine of 11 patients with suspected neurally mediated syncope (approximate sensitivity, 82%). On the other hand, among nine patients in whom conventional EPS testing provided a diagnosis (i.e. PES-positive), only two (22%) developed symptoms during tilt testing.

Tilt testing in older patients

To date, the specific utility of tilt table testing as a diagnostic technique in older patients has only received limited study. Lipsitz et al. (143) reported the results of 60° upright tilt (maximum duration 15 minutes) in 22 elderly individuals (83 ± 6 years of age). Six of these individuals had had a history of unexplained syncope despite previous evaluation. Of these six symptomatic patients, one had a positive tilt table test while the remaining five were negative. Of the 16 asymptomatic subjects, all were tilt table test-negative. By contrast, four of nine younger patients had positive responses during the same protocol; two of the four positive tests occurred in individuals with previous history of unexplained syncope. Based on these findings it was suggested that elderly patients may be less susceptible to neurally mediated hypotension–bradycardia during postural stress than are younger subjects. However, recently Calkins et al. (144) reported findings during 70° (15 minutes duration) tilt testing in 52 older patients (> 60 years) and 59 younger patients (< 60 years). The frequency of positive tilt table responses were comparable in both groups (61% and 71%, respectively). The principal difference noted between the two groups was that the older patients tended to exhibit a predominant vasodepressor response more frequently than did younger individuals. In summary, further study is needed to determine whether tilt table testing is as useful in the elderly syncope patient as it is in the younger patient.

TREATMENT

Prevention of recurrent syncope and presyncope, and thereby elimination of associated morbidity, is the ultimate treatment goal. Clearly, however, the therapeutic direction to be pursued, and the effectiveness of the selected treatment(s), are determined by the accuracy of the diagnostic evaluation and limited by patient-related acceptance and tolerance of various available therapeutic modalities. The latter is a particular problem in older patients, where multiple potential aetiologies may coexist and where side-effects of treatment (particularly drugs) often prove unacceptable.

A detailed review of available treatments for all conditions which may be associated with syncope in the elderly patient is beyond the scope of this discussion. However, a number of general treatment considerations should receive attention in all cases. Priority should be given to identification and correction of anaemia and/or metabolic derangements, thereby reducing the potential impact of any subsequent transient circulatory disturbance. Thus, for example, optimization of pulmonary and cardiac status to minimize risk of hypoxaemia and marginal cerebral blood flow may tend to ameliorate the effect of a non-sustained dysrhythmia, and perhaps avert frank syncope. Similarly, diminution of susceptibility to posturally induced transient hypotension may be achieved by emphasizing the benefits of regular exercise (including prescription of supervised exercise programmes when appropriate), cautionary warnings regarding abrupt postural change, and avoidance of tight collars and exposure to isometric stress. The addition of support hose (preferably to waist height) and a more liberal salt intake may also be advantageous in selected individuals. As a consequence of these general measures, cerebrovascular O_2 delivery may be less tenuous and the patient thereby in a better position to tolerate other unpredictable cardiovascular stresses. Finally, careful scrutiny for and elimination of potentially contributory drugs or drug interactions may further reduce the older patients' susceptibility to syncope.

Treatment of syncope of cardiovascular origin may necessitate attempted reversal of a structural abnormality (e.g. valvular stenosis, ventricular aneurysm, severe coronary artery lesion) or prevention of an arrhythmic recurrence. In regard to structural disturbances, careful invasive haemodynamic studies are essential, and electrophysiological studies may also be required in order to document the problem and guide treatment selection. In some cases, medical management to improve cardiac output or reduce dynamic outflow obstruction may be sufficient. In other cases, appropriate treatment may be associated with considerable operative risk in elderly patients. However, at least in the case of valvular aortic stenosis, correction can be achieved at modest operative risk (3–11%) in the elderly patient. Clearly, this diagnosis must be carefully considered given the high mortality associated with the untreated state (148–150).

In regard to cardiac arrhythmias, prevention of tachy- and bradyarrhythmias also entails acceptance of risks, specifically the risks associated with use of antiarrhythmic drug and/or implanted device therapy. In such cases, careful invasive electrophysiological testing may prove useful not only to define the problem, but also to maximize the chance of selecting an effective therapeutic agent or device. Drugs present special problems since the older patient is more susceptible than the younger individual to drug toxicity due to age-dependent alterations of drug metabolism and excretion, more limited capacity for protein binding, decreased volume of distribution, and greater propensity for adverse drug interactions. Pacemakers, on the other hand, although of low risk to implant, are expensive and if used inappropriately may aggravate the problem (e.g. 'pacemaker syndrome', pacemaker-mediated tachycardia). Furthermore, many physicians tend to underestimate the need for physiological pacing modalities (i.e. rate-adaptive and/or dual-chamber systems) in older subjects who have limited intrinsic compensatory haemodynamic reserves (40). As a result, pacemaker system selection may be suboptimal and fail to achieve desired results.

The treatment value of implanted cardiac pacemakers is well established when documentation of symptomatic bradycardia (e.g. complete or high-grade AV blocks, sinus pauses or arrest) is in hand. As noted above, however, the role of cardiac pacing for syncope prevention is less certain for those patients with apparent conduction system disease (e.g. chronic bundle branch block) but in whom a bradycardic basis for syncope is not proven (151,152). Even more controversial is the empirical use of cardiac pacemakers in patients with recurrent syncope of unknown origin despite multiple extensive evaluations. By way of example, Rattes *et al.* (153) recently reported the outcome of pacemaker implantation in three groups of individuals: (i) 31 patients (mean age 73 years) with documented symptomatic bradycardia; (ii) 42 patients (mean age 71 years) with known bradycardia but without clear-cut symptom correlation; and (iii) 31 patients (mean age 69 years) with only a history 'suggestive' of bradycardia but without any documentation. Subsequent follow-up (mean, 43, 45, and 26 months respectively in the three groups) was associated with syncope recurrence in 6.3%, 7.3% and 32.2% of patients in each group, respectively. The authors concluded that, while clearly less efficacious than in patients with evident bradycardia, empirical cardiac pacing may nonetheless be warranted in an attempt to protect older individuals in whom it is not possible to establish a diagnosis despite extensive clinical studies. While this view is supported by other smaller experiences (98,99,154), further assessment with parallel control groups would be highly desirable.

Although neurally mediated syncopal syndromes are not thought to be as common a problem among older individuals as they are in the young, treatment of these conditions in the elderly poses several problems. Recently, apart from some of the general therapeutic strategies noted above, certain drugs have been reported to be helpful in controlling attacks. However, among the agents thought to be useful in certain forms of neurally mediated hypotension–bradycardia, the

β-adrenergic blockers (52) and disopyramide (55) may be difficult to use in older individuals. The former often aggravate bradycardia, reduce exercise tolerance, adversely impact pulmonary function and exacerbate already commonly existing problems with mental acuity. Disopyramide, due to its marked vagolytic effects, poses problems in patients with glaucoma or prostatic hypertrophy. Other, less widely used drugs such as scopolamine and ephedrine may be similarly difficult to use in the older patient. Additionally, it should be noted that the efficacy of pharmacological treatment for these syndromes has primarily been examined in younger patients, and it is uncertain whether their as yet incompletely substantiated benefits outweigh the risks/side-effects in the older population.

Pacemaker therapy may be warranted in those cases of neurally mediated syncope where marked bradycardia is clearly documented. Dual-chamber pacing systems appear to be the better choice in patients with carotid sinus syndrome (24,61). Further, special forms of pacing have reported to be beneficial in a few patients with neurally mediated syncope (155). However, it should be kept in mind that prevention of bradycardia alone by conventional pacing techniques may not be completely effective in many patients with neurally mediated syncopal syndromes. Peripheral vasodilation is an important and almost universal feature of these syndromes, and in many patients it is this 'vasodepressor' component of the syndrome which is the principal cause of the systemic hypotension. Consequently, patients should be warned that dizziness and presyncope may recur despite pacing alone, although it is likely that frank syncope can be averted. In such circumstances, it is probably best to employ pacing therapies in concert with the the general treatment measures discussed above, and when necessary in conjunction with pharmacological treatment.

CONCLUSION

Faints and falls occur commonly in elderly patients, in part contributed to by various age-related processes, including coexisting diseases, sensitivity to medications, diminution of compensatory reserves, and diminished physical strength and agility. Such events not only pose an important source of morbidity for older individuals, but may also result in a substantial economic burden and may mark the end of an independent lifestyle. Not infrequently, it is difficult to discern from description alone whether the event was an accident, a seizure disturbance, or a true syncopal episode contributed to by one or more of the many causes discussed above. Indeed, although it is commonly stated that the history alone provides a diagnosis in 50–70% of syncope cases, such a diagnosis should be at best considered as tentative. An unequivocal diagnosis should be sought, bearing in mind that, in the elderly patient especially, many disease states present in an 'atypical' fashion. Thus, systemic infections may occur without fever or leucocytosis, myocardial infarction may occur without chest pain, and anaemia may develop sufficiently insidiously to be overlooked. Consequently, it is unwise to rely solely upon an unsubstantiated diagnosis. Careful diagnostic assessment of even single syncopal episodes, while difficult and often unrewarding, is even more essential in the elderly patient than is the case in the younger individual. Exclusion of cardiac causes of syncope should receive a particularly high priority in view of their relative frequency and the high subsequent mortality associated with such causes when untreated.

In the older patient, the approach to treatment of faints and falls must be multifactorial. General improvements in health and nutritional status, avoidance of behavioural and/or environmental 'triggers' when possible, elimination of contributory medications, and direct attention to substantial causal factors, all play a role in reducing susceptibility to recurrence. Such effort is warranted in an attempt to prevent potentially serious complications, and permit the elderly patient to maintain an independent and active lifestyle for as long as possible.

Acknowledgements

The authors would like to thank Barry L. S. Detloff and Renee Haugh for valuable technical assistance, and Wendy Markuson and Stephanie Colbert for preparing the manuscript. This work was supported by grants-in-aid from the American Heart Association–Minnesota Affiliate (S.R.) and the American Heart Association, Dallas, Texas (D.G.B.).

REFERENCES

1. Brody JA (1984) Facts, projections, and gaps concerning data on ageing. *Public Health Rep* **99**: 468–475.
2. Brody JA (1985) Prospects for an ageing population. *Nature* **315**: 463–466.
3. Ross RT (1988) *Syncope*. Saunders, London.
4. Savage DD, Corwin L, McGee DL *et al.* (1985) Epidemiologic features of isolated syncope: the Framingham Study. *Stroke* **16**: 626–629.
5. Kapoor WN, Karpf M, Wieand S *et al.* (1983) A prospective evaluation and follow-up of patients with syncope. *N Engl J Med* **309**: 197–204.
6. Kapoor WN, Peterson J, Wieand HS, Karpf M (1987) Diagnostic and prognostic implications of recurrences in patients with syncope. *Am J Med* **83**: 700–708.
7. Kapoor WN, Hammill SC, Gersh BJ (1989) Diagnosis and natural history of syncope and the role of invasive electrophysiologic testing. *Am J Cardiol* **62**: 730–734.
8. Day SC, Cook EF, Funkenstein H, Goldman L (1982) Evaluation and outcome of emergency room patients with transient loss of consciousness. *Am J Med* **73**: 15–23.
9. Lipsitz LA, Wei JY, Rowe JW (1985) Syncope in an elderly, institutionalized population: prevalence, incidence and associated risk. *Q J Med* **55**: 45–54.
10. Silverstein MD, Singer DE, Mulleyag *et al.* (1982) Patients with syncope admitted to medical intensive care units. *JAMA* **218**: 1185–1189.
11. Gibson GE, Pulsinelli W, Blass JP, Duffy TE (1981) Brain dysfunction in mild to moderate hypoxia. *Am J Med* **70**: 1247–1254.
12. McHenry LC, Fazekas JF, Sullivan JF (1961) Cerebral hemodynamics of syncope. *Am J Med Sci* **214**: 173–178.
13. Rowell LB (1986) *Human Circulation: Regulation during Physical Stress*. Oxford University Press, New York.

14. Cook P, James I. Cerebral vasodilators. *N Engl J Med* **305**: 1508–1513.

15. Scheinberg P, Blackburn I, Rich M, Saslaw M (1953) Effects of aging on cerebral circulation and metabolism. *Arch Neurol Psychiat* **70**: 77–85.

16. Dandona P, James IM, Newbury PA *et al.* (1978) Cerebral blood flow in diabetes mellitus: evidence of abnormal cerebral vascular reactivity. *Br Med J* **2**: 325–326.

18. Weiss S, Baker JP (1933) The carotid sinus reflex in health and disease: its role in the causation of fainting and convulsions. *Medicine* **12**: 297–354.

19. Nathanson MH (1946) Hyperactive cardioinhibitory carotid sinus reflex. *Arch Intern Med* **77**: 491–502.

20. Heidorn GH, McNamara AP (1956) Effect of carotid sinus stimulation on the electrocardiograms of clinically normal individuals. *Circulation* **14**: 1104–1113.

21. Lown B, Levine JA (1961) The carotid sinus: clinical value of its stimulation. *Circulation* **23**: 766–789.

22. Thomas JE (1969) Hyperactive carotid sinus reflex and carotid sinus syncope. *Mayo Clin Proc* **44**: 127–139.

23. Brown KA, Maloney JD, Smith HC *et al.* (1980) Carotid sinus reflex in patients undergoing coronary angiography: relationship of degree and location of coronary artery disease to response to carotid sinus massage. *Circulation* **62**: 697–703.

24. Almquist A, Gornick CC, Benson DW Jr *et al.* (1985) Carotid sinus hypersensitivity: evaluation of the vasodepressor component. *Circulation* **67**: 927–936.

25. Wood E (1990) Hydrostatic homeostatic effects during changing force environments. *Aviat Space Environ Med* **61**: 366–373.

26. Lipsitz LA (1983) Syncope in the elderly. *Ann Intern Med* **99**: 92–105.

27. Lombard JT, Selzer A (1987) Valvular aortic stenosis. *Ann Intern Med* **106**: 292–298.

28. Atwood JE, Kawanishi S, Myers J, Froelicher VF (1988) Exercise testing in patients with aortic stenosis *Chest* **93**: 1083–1087.

29. Topol EJ, Traill TA, Fortuin NJ (1985) Hypertensive hypertrophic cardiomyopathy of the elderly. *N Engl J Med* **312**: 277–283.

30. Pathy MS (1967) Clinical presentation of myocardial infarction in the elderly. *Br Heart J* **29**: 190–199.

31. Dixon MS, Thomas P, Sheridon DJ (1988) Syncope is the presentation of unstable angina. *Int J Cardiol* **19**: 125–129.

32. Ferrer MI (1968) The sinus syndrome in atrial disease. *JAMA* **206**: 645–646.

33. Ferrer MI (1973) The sick sinus syndrome. *Circulation* **47**: 635–641.

34. Strauss HC, Prystowsky EN, Scheinman MM (1977) Sino-atrial and atrial electrogenesis. *Prog Cardiovasc Dis* **19**: 385–404.

35. Scheinman MM, Strauss HC, Abbott JA (1979) Electrophysiologic testing for patients with sinus node dysfunction. *J Electrocardiol* **12**: 211–216.

36. Benditt DG, Milstein S, Goldstein MA *et al.* (1990) Sinus node dysfunction: pathophysiology, clinical features, evaluation and treatment. In *Cardiac Electrophysiology: From Cell to Bedside*, Zipes DP, Jalife J (eds). Saunders, Philadelphia, pp. 708–734.

37. Chin C-F, Messenger JC, Greenberg PS, Ellestad MD (1979) Chronotropic incompetence in exercise testing. *Clin Cardiol* **2**: 12–18.

38. Buetikofer J, Fetter J, Milstein S *et al.* (1988) Variability of sinoatrial rate—response during exercise: impact on assessment of chronotropic competence in sinus node dysfunction (Abstract). *PACE* **11**: 531.

39. Corbelli R, Masterson M, Wilkoff B (1990) Chronotropic response to exercise in patients with atrial fibrillation. *PACE* **13**: 179–187.

40. Rickards AF, Donaldson RM (1983) Rate responsive pacing. *Clin Prog Pacing Electrophysiol* **1**: 21–29.

41. Parsonnet V, Bernstein A, Galasso D (1988) Cardiac pacing practices in the United

States in 1985. *Am J Cardiol* **62**: 71–77.

42. Manolis AS. Syncope in the elderly. *Compr Ther* **15**: 31–42.
43. Ezri M, Lerman BB, Marchilinski FE *et al.* (1983) Electrophysiologic evaluation of syncope with bifascicular block *Am Heart J* **106**: 693–697.
44. Morady F, Higgins J, Peters RW *et al.* (1984) Electrophysiologic testing in bundle branch block and unexplained syncope. *Am J Cardiol* **54**: 587–591.
45. Dhingra RC, Denes P, Wu D *et al.* (1974) Syncope in patients with chronic bifascicular block: significance, causative mechanisms, and clinical implications. *Ann Intern Med* **81**: 302–306.
46. Sugrue DD, Holmes DR Jr, Gersh DJ *et al.* (1987) Impact of intracardiac electrophysiologic testing on the management of elderly patients with recurrent syncope or near syncope. *J Am Geriatr Soc* **35**: 1070–1083.
47. Camm A John, Lau CP (1988) Syncope of undetermined origin: diagnosis and management. *Prog Cardiol* **1**: 139–156.
48. Camm AJ, Evans KE, Ward DE, Martin A (1981) The rhythm of the heart in active elderly subjects. *Am Heart J* **99**: 598–603.
49. Fleg JL, Kennedy HL (1982) Cardiac arrhythmias in a healthy elderly population: detection by 24-hour ambulatory electrocardiography. *Chest* **81**: 302–307.
50. Robbins AS, Rubenstein LZ (1984) Postural hypotension in the elderly. *J Am Geriatr Soc* **32**: 769–774.
51. Langford FPJ, Langford HG (1987) Management of orthostatic hypotension in the geriatric patient. *Geriatr Med* **6**: 67–73.
52. Almquist A, Goldenberg IF, Milstein S *et al.* (1989) Provocation of bradycardia and hypotension by isoproterenol and upright posture in patients with unexplained syncope. *N Engl J Med* **320**: 346–351.
53. Abboud FM (1989) Ventricular syncope: is the heart a sensory organ? (Editorial). *N Engl J Med* **320**: 390–392.
54. Milstein S, Buetikofer J, Lesser J *et al.* (1989) Cardiac asystole: a manifestation of neurally mediated hypotension–bradycardia. *J Am Coll Cardiol* **14**: 1626–1632.
55. Milstein S, Buetikofer J, Lesser J *et al.* (1990) Usefulness of disopyramide for prevention of upright tilt induced hypotension-bradycardia. *Am J Cardiol* **65**: 1339–1344.
56. Wallin BG, Sundlof, G (1982) Sympathetic outflow in muscles during vasovagal syncope. *J Auton Nerv Syst* **6**: 287–291.
57. Chen M-Y, Goldenberg IF, Milstein S *et al.* (1989) Cardiac electrophysiologic and hemodynamic correlates of neurally-mediated syncope. *Am J Cardiol* **63**: 66–72.
58. Parry CH (1979) An inquiry into the symptoms and causes of the syncope anginosa. Cutwell, Bath, p. 102.
59. Leatham A (1982) Carotid sinus syncope. *Br Heart J* **47**: 409–410.
60. Sugrue DD, Wood DL, McGoon MD (1984) Carotid sinus hypersensitivity and syncope. *Mayo Clin Proc* **59**: 637–640.
61. Strasberg B, Sagie A, Erdman S *et al.* (1989) Carotid sinus hypersensitivity and the carotid sinus syndrome. *Prog Cardiovasc Dis* **31**: 379–391.
62. Rowe JW (1980) Ageing and renal function. *Annu Rev Gerontrol Geriatr* **1**: 161–179.
63. Weissler AM, Warren JV, Estes EH Jr *et al.* (1957) Vasodepressor syncope: factors influencing cardiac output. *Circulation* **15**: 875–882.
64. Come PC, Pitt B (1976) Nitroglycerin-induced severe hypotension and bradycardia in patients with acute myocardial infarction. *Circulation* **54**: 624–628.
65. Rosoff MH, Cohen MV (1986) Profound bradycardia after amyl nitrite in patients with a tendency to vasovagal episodes. *Br Heart J* **55**: 97–100.
66. Charcot JM (1876) Discussion on a paper by M. Levan. *Gaz Med Paris* **5**: 588.
67. Sharpey-Schafer EP (1953) The mechanism of syncope after coughing. *Br Med J* **2**:

860–863.

68. Faulkner M, Sharpey-Schafer EP (1959) Circulatory effects of trumpet playing. *Br Med J* **1**: 685–686.

69. Klein LJ, Saltzman AJ, Heyman A, Sieker HO (1964) Syncope induced by the valsalva maneuver. *Am J Med* **37**: 263–268.

70. Kapoor WN, Peterson JR, Karpf M (1985) Micturition syncope: a reappraisal. *JAMA* **253**: 796–798.

71. Guttman L, Whitteridge D (1947) Effects of bladder distension on autonomic mechanisms after spinal cord injuries. *Brain* **70**: 361–404.

72. Mathias CJ, Christensen NJ, Corbett JL *et al.* (1976) Plasma catecholamines during paroxysmal neurogenic hypertension in quadriplegic man. *Circ Res* **39**: 204–208.

73. Lyle CB, Monroe JT, Flinn DE, Lamb LE (1961) Micturition syncope: report of 24 cases. *N Engl J Med* **265**: 982–986.

74. Lukash WM, Sawyer GT, Davies JE (1964) Micturition syncope produced by orthostasis and bladder distention. *N Engl J Med* **270**: 341–344.

75. Johnson RH, Lambie DG, Spalding JMK (1984) *Neurocardiology: The Interrelationships Between Dysfunction in the Nervous and Cardiovascular Systems.* Saunders, London.

76. Iggo A (1957) Gastrointestinal tension receptors with unmyelinated afferent fibres in the vagus of the cat. *Q J Exp Physiol* **42**: 130–143.

77. Pathy MS (1978) Defecation syncope. *Age Ageing* **7**: 233–236.

78. Levin B, Posner JB (1972) Swallow syncope: report of a case and review of the literature. *Neurology* **22**: 1086–1093.

79. Palmer ED (1976) The abnormal upper gastrointestinal vasovagal reflexes that affect the heart. *Am J Gastroenterol* **66**: 513–522.

80. Elam MP, Laird JR, Johnson S, Stratton JR (1989) Swallow syncope associated with complete atrioventricular block: a case report and review of the literature. *Military Med* **154**: 465–466.

81. Bortolotti M, Cirignotta F, Lobo G (1982) Atrioventricular block induced by swallowing with documentation by His bundle recordings. *JAMA* **248**: 2297–2299.

82. Mehta D, Saverymutta SH, Camm AJ (1988) Recurrent paroxysmal complete heart block induced by vomiting. *Chest* **94**: 433–435.

83. Garretson HD, Elvidge AR (1963) Glossopharyngeal neuralgia with asystole and seizures. *Arch Neurol* **8**: 26–31.

84. Dykman TR, Montgomery EB Jr, Gerstenberger PB *et al.* (1981) Glossopharyngeal neuralgia with syncope secondary to tumour. *Am J Med* **71**: 165–168.

85. Wallin BG, Westerberg C-E, Sundlof G (1984) Syncope induced by glossopharyngeal neuralgia: sympathetic outflow to muscle. *Neurology* **34**: 522–524.

86. Fleg JL, Asante AVK (1983) Asystole following treadmill exercise in a man without organic heart disease. *Arch Intern Med* **143**: 1821–1822.

87. Hirata T, Yano K, Okui T *et al.* (1987) Asystole with syncope following strenuous exercise in a man with organic heart disease. *J Electrocardiol* **20**: 280–283.

88. Huycke EC, Card HG, Sobol SM *et al.* (1987) Post-exertional cardiac asystole in a young man without organic heart disease. *Ann Intern Med* **106**: 844–845.

89. Pedersen WR, Janosik DL, Goldenberg IF *et al.* (1989) Post-exercise asystolic arrest in a young man without organic heart disease: utility of head-up tilt testing in guiding therapy. *Am Heart J* **118**: 410–413.

90. Tamura Y, Onodera O, Kodera K *et al.* (1990) Atrial standstill after treadmill exercise test and unique response to isoproternol infusion in recurrent postexercise syncope. *Am J Cardiol* **65**: 533–535.

91. Kapoor WN (1989) Syncope with abrupt termination of exercise. *Am J Med* **87**: 597–599.

92. Barcroft H, Edholm OG, McMichael J, Sharpey-Shafer EP (1944) Posthaemorrhagic fainting. *Lancet* **i**: 489–491.

93. Barcroft H, Edholm OG (1945) On the vasodilatation in human skeletal muscle during post-hemorrhagic fainting. *J. Physiol (Lond)* **104**: 161–175.

94. Oberg B, Thoren P (1972) Increased activity in left ventricular receptors during hemorrhage or occlusion of caval veins in the cat: a possible cause of the vaso-vagal reaction. *Acta Physiol Scand* **85**: 164–173.

95. Secher NH, Sander-Jensen K, Werner C *et al.* (1984) Bradycardia, a severe but reversible hypovolemic shock in man. *Circ Shock* **14**: 267–274.

96. Hauser WA, Kurland LT (1975) The epidemiology of epilepsy in Rochester, Minnesota 1935–1967. *Epilepsila* **16**: 1–66.

97. Godfrey JBW (1989) Misleading presentation of epilepsy in elderly people. *Age Ageing* **18**: 17–20.

98. DiMarco JP, Garan H, Harthorne JW, Ruskin JN (1981) Intracardiac electrophysiologic techniques in recurrent syncope of unknown cause. *Ann Intern Med* **95**: 542–548.

99. Gulamhusein S, Naccarelli GV, Ko PT *et al.* (1983) Value and limitations of clinical electrophysiologic study in assessment of patients with unexplained syncope. *Am J Med* **73**: 700–705.

100. Akhtar M, Shenasa M, Denker S *et al.* (1983) Role of cardiac electrophysiologic studies in patients with unexplained recurrent syncope. *PACE* **6**: 192–201.

101. Doherty JU, Pembroke-Rogers D, Grogan EW *et al.* (1985) Electrophysiologic evaluation and follow-up characteristics of patients with recurrent unexplained syncope and presyncope. *Am J Cardiol* **55**: 703–708.

102. Denes P, Uretz E, Ezri MD, Borbola J (1988) Clinical predictors of electrophysiologic findings in patients with syncope of unknown origin. *Arch Intern Med* **148**: 1922–1928.

103. Kudenchuk PJ, McAnulty JH (1985) Syncope: evaluation and treatment. *Mod Conc Cardiovasc Dis* **54**: 25–29.

104. Olshansky B, Mazuz M, Martins JB (1985) Significance of inducible tachycardia in patients with syncope of unknown origin: a long-term follow-up. *J Am Coll Cardiol* **5**: 216–223.

105. Morady F, Shen E, Schwartz A *et al.* (1983) Long-term follow-up of patients with recurrent unexplained syncope evaluated by electrophysiologic testing. *J Am Coll Cardiol* **2**: 1053–1059.

106. Bass EB, Elson JJ, Fogoros RN *et al.* (1988) Long-term prognosis of patients undergoing electrophysiologic studies for syncope of unknown origin. *Am J Cardiol* **62**: 1186–1191.

107. Fujimura O, Yee R, Klein GJ *et al.* (1989) The diagnostic sensitivity of electrophysiologic testing in patients with syncope caused by transient bradycardia. *N Engl J Med* **321**: 1703–1707.

108. Talan DA, Bauernfeind RA, Ashley WW *et al.* (1982) Twenty-four hour continuous ECG recordings in long-distance runners. *Chest* **82**: 19–24.

109. Viitaslao MT, Kalar D, Eisaio A (1982) Ambulatory electrocardiographic recordings in endurance athletes. *Br Heart J* **47**: 213–220.

110. Hattori M, Toyama J, Ito A *et al.* (1983) Comparative evaluation of depressed automaticity in sick sinus syndrome by Holter monitoring and overdrive suppression test. *Am Heart J* **105**: 587–592.

111. Johansson BW (1977) Long-term ECG in ambulatory clinical practice. *Eur J Cardiol* **5**: 39–48.

112. Winkle RA (1980) Ambulatory electrocardiography. *Mod Conc Cardiovasc Dis* **49**: 7–12.

113. Ector H, Rolies L, De Geest H (1983) Dynamic electrocardiography and ventricular pauses of 3 seconds and more: etiology and therapeutic implications. *PACE* **6**: 548–551.
114. Hilgard J, Ezri MD, Denes P (1985) Significance of ventricular pauses of 3 seconds or more detected on twenty-four hour Holter recordings. *Am J Cardiol* **55**: 1005–1008.
115. Grodman RS, Capone RJ, Most AS (1979) Arrhythmia surveillance by transtelephonic monitoring: comparison with Holter monitoring in symptomatic ambulatory patients. *Am Heart J* **98**: 459–464.
116. Rahimtoola SH, Zipes DP, Akhtar M *et al.* (1987) Consensus statement of the conference on the state of the art of electrophysiology testing in the diagnosis and treatment of patients with cardiac arrhythmias. *Circulation* (Suppl. III) **75**: 3–11.
117. Fisher J (1981) Role of electrophysiologic testing in the diagnosis and treatment of patients with known and suspected bradycardias and tachycardias. *Prog Cardiovasc Dis* **24**: 25–90.
118. Josephson ME, Seides S (1971) *Clinical Cardiac Electrophysiology.* Lea & Febiger, Philadelphia.
119. Hammill SC, Holmes DR, Wood DL *et al.* (1984) Electrophysiologic testing in the upright position: improved evaluation of patients with rhythm disturbances using a tilt table. *J Am Coll Cardiol* **4**: 65–71.
120. Crozier I, Ikram H (1986) Electrophysiological evaluation and natural history of unexplained syncope (Abstract). *Aust N Z J Med* **16**: 587.
121. Strauss HC, Grant AO, Scheinman MM, Wallace AG (1980) The use of cardiac stimulation techniques to evaluate sinus node dysfunction. In *Physiology of Atrial Pacemakers and Conductive Tissues*, Little RC (ed.). Futura, Mt Kisco, pp. 339–365.
122. Gann D, Tolentino A, Samet P (1979) Electrophysiologic evaluation of elderly patients with sinus bradycardia: a long-term follow-up study. *Ann Intern Med* **90**: 24–29.
123. Scheinman MM, Peters, R, Sauve MJ *et al.* (1982) Value of the H–Q interval in patients with bundle branch block and the role of prophylactic permanent pacing. *Am J Cardiol* **50**: 1316–1322.
124. Dhingra RC, Wyndham C, Baurenfeind R *et al.* (1979) Significance of block distal to the His bundle induced by atrial pacing in patients with chronic bifascicular block. *Circulation* **60**: 1455–1464.
125. McKenna WJ, Rowland E, Davies J (1980) Failure to predict development of atrial ventricular block with electrophysiological testing supplemented by Ajamalime. *PACE* **3**: 666–669.
126. Brugada P, Abdollah H, Heddle B, Wellens HJJ (1983) Results of a ventricular stimulation protocol using a maximum of 4 premature stimuli in patients without documented or suspected ventricular arrythmies. *Am J Cardiol* **52**: 1214–1218.
127. Brugada P, Green M, Abdollah H, Wellens HJJ (1984) Significance of ventricular arrhythmias initiated by programmed ventricular stimulation: the importance of the type of ventricular arrythmia induced and the number of premature stimuli required. *Circulation* **69**: 87–92.
128. Buxton AE, Waxman, HL, Marchlinski FE *et al.* (1984) Role of triple extrastimuli during electrophysiologic study of patients with documented sustained ventricular tachyarrythmias. *Circulation* **69**: 532–540.
129. Morady F, DiCarlo L, Winston S, Davis JC, Scheinman MM (1984) A prospective comparison of triple extrastimuli and left ventricular stimulation in studies of ventricular tachycardia induction. *Circulation* **70**: 52–57.
130. Wellens HJJ, Brugada P, Stevenson WG (1985) Programmed electrical stimulation of the heart in patients with life-threatening ventricular arrhythmias: what is the

significance of the induced arrhythmias and what is the correct stimulation protocol? *Circulation* **72**: 1–7.

131. Jaegar F, Fouad-Tarazi F, Maloney J (1990) Vasovagal syncope: lack of relationship between baseline blood volume and presyncopal chronotropic orthostatic response (Abstract). *Rev Europ Technol Biomedicale* **12**: 92.

132. Kenny RA, Ingram A, Bayliss J, Sutton R (1986) Head-up tilt: a useful test for investigating unexplained syncope. *Lancet* **i**: 1351–1355.

133. Kenny RA, Ingram I, Vardas P, Sutton R (1987) Unexplained cardiac syncope: the role of the vasovagal syndrome. In *Cardiac Pacing and Electrophysiology. Proceedings of the VIIIth World Symposium on Cardiac Pacing and Electrophysiology.* Belhassen B, Feldman S, Copperman Y (ed.). R & L Creative Communications, Tel Aviv, pp. 233–235.

134. Abi-Samra F, Maloney JD, Fouad-Tarazi FM, Castle L (1988) The usefulness of head-up tilt testing and hemodynamic investigations in the workup of syncope of unknown origin. *PACE* **11**: 1202–1214.

135. Waxman MB, Yao L, Cameron DA *et al.* (1989) Isoproterenol induction of vasodepressor-type reaction in vasodepressor-prone persons. *Am J Cardiol* **63**: 58–65.

136. Fitzpatrick A, Sutton R (1989) Tilting towards a diagnosis in unexplained syncope. *Lancet* **i**: 658–660.

137. Fitzpatrick A, Theodorakis G, Ahmed R, Sutton R (1990) Clinical features of patients with unexplained syncope (Abstract). *Rev Europ Technol Biomedicale* **12**: 91.

138. Fitzpatrick A, Williams S, Ahmed R *et al.* (1990) A randomised trial of medical therapy for vasodepressor vasovagal syncope (Abstract). *J Am Coll Cardiol* **15**: 97.

139. Fitzpatrick A, Williams T, Jeffrey C *et al.* (1990) Pathogenic role for arginine vasopressin (AVP) and catecholamines (EP & NEP) in vasovagal syncope (Abstract). *J Am Coll Cardiol* **15**: 98.

140. Fitzpatrick A, Theodorakis G, Ahmed R *et al.* (1990) Methodology of head-up tilt testing in the investigation of unexplained syncope (Abstract). *PACE* **13**: 561.

141. Raviele A, Gasparini G, Di Pede F *et al.* (1990) Sincopi di natura indeterminata dopo studio elettrofisiologico. Utilita dell'head-up tillt test nella diagnosi di origine vaso-vagale e nella scelta della terapia. *G Ital Cardiol* **20**: 185–194.

142. Raviele A, Gasparini G, Di Pede F *et al.* (1990) Usefulness of head-up tilt test in evaluating patients with syncope of unknown origin and negative electrophysiologic study. *Am J Cardiol* **65**: 1322–1327.

143. Lipsitz LA, Marks ER, Coestner J *et al.* (1989) Reduced susceptibility to syncope during postural tilt in old age. *Arch Intern Med* **149**: 2709–2712.

144. Calkins H, Sousa J, El-Atassi R *et al.* (1991) Comparison of responses to head up tilt table testing of elderly and young patients with syncope of unknown origin (Abstract). *J Am Coll Cardiol* **17**: 294A.

145. Fitzpatrick AP, Sutton R (1989) Tilt-induced syncope. (Letter) *N Engl J Med* **321**: 331.

146. Benditt DG, Milstein S, Goldenberg IF, Gornick CC (1989) Tilt-induced syncope (Letter). *N Engl J Med* **331**: 331.

147. Vardas P, Vemmos C, Vrouchos G, Moulopoulos S (1990) The tilting test in asymptomatic individuals with severe and unexplained sinus bradycardia (Abstract). *Rev Europ Technol Biomediale* **12**: 91.

148. Carabello BA, Green LH, Grossman W *et al.* (1980) Hemodynamic determinants of prognosis of aortic valve replacement in critical aortic stenosis and advanced congestive heart failure. *Circulation* **62**: 42–48.

149. Jamieson WRE, Dooner J, Munro AI *et al.* (1981) Cardiac valve replacement in the

elderly: a review of 320 cases. *Circulation* **64** (Suppl. II): 177–183.
150. Hochberg MS, Morrow AG, Michaelis LL *et al.* (1977) Aortic valve replacement in the elderly: encouraging post-operative clinical and hemodynamic results. *Arch Surg* **112**: 1475–1480.
151. Peters RW, Scheinman MM, Modin G *et al.* (1979) Prophylactic permanent pacemakers for patients with chronic bundle-branch block. *Am J Med* **66**: 978–985.
152. McAnulty JH, Rahimtoola SH, Murphy E *et al.* (1982) Natural history of 'high-risk' bundle-branch block: final report of a prospective study. *N Engl J Med* **307**: 137–143.
153. Rattes NF, Klein GJ, Sharma AD *et al.* (1989) Efficacy of empirical cardiac pacing in syncope of unknown cause. *Can Med Assoc J* **140**: 381–385.
154. Hess DS, Morady F, Scheinman MM (1982) Electrophysiologic testing in the evaluation of patients with syncope of undetermined origin. *Am J Cardiol* **50**: 1309–1315.
155. McGuinn WP, Wilkoff BL, Maloney JD *et al.* (1991) Treatment of autonomically-mediated syncope with rapid AV sequential pacing on demand (Abstract). *J Am Coll Cardiol* **17**: 271A.
156. Teichman SL, Felder SD, Matos JA *et al.* (1985) The value of electrophysiologic studies in syncope of undetermined origin: report of 150 cases. *Am Heart J* **110**: 469–479.

23 The Heart and Stroke Disease

ANTHONY MARTIN
The General Hospital, Jersey, Channel Islands

Strokes are the third most common cause of death in the USA and the UK. The American Heart Association estimated that there were about 160 000 deaths from stroke and about 2 million survivors of stroke in 1982 (AHA Heart Facts 1985). Of the survivors of stroke about one-third will be severely handicapped, many requiring institutional care. Since heart disease is associated with a significant proportion of strokes (1,2), and double that in the very elderly (3,4), the importance of the subject needs no exaggeration.

Hypertension is the most common risk factor for stroke disease, but in recent years there has been much discussion about the role of hypertension in the elderly, its treatment and the association of strokes. Similarly, the existence of atrial fibrillation, either established or paroxysmal and with or without the coexistence of valvular disease, as a major risk factor for strokes has been the subject of much debate. Furthermore, the 1 month mortality in acute stroke with atrial fibrillation is much greater than in those with sinus rhythm (5). The role of atrial fibrillation and other disorders of heart rhythm in the production of non-focal neurological lesions other than stroke or transient ischaemic attacks (TIAs) is clearly important, since they are potentially treatable (6). Myocardial infarction and coronary artery bypass surgery are other risk factors for stroke that need to be elucidated, especially concerning the role of anticoagulant and antiplatelet treatment. In addition, paradoxical embolism in the presence of a patent foramen ovale is known to be an important cause of strokes in younger people, and the situation in elderly people is rather less clear.

The management of strokes related to heart disease in elderly people has special problems. As in all elderly people the multifactorial nature of the problem is manifest; arteriosclerotic cerebrovascular disease may be associated with past or present hypertension, cardiac and carotid artery disease or degenerative change in other organ systems, especially of the lungs and kidneys. Thus the exact cause of an ischaemic cerebral episode may be blurred and the presence of a potential cardioembolic source alone does not establish the stroke mechanism. Similarly the potential unwanted effects of treatment for cardiogenetic stroke may pose problems in older people and thus limit the range of invasive investigations that the physician might choose.

Geriatric Cardiology. Principles and Practice.   Edited by A. Martin and A. J. Camm
© 1994 John Wiley & Sons Ltd

MECHANISMS AND PATHOLOGY OF STROKE

Individual neurological features of stroke are neither sensitive nor specific indicators of the stroke mechanism. For example, sudden neurological deficit has been reported in 25–82% of people with potential cardioembolic sources, but also in 14–66% of patients with other causes of ischaemic stroke (2). Specific neurological features do not seem to be predictive of a cardiogenic mechanism of stroke.

The lack of specific neurological features in stroke disease may be due to the overlap between arterial sources (7). It is likely that emboli arising from proximal arteries may be smaller than those emanating from the heart, although those from the latter source are far from uniform (2).

Characteristically, small cardiogenic emboli arise from mitral valve prolapse (8), infective endocarditis (9), calcific aortic stenosis (10) and prosthetic heart valves (2). Smaller emboli are likely to cause amaurosis fugax or subcortical infarcts (lacunar strokes). Large cardiogenic emboli usually involve the cerebral arteries and cause obstruction of the large branch arteries producing, for example, posterior cerebral artery syndromes (11).

Cardiogenic brain embolism may cause haemorrhagic transformation deep within the infarct. About 20% of such infarcts show secondary haemorrhage 2–4 days after the acute event; the frequency of such haemorrhage is probably higher in large infarcts (12). Haemorrhagic transformation of infarcts caused by non-cardiac sources of emboli occurs less frequently, is usually less dense and confined to the periphery of the infarct (12).

EPIDEMIOLOGY OF CARDIOGENIC STROKE

Cardiogenic stroke is not confined to older persons. Indeed, the age of the patient with stroke due to prosthetic heart valve, infective endocarditis or rheumatic mitral stenosis averages between 50 and 60 years (13). The incidence of rheumatic valvular disease is rapidly decreasing in the Western world, and infective endocarditis is becoming a disease of much older people.

Prosthetic heart valves are increasingly being inserted into people over the age of 65 years. One might therefore expect the historical age pattern of cardiogenic stroke to change to a much older age group in the future. With the improved detection and management of hypertension one might also expect to see the incidence of hypertensive stroke to fall in both middle-aged and elderly people.

Atrial fibrillation of non-rheumatic origin is the most common substrate of true cardiogenic stroke and tends to affect people over the age of 70 years. The possible age-related sources of cardiogenic stroke are shown in Figure 1.

Davis and Hart (13) have recently published a suggested schematic concept of the importance of cardiogenic stroke, particularly stroke associated with atrial fibrillation in older patients (Figure 2).

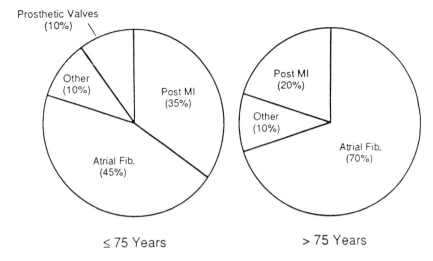

Figure 1. Age-related changes in the sources of cardiogenic embolism. After Davis and Hart (13) with permission from W. B. Saunders Co.

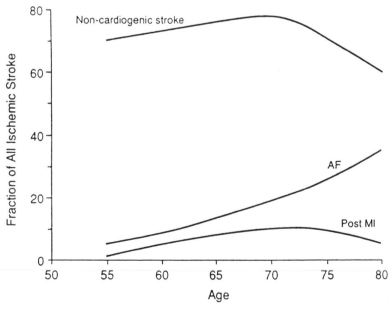

Figure 2. Schematic diagram showing the increasing importance of atrial fibrillation in cardiogenic stroke. After Davis and Hart (13) with permission from W. B. Saunders Co.

THE DIAGNOSIS OF CARDIOGENIC STROKE

As has been observed above, the clinical presentation and neurological findings are of little help in accurately identifying cardiogenic stroke. It is therefore incumbent on the physician always to consider the potential for a cardiac cause of stroke. The major cardiac sources include atrial fibrillation, mitral valve disease, prosthetic heart valves, myocardial infarction and left ventricular aneurysm.

A history of hypertension of carotid artery bruits should alert one to the possibility of cardiogenic stroke. The presence of an acute or prior cortical infarct or large subcortical infarct on either computed tomography (CT) or magnetic resonance imaging (MRI) are also signs of a potential cardiac source.

Isolated Wernicke's (receptive) dysphasia, posterior cerebrellar artery syndromes and amaurosis fugax are often associated with cardiogenic emboli that are small. These small emboli often arise from calcific aortic stenosis, mitral valve prolapse and infective endocarditis. Investigation of all stroke patients should include an electrocardiogram (ECG) to exclude established atrial fibrillation and silent myocardial infarction. CT and/or MRI is essential to localize the anatomical position and extent of the lesion. Since at least 20% of cardioembolic strokes undergo haemorrhagic transformation, CT imaging should be repeated 2–4 days after the acute event.

Prolonged ECG monitoring by telemetry will help uncover cases of paroxysmal atrial fibrillation, although paroxysmal atrial fibrillation on its own is probably not an important cause of cardiogenic embolism.

Echocardiography, especially using transoesophageal techniques, is essential to diagnose septal defects, atrial and ventricular thrombi and mitral valve stenosis or prolapse. Unfortunately the finding of a cardiac abnormality does not necessarily imply a definite cardiac causation for the stroke, although the detection of atrial fibrillation, rheumatic valvular disease and intracardiac thrombi is more suggestive of a direct cause than are mitral valve prolapse and mitral annulus calcification, which are seen in a large number of elderly people without stroke.

SPECIFIC DISEASES ASSOCIATED WITH STROKE

Hypertension

Data collected from the Framingham Study have confirmed beyond any reasonable doubt that both systolic and diastolic hypertension are the dominant risk factors for strokes of all types; furthermore the risk factor for strokes rises with the level of the blood pressure in both men and women (4). However, the situation in elderly people is not so clear-cut, partly because of the potential inaccuracies of measuring blood pressure by the indirect method in older people with arteriosclerosis (14).

Table 1. Standardized multivariate and regression coefficients of risk factors for atherosclerotic brain infarction, men and women, aged 35–64 and 65–94 (30-year follow-up, the Framingham Study)

	Men (age, years)		Women (age, years)	
Hypertension	0.914***	0.429***	0.419***	0.256*
Systolic BP	0.646***	0.470***	0.416***	0.267**
Diastolic BP	0.634***	0.226	0.395***	0.077

From Wolf PA, Kannel WB, Cupples LA, D'Agostino R (1986) Update on epidemiology of stroke. In *Stroke: Epidemiological, Therapeutic and Socio-economic Aspects*, Rose FC (ed.). Symposium series 99, Royal Society of Medicine, London.
*$p = 0.05$; **$p = 0.01$; ***$p = 0.001$.
+ multivariate contains systolic blood pressure (BP), left ventricular hypertension by ECG, cigarette smoking, glucose intolerance, total serum cholesterol and the other appropriate variable.

The Framingham Study has shown that there is a highly significant relationship between hypertension and systolic hypertension, but not between diastolic hypertension and atherosclerotic brain infarction in men aged 65–94 years (see Table 1). The relationship between hypertension and systolic hypertension and atherosclerotic brain infarction in older women is much less strong and there is little relationship between diastolic hypertension and strokes in older women (15).

The data from the Framingham Study contradicts the widely held belief that the effect of increased blood pressure on stroke incidence wanes with advancing age and that elevation of systolic blood pressure is innocuous in elderly people.

MacMahon *et al.* (16) have reviewed seven studies that provided data on cerebrovascular disease; a total of 843 strokes (599 fatal and 244 non-fatal) were recorded. These studies included MRFIT (17), Chicago Heart Association stroke deaths (18), Whitehall stroke deaths (19), Honolulu stroke incidence (20), Framingham (21), Western Electric (22) and the Chicago Poeple's Gas Company (23). The authors found that a 7.5 mmHg difference in usual diastolic blood pressure was estimated to be associated with a 45% difference in the risk of stroke. There were no significant differences between the sizes of the effects in different studies, between the sizes of the effects in men and women, or between the sizes of the effects in those studies that reported fatal strokes alone and in those that reported both fatal and non-fatal strokes (Figure 3).

The combined results of these prospective studies indicated that the usual diastolic blood pressure was positively related to the risks of stroke not only among those individuals who might have been considered 'hypertensive' but also among those who would have usually been considered 'normotensive'.

The trial of the European Working Party on High Blood Pressure in the Elderly (EWPHE) has revealed important information that not only confirms the risks of hypertension and systolic hypertension in stroke disease but has indicated that treatment can reduce the risks (24). The EWPHE trial showed a significant reduction in cerebrovascular events in the treated group (24). All these

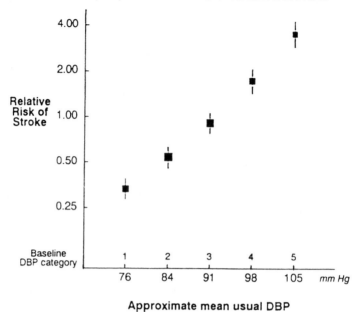

Stroke and usual DBP
(in 5 categories defined by baseline DBP)
7 prospective observational studies: 843 events

Approximate mean usual DBP

Figure 3. The relative risk of stroke and usual diastolic blood pressure. From MacMahon *et al.* (16) with permission from *The Lancet*

patients were over 60 years of age, had diastolic pressure between 90 and 119 mmHg and did not have a history of diabetes, congestive cardiac failure or cerebral haemorrhage. Treatment consisted of hydrochlorothiazide and triamterene, with the addition of methyldopa if the blood pressure was not controlled.

This method of treatment might be regarded now as being rather old-fashioned but, despite this and the high incidence of glucose intolerance and hyperuricaemia, the treated group showed a significantly beneficial effect with regard to the reduced incidence of stroke and cerebrovascular events.

The question of treatment of raised blood pressure has not yet been completely answered since over-aggressive treatment of hypertension may itself produce strokes (25). It is well known that the abrupt reduction in blood pressure below the level at which autoregulation of cerebral blood flow occurs leads to a generalized reduction in cerebral blood flow, which most commonly leads to syncopal attacks. Abrupt lowering of blood pressure can produce focal cerebral ischaemia (26). This probably occurs in 'watershed' areas of the brain, where blood supply is already compromised, such as distal to significant major arterial stenosis.

Atrial fibrillation

Atrial fibrillation is a frequently found arrhythmia in healthy elderly people. Camm and his colleagues (27) found that this was present in 12% of people over 75 years living in their own homes when evaluated by dynamic electrocardiography. In sick elderly people the incidence is much higher, and Patel (28) found on routine electrocardiography of 300 patients admitted to an acute geriatric unit that the incidence of atrial fibrillation was 21.6%. In a large Welsh study of patients admitted to a geriatric unit 10% were found to have atrial fibrillation and of these 33% had paroxysmal atrial fibrillation on the basis of two ECGs performed at 24-hour intervals (29). Using dynamic 24-hour electrocardiography Camm *et al.* (27) found that the paroxysms of atrial fibrillation were very brief and would almost certainly have been missed by routine resting ECGs. Thus it is likely that the true incidence of atrial fibrillation in the Welsh study would have been substantially higher than the figures reported.

Chronic atrial fibrillation is undoubtedly associated with a significantly greater risk of stroke than a similar population in sinus rhythm. Data from the Framingham Study in which 5184 men and women were followed up suggested that those in atrial fibrillation had a significant increase in the incidence of stroke compared to those in sinus rhythm (4). The same study group identified 32 men and 11 women who were supposed to have lone atrial fibrillation, i.e. without pre-existing or coexisting coronary heart disease, congestive heart failure, rheumatic heart disease or hypertensive cardiovascular disease, and in these patients the incidence of stroke was four times higher than in the control group (30). Whether these cases were truly lone fibrillators is a matter of some dispute since thyrotoxicosis was not excluded and the incidence of S–T segment and T wave abnormalities in these patients was higher than in the matched control group in sinus rhythm. However, even if it exists as a true entity, lone atrial fibrillation would appear far from being benign.

The presence of rheumatic valvular disease with atrial fibrillation increases the risk of stroke considerably—approximately threefold over those with atrial fibrillation and no evidence of valvular disease (4). Work from the Oxford Community Stroke Project suggests that the greatest danger of death in those with atrial fibrillation without rheumatic valvular disease is in the first 30 days after the first stroke; thereafter there seems to be little effect of the risk of recurrent stroke (31).

However, other reports have suggested that the risk of subsequent strokes after a stroke due to non-rheumatic atrial fibrillation exceeds 8% per annum (32).

Chronic atrial fibrillation appears to be a much greater risk factor for stroke than paroxysmal atrial fibrillation. In the Welsh study of 4100 patients admitted to a geriatric unit, 414 had atrial fibrillation (276 chronic and 138 paroxysmal). Of the patients with chronic atrial fibrillation, 41.7% had a stroke compared with 26.8% with paroxysmal atrial fibrillation (29).

Atrial fibrillation is increasingly seen as an accompaniment to thyrotoxicosis as age advances and after the age of 70 years it is almost always present (33). Less than one half of patients revert to sinus rhythm following treatment of thyrotoxicosis. The embolism rate seems to be between 5% and 10% in the first 4 months of established atrial fibrillation in thyrotoxic patients (34) but may be higher in those patients with cardiomegaly and with heart failure (35).

The occurrence of 'silent' or subclinical cerebral infarcts in non-rheumatic atrial fibrillation appears to be about 15% (36,37).

Specific increased risk factors in patients with non-rheumatic atrial fibrillation are somewhat controversial, but congestive heart failure appears to increase the embolism risk (35). Left ventricular dysfunction and segmental wall motion abnormalities detected by echocardiography have been associated with a higher embolism risk (38). There is also evidence that left atrial chamber enlargement increases the risk of stroke (39).

Management of patients with chronic atrial fibrillation

The risk of embolism in patients with rheumatic valvular disease and atrial fibrillation is so high that long-term anticoagulation should be used in all cases unless there are major contraindications.

In those with non-rheumatic atrial fibrillation the picture is not so clear-cut. The results of important trials, such as the Copenhagen (40), the SPAF (41,42), the Boston (44), the Canadian (45) and the Veterans (46) studies, are now available.

The Copenhagen Study involved patients with a mean age of 74 years and reported a significant reduction of 59% in strokes and transient ischaemic attacks in those patients given warfarin in full doses, but a reduction of only 14% in those given aspirin in a dose of 75 mg per day (40).

The SPAF trial reported a 67% reduction in stroke in those given low-dose warfarin (mean North American prothrombin time 1.45 × control, INR 1.5–3.0) (41,42). However, in this North American multicentre trial patients over the age of 75 years with atrial fibrillation were excluded from warfarin therapy and the mean age of the patients given warfarin in the first phase of the trial was 65 years. The concurrent but more recently reported Veterans Affairs Study (46) included male patients over 70 years in the low-dose warfarin-treated group and showed a risk reduction of 0.79.

A smaller, but highly significant, trial was carried out in the Boston area (44). Low-dose warfarin was used (target prothrombin time 1.2–1.5) in 212 patients against 208 on placebo. There were only two strokes in the warfarin group (incidence 0.41% per year) as opposed to 13 strokes in the placebo group (2.98% per year), giving a reduction in stroke risk of 0.86. Only 15% of the patients were below 60 years and almost 10% were over the age of 80 years.

The Canadian Trial (45) using low-dose warfarin was stopped early because of the 'positive' results of other trials. Only 378 of the projected 630 patients were recruited. In this study the annual rate of stroke was 3.5% in the warfarin group compared with 5.3% in the placebo group. The relative risk reduction of stroke on active treatment was 37%.

In all the five trials mentioned above the incidence of major bleeding was very low (0.5–1.5% per annum). Thus warfarin therapy, either in full or low dosage, appeared to be both effective and safe (Table 2).

Alternative prophylactic treatment in the prevention of stroke has largely involved trials with aspirin. In the Copenhagen study the dose of aspirin used was 75 mg per day and this failed to show any significant reduction in the rate of stroke (40). However, in the SPAF study the dose of aspirin used was 325 mg per day and in these patients there was a significant reduction of 42% in stroke and a 32% reduction in stroke or death in the aspirin-treated patients (41,42). In patients over 75 years there appears to be no benefit in giving aspirin, although these age-related analyses in the SPAF study were secondary and require confirmation. Further information may come from the ESPS11 study currently in progress, where aspirin 50 mg and/or dipyridamole 300 mg per day are compared with placebo in the prevention of strokes or transient ischaemic attacks following a previous cerebrovascular event, although this study does not only concern patients with atrial fibrillation.

In summary, the role of warfarin started 4–5 days after the stroke, at least in low dosage, is indicated in patients with non-rheumatic atrial fibrillation unless there are major contraindications to anticoagulation therapy. The role of aspirin is still unclear, but there are no studies that show the benefit of aspirin in doses of less than 325 mg per day in patients aged 75 years and below. We shall have to wait for further evidence to demonstrate the usefulness of low-dose aspirin in all patients and especially those over 75 years in any dose.

The Dutch TIA Trial has recently been reported (43) in which aspirin in two different dosages (30 mg and 283 mg) was used to assess the effect on the

Table 2. Anticoagulant and antithrombotic therapy in chronic atrial fibrillation: results of five randomized trials with placebo

Trial	Total no. patients	Agent	Reduction in stroke (%)	
Copenhagen (40)	1007	Warfarin	59	$p = 0.01$
		Aspirin 75 mg/d	14	$p = NS$
SPAF (41, 42)	1244	Warfarin	67	$p = 0.01$
		Aspirin 325 mg/d	42	$p = 0.02$
Boston (BAATAF) (44)	420	Warfarin	86	$p = 0.002$
Canadian (CAFA) (45)	378	Warfarin	37	$p = 0.17$
Veterans (46)	571	Warfarin	79	$p = 0.001$

Intention to treat analysis for ischaemic stroke and systemic embolism (excluding TIA).

occurrence of death from all vascular causes and non-fatal stroke or non-fatal myocardial infarction in patients who had suffered a transient ischaemic attack or minor stroke. A total of 3131 patients were included in this study and the mean follow-up was 2.6 years. The results indicated that 30 mg aspirin was no less effective than 283 mg in the prevention of vascular events and has fewer adverse side-effects in terms of both major and minor bleeding episodes. Patients with atrial fibrillation were specifically excluded.

Myocardial infarction

Acute myocardial infarction may be associated with stroke in about 2.5% of patients in the first 4 weeks after infarction (47,48). Anterior wall infarction appears to be of much greater potential risk of subsequent stroke than other areas of infarction (2,47,48).

Left ventricular thrombus formation usually occurs in the presence of ventricular wall motion abnormalities and is thus more likely to be associated with anterior infarction. Several studies have shown that left ventricular thrombi occur in 28–37% of patients with anterior myocardial infarction (49,50) compared with only 0–5% in inferior infarction (49). Left ventricular thrombi are much more likely to increase the risk of embolism (48,51). However, the

Table 3. Major sources of cardiogenic cerebral embolism

Arrythmias
    Atrial fibrillation
    Sinus node disease
Valvular disease
    Rheumatic mitral stenosis
    Prosthetic heart valves
    Calcific aortic stenosis
    Mitral valve prolapse
    Infective endocarditis
    Non-bacterial endocarditis
    Mitral annulus calcification
Ischaemic heart disease
    Acute myocardial infarction
    Ventricular aneurysm
    Left ventricular wall motion disorders
Non-ischaemic cardiomyopathy (especially with atrial fibrillation)
    Hypertrophic cardiomyopathy
    Cardiac amyloidosis
    Alcoholic cardiomyopathy
Intracardiac thrombi related to thrombotic states
    Myeloproliferative disorders
    Malignancy
Cardiac tumours
    Primary
    Secondary

current widespread use of thrombolytic and subsequent anticoagulant therapy is likely to have a markedly beneficial effect on the reduction of brain embolism after acute myocardial infarction (52).

Most authors recommend 6 months anticoagulation for identified left ventricular thrombi, especially if protrusion or mobility is present (2). Less is known about platelet antiaggregant therapy, but the ISIS-2 trial showed that aspirin halved the stroke prevalence in patients given aspirin within 5 hours of acute myocardial infarction (52).

Left ventricular thrombus occurring late after myocardial infarction is probably of much less risk of embolism, although the data are inconclusive. Most emboli occur within 4 months of an acute infarction but the risk of later discovery of left ventricular thrombus may still carry a significant risk of embolism, and there is certainly an indication for anticoagulation as secondary prevention after a stroke associated with long-standing left ventricular thrombus (2).

Non-ischaemic cardiomyopathy

Any myocardial disorder that affects left ventricular contractility may predispose to thrombus formation and embolism. Indeed, cerebral embolism has been described as the presenting feature of cardiac amyloidosis (53). The risk of embolism is low in hypertrophic cardiomyopathy unless atrial fibrillation is present (54).

Left ventricular thrombus may also occur in the absence of demonstrable myocardial disease and has been described in myeloproliferative disorders (55), polycystic disease (56) and in malignancy (57) (Table 3).

Valvular disease

It has long been recognized that rheumatic mitral valvular disease, especially when associated with atrial fibrillation, is a major source of embolism. However, emboli can occur in a significant number of patients with rheumatic valvular disease and continual sinus rhythm (2). These patients should be anticoagulated unless there are major contradictions to this therapy. Mitral ring calcification is often seen in old age and may be associated with embolism, although many of these patients have established atrial fibrillation and other manifestations of atherosclerosis.

Degenerative calcific aortic stenosis may occasionally give rise to emboli, usually of a small type, which can cause amaurosis fugax. The risks, however, are greatly increased when cardiac catheterization and valvuloplasty are attempted in patients with calcific aortic stenosis (58).

Infective and non-bacterial thrombotic endocarditis are both frequently associated with embolic strokes. Infective endocarditis is often missed in older people despite the fact that this condition now occurs predominantly in older people and is clinically more acute than the classical rheumatic form previously seen in young and middle-aged people (59). Embolism tends to occur early in infective endocarditis and is seen in 15–20% of cases (9). In *Staphylococcus aureus* endocarditis involving either a native or mechanical prosthetic valve, cerebral haemorrhage is a particularly lethal complication (9).

In non-bacterial thrombotic endocarditis clinical emboli occur in at least 30% of cases and in autopsy studies are present in the majority of cases due to cancer (2). Non-bacterial thrombotic endocarditis may not be associated with underlying valvular abnormalities and may also appear as part of the syndrome of diffuse intravascular coagulation. In these instances the emboli are usually multiple and neurologically devastating.

Prosthetic cardiac valves, whether mechanical (Starr–Edwards, Bjork–Shiley, etc.) or bioprosthetic (Hancock, Carpentier–Edwards, etc.), may give rise to emboli, especially if associated with atrial fibrillation. Mechanical valves require long-term anticoagulation, but even then the embolism rate is of the order of 3% per annum for mitral and 1.5% for aortic valves (2,60).

The embolism rate for non-anticoagulated bioprosthetic valves is probably of the same order. In anticoagulated patients the emboli are small and may leave permanent neurological deficit in only about 1% per annum (2). The haemorrhagic risk in anticoagulated patients is about 1–2% per annum. Low-dose anticoagulation may reduce this risk and be made more effective if combined with aspirin or dipyrimadole (2).

Coronary artery surgery

Coronary artery bypass surgery may be followed by stroke in about 2% of cases (61). Despite long-term interest in this phenomenon the causes of stroke remain largely unknown, although atrial fibrillation and a history of previous stroke have been implicated as major risk factors (62). It has also been suggested that the presence of carotid artery bruits increases the risk of postoperative stroke fourfold (63), although others have questioned the validity of these results (64). There appears to be no benefit in performing carotid endarterectomy prior to bypass in these patients.

Mitral valve prolapse

Mitral valve prolapse or 'floppy mitral valve' is well recognized in diseases of collagen, such as the Ehlers–Danlos syndrome, but has been found increasingly in ageing individuals (65). The collagen in the mitral valve cusp becomes soft and stretched and allows the cusp to prolapse. Mitral valve prolapse may lead to both some degree of mitral regurgitation and to an increased susceptibility to infective endocarditis in older people. Mitral valve prolapse may be associated with ischaemic stroke in younger people (66), presumably of a thromboembolic nature.

However, the widespread coexistence of mitral valve prolapse, atrial fibrillation and atherosclerosis in older people probably indicates that mitral valve prolapse is not a major risk factor for stroke in old age.

It has been recognized in recent years that paradoxical embolism through a patent foramen ovale may lead to stroke in young patients (67,68). Any vascular shunt that bypasses the pulmonary capillary bed will allow venous or right heart chamber thrombi to pass into the systemic circulation. It is now known that patent foramen ovale may be compatible with old age and its presence thus provides a potential source of embolism in older people.

REFERENCES

1. Cerebral Embolism Task Force (1986) Cardiogenic brain embolism. *Arch Neurol* **43**: 71–84.
2. Cerebral Embolism Task Force (1989) Cardiogenic brain embolism: the second report of the Cerebral Embolism Task Force. *Arch Neurol* **46**: 727–743.
3. Wolf PA, Kannel WB, Verter J (1983) Current status of risk factors for stroke. *Neurol Clin* **1**: 317–343.
4. Wolf PA, Abbott RD, Kannel WB (1987) Atrial fibrillation: a major contribution to stroke in the elderly. *Arch Intern Med* **147**: 1561–1564.
5. Candelise L, Pinardi G, Morabito A (1990) The Italian Stroke Study Group: mortality in acute stroke with atrial fibrillation. *Stroke* **22**: 169–174.
6. DeBono DP, Warlow CP, Hyman NM (1982) Cardiac rhythm abnormalities in patients presenting with transient non-focal neurological symptoms: a diagnostic grey area? *Br Med J* **284**: 1437–1439.
7. Caplan LR, Hier DB, D'Cruz I (1983) Cerebral embolism in the Michael Reese Stroke Registry. *Stroke* **14**: 530–537.
8. Jackson AC, Boughner DR, Barnett HJM (1984) Mitral valve prolapse and cerebral ischaemic events in young patients. *Neurology* **34**: 784–787.
9. Hart RG, Foster JW, Luther MF (1987) Bacterial endocarditis, stroke and brain haemorrhage (Abstract). *Stroke* **18**: 298.
10. Kapila A, Hart RG (1986) Calcific cerebral emboli and aortic stenosis: detection by computed tomography. *Stroke* **17**: 619–621.
11. Fisher CM (1987) The posterior cerebellar artery syndrome. *Can J Neurol Sci* **13**: 232–239.
12. Hart RG, Easton JD (1986) Haemorrhagic infarcts. *Stroke* **17**: 586–588.
13. Davis WD, Hart RG (1991) Cardiogenic stroke in the elderly. *Clin Geriatr Med* **7**: 429–442.
14. Martin A (1984) Hypertension. In *Heart Disease in the Elderly*, Martin A, Camm AJ (eds). Wiley, Chichester, pp. 59–77.
15. Wolf PA, Kannel WB, Cupples LA, D'Agostino R (1986) Update: on epidemiology of stroke. In *Stroke: Epidemiological, Therapeutic and Socio-economic Aspects*, Rose FC (ed.). Symposium Series 99, Royal Society of Medicine, London.
16. MacMahon S, Peto R, Cutler J et al. (1990) Blood pressure, stroke and coronary heart disease. Pt I. Prolonged differences in blood pressure: prospective observational studies corrected for the regression dilution bias. *Lancet* **335**: 765–774.
17. Stamler J, Neaton JD, Wentworth DN (1989) Blood pressure (systolic and diastolic) and risk of fatal coronary heart disease. *Hypertension* **13** (Suppl. I): 2–12.
18. Stamler J, Rhomberg P, Schoenberger JA et al. (1975) Multivariate analysis of the relationship of seven variables to blood pressure: findings of the Chicago Heart Association Detection Project in Industry 1967–1972. *J Chronic Dis* **28**: 527–548.
19. Reid DD, Hamilton PJS, McCartney P, Rose G (1976) Smoking and other risk

factors for coronary heart disease in British civil servants. *Lancet* **ii**: 979–984.

20. Kagan A, Harris BR, Winkelstein W (1974) Epidemiologic studies of coronary disease and stroke in Japanese men living in Japan, Hawaii and California: demographic, physical, dietary and biochemical characteristics. *J Chronic Dis* **27**: 345–364.
21. Dawber TR (1980) *The Framingham Study: The Epidemiology of Atherosclerotic Disease.* Harvard University Press, Cambridge, MA.
22. Paul O, Lepper MJ, Phelan WH *et al.* (1963) A longitudinal study of coronary heart disease. *Circulation* **28**: 20–31.
23. Dyer AR (1975) An analysis of the relationship of systolic blood pressure, serum cholesterol and smoking to 14 years mortality in the Chicago People's Gas Company. *J Chronic Dis* **28**: 571–578.
24. Amery A, Birkeenhager W, Brixto P *et al.* (1985) Mortality and morbidity results from the European Working Party in High Blood Pressure in the Elderly Trial. *Lancet* **i**: 1349–1354.
25. McLaren GD, Danta G (1987) Cerebral infarction due to the presumed haemodynamic factors in ambulant hypertensive patients. In *Clinical and Experimental Neurology*, Eadie M (ed.). Williams & Williams, Sydney.
26. Moulds RFW (1987) Strokes and hypertension: the effect of treatment. *Med J Austr* **146**: 406–407.
27. Camm AJ, Evans KE, Ward DE, Martin A (1980) The rhythm of the heart in elderly active subjects. *Am Heart J* **79**: 598–602.
28. Patel KP (1977) Electrocardiographic abnormalities in the sick elderly. *Age Ageing* **6**: 163–167.
29. Treseder AS, Sastry BSD, Thomas TPL *et al.* Atrial fibrillation and stroke in elderly hospitalised patients. *Age Ageing* **15**: 89–92.
30. Brand FN, Abbott RD, Kannel WB, Wolf PA (1985) Characteristics and prognosis of lone atrial fibrillation. *JAMA* **254**: 3449–3453.
31. Sandercock P, Warlow C, Bamford J *et al.* (1986) Is a controlled trial of long-term oral anticoagulants in patients with stroke and non-rheumatic atrial fibrillation worthwhile? *Lancet* **i**: 788–792.
32. Lodder J, Dennis MS, Van Raak L, Jones LN, Warlow CP (1988) Cooperative study on the value of long-term anticoagulation in stroke patients with non-rheumatic atrial fibrillation. *Br Med J Clin Res* **296**: 1435–1438.
33. Martin A (1974) *The Natural History of Atrial Fibrillation in the Elderly.* MD thesis, London.
34. Preste CF, Hart RG (1989) Thyrotoxicosis, atrial fibrillation and embolism revisited. *Am Heart J* **117**: 976–977.
35. Yuen RWM, Gutteridge DH, Thompson PL, Robinson JS (1979) Embolism in thyrotoxic atrial fibrillation. *Med J Aust* **1**: 630–631.
36. Petersen P, Masden EB, Brun B *et al.* (1987) Silent cerebral infarction in patients with chronic atrial fibrillation. *Stroke* **18**: 1098–1100.
37. Kempster PA, Gerraty RP, Gates PC (1988) Asymptomatic cerebral infarction in patients with chronic atrial fibrillation. *Br Med J Clin Res* **296**: 1435–1438.
38. Ruocco NA, Most AS (1986) Clinical and echocardiographic risk factors for systemic embolisation in patients with atrial fibrillation in the absence of mitral stenosis (Abstract) *J Am Coll Cardiol* **7**: 165.
39. Aranow WS, Gutstein H, Hsieh FY (1989) Risk factors for thromboembolic stroke in elderly patients with chronic atrial fibrillation. *Am J Cardiol* **63**: 366–367.
40. Petersen P, Boysen G, Godtfredson J, Andersen ED (1989) Placebo controlled, randomised trial of warfarin and aspirin for prevention of thromboembolic complications in chronic atrial fibrillation. *Lancet* **i**: 175–179.
41. Stroke Prevention in Atrial Fibrillation Study Investigators (1990) Report of the

stroke prevention in atrial fibrillation study. *N Engl J Med* **322**: 863–867.

42. Stroke Prevention in Atrial Fibrillation Study Investigators (1991). The stroke prevention in atrial fibrillation study: patient characteristics and final results of placebo comparisons. *Circulation* **84**: 527–539.

43. The Dutch TIA Trial Study Group (1991) A comparison of two doses of aspirin (30 mg and 283 mg a day) in patients after a transient ischaemic attack or minor ischaemic stroke. *N Engl J Med* **325**: 1261–1266.

44. The Boston Area Atrial Fibrillation Investigators (1990) The effect of low-dose warfarin on the risk of stroke in patients with nonrheumatic atrial fibrillation. *N Engl J Med* **323**: 1505–1511.

45. Connolly SJ, Laupacis A, Gent M *et al.* (1991) Canadian atrial fibrillation anticoagulation (CAFA) study. *J Am Coll Cardiol* **18**: 349–355.

46. The Veterans Affairs Stroke Prevention on Nonrheumatic Atrial Fibrillation Investigators (1992) Warfarin in the prevention of stroke associated with non-rheumatic atrial fibrillation. *N Engl J Med* **327**: 1406–14122.

47. Pulatti MM, Cusmano E, Testa MG *et al.* (1986) Incidence of systemic thromboembolic lesions in acute myocardial infarction. *Clin Cardiol* **3**: 331–333.

48. Johannessen KA, Nordrehaug JF, von der Lippe G, Vollsett SE (1988) Risk factors for embolisation in patients with left ventricular thrombi and acute myocardial infarction. *Br Heart J* **60**: 104–110.

49. Visser CA, Kan G, Maltzer RS *et al.* (1984) Long-term follow-up of left ventricular thrombus after acute myocardial infarction, *Chest* **86**: 532–536.

50. Turpie AGG, Robinson JG, Doyle DJ *et al.* (1989) Comparison of high dose with low dose subcutaneous heparin to prevent left ventricular mural thrombosis in patients with acute transmural myocardial infarction. *N Engl J Med* **320**: 352–357.

51. Haughland JM, Asinger RW, Mikell FL *et al.* (1984) Embolic potential of left ventricular thrombi detected by two-dimensional echocardiography. *Circulation* **70**: 588–594.

52. ISIS-2 (Second International Study of Infarct Survival) Collaborative Group (1988) Randomised controlled trial of intravenous streptokinase, oral aspirin, both or neither among 17,187 cases of suspected acute myocardial infarction: ISIS-2. *Lancet* **ii**: 349–360.

53. Botke HE, Rasmussen OB (1986) Recurrent cerebral embolism in cardiac amyloidosis. *Int J Cardiol* **13**: 81–83.

54. Kogure S, Yamamoto Y, Tomono S (1986) High risk of systemic embolism in hypertrophic cardiomyopathy. *Jpn Heart J* **27**: 475–480.

55. Toto AS, Parameswaran R, Kotler MN, Parry W (1987) Rapid development of left ventricular thrombus in a patient with myeloproliferative disorder. *Am Heart J* **114**: 436–437.

56. Schmaier AH, Denenberg B (1984) Left ventricular thrombus with normal left ventricular function and hyperaggregable platelets in a patient with polycystic disease of multiple organs. *Am J Med Sci* **288**: 223–227.

57. De Groat TS, Parameswaran R, Popper P, Kotler MN (1985) Left ventricular thrombi in association with normal left ventricular wall motion in patients with malignancy. *Am J Cardiol* **56**: 827–828.

58. Davidson CJ, Skelton TN, Kisslo KB *et al.* (1988) The risk of systemic embolisation associated with percutaneous balloon valvuloplasty in adults. *Ann Intern Med* **108**: 557–560.

59. Hayward GW (1973) Infective endocarditis: a changing disease I, II. *Br Med J* **ii**: 706–709, 764–766.

60. Kuntze CE, Ebels T, Eijgelaar A, van der Heide JNH (1989) Rates of thromboembolism with three different mechanical heart valve prostheses: randomised study. *Lancet*

i: 514–517.

61. Loop FD, Cosgrove DM, Lytle BW *et al.* (1979) An 11 year evolution of coronary arterial surgery (1968–1978). *Ann Surg* **190**: 444–455.

62. Taylor GJ, Malik SA, Colliver JA *et al.* (1987) Usefulness of atrial fibrillation as a predictor of stroke after isolated coronary artery bypass grafting. *Am J Cardiol* **60**: 905–907.

63. Reed GL, Singer DE, Picard EH, De Sanctis RW (1988) Stroke following coronary artery bypass surgery: a case–control estimate of risk from carotid bruits. *N Engl J Med* **319**: 1246–1250.

64. Furlan AJ (1989) Risk of stroke from carotid bruits. *N Engl J Med* **320**: 937.

65. Davies MJ, Moore BN, Braimbridge MB (1978) The floppy mitral valve: study of incidence, pathology and complications in surgical necroscopy and forensic material. *Br Heart J* **40**: 468–481.

66. Wolf PA, Sila CA (1987) Cerebral ischaemia with mitral valve prolapse. *Am Heart J* **113**: 1308–1315.

67. Lechat P, Mas JL, Lascault G *et al.* (1988) Prevalence of patent foramen ovale in patients with stroke. *N Engl J Med* **318**: 1148–1152.

68. Webster MWI, Chancellor AM, Smith HJ *et al.* (1988) Patent foramen ovale in young stroke patients. *Lancet* **ii**: 11–12.

24 Congestive Heart Failure in the Elderly

JEROME L. FLEG

Gerontology Research Center, National Institute on Aging, and Johns Hopkins Medical Institutions, Baltimore, Maryland, USA

It is paradoxical that while coronary artery disease mortality in the USA has plummeted by about 42% over the past two decades, deaths due to congestive heart failure (CHF) have risen by about one-third during this same period (1). The dramatic ageing of the general population plus improved survival rates after myocardial infarction probably account for much of this increase in CHF. Indeed heart failure is the most common discharge diagnosis for hospitalized patients older than 65 years and accounts for over 500 000 hospital admissions yearly (2). Between 1973 and 1986, the number of discharges due to heart failure more than doubled, with the largest increase seen in the subset older than 75 years (Figure 1). Approximately 2.5 million Americans have CHF, of whom 75% or more are over 60 years of age. The prevalence of CHF rises some 200-fold between the second and eighth decades (4). Thus heart failure is unequivocally a disorder dominated by the elderly.

PROGNOSIS

Despite recent therapeutic advances, the long-term survival of patients with CHF remains poor. During the late 1960s, the Framingham Study observed 5-year survival rates of approximately 50% in patients wth CHF of onset after age 45 years (5); there is little evidence that survival rates have improved over time. For example, mortality in the recent SOLVD Study averaged 37.5% over a mean follow-up of 41.4 months (6). In patients with New York Heart Association (NYHA) class 4 symptoms, 1-year mortality approaches 50% (7). Several additional adverse prognostic factors have been identified, including the magnitude of left ventricular (LV) ejection fraction reduction (8), low maximal aerobic capacity (9,10), hyponatraemia (11), elevated plasma noradrenaline (norepinephrine) (12) non-sustained ventricular tachycardia on ambulatory electrocardiogram (ECG) (13), an S3 gallop (10) and an ischaemic aetiology (10) (Figure 2). It is noteworthy that age *per se* has not been identified as an adverse

Geriatric Cardiology. Principles and Practice. Edited by A. Martin and A.J. Camm
© 1994 John Wiley & Sons Ltd

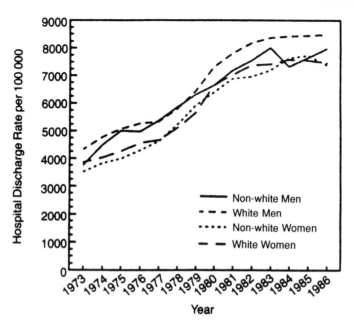

Figure 1. Increase in annual hospital discharge rates for congestive heart failure from US hospitals in patients over 75 years old by sex and race. Reproduced from Ghali *et al.* (3) with permission, copyright 1990, American Medical Association

prognostic factor. In the elderly CONSENSUS Trial population, there was a positive association between mortality and serum levels of noradrenaline, adrenaline (epinephrine), angiotensin II, aldosterone and atrial natriuretic peptide in the placebo group; no such association was seen in enalapril-treated patients (14).

PATHOPHYSIOLOGICAL CONSIDERATIONS

Until this decade, impaired LV systolic function was considered essential for the development of CHF. It is now recognized that as many as 40% of heart failure patients have intact systolic function (i.e. ejection fraction >45%) (15). In these individuals, CHF is thought to be due to diastolic dysfunction. Such 'diastolic' heart failure may be more prevalent with advanced age. For example, Wong *et al.* found ejection fractions ≥45% in only 6% of patients aged 60 or younger versus 41% of those of age >70 years (16).

At least two factors may contribute to a high prevalence of CHF despite perceived systolic function in the elderly. First of all, a well-documented increase in LV wall thickness and decrease in early diastolic filling rate is found with age even in healthy normotensive populations (17). Furthermore, there is a dramatic age-associated increase in the prevalence of hypertension, a condition strongly associated with diastolic dysfunction (18). The critical importance of separating 'systolic' versus 'diastolic' CHF lies in the fact that traditional drug therapy for

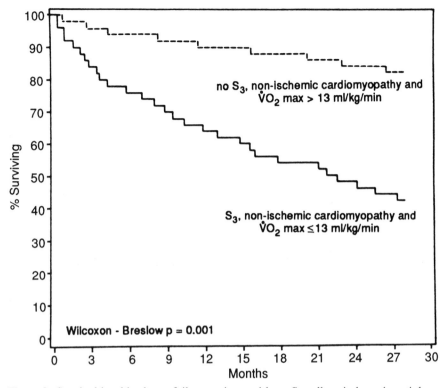

Figure 2. Survival in older heart failure patients with an S₃ gallop, ischaemic aetiology and maximal oxygen consumption ≤ 13 ml/kg per minute compared with patients without these adverse prognostic indicators. Reproduced from Likoff *et al.* (10) with permission

the former may actually aggravate the latter. This therapeutic difference will be discussed in detail later.

AETIOLOGY

Although classic systolic dysfunction CHF can be produced by a large variety of diseases, coronary artery disease, hypertension and valvular disorders are by far the most common. Coronary artery disease (CAD) was the dominant precursor to CHF development in 39% of cases in the Framingham study (5). A history of angina pectoris or myocardial infarction is helpful in diagnosis but may be absent in a sizeable percentage of elderly patients. Diagnostic Q waves of infarction are often present in the elderly despite complete absence of a clinical event; some 30–40% of infarctions are painless in this age group (19). The demonstration of regional LV wall motion abnormalities on echocardiography, often with LV aneurysm formation, is virtually diagnostic for CAD. If CAD is mild, systolic function may be preserved, with an impairment only in early diastolic filling.

Hypertension was the most frequent precursor to CHF in Framingham, contributing to 75% of cases (5). Aggressive programmes to detect and treat hypertension begun in the early 1970s have undoubtedly lowered this figure. Concentric LV hypertrophy on two-dimensional echocardiography, without regional wall motion abnormalities or valvular lesions, strongly suggest a hypertensive aetiology. Systolic function may be reduced or preserved, as in CAD.

Left ventricular hypertrophy may sometimes be extreme and may give rise to LV outflow obstruction. Although frequently conceived of as a disease of younger persons, hypertrophic cardiomyopathy is not uncommon in the elderly (20). Patients with marked LV hypertrophy, whether symmetric or asymmetric, frequently have diastolic dysfunction with well-preserved systolic function.

Rheumatic or other primary valvular diseases are recognized by significant valvular thickening and deformity and diminished leaflet mobility on echocardiographic examination, accompanied by the expected chamber dilatation and/or hypertrophy without regional LV wall motion abnormality. Doppler echocardiography has proved a valuable tool, both to quantify transvalvular gradients in mitral and aortic stenosis and to demonstrate regurgitant jets from these valves.

Although rheumatic heart disease was a precursor to CHF in 21% of Framingham cases of CHF, the percentage may be lower today, given the continuing decline in the incidence of acute rheumatic fever. Myxomatous degeneration of the mitral valve and idiopathic chordal rupture now represent the most common causes of severe mitral regurgitation, and both are common in old age. Recent reports of mitral valve prolapse in elderly subjects emphasize that CHF is often the dominant clinical manifestation, particularly in men (21).

The demonstration of biventricular dilatation and systolic dysfunction without discrete wall motion abnormalities is highly suggestive of a dilated cardiomyopathy. Such myopathies are frequently without identifiable cause. Nevertheless, toxic aetiologies, especially ethanol, should be sought in elderly as in younger patients.

Restrictive cardiomyopathy should be suspected in any patient with small, thick-walled ventricles, reduced systolic function and dilated atria. In the elderly, such findings are most commonly due to amyloidosis, which can frequently be diagnosed by the presence of characteristic 'granular sparkling' myocardial echoes on two-dimensional echocardiographic study. Despite the frequent occurrence of amyloid deposition in senescent hearts (usually within the atria), extensive deposits in ventricular myocardium occur in only 5% of unselected elderly persons (22).

HAEMODYNAMICS AND NEUROHORMONAL PROFILE

Despite the many studies which have assessed haemodynamics and neurohormonal activation in CHF, there has been little attention to the effect of age on these important variables. In a recent study by Cody *et al.*, in 128 hospitalized heart failure patients aged 28–80 years, heart rate was lower and systemic vascular resistance was higher in older patients (23). Mean arterial pressure, right and left heart pressures, cardiac index and stroke volume index were unrelated to age. Plasma noradrenaline increased modestly with age, with highest values in the 56–65-year-old group. No clear-cut age trends were demonstrable for plasma renin activity, serum sodium, urinary aldosterone or urinary sodium excretion (23).

Notable age-associated changes in renal function were noted in these heart failure patients (23). Both glomerular filtration rate and filtration fraction diminished progressively with age, while renal vascular resistance increased. As a result both serum urea nitrogen and serum creatinine were higher in older patients. Thus, renal function declines with age in CHF patients as in healthy adults; the combined effects of age and CHF on renal function must be considered when prescribing digitalis, diuretics and certain vasodilators.

PRECIPITANTS OF CONGESTIVE HEART FAILURE

Reliable data for the relative importance of specific heart failure precipitants in the elderly are lacking. In this author's experience, non-compliance with dietary or drug regimens is the most common precipitant of CHF in this age group. The ubiquity of salt in commercially prepared food coupled with dependence of many elderly patients on such food sources may make strict sodium restriction difficult to achieve. Similarly, a high rate of pharmacological non-compliance in the elderly has been shown by many investigators, particularly when multiple drugs are prescribed. The frequent use of sodium-retaining non-steroidal anti-inflammatory drugs (NSAIDs) for arthritis is certainly a more common contributor to CHF exacerbations in older than in younger patients.

Given the dramatic age-associated increase in atrial fibrillation, this arrhythmia is an important precipitant of CHF in the elderly. In a large series from the 1950s this arrhythmia was present in 47% of elderly heart failure patients (24)—a nearly identical percentage to that in the recent CONSENSUS trial (25). In another study, atrial fibrillation was present in 35% of heart failure patients older than 70 years, but only 6% of those aged 60 and under (16). Furthermore, within the former group, atrial fibrillation was found in 22% of those with decreased systolic function but 54% of those with normal systolic function; this suggests that atrial fibrillation plays a particularly important role in precipitating heart failure in patients with preserved LV systolic function. Atrial fibrillation may be more likely to precipitate CHF in the senescent heart because of the increased dependence on the atrial contribution to LV filling (i.e. 'atrial kick') with advancing age (26). Tachycardia of any type will decrease early diastolic filling time and increase myocardial oxygen demand, causing a greater rise in LV filling pressure in the thicker, stiffer LV of senescence than in a younger, more compliant ventricle.

Myocardial ischaemia or infarction may present as acute CHF, often with little or no chest pain (27). The incidence of CHF accompanying acute infarction increases strikingly with age, approximating 35% over age 75, even in the late 1980s (28). Similarly, acute pulmonary oedema may be the dominant manifestation of ischemic LV dysfunction in older subjects, often with associated mitral regurgitation. In a recent series of 40 such elderly patients with acute pulmonary oedema, moderate or severe mitral regurgitation was present in 35%, and was most often clinically silent (29).

Systemic sources for an acute bout of CHF should also not be overlooked. Anaemia, systemic infection, particularly of pulmonary origin, and thyroid disease may precipitate CHF because of the associated increase in metabolic demands. Thyrotoxicosis is particularly worthy of mention in the elderly because it often appears without typical clinical manifestations and may precipitate atrial fibrillation (30).

DIAGNOSIS

Although dyspnoea, fatigue and oedema remain hallmarks of CHF in older as in younger patients, the diagnosis of heart failure may be elusive in the elderly. For example, an unrelated dementia or confusion due to CHF itself may limit the examiner's ability to obtain a reliable history. Because older individuals may be relatively immobile for a variety of reasons, assessment of exertional dyspnoea or fatigue may be problematic. Furthermore, these symptoms may be due to chronic pulmonary disease, obesity or generalized deconditioning.

Physical findings may also be difficult to interpret in the elderly. Basilar rales are common in this age group, secondary to atelectasis or chronic lung disease. Ankle oedema is also a frequent finding, due to venous insufficiency. Jugular venous distension on the left side only may be caused by compression from an elongated unfolded aortic arch. Finally, a low diaphragm due to obstructive lung disease may displace the liver inferiorly and erroneously suggest hepatomegaly. The S3 gallop, however, remains a specific indicator of LV volume overload and dysfunction in old age.

LABORATORY WORK-UP

The hallmark of the laboratory work-up for any CHF patient is assessment of LV function. The presence of abnormal ejection fraction would lead away from traditional heart failure drug therapy and towards a regimen to improve diastolic relaxation. Two-dimensional echocardiography is probably the imaging procedure of choice in all CHF patients because it delineates both LV function and structure. The presence and extent of wall motion abnormalities, LV hypertrophy, valvular calcification and pericardial effusion are readily detected by two-dimensional echocardiography. The addition of Doppler to the echo examination allows accurate quantification of valvular lesions and diastolic LV function.

For the minority of older CHF patients in whom conventional echo Doppler examination is technically suboptimal, radionuclide ventriculography remains an excellent tool to assess LV systolic function and wall motion. If more anatomical information is required, transoesophageal echocardiography should be performed. This procedure is particularly valuable in the older CHF patient in whom atrial thrombi, endocarditis or prosthetic value dysfunction is suspected. Exercise testing, especially with measurement of oxygen consumption, although not absolutely necessary for diagnosis or treatment, may be a useful means of quantifying the patient's functional status and monitoring the response to therapy. In addition, peak oxygen consumption has been down to be a strong independent predictor of mortality in CHF patients (9,10).

As previously mentioned, the resting electrocardiogram (ECG) remains a valuable diagnostic tool, defining cardiac rhythm disturbances as well as evidence of prior infarctions, LV hypertrophy and conduction system abnormalities. Given the high density of complex ventricular ectopic activity usually found in CHF patients, routine ambulatory electrocardiography is probably not useful unless syncope in present or paroxysmal tacharrhythmias are suspected. Chest X-ray, although supplanted by echocardiography for assessment of heart size and specific cardiac chamber anatomy, provides unique information regarding the presence of pulmonary congestion or infiltrates or pleural effusions.

Routine blood work should also not be overlooked. A low haemoglobin may identify the underlying precipitant for an episode of CHF and possibly indicate an occult source of bleeding or a nutritional deficiency. Thyroid function tests should probably be performed on all elderly CHF patients without an obvious underlying aetiology, especially if atrial fibrillation is present. Serum electrolytes are essential in monitoring the effects of diuretic therapy; in addition, hyponatraemia indicates elevated plasma renin levels and reduced long-term survival (11).

TREATMENT

Non-pharmacological measures

Although pharmacological therapy is the cornerstone of treatment for CHF in all age groups, the importance of modifying lifestyle variables should not be overlooked. Moderate restriction of dietary sodium will frequently allow a minimization of diuretic dosage, thus reducing the incidence of biochemical side-effects so prevalent in the elderly. Alcoholic beverages should be avoided because of their myocardial depressant and arrhythmogenic effects. The additive negative effects of ageing and heart failure on pulmonary function should discourage cigarette smoking in elderly CHF patients.

The optimal level of physical activity for CHF patients is not firmly established. Although prolonged bed rest was advocated for some forms of CHF in the early 1970s, the efficacy of this approach was largely anecdotal. On the other hand, the negative effects of bed rest on aerobic capacity, muscle mass, bone mineral density and metabolic function, already reduced by ageing *per se*, are widely documented. Current wisdom therefore dictates that complete or prolonged bed rest be particularly avoided in geriatric CHF patients. In fact, several recent studies have demonstrated significant improvement in aerobic capacity in heart failure patients after exercise training, even those with severe LV dysfunction (31,32). The efficacy of this approach in elderly CHF patients is still largely unexplored.

Drug therapy

General considerations

Given the multiple medical conditions present in many elderly CHF patients, polypharmacy is the rule; the average hospitalized Medicare patient receives 10 medications daily (33). Recent surveys indicate that at least half of patients taking digitalis have serum levels outside the therapeutic range (34). Thus, the treatment regimen should be made as simple as possible. Regimens of once- or twice-daily diuretic and vasodilator administration should be used whenever possible. Coupling medication doses with regular activities such as arising from bed or meals may enhance compliance. The potential for digitalis toxicity should be minimized by monitoring serum digoxin levels and avoiding hypovolaemia and hypomagnesaemia. Digoxin dosage should be reduced in the presence of quinidine, verapamil or amiodarone, all of which interfere with renal excretion of this drug. Frequent follow-up visits and electrolyte determinations may prevent an iatrogenic hospitalization. The often-quoted dictum 'start low, go slow' is particularly appropriate in the drug treatment of elderly CHF patients. Initial doses of diuretics and vasodilators should be small to minimize the risk of azotaemia and hypotension.

Diuretics

Diuretics continue to be the mainstay for treatment of CHF symptoms, particularly those due to pulmonary and systemic venous congestion. Diuretics should be slowly titrated, starting with a low initial dosage. A thiazide may be preferred initial treatment for those with mild CHF and preserved renal function. Loop diuretics such as furosemide or bumetanide are necessary for patients with more severe heart failure or renal disease. Thiazide and loop diuretics share similar biochemical side effects: hypovolaemia, hyponatraemia, hypomagnesaemia, azotaemia, hyperglycaemia and hyperuricaemia. The age-associated reductions in renal function and dietary intake increase the risk of these side-effects in older CHF patients. In one study of 200 elderly medical and surgical patients, furosemide was responsible for 49% of all drug-induced complications (35). These drugs should be carefully monitored in older CHF patients, with frequent determination of serum electrolytes and renal function. In some patients, a modest degree of peripheral oedema may be preferable to attainment of dry weight at the expense of major biochemical derangement. Patients refractory to large doses of loop diuretics often respond to the addition of metolazone or a potassium-sparing diuretic.

Inotropic agents

For over 200 years, digitalis has been the pharmacological cornerstone for CHF. Nevertheless, the benefit of chronic digitalis therapy in CHF continues to be debated, prticularly in elderly patients in sinus rhythm. In three recent studies, comprising 64 such patients receiving digitalis and diuretics for stable heart failure, withdrawal of digoxin caused no exacerbation of symptoms or deterioration of exercise performance (35–37). However, other studies in somewhat younger, and probably sicker, populations, have shown sustained clinical benefit from digitalis (39,40). Older patients with CHF poorly responsive to diuretics and vasodilator therapy as well as those with atrial fibrillation are unequivocal candidates for digitalis glycosides. When employed for CHF, digitalis should be started in maintenance doses without a loading dose to decrease the risk of toxicity. The age-related reduction in renal function dictates a generally lower maintenance dose of digoxin in elderly patients, typically 0.125 mg daily. An ongoing NIH trial will hopefully resolve the still unanswered question of whether long-term digitalis therapy affects mortality in CHF.

Several newer and more powerful inotropic agents have been evaluated for CHF in the past decade. Intermittent intravenous infusions of dobutamine have caused sustained haemodynamic improvement in small pilot studies (41,42). The oral dopamine congener, L-dopa, has also shown immediate and long-term benefits (43). The phosphodiesterase inhibitors amrinone and milrinone have been employed in several clinical trials across a broad age spectrum (44–49). Although immediate haemodynamic improvement is usually seen, maintenance therapy with these agents has generally been disappointing. In some of these trials, a suggestion of accelerated mortality has arisen (47,48), possibly mediated by an exacerbation of ventricular arrhythmias.

In the recently completed PROMISE trial, milrinone therapy was associated with a 34% increase in cardiovascular mortality in patients with NYHA class 3 and 4 heart failure (49). Identical increases in mortality were seen in patients older than 65 years, as in younger patients. Similar disappointing results have been observed with newer β-adrenergic agonists such as pirbuterol (50) and xamoterol (51). Thus, none of these newer inotropic drugs is approved for oral use.

Vasodilators

The greatest pharmacological advance in the past decade in the treatment of heart failure has been the introduction of vasodilator therapy. Several subclasses of these drugs have been employed. Although many early vasodilator trials included a predominance of younger patients with non-ischaemic aetiologies, most recent trials have included patients in their 70s or older. Most studies, however, have not specifically examined the effect of age on the response to therapy.

α-Adrenergic blockers have not been found to reduce morbidity or mortality in CHF patients, perhaps related to the development of haemodynamic tolerance (52). Long-acting nitrates are similarly limited by the rapid development of tolerance (53,54) despite some evidence of improved exercise capacity with these agents (54). Several pure arterial vasodilators such as hydralazine (55), minoxidil (56) and nifedipine (57) have been employed in chronic CHF; these agents have generally proved disappointing, due both to attenuation of their haemodynamic effects and precipitation of side-effects such as dizziness, angina pectoris or ventricular arrhythmias. However, the combination of hydralazine and in-sosorbide dinitrate reduced cardiac mortality by 23% over 3 years in the multicentre V-HeFT I, a population of male veterans aged 18–75 years with NYHA class 2 and 3 heart failure (8). This reduction in mortality occurred regardless of heart failure aetiology, ejection fraction, exercise capacity or age above versus below the mean of 60 years. The V-HeFT I trial, in fact, provided the first demonstration that any therapy for CHF could improve survival.

Of all vasodilating agents used in CHF, the angiotensin-converting enzyme (ACE) inhibitors have proven the most efficacious. Captopril, the first ACE inhibitor available, demonstrated clinical improvement, enhanced exercise tolerance and decreased hospitalization rate in early studies (58,59), comprised largely of patients younger than 70 years. The landmark CONSENSUS trial, however, is particularly relevant to the elderly. In this study, elderly (mean age 70 years) patients with severe CHF (NYHA class 4) who were receiving digitalis, high-dose diuretics and, in about half, long-acting nitrates, were randomized to enalapril or placebo. The trial was stopped prematurely at 12 months because mortality in the enalapril group was 36% versus 52% in the placebo group (Figure 3). The reduction in death rate with enalapril was due solely to a decrease in mortality from progressive CHF; sudden death rates were unaffected. Functional capacity was also improved with enalapril and side-effects were uncommon, requiring drug withdrawal in 17% of patients versus 14% in the placebo group. The principal side-effects, hypotension and azotaemia, were minimized by lowering the starting dose to 2.5 mg daily in patients with hypovolaemia, pre-existing azotaemia or hyponatraemia.

A recent risk–benefit analysis of ACE inhibitors has shown similar rates of clinical improvement and similar risks of adverse effects in CHF patients younger versus older than 65 years (60). Haemodynamic responses to these agents were also similar between age groups (Table 1). The recently completed V-HeFT II trial in men aged 18–75 years demonstrated that 2-year mortality was 18% lower with enalapril than with the combination of hydralazine and isosorbide dinitrate (61). Thus, ACE inhibitors are currently the vasodilators of choice in chronic

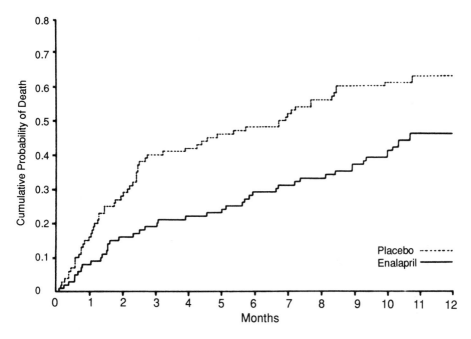

Figure 3. Reduction in mortality in elderly patients with New York Heart Association class IV congestive heart failure treated with enalapril in the CONSENSUS trial. By 6 months, mortality in the enalapril group was 40% lower than in the placebo group ($p < 0.002$). Reproduced from CONSENSUS Trial Study Group (25) by permission of the *New England Journal of Medicine*

Table 1. Converting enzyme inhibitors in chronic heart failure: effect of age

	<65 years ($n = 15$)		≥65 years ($n = 53$)	
	Pre	Post	Pre	Post
Cardiac index (1/min per square metre)	1.7	2.0*	1.8	2.0*
Heart rate (beats/min)	87	78*	80	74*
Mean arterial pressure (mmHg)	84	68*	84	67*
Systemic vascular resistance (dyne s/cm⁵)	2012	1441*	2036	1518*
Pulmonary wedge pressure (mmHg)	26	16*	27	16*
Right atrial pressure (mmHg)	12	8*	11	6*
Blood urea nitrogen (mm/dl)	35	44*	47†	60*
Serum creatinine (mg/dl)	1.5	1.6*	1.9†	2.1*

Adapted from Pinsky *et al.* (60) with permission from the American College of Cardiology.
*$p < 0.05$ pre- versus post-drug.
†$p < 0.05$ versus younger patients.

heart failure, regardless of age. Furthermore, these agents have been shown to reduce ventricular dilatation after anterior myocardial infarction (62). Whether these drugs will reduce the incidence of *de novo* heart failure and prolong survival in asymptomatic elderly patients with LV dysfunction must await the results of the ongoing SOLVD and SAVE prevention trials. Several once-a-day ACE inhibitors have been introduced within the past few years; other than facilitating compliance, they probably offer no significant advantage over captopril or enalapril.

Treatment of congestive heart failure when systolic function is normal

The surprisingly high prevalence of CHF associated with preserved LV systolic function in older heart failure populations has been previously mentioned. Such patients would not be expected to benefit from inotropes or vasodilators, used primarily to improve systolic LV performance. Although diuretics may be useful in relieving symptoms of pulmonary congestion in such patients, over-diuresis may further reduce an already low preload, resulting in hypotension. Indeed, inappropriate therapy of 'diastolic' CHF with diuretics, digitalis or vasodilators has caused significant morbidity and mortality (63).

In patients with CHF and preserved systolic function, it is assumed that heart failure signs and symptoms are due to diastolic dysfunction. Thus, appropriate initial therapy for these patients consists of drugs which improve diastolic filling characteristics, i.e. calcium channel blockers or β-blockers. Both of these agents have been extensively used in younger patients with hypertrophic cardiomyopathy. Recently, Setaro *et al.* demonstrated improved peak filling rate, exercise capacity and clinicoradiographic CHF score in 20 older patients (mean age 68 years) with CHF and ejection fraction >45% who were treated with verapamil (64). Maintenance therapy with verapamil, diltiazem or β-blockers has the added benefit of slowing conduction within the atrioventricular mode—beneficial in controlling ventricular rate in atrial fibrillation or preventing episodes of paroxysmal supraventricular tachycardia.

Surgical therapy

Although drugs are certainly the mainstay of heart failure treatment, the role of surgery should not be overlooked. Calcific aortic stenosis—a not uncommon cause of CHF in the elderly—is curable by valve replacement with a mortality rate < 15%, even in octogenarians (65). Aortic valvuloplasty increases valve area and decreases symptoms acutely but is associated with a high relapse rate (66); this procedure should be reserved for patients who are not surgical candidates. Coronary artery revascularization may occasionally improve LV function dramatically by improving blood flow to hibernating myocardium. Finally, cardiac transplantation is now being performed in patients age 60–70 years old in many centres, with excellent results. Rejection may actually be less common in older than younger transplant recipients (67), and survival appears unrelated to age (67,68). The scarcity of donors and the multisystem disease so common in elderly CHF patients will severely limit the application of cardiac transplantation to this age group.

CONCLUSION

The dramatic ageing of the American population, coupled with other factors such as improved survival after myocardial infarction, has resulted in a dramatic increase in the prevalence of heart failure over the past two decades. CAD is responsible for the majority of CHF in the elderly as in younger patients, but specific entities like calcific aortic stenosis and non-obstructive hypertensive hypertrophic cardiomyopathy are important additional causes of heart failure which are uncommon in younger populations. Medical therapy of CHF in the elderly is generally similar to that of younger patients, but lower initial drug doses and slow, careful titration are essential to avoid azotaemia, electrolyte imbalance and hypotension. Despite the improvement in survival recently demonstrated with vasodilator therapy, long-term survival in CHF remains poor in all age groups. Hopefully, the more aggressive treatment of coronary risk factors and widespread use of ACE inhibitors to prevent ventricular dilatation after myocardial infarction will reduce the future incidence of this malignant disorder.

REFERENCES

1. Thomas P (Nov. 13, 1989) Heart failure: a grim trend. *Medical World News* 32–38.
2. Kozak IJ, Molen M (1985) Detailed diagnoses and surgical procedures for patients discharged from short-stay hospitals: United States, 1983. National Center for Health Studies, Hyattsville, MD, DHHS publication no. (PHS)85-1743 (Vital and health statistics, series 13, no. 82).
3. Ghali JK, Cooper R, Ford I (1990) Trends in hospitalization rates for heart failure in the United States, 1973–1986. *Arch Int Med* **150**: 769–773.
4. Klainer LM, Gibson TD, White KL (1965) The epidemiology of cardiac failure. *J Chronic Dis* **18**: 797–814.
5. McKee PA, Castelli WP, McNamara PM *et al.* (1971) The natural history of congestive heart failure in the Framingham Study. *N Engl J Med* **285**: 1441–1445.
6. The SOLVD Investigators (1991) Effect of enalapril on survival in patients with reduced left ventricular ejection fractions and congestive heart failure. *N Engl J Med* **325**: 293–302.
7. Califf RM, Baunous P, Harrel FE *et al.* (1982) The prognosis in the presence of coronary artery disease. In *Congestive Heart Failure: Current Research and Clinical Application*, Braunwald E, Mock MB, Watson JT (eds). Grune & Stratton, New York, pp. 31–40.
8. Cohn JN, Archibald DG, Ziesche S *et al.* (1986) Effect of vasodilator therapy on mortality in chronic congestive heart failure *N Engl J Med* **314**: 1547–1552.
9. Szlachcic J, Massie BM, Kramer BL *et al.* (1985) Correlates and prognostic implications of exercise capacity in chronic congestive heart failure. *Am J Cardiol* **55**:

1037–1042.

10. Likoff MJ, Chandler SL, Kay HR (1987) Clinical determinants of mortality in chronic congestive heart failure secondary to idiopathic dilated or ischemic cardiomyopathy. *Am J Cardiol* **59**: 634–638.

11. Mettauer B, Rouleau JL, Bichot D *et al.* (1986) Sodium and water excretion abnormalities in congestive heart failure. *Ann Intern Med* **105**: 161–167.

12. Cohn JN, Levine TB, Olivari MT *et al.* (1984) Plasma norepinephrine as a guide to prognosis in patients with chronic congestive heart failure. *N Engl J Med* **311**: 819–823.

13. Bigger JT (1987) Why patients with congestive heart failure die: arrhythmias and sudden cardiac death. *Circulation* **75** (Suppl. IV): IV-28–IV-35.

14. Swedberg K, Eneroth P, Kjekshus J, Snapinn S, for the Consensus Trial Study Group (1990) Efffects of enalapril and neuroendocrine activation on prognosis in severe congestive heart failure (follow-up of the Consensus trial). *Am J Cardiol* **66**: 40D–45D.

15. Souger R, Wohlgelernter D, Vita N *et al.* (1985) Intact systolic left ventricular functional in clinical congestive heart failure. *Am J Cardiol* **55**: 1032–1036.

16. Wong WF, Gold S, Fukuyama O, Blanchett PL (1989) Diastolic dysfunction in elderly patients with congestive heart failure. *Am J Cardiol* **63**: 1526–1528.

17. Gerstenblith G, Fredericksen J, Yin FC *et al.* (1977) Echocardiographic assessment of a normal adult aging population. *Circulation* **56**: 273–278.

18. Inouye I, Massie B, Loge D *et al.* (1984) Abnormal left ventricular filling: an early finding in mild to moderate systemic hypertension. *Am J Cardiol* **53**: 120–126.

19. Aronow WS (1987) Prevalence of presenting symptoms of recognized acute myocardial infarction and of unrecognized healed myocardial infarction in elderly patients. *Am J Cardiol* **60**: 1182.

20. Fay WP, Taliercio CP, Ilstrup DM *et al.* (1990) Natural history of hypertrophic cardiomyopathy in the elderly. *J Am Coll Cardiol* **16**: 821–826.

21. Tresch DD, Siegel R, Keelan MH Jr *et al.* (1979) Mitral value prolapse in the elderly. *J Am Geriatr Soc* **27**: 421–424.

22. Hodkinson HM, Pomerance A (1977) The clincal significance of senile cardiac amyloidosis: a prospective clinical–pathological study. *Q J Med* **46**: 381–387.

23. Cody RJ, Torre S, Clark M, Pondolfino K (1989) Age-related hemodynamic, renal and hormonal differences among patients with congestive heart failure. *Arch Int Med* **149**: 1023–1028.

24. Bedford PD, Caird FI (1956) Congestive heart failure in the elderly. *Q J Med* **25**: 407–426.

25. The Consensus Trial Study Group (1987) Effects of enalapril on mortality severe congestive heart failure. *N Engl J Med* **316**: 1429–1435.

26. Miyatake K, Okomoto J, Kimoshita N *et al.* (1984) Augmentation of atrial contribution to left ventricular flow with aging as assessed by intracardiac Doppler flowmetry. *Am J Cardiol* **53**: 586–589.

27. Pathy MS (1976) Clinical features of ischemic heart disease. In *Cardiology in Old Age*, Caird FI, Dall JLC, Kennedy RD (eds). Plenum Press, New York, pp. 193–208.

28. Weaver WD, Litwin PE, Martin JS *et al.* (1991) Effect of age on use of thrombolytic therapy and mortality in acute myocardial infarction. *J Am Coll Cardiol* **18**: 657–662.

29. Stone GW, Griffin B, Shah PK *et al.* (1991) Prevalence of unsuspected mitral regurgitation and left ventricular diastolic dysfunction in patients with coronary artery disease and acute pulmonary edema associated with normal or depressed left ventricular systolic function. *Am J Cardiol* **67**: 37–41.

30. Williams BO (1981) Atrial fibrillation and congestive heart failure in the elderly. *Intern Med* **2**: 29–36.

31. Conn EH, Williams RS, Wallace AG (1982) Exercise responses before and after physical conditioning in patients with severely depressed left ventricular function. *Am J Cardiol* **49**: 296–300.
32. Sullivan MJ, Higginbotham MB, Cobb FR (1989) Exercise training in patients with chronic heart failure delays ventilatory and aerobic threshold and improves submaximal exercise performance. *Circulation* **79**: 324–329.
33. Ouslander J (1981) Drug prescribing for the elderly. *West J Med* **135**: 455–462.
34. Liverpool Therapeutics Group (1978) Use of digitalis in general practice. *Br Med J* **2**: 673–675.
35. Spino DH, Sellers EM, Kaplan HL *et al.* (1978) Adverse biochemical and clinical consequences of furosemide administration. *Can Med Assoc J* **118**: 1513–1518.
36. Fleg JL, Gottlieb SH, Lakatta EG (1982) Is digoxin really important in treatment of compensated heart failure? A placebo-controlled crossover study in patients with sinus rhythm. *Am J Med* **73**: 244–250.
37. Gheorghiade M, Beller EA (1983) Effects of discontinuing maintenance digoxin therapy in patients with ischemic heart disease and congestive heart failure in sinus rhythm. *Am J Cardiol* **51**: 1243–1250.
38. Aronow WS, Starling L, Etienne F (1986) Lack of efficacy of digoxin in treatment of compensated CHF with third heart sound and sinus rhythm in elderly patients receiving diuretic therapy. *Am J Cardiol* **58**: 168–169.
39. Captopril–Digoxin Multicenter Research Group (1988) Comparative effects of therapy with captopril and digoxin in patients with mild to moderate heart failure. *JAMA* **259**: 539–544.
40. DiBianco R, Shabetai R, Kostuk W *et al.* (1989) A comparison of oral milrinone, digoxin and their combination in the treatment of patients with chronic heart failure. *N Engl J Med* **320**: 677–683.
41. Leier CV, Huss P, Lewis RP *et al.* (1982) Drug induced conditioning in congestive heart failure. *Circulation* **65**: 1382–1387.
42. Applefeld MM, Newman KA, Grove WR *et al.* (1983) Intermittent, continuous outpatient dobutamine infusion in the management of congestive heart failure. *Am J Cardiol* **51**: 455–458.
43. Rajfer S, Anton A, Rossen *et al.* (1984) Beneficial hemodynamic effects of oral levodopa in heart failure. *N Engl J Med* **31**: 1357–1362.
44. Benotti JR, Grossman W, Braunwald E *et al.* (1978) Hemodynamic assessment of amrinone. *N Engl J Med* **299**: 1373–1377.
45. DiBianco R, Shabetai R, Silverman B *et al.* (1984) Oral amrinone for the treatment of chronic congestive heart failure: results of a multicenter randomized double-blind and placebo-controlled withdrawal study. *J Am Coll Cardiol* **4**: 855–856.
46. Timmis AD, Smyth P, Jewitt DE (1985) Milrinone in heart failure: effects on exercise hemodynamics during short-term treatment. *Br Heart J* **54**: 42–47.
47. Wilmshurst PT, Webb-Peploe MM (1983) Side effects of amrinone therapy. *Br Heart J* **49**: 447–451.
48. Packer M, Medina N, Yushak M (1984) Hemodynamic and clinical limitations of long-term inotropic therapy with amrinone in patients with severe chronic heart failure. *Circulation* **70**: 1038–1047.
49. Packer M, Carver JR, Rodeheffer RJ *et al.* (1991) Effect of oral milrinone on mortality in severe chronic heart failure. *N Engl J Med* **325**: 1468–1475.
50. Weber KT, Andrews V, Janicki JS *et al.* (1982) Pirbuterol, an oral beta-adrenergic receptor agonist, in the treatment of chronic cardiac failure. *Circulation* **66**: 1262–1267.
51. Xamoterol In Severe Heart Failure Study Group (1990) Xamoterol in severe heart failure. *Lancet* **336**: 1–6.

52. Packer M, Meller J, Gorlin R et al. (1979) Hemodynamic and clinical tachyphylaxis to prazosin-mediated afterload reduction in severe chronic heart failure. *Circulation* **59**: 531–539.
53. Roth A, Kulick D, Freidenberger L et al. (1987) Early tolerance to hemodynamic effects of high dose transdermal nitroglycerin in responders with severe chronic heart failure. *J Am Coll Cardiol* **9**: 858–864.
54. Leier CV, Huss P, Magorien RD et al. (1983) Improved exercise capacity and differing arterial and venous tolerance during chronic isosorbide dinitrate therapy for congestive heart failure. *Circulation* **67**: 817–822.
55. Chatterjee K, Parmley WW, Massie B et al. (1976) Oral hydralazine therapy for chronic refractory heart failure. *Circulation* **54**: 879–883.
56. Franciosa JA, Cohn JN (1981) Effects of minoxidil on hemodynamics in patients with congestive heart failure. *Circulation* **63**: 652–657.
57. Matsumoto S, Ito T, Sada T et al. (1980) Hemodynamic effects of nifedepine in congestive heart failure. *Am J Cardiol* **46**: 476–480.
58. Levine TB, Franciosa JA, Cohn JN (1980) Acute and long-term response to a converting-enzyme inhibitor, captopril, in congestive heart failure. *Circulation* **62**: 35–41.
59. Cannon PT, Powers ER, Reison DS et al. (1983) A placebo controlled trial of captopril in refractory chronic congestive heart failure: Captopril Multicenter Research Group. *J Am Coll Cardiol* **2**: 755–763.
60. Pinsky DJ, Kukin ML, Packer M (1989) Does age modify the hemodynamic and clinical response to converting enzyme inhibitors in patients with chronic heart failure? *J Am Coll Cardiol* **13**: 57A.
61. Cohn JN, Johnson G, Ziesche S et al. (1991) A comparison of enalapril with hydralazine–isosorbide dinitrate in the treatment of chronic congestive heart failure. *N Engl J Med* **325**: 303–310.
62. Pfeffer MA, Lamas G, Vaughan DE et al. (1988) Effects of captopril on progressive ventricular dilatation after anterior myocardial infarction. *N Engl J Med* **319**: 80–86.
63. Topol E, Trail T, Fortuin N (1985) Hypertensive hypertrophic cardiomyopathy of the elderly. *N Engl J Med* **312**: 277–283.
64. Setaro JF, Zaret BL, Schulman DS et al. (1990) Usefulness of verapamil for congestive heart failure associated with abnormal left ventricular diastolic filling and normal left ventricular systolic performance. *Am J Cardiol* **66**: 981–986.
65. Culiford AT, Galloway AC, Colvin SB et al. (1991) Aortic valve replacement for aortic stenosis in persons aged 80 years and older. *Am J Cardiol* **67**: 1256–1260.
66. Davidson CJ, Harrison JK, Leithe ME et al. (1990) Failure of balloon aortic valvuloplasty to result in sustained clinical improvement in patients with depressed left ventricular function. *Am J Cardiol* **65**: 72–77.
67. Renlund DE, Gilbert EM, O'Connell JB et al. (1988) Age-associated decline in cardiac allograft rejection. *Am J Med* **83**: 391–398.
68. Frazier OH, Marcris MP, Duncan JM et al. (1988) Cardiac transplantation in patients over 60 years of age. *Ann Thorac Surg* **45**: 129–132.

25 Chest Pain

Gartnavel General Hospital, Glasgow, UK

The analysis of chest pain or discomfort in older patients is often more difficult than in their younger counterparts. Accurate history taking may be confounded by the patient's poor memory, multiple pathology manifest by multiple symptoms or atypical presenting features of the underlying condition. Altered pain perception may be a feature of the ageing process. Physicians should attempt whenever possible to characterize the pain in terms of its site, radiation, frequency, duration, quality, associated clinical features, precipitants and factors which appear to aggravate or relieve the symptom. Pain may signal pathology or abnormal function in several systems (Table 1).

CARDIAC PAIN

Angina

Angina is a common symptom in both sexes in older populations (1–3). Many elderly angina patients have a considerable degree of disability and dependency and they make important demands on medical and other resources (3). Most cases are due to coronary heart disease, severe aortic stenosis or regurgitation and rarely hypertrophic cardiomyopathy.

Anginal pain is usually midline and on both sides of the chest. The pain is usually substernal but may on occasion be confined to either the right or left side of the midline. It may radiate to the patient's arms, back, neck or jaws and it may be manifest by headache or epigastric pain in the absence of chest pain. Angina may be present for periods of 2–15 minutes and it is characteristically described as a deep visceral sensation. It may not be described by the patient as a pain but as an unpleasant feeling, and it is variously described as a sensation which is choking, pressing, squeezing, strangling, constricting, bursting or burning. The patient may report a feeling of a band across the chest or a weight on the chest. Some patients attribute the pain of angina to indigestion and they may have associated symptoms of flatulence and a sensation of abdominal distension. Transient myocardial ischaemia may be manifest by symptoms other than anginal pain, i.e. anginal equivalents. These can include breathlessness, palpitations, excess fatigue, lightheadedness or focal neurological symptoms.

Geriatric Cardiology. Principles and Practice. Edited by A. Martin and A. J. Camm
© 1994 John Wiley & Sons Ltd

Table 1. Sources of chest pain or discomfort

Intrathoracic
  Heart
  Aorta
  Pulmonary artery
  Tracheobronchial tree
  Pleura
  Oesophagus
  Diaphragm

Extrathoracic
Above the diaphragm
  Neck and thoracic wall
    Breasts
    Skin
    Muscles
    Spine
    Sensory nerves
    Costochondral junction

Below the diaphragm
  Stomach
  Duodenum
  Gallbladder
  Pancreas

Psychological

Angina is classically provoked by effort or psychological stress and relieved by rest or nitrates. The intensity of exertion required to induce anginal symptoms may be very variable in individuals from day to day. Patients often describe their symptoms as being induced by walking uphill, during cold weather or after a heavy meal.

Prinzmetal or variant angina is atypical in its presentation in that it usually occurs at rest at night and it may not be influenced by exertion. This form of angina may be due to coronary artery spasm in normal or diseased vessels. The spasm may be localized or diffuse and some affected individuals may have spontaneous exacerbations and remissions and may remain asymptomatic without treatment for periods of up to 5 years.

Unstable angina pectoris is a syndrome in the continuum between stable angina and acute myocardial infarction. This condition may be manifest by the occurrence of rest pain or a significant increase in the frequency or severity of the angina in a patient with chronic stable angina, severe prolonged chest pain incompletely relieved by nitrates lasting 15 minutes or more but without electrocardiogram (ECG) or cardiac enzyme evidence of acute myocardial infarction or new-onset angina at rest or on mininal effort (4).

Syndrome X has been described in patients who have symptoms of angina but apparently normal coronary arteries. The natural history of this disorder is benign and symptoms often subside with time. Some patients gain pain relief with nitrates.

Patients with anginal symptoms often have no abnormal physical signs. Some of those affected may have demonstrable clinical signs of underlying anaemia, hypothyroidism, left ventricular dysfunction or aortic valve disease.

Investigation

Basic studies should include a full blood count, thyroid function tests, 12-lead ECG and chest radiograph. Serum lipid studies may help to characterize the patient's vascular risk profile.

The resting ECG is often of little diagnostic help in elderly people with anginal symptoms as it may well be entirely normal. Diagnostic difficulties also occur because many asymptomatic older people have abnormnal ECG tracings (5). Non-invasive tests which may prove valuable include exercise electrocardiography using a standard treadmill or bicycle protocol, echocardiography and radionuclide perfusion studies. Invasive investigations including coronary arteriography and cardiac catheterization are necessary prerequisites for cardiac surgical intervention.

Management

Patients with stable angina should be advised about weight reduction, tobacco avoidance and appropriate regular exercise. Sudden exertion or isometric strain should be avoided.

Medical treatment

Nitrates are the drugs of first choice in angina. Various forms are available for use and include ointments, sublingual and long-acting oral preparations. Tolerance to nitrates or failure of pain control are indications for β-adrenergic blockade or calcium entry-blocking drugs.

The treatment of unstable angina should initially include bed rest, aspirin and nitrates with additional calcium entry blockers and β-blockade if required. If the pain is not satisfactorily controlled by these measures then coronary arteriography is indicated and thrombolytic therapy or coronary artery surgery may be indicated.

The pain of variant angina often responds to nitrates. β-Blocking drugs are not usually indicated but calcium entry blockers may give relief.

Surgical treatment

Coronary artery bypass grafting (CABG) can offer dramatic relief of symptoms in older patients with intractable stable or unstable angina not responsive to medical treatment. Symptomatic improvement can be expected in most patients and the benefits of surgery are probably greater in the high-risk groups, e.g. those with the most severe angina, poor left ventricular function and left main coronary artery disease (6,7).

Percutaneous transluminal coronary angioplasty (PTCA) is less invasive than coronary artery surgery and it may be an ideal treatment option in older patients with symptomatic coronary heart disease that is unresponsive to medical treatment (8–10).

Acute myocardial infarction

Acute myocardial infarction may present in a variety of ways in old age. The clinical presentation may be classical, atypical or silent. Classical acute myocardial infarction is usually associated with severe prolonged pain and/or breathlessness with sweating. The pain is similar in character and radiation to angina but more intense and it lasts for more than half an hour. It may last for several hours and it is not usually relieved by sublingual nitrates. The patient often experiences a fear of impending doom or death.

The earlier published studies on myocardial infarction reported a wide variation in the incidence of painless infarction in elderly people (11,12). This may be explained by different interpretations of what constitutes pain, the inclusion in studies of subjects unable to give a reliable history and varying criteria for the diagnosis of acute myocardial infarction (13). More recent studies have confirmed that chest pain is present in the majority of patients over the age of 65 with acute myocardial infarction (14,15). The incidence of painless infarction increases with advancing age (16). It is not clear why older patients appear to report less chest pain although a number of explanatory hypotheses have been suggested (17,18) (Table 2).

The diagnosis of acute myocardial infarction may be based on the history and physical examination in an extremely ill patient. Clinical signs may be absent but a variety may be detected and these include mild pyrexia, sweating, tachycardia or bradycardia. The blood pressure may be raised initially and fall over the first

Table 2. Hypotheses for reduced chest pain in myocardial ischaemia

---

Age-associated increased pain threshold
Overriding symptoms of dyspnoea or of other medical disorders
Confusion
Communication disorder
Denial of symptoms
Defective anginal warning system
Inappropriate endorphinergic mechanism
Autonomic nervous system dysfunction with sensory nerve damage
    Diabetes mellitus
    Previous ischaemic damage

---

few days. Only the minority of elderly patients are shocked. Left ventricular enlargement may be indicated by displacement of the apex beat, and abnormal systolic pulsation at the left sternal border may be due to paradoxical protrusion of the infarcted anterior wall of the left ventricle. The heart sounds may be normal or quiet and a fourth atrial sound may be present. A transient pericardial friction rub may be heard on the second or third day and a soft pansystolic mitral murmur is often present due to papillary muscle dysfunction or left ventricular dilatation.

Investigations

The diagnosis is most usefully confirmed by standard 12-lead ECGs and serum cardiac enzyme studies taken serially over 3 days. The most sensitive marker of acute infarction at any age is an elevated serum myocardial-derived creatine kinase (MB-CK) enzyme.

Management

Modern management of acute myocardial infarction now includes thrombolytic regimens to limit myocardial damage, improve left ventricular function and reduce mortality. Older patients benefit as much as their younger counterparts from admission to coronary care units, and age alone does not militate against the success of thrombolytic treatment in suspected acute myocardial infarction. The benefits of thrombolysis are most apparent in those patients at greatest risk (19–22). In patients with suspected myocardial infarction within 24 hours of onset of symptoms, thrombolytic treatment is nearly always indicated under 70 and may be of benefit over 75 years of age (23). The treatment options are all effective in older patients but streptokinase is the most widely used and least expensive thrombolytic agent.

Chest pain relief is an important objective in coronary care. It is most often attempted using opiates, e.g. morphine or heroin. Although these narcotic analgesics are still the usual treatment in many hospitals, knowledge of optimal doses, duration of pain relief, and time between administration and pain relief is not yet complete. The relief of pain is often inadequate and improved analgesia may be obtained with the use of a variety of other agents (24) (Table 3).

Other cardiac causes of chest pain

Pericarditis

Acute pericarditis occurs in 10% of elderly patients with classical acute myocardial infarction (25). It is usually transient during the first few days of the illness and it is often asymptomatic. Other forms of acute pericarditis are rare in old age (Table 4).

Table 3. Treatment options for pain relief in myocardial infarction (24)

Opiates
β-Blockers
Gylceryl trinitrate
Thrombolysis
Sedatives
Anti-inflammatories
Nitrous oxide
Epidural or intrathecal anaesthesia

Table 4. Causes of acute pericarditis

More common	Less common
Acute myocardial infarction	Infections
Idiopathic	Radiation
Neoplastic	Connective tissue disorders
Uraemia	Autoimmune, e.g. Dressler's syndrome
Trauma	Drug-induced, e.g. hydralazine
	Hypothyroidism

Chest pain may be a feature of acute pericarditis and it is classically precordial or substernal, although on occasion it may be localized in the epigastrium. It may radiate to the neck, shoulder and arm on the left side. Characteristically, the pain is sharper in quality than angina and it may last for hours. It is not provoked by effort and it may be aggravated by lying in the supine position, deep inspiration, coughing, swallowing, twisting movements of the trunk or turning in bed. It may be relieved by sitting up and leaning forward. Pain may be accompanied by breathlessness, fever, chills and fatigue. Auscultation may reveal a pericardial friction rub which is superficial and varies in intensity with respiratory manoeuvres. Classical ECG abnormalities occcur within hours or days of the onset of pain and these include diffuse ST elevation, concave upwards, followed by return of the ST segment to normal with upright T waves, then T wave inversion followed by a return to normal. A pericardial effusion may develop during the course of acute pericarditis and this is best confirmed by echocardiography. Treatment of acute pericarditis is symptomatic and directed at the management of any underlying conditions.

Postmyocardial infarction syndrome (Dressler's syndrome)

This condition is an uncommon complication of acute myocardial infarction. Its cause is unknown and it appears to be the result of an autoimmune antibody response to pericardial and myocardial antigens exposed to the immune system at the time of the infarction. The onset is usually within 2–10 weeks of the acute myocardial infarction. Presenting features include fever, pericarditis, pleuritis and severe malaise. Chest pain can be severe and it may mimic the pain of acute infarction or it may be mild with vague discomfort not relieved by nitrates. Clinical signs include pericardial and/or pleural friction rubs. The chest radiograph will demonstrate cardiomegally due to pericardial effusion and also pleural effusions. Electrocardiographic evidence of acute pericarditis will be present and the affected patient will have an elevated white cell count and erythrocyte sedimentation rate (ESR). This syndrome should be managed by discontinuing any anticoagulant therapy, and non-steroidal anti-inflammatory agents or steroid drugs may be effective therapeutic options. Some patients suffer recurrent episodes of the postmyocardial infarction syndrome and they may suffer prolonged periods of considerable disability.

Mitral stenosis

Rheumatic heart disease is usually acquired before the third decade but related clinical problems predominate in middle age. Mild or moderate chronic rheumatic heart disease in old age is usually associated with minimal valvular lesions, dyspnoea, fatigue and cyanosis. The mitral valve is most often involved, the aortic valve next and the other valves are rarely affected. Mitral stenosis usually presents with exertional dyspnoea and episodes of haemoptysis, winter bronchitis and paroxysmal nocturnal dyspnoea. A minority of patients experience chest pain or discomfort which is indistinguishable from angina. The mechanism of this pain is not clear but it may be due to right ventricular hypertension, coronary artery obstruction due to emboli or coexistent coronary heart disease. Chest pain or back pain aggravated by effort may occasionally be due to aneurysmal enlargement of the left atrium in mitral valve disease.

Mitral valve prolapse: the floppy mitral valve

In this common valve disorder, mucoid degeneration results in softening of the fibrosa with expansion of the valve cusps, stretching of the chordae tendineae and systolic prolapse of the valve into the left atrium with associated mitral regurgitation. The incidence of this disorder increases with age (26). It is often asymptomatic but some patients may develop chest pain like angina, palpitations or syncope, and infective endocarditis and congestive cardiac failure may occur (27). The cause of the pain is obscure and affected patients often have normal coronary arteriograms. Mitral valve prolapse can be confirmed by echocardiography, and the natural history and prognosis of this condition are not yet clear.

Myocarditis

This inflammatory disorder is usually viral or rickettsial in origin. Symptoms may include chest discomfort, skeletal myalgia, dyspnoea and palpitation. The patient has a tachycardia and fever. The ECG may show transient repolarization changes and occasionally conduction defects. Cross-sectional echocardiography will demonstrate poor contraction of normal-sized or minimally dilated ventricles. Treatment with steroids or other forms of immunosuppressant therapy may be indicated.

Hypertrophic obstructive cardiomyopathy

In this relatively rare condition the anterior mitral valve leaflet apposes to the hypertrophied interventricular septum during systole, with resultant obstruction of the left ventricular outflow tract. A subgroup of elderly patients with this disorder have severe concentric hypertrophy of the left ventricle associated with diastolic dysfunction and mild, moderate or severe hypertension, namely hypertensive hypertrophic cardiomyopathy (28). Symptoms may include angina, in the absence of coronary heart disease, syncope, dizziness and palpitation. The chest pain may be due to narrowing or compression of intramural coronary arteries or subendocardial ischaemia related to high diastolic pressure, increased ventricular wall thickness and increased myocardial oxygen requirements. Clinical signs include a fourth heart sound, a systolic murmur and pulmonary congestion or other features of heart failure. The diagnosis can be confirmed by echocardiography. Symptomatic patients can be successfully treated with a β-blocking agent combined with a calcium entry blocker. Diuretics and vasodilators are poorly tolerated and contraindicated. Surgical procedures, e.g. myotomy and myectomy, may provide benefit in cases resistant to medical treatment (29).

Congenital absence of the pericardium

Only a few patients with major congenital heart lesions will survive into old age without earlier corrective surgery. Occasional cases of atrial septal defect, patent ductus arteriosus, coarctation of the aorta and pulmonic stenosis survive into old age, but most affected individuals have symptoms before the age of 60 years. Congenital absence of the pericardium is a rare disorder which may occur in association with other forms of congenital heart disease. Clinical features include non-specific chest pain and bradycardia. The chest pain lasts for seconds, is provoked by lying on the left side and it is relieved by changing position. The ECG demonstrates right axis deviation and the chest radiograph characteristically shows a shift of the heart to the left and prominence of the pulmonary artery.

Aortic aneurysms

Aneurysmal dilatation of the thoracic aorta occurs most often in the fifth, sixth and seventh decades. Males are predominantly affected and in most cases the underlying pathology is atherosclerosis or occasionally tertiary or late syphilis.

Thoracic aneurysms

Most patients with thoracic aneurysms are asymptomatic and the diagnosis is made on routine chest radiography. Large aneurysms will cause symptoms by compression of adjacent structures. Chest pain can be produced by stretching of surrounding soft tissues, by the erosion of overlying bone or as the result of involvement of the aortic valve and obstruction of the coronary arteries. Other symptoms due to compression include dysphagia, dyspnoea and stridor, hoarseness, superior vena cava syndrome and Horner's syndrome. If an aneurysm ruptures then death is an almost inevitable consequence.

The diagnosis is made by chest radiography, syphilis serology, computed tomography (CT) and aortography. Appropriate antibiotic therapy is indicated in syphilitic disease of the aorta, and elective surgical resection should be considered in an otherwise fit elderly patient with symptoms of compression or a rapidly enlarging aneurysm. This operation is associated with a high mortality.

Dissecting aortic aneurysm

In this condition the underlying pathology is usually medial degeneration with separation of the intima from the media in the aortic wall in a patient with hypertensive disease. The clinical presentation may be very dramatic, with severe chest pain of a tearing or ripping character. It is either substernal and may mimic acute myocardial infarction, or it presents in the back between the scapulae and it can radiate to the neck, arms, abdomen, flanks or extremities. In some patients the presentation is more insidious, with less severe pain or intermittent symptoms, and the diagnosis may be obscure. Pain may be accompanied by nausea and vomiting, and up to one-third of patients have transient or established neurological deficits (30).

The diagnosis can be confirmed and the extent of the lesion can be assessed using a number of investigations. CT is probably as or more accurate than aortography and it has largely superseded the latter invasive technique. Magnetic resonance imaging may be useful, but the most accurate diagnostic tool currently available is transoesophageal echocardiography (31). Urgent management in the emergency situation should combine a medical and surgical approach. Hypertensive blood pressure levels require intensive treatment, and when pressures are stabilized surgical resection is indicated (32).

Primary pulmonary hypertension

This disorder of unknown aetiology occurs predominantly in young women but it also affects significant numbers of middle-aged and elderly men and women (33). A number of underlying pathological processes have been identified, and these include pulmonary arteriolar vasoconstriction due to hyperactivity of the pulmonary arterioles, with resultant irreversible obliterative vascular changes, microthrombosis and vasoconstriction. The onset is usually insidious, and breathlessness is the commanding symptom. Fatigue is common and chest pain is present in up to 75% of affected patients. The pain is precordial and may radiate to the neck but not the arms. Several mechanisms contribute to the development of pain and these include hypoxaemia, low cardiac output, ischaemia of the right ventricular subendocardium and distension of the pulmonary artery. Clinical signs are usually in keeping with right ventricular overload, with a loud pulmonary second heart sound, right ventricular heave, tricuspid valve insufficiency and raised jugular venous pressure.

Causes of secondary pulmonary hypertension should be excluded and these include pulmonary vascular diseases, e.g. pulmonary thromboembolism, pulmonary parenchymal diseases, e.g. chronic obstructive airways disease, pleural fibrosis or a variety of cardiac disorders, e.g. left heart failure due to mitral valve disease. In primary pulmonary hypertension the ECG will demonstrate right ventricular hypertrophy and right axis deviation. Chest radiography will characteristically show prominence of the main pulmonary artery, and the echocardiogram will confirm the presence of right ventricular enlargement and tricuspid incompetence. A lung perfusion scan may show signs of patchy perfusion defects, and pulmonary function tests will demonstrate hypoxaemia, hypocapnia and a reduction in diffusion capacity. The diagnosis is confirmed by right heart catheterization.

This disease carries a uniformly poor prognosis. In view of the underlying pathological processes, treatment with long-term oral anticoagulants and various vasodilators has been attempted but the long-term results of these treatment strategies have been inconsistent and disappointing (33). A potential curative treatment for younger patients is heart–lung transplantation.

Pulmonary embolism

Venous thrombosis and pulmonary embolism is a frequent cause of death in elderly hospital inpatients. Predisposing factors include obesity, immobility, recent surgery, malignant disease, anaemia, polycythaemia, fractured femur, cardiac failure, hemiplegia and chronic venous disease of the legs. The sources of emboli are usually thrombi in the pelvic or leg veins or the right atrium in atrial fibrillation. The majority of cases of minor pulmonary embolism are silent and, when present, the clinical features may be non-specific in elderly people (34). Some patients may present more classically with varying degrees of breathlessness, syncope, haemoptysis or fever. Pulmonary infarction is manifest by pleuritic pain which is sharp and stabbing, often described by patients as knife-like, and it is accentuated by movement, coughing or respiratory manoeuvres. Massive pulmonary embolism occurs when more than half of the pulmonary circulation is obstructed.

Clinical signs may include an increase in the respiratory rate, unexplained sinus tachycardia or atrial fibrillation of sudden onset, a pleural rub or segmental lung collapse, consolidation or pleural effusion.

Acute massive pulmonary embolus presents with collapse, severe breathlessness, acute central chest pain which may mimic acute myocardial infarction and acute right ventricular failure. Affected patients prefer to lie down as venous return is at its maximum in the supine position, and if they sit up they may lose consciousness owing to severe hypotension. The ECG may show no abnormality or the classical S1Q3T3 pattern may be present. Increasing clockwise rotation of the heart in association with an RSR pattern in leads V1 and V2 may occur. The chest radiograph may be normal or linear, or wedge-shaped shadows may be seen in association with pleural effusion. Arterial blood gas analysis may demonstrate hypoxaemia and hypocapnia with reduced gas transfer. Pulmonary arteriography and non-invasive lung scanning are useful diagnostic techniques.

Anticoagulants are indicated for venous thrombosis and pulmonary embolus and they are usually well tolerated in elderly patients (34). Drug regimens should combine intravenous heparin and oral warfarin. Heparin should be administered over 3–4 days until warfarin takes its effect. Warfarin maintenance should be continued for 3 months under careful control of the prothrombin time.

Chest diseases

The lower respiratory tract is largely insensitive to pain, and many lung disorders can develop to an advanced stage without any sensation of pain. The tracheobronchial tree and parietal pleura are, however, very sensitive to pain. Pleuritic pain probably arises due to stretching of inflamed pleura and it may be the result of infection, pulmonary infarction or connective tissue disorders, e.g. rheumatoid disease or systemic lupus erythematosus. If pleurisy progresses to pleural effusion, the pain tends to reduce to a dull, aching sensation.

Respiratory infections

Most respiratory infections present with systemic features of infection in association with localized signs within the respiratory system, and pain or discomfort may accompany a number of disorders. Acute tracheobronchitis is usually viral in origin and the patient presents with a dry cough and retrosternal discomfort. Classical lobar pneumonia may occur in older people but it is uncommon compared with the incidence of bronchopneumonia. Any of the classical features of lobar pneumonia, e.g. high fever, cough, spit, breathlessness, haemopytysis or pleuritic pain, may occur in older patients but the clinical presentation is usually much less dramatic and the illness is often insidious in onset and it may present as a toxic confusional state or a non-specific deterioration in health, in much the same way as many other acute illnesses present in old age. In lobar pneumonia, the physical examination may reveal dehydration, tachycardia or increased respiratory rate with little or no increase in the temperature. The percussion note is dull and movement of the chest is impaired on the affected side. Auscultation will detect bronchial breath sounds and fine or coarse crepitations. The diagnosis rests on chest radiography, bacteriological culture of sputum or laryngeal swabs and blood cultures. Immunofluorescent techniques may help in the diagnosis of viral infections. Appropriate antimicrobial treatment should be started as soon as possible and parenteral therapy may be required in patients who are severely ill. The differential diagnosis of chest pain and breathlessness in the absence of any significant cough should include early pneumonia, pneumothorax, pleural effusion and pulmonary embolus.

Pneumothorax

Most cases of pneumothorax are spontaneous, due to a small apical lung bulla and occur mainly in younger men. A smaller proportion are traumatic or secondary to pulmonary disease, e.g. tuberculosis, emphysema, lung abscess or carcinoma, and the latter are more often encountered in older patients. In a pneumothorax, air leaks into the pleural space and patients present with pain which may range from mild discomfort to a sharp, tearing sensation. It can mimic the pain of acute infarction. Breathlessness is usually the commanding feature and the principal physical signs over the affected area are of hyper-resonance and quiet or absent breath sounds.

The diagnosis is usually confirmed by chest radiography. The natural history of pneumothorax follows three courses. It may be due to a small tear and it can often seal spontaneously, i.e. closed pneumothorax. Recovery is normally gradual and complete. The second form is due to a persistent escape of air into the pleural space with the development of a bronchopleural fistula, i.e. open pneumothorax. The lung remains collapsed, and active intervention by insertion of a pulmonary drain is indicated. The most severe form of pneumothorax is complicated by a valve effect at the site of the air leak, i.e. tension pneumothorax. This is a medical emergency and requires urgent intervention with drainage. Persistent or recurrent pneumothorax may require thoracic measures, e.g. pleuradesis or pleurectomy, and these measures are usually curative.

Pleural effusion

Pain is often absent in a slowly developing pleural effusion. Discomfort may occur due to the physical presence of a very large collection of exudate or transudate. Physical signs will usually include dullness to percussion and quiet or absent breath sounds, and the diagnosis is confirmed by chest radiography. Samples of pleural fluid should be examined by the cytologist, microbiologist and biochemist to elucidate the underlying cause of the effusion.

Lung tumours

Bronchogenic carcinoma

Many older people with bronchogenic carcinoma present clinically with symptoms due to secondary metastatic disease of the brain, liver or skeleton. The disease can also present with classical features of dry persistent cough, hemoptysis, weakness, weight loss, breathlessness or chest pain. Pain or discomfort is a feature in up to 40% of affected patients at the time of diagnosis. It may be ill defined in character or an intermittent ache. Pleural pain may accompany superadded infection and direct invasion of the ribs or rib metastases may produce bone pain.

A tumour in the superior pulmonary sulcus (Pancoast tumour) will produce progressive constant pain in the shoulder, upper anterior chest region or between the scapulae. The pain may spread to the arm on the affected side if the brachial plexus is involved. A Pancoast tumour may produce weakness and atrophy of the muscles in the hand, and associated features can include hoarseness, spinal cord compression and Horner's syndrome, with ptosis, sunken eyeball, narrow palpebral fissure, contracted pupil and lack of thermal sweating on the affected side of the face.

Diagnosis is made by chest radiography, CT, sputum cytology, bronchoscopy and biopsy. Active management of bronchogenic carcinoma in the older patient includes surgery, radiotherapy and cytotoxic drugs. The treatment with the best chance of cure is surgical excision of the lesion, but few affected patients are candidates for surgery because of the inoperable site of the tumour, intrathoracic spread, metastatic disease or coexisting major illness. Radiotherapy is essentially a palliative treatment if superior vena cava obstruction, tracheal compression, recurrent haemoptysis, chest wall involvement or painful skeletal metastases are present. Cytotoxic drugs have a limited role in the treatment of elderly patients but they may be of particular value in large malignant pleural effusions. Pain relief may be obtained with combined regimens including opiate analgesics and phenothiazines, and radiotherapy and non-steroidal anti-inflammatory drugs may be effective in the management of bone pain.

Other less common lung tumours which may present with varying degrees of chest pain or discomfort include pleural fibroma and pleural mesothelioma.

Chest wall disorders

Chest pain or discomfort may be the result of trauma, e.g. after a fall. Pain may accompany muscle sprains or tears or fractures of the ribs or spine. Rib fractures are characterized by local bony tenderness and bruising, and they are aggravated by rib-cage springing. The diagnosis is confirmed by radiographic examination of the affected area.

Intercostal muscle pain may be produced by simple myalgia, which usually presents with a localized tender spot or epidemic myalgia.

Epidemic myalgia (Bornholm's disease)

This disorder may occur in minor epidemics and is the result of a viral myositis due to Coxsackie B virus or other viruses. Intercostal muscle pain may be very severe and it tends to be aggravated by all chest wall movements. Systemic features may be absent and physical examination occasionally reveals a pleural rub or small pleural effusion. The diagnosis is confirmed by isolation of the causal virus from the throat or stools or by demonstrating a rising serum antibody titre to the virus. In some patients this condition tends to be recurrent for a time before it settles. Treatment is symptomatic and pain relief is usually obtained using adequate doses of simple analgesics.

Herpes zoster

This disorder, caused by the varicella zoster virus, is an infectious process associated with the appearance of a circumscribed vesicular eruption of the skin or mucous membranes. The localized eruption, often involving one or more dermatomes, reflects an inflammatory process in related dorsal root ganglia. Reactivation of latent virus may be precipitated by physical trauma to the affected dermatome. Zoster is characteristically a disease affecting adults, and attack rates increase with age. Shooting pains and paraesthesia often precede the appearance of the rash by several days, and when the thoracic dermatomes are involved the pain may mimic severe pleuritic pain. Systemic features may be absent and the diagnosis becomes apparent when the characteristic unilateral rash appears in a dermatome distribution. The rash may not appear and in these circumstances the diagnosis may remain obscure, i.e. zoster *sine herpete*. Post-herpetic neuralgia in affected dermatomes may be a commanding problem in older patients and pain relief may be difficult to achieve.

Costochondritis (Tietze's syndrome)

This disorder usually presents with pain in the second costochondral junction on one or both sides. On occasion other costochondral joints or the sternoclavicular joint may be involved. The pain is aggravated by respiration or coughing, and the affected joint is tender or swollen; the overlying skin may be inflamed. The cause of this clinical syndrome is not known and biopsy shows no abnormality. There is no established effective treatment and the condition is usually self-limiting. Patients should be reassured that they do not have serious cardiac or pulmonary disorders.

Pleurodynia

This condition occurs in patients who have experienced previous pleural diseases, e.g. tuberculosis, empyema or chest trauma or thoracic surgery. Affected patients may present with pleural pain of a dull aching nature with no demonstrable active pathology.

Rib tip syndrome (clicking rib)

This rare condition is caused by undue mobility of the anterior ends of the lower ribs where they attach to each other. The associated pain is sharp, can be very severe and is aggravated by movement. Symptomatic treatment with analgesics may offer relief, and permanent cure is achieved by surgical removal of the affected rib portion.

Oesophageal disorders

Chest pain may be a major presenting symptom in disorders of the oesophagus in elderly patients (35,36). Oesophageal pain may have the characteristics of heartburn, i.e. a burning sensation with a typically upward moving character, or it may closely resemble angina pectoris. It is characteristically substernal and radiates to the back, neck, jaws, shoulders or one or both arms. It may be transient or last for up to 6 hours. It can be precipitated by exercise, drinking very cold or hot liquids, and emotional stress. Pain due to acid sensitivity is relieved by antacids, and the pain of motor disorders may be relieved by nitrates. Dysphagia is the other major symptom of oesophageal disease and it may present in association with chest pains or heartburn. Intermittent dysphagia for solids and liquids in association with chest pain suggests an underlying motility disorder, e.g. diffuse oesophageal spasm. Progressive dysphagia for solids and liquids in the absence of heartburn may indicate the presence of achalasia, and progressive dysphagia for solid food only in association with heartburn suggests a mechanical obstruction, e.g. stricture (35).

Gastro-oesophageal reflux

Symptoms associated with reflux of gastric acid are common in the general population and perhaps even more prevalent in older people owing to an age-associated reduction in oesophageal motility, a less efficient lower oesoph-agel sphincter (LOS) mechanism and an increased prevalence of hiatus hernia (35). A number of drugs may induce or aggravate reflux by reducing LOS pressure, e.g.theophylline, nitrates, calcium entry blockers, benzodiazepines and anticholinergic agents.

Typical symptoms include heartburn and acid regurgitation, and atypical presentations may include angina-like pain, hoarseness, bronchospasm and hiccup. The diagnosis is confirmed by characteristic findings on endoscopy in association with oesophageal pH monitoring studies. Management includes prudent lifestyle changes, antacids, motility-modifying drugs which increase LOS tone, increase oesophageal peristalsis and improve gastric emptying, acid

Table 5. Management of gastro-oesophageal reflux

Lifestyle changes
   Regular small meals
   Weight loss if appropriate
   Elevation of the head of the bed
   Reduced fat in the diet
   Avoid mucosal irritants, e.g. citrus juices, tomato products, coffee, alcohol
   Stop tobacco smoking

Antacids

Motility-modifying drugs
   Metoclopramide
   Bethanecol
   Domperidone
   Cisapride

Acid suppressants
   H2-blockers
   Omeprazole

Enhanced mucosal resistance
   Sucralfate
   Alginates

Surgical treatment
   Nissen fundoplication

---

suppressants and drugs which enhance mucosal resistance to injury. Surgical treatment, e.g. Nissen fundoplication, is occasionally indicated in patients whose symptoms are resistant to medical measures (Table 5).

Oesophageal cancer

Squamous cell carcinoma accounts for 98% of cases of oesophageal cancer and the remainder are adenocarcinomatous in type. This condition classically affects males over 60 years of age, and important aetiological factors include excessive use of tobacco and alcohol. Affected patients classically present with rapidly progressive dysphagia occasionally preceded by transient symptoms of substernal oppression, discomfort or fullness. Three different types of pain may accompany dysphagia. The first is a pressure or aching feeling due to impaction of food at the site of the tumour. This may occur at any level of the oesophagus and may radiate to the neck, jaws or between the scapulae. It may be retrosternal and mimic cardiac pain. The second type of pain is of a burning character and is due to the local effect of swallowed substances, e.g. alcohol, citrus juices, potassium chloride or ferrous sulphate. The third type of pain may develop as a steady ache in the middle of the chest or back at a more advanced stage of the disease.

Physical examination usually reveals evidence of undernutrition and severe weight loss. The diagnosis is confirmed by double-contrast barium swallow examination and endoscopy with biopsy. A diagnosis of oesophageal cancer is rarely made early enough to allow for a cure, and management is essentially palliative. Surgical resection and radiotherapy may be indicated in selected cases and symptomatic relief may be achieved by transendoscopic laser recanalization of the tumour.

Oesophageal motility disorders

Primary motor disorders of the oesophagus may present with chest pain and dysphagia. The pain may be severe and is due to muscle contraction, luminal distension and mucosal acid damage. Usually midline and retrosternal, it may radiate to the suprasternal notch but not typically to the arms. Unlike angina, it is not related to effort, may frequently occur spontaneously, and after an acute episode patients may experience a dull, persisting discomfort.

Presbyoesophagus

The incidence of non-peristaltic contractions of the oesophagus increases with age, and cineradiography may demonstrate impaired peristalsis in most non-agenarians. Symptoms of dysphagia or pain are rarely encountered in elderly people with this disorder (37).

Achalasia

This motor disorder, defined as an aperistalsis of the oesophageal body and defective relaxation of the LOS, is usually of unknown cause and it may develop for the first time in old age. Less common secondary causes include malignant tumours of the pancreas, lung and stomach or lymphoma in the oesophagus.

Dysphagia for liquids and solids is the commanding symptom and this may be accompanied by weight loss, regurgitation and oesophageal pain, which may be less pronounced in elderly people. The diagnosis is confirmed by demonstrating an absence of peristalsis on cineradiography and typical manometric features of aperistalsis of the body of the oesophagus and defective LOS relaxation.

Management is essentially palliative and the objective is to improve oesophageal emptying and reduce lower oesophageal obstruction. Some patients may benefit from the use of anticholinergics, nitrates or calcium entry blockers, and surgical measures include dilatation and bouginage or myotomy.

Diffuse oesophageal spasm

This is a disorder of smooth muscle characterized by spontaneous, high-altitude, aperistaltic and prolonged contractions with normal relaxation of the LOS. Affected patients are usually over 50 years of age and may be symptom-free

Table 6. Drugs which may cause mucosal injury in the oesophagus

---

Non-steroidal anti-inflammatory drugs
Emepronium bromide
Tetracyclines
Quinidine
Potassium chloride

---

or they may suffer intermittent chest pain, dysphagia or both. The diagnosis is confirmed by oesophageal manometry and pH monitoring, and radiology shows segmental spasm or a 'corkscrew' oesophagus. Treatment of this disorder is generally disappointing and variable results may be obtained with anticholinergics, nitrates, calcium entry blockers and surgical dilatation or myotomy.

Mucosal injury to the oesophagus
Oesophageal pain and dysphagia may result from direct mucosal injury due to the adverse effects of drugs which are commonly prescribed in older patients (Table 6). Management includes stopping the offending drug and the liberal use of antacids. This condition is usually temporary and responds to short-term treatment.

Disorders below the diaphragm

A number of disorders arising below the diaphragm and common in old age may present with pain referred to the chest. Most of these conditions, e.g. acute pancreatitis, perforated peptic ulcer or gallstone disease, will be characterized by predominantly upper abdominal symptoms and signs, but some older patients may have less classical presentations, and vague pain or discomfort in the lower chest may accompany partial obstruction of the biliary tract.

CHEST PAIN AND PSYCHOLOGICAL DISORDERS

Chest pain is one of several physical symptoms which may have no demonstrable organic basis. In most patients chest pain of this nature is transient but some affected individuals may have prolonged symptoms and associated disability despite negative investigations and reassurance (38). Many patients do not have any underlying psychiatric disorder, although psychological factors may influence the interpretation of minor physiological sensations or may lead to the misinterpretation of physical symptoms (Table 7). Organic causes of chest pain may coexist with pain of predominantly psychological origin, e.g. many patients with a history of angina or acute myocardial infarction are particularly aware and often very concerned if they experience any chest discomfort.

Table 7. Psychological factors and chest pain without organic cause (38)

Personality
Life stresses
Previous experience of illness
Attitudes to medical care
Personal expectations
Behaviour

Da Costa's syndrome

Variously known as effort syndrome, neurocirculatory asthenia, disorderly action of the heart, soldier's heart, functional or psychogenic disorder, this condition can affect both sexes and is especially prevalent amongst young male recruits to the armed forces during time of war. It has been described as a disorder of the autonomic nervous system control of the cardiovascular system and appears to be the result of repetitive, intense emotional stimuli. The affected individual has a fear and anxiety about his safety and future security. Symptoms include chest pain, breathlessness on minimal exertion, palpitation, exhaustion and dizziness. The pain is invariably localized to the cardiac apex and has a dull, aching quality or it may be cramping or knife-like. It may last for hours and can radiate to the left arm. Not induced by effort, it is often apparently precipitated by fatigue or emotional stress. Management includes appropriate investigation, sympathetic explanation and reassurance. Troublesome palpitation may respond to treatment with small doses of β-blocking agents.

A number of psychiatric illnesses may present with chest pain (Table 8), and after organic causes have been excluded specific psychiatric treatment may be indicated.

Panic disorder

In this condition, affected patients have recurrent episodes of intense fear or emotional discomfort. Symptoms may last for several minutes and include chest pain, breathlessness, dizziness, trembling, sweating, nausea or abdominal distress, paraesthesia or a fear of dying. There is evidence of an association between panic disorder and chest pain with negative cardiac investigations (40). Panic disorder and atypical chest pain characteristically affect young females but it is not unknown in older subjects or in patients with known heart disease. The mechanism for pain in panic disorder may be related to a hyperventilation effect producing an increase in myocardial contractility, stroke volume and cardiac output. ST–T segment and T wave abnormalities may occur on the ECG, and coronary arteriography shows no abnormality. Treatment with tricyclic antide-

Table 8. Chest pain presenting in psychiatric illnesses (39)

Anxiety disorders
    Generalized anxiety disorder
    Panic disorder $\pm$ agoraphobia
    Agoraphobia
    Obsessive-compulsive disorder

Somatoform disorders
    Conversion disorder
    Hypochondriasis
    Somatization disorder
    Somatoform pain disorder

Depressive illness

Schizophrenia

---

pressants, benzodiazepines and monoamine oxidase inhibitors may be effective in selected patients.

Hypochondriasis

This somatoform disorder may affect patients of either sex at any age. The condition may be manifest as a cardiac neurosis with chest pain, or multiple symptoms may occur. Affected individuals tend to be preoccupied with a fear of having a serious cardiac illness despite medical reassurance and advice to the contrary.

Depressive illness

The diagnosis of major depressive illness is often missed in older patients. The presentation may be distorted by the overlap of physical symptoms and classical depressive features of sadness, sleep disturbance, diurnal mood variation and feelings of unworthiness. Elderly patients may have hypochondriacal features, and chest pain or abdominal pain with no organic basis may be a commanding symptom. Depression may be difficult to treat in this age group but some patients will respond to tricyclic antidepressant drugs, cognitive psychotherapy or electroconvulsant therapy.

REFERENCES

1. Cannon PJ, Connell PA, Stockley IH *et al.* (1988) Prevalence of angina as assessed by a survey of prescriptions for nitrates. *Lancet* **i**: 979–981.
2. LaCroix AZ, Guralnik NM, Curb JD *et al.* (1990) Chest pain and coronary heart

disease mortality among older men and women in three communities, *Circulation* **81**: 437–446.

3. Vetter NJ, Ford D (1990) Angina among elderly people and its relationship with disability. *Age Ageing* **19**: 159–163.

4. Luchi RJ, Woolbert SC, McIntosh HD (1989) Atherosclerotic heart disease. In *Clinical Geriatric Cardiology*, Luchi RJ (ed.). Churchill Livingstone, Edinburgh, pp. 127–168.

5. Fisch C (1981) The electrocardiogram in the aged. In *Geriatric Cardiology*, Noble RJ, Rothbaum DA (eds.). Davis, Philadelphia.

6. Gersh BJ, Kronmal RA, Frye RL *et al.* (1983) Coronary arteriography and coronary artery bypass surgery: morbidity and mortality in patients aged 65 years or older. *Circulation* **67**: 483–491.

7. Horneffer PJ, Gardner TJ, Manolio TA *et al.* (1987) The effects of age on outcome after coronary bypass surgery. *Circulation* **76** (Suppl. IIA): 6–12.

8. Simpfendorfer C, Raymond R, Schraider J *et al.* (1988) Early and longterm results of percutaneous transluminal coronary angioplasty in patients 70 years of age and older with angina pectoris. *Am J Cardiol* **62**: 959–961.

9. Holt GW, Sugrue D, Bresnahan J *et al.* (1988) Results of percutaneous transluminal coronary angioplasty for unstable angina pectoris in patients 70 years of age and older. *Am J Cardiol* **61**: 994–997.

10. Royal College of Physicians (1991) Report on cardiological intervention in elderly patients. *J R Coll Physicians Lond* **25**: 197–205.

11. Rodstein M (1956) The characteristics of non-fatal myocardial infarction in the elderly. *Arch Intern Med* **98**: 84–90.

12. Pathy MS (1967) Clinical presentation of myocardial infarction in the elderly. *Br Heart J* **29**: 190–199.

13. MacDonald JB (1984) Presentation of acute myocardial infarction in the elderly: a review. *Age Ageing* **13**: 196–200.

14. MacDonald JB, Baillie J, Williams BO, Ballantyne D (1983) Coronary care in the elderly. *Age Ageing* **12**: 17–20.

15. Bayer AJ, Chandra JS, Farag RR, Pathy MS (1986) Changing presentation of myocardial infarction with increasing age. *J Am Geriatr Soc* **34**: 263–266.

16. Bayer AJ (1988) Presentation and management of myocardial infarction in the elderly. *Br J Hosp Med* **40**: 300–360.

17. Glazier JJ, Piessens J (1991) Mechanisms of painless myocardial ischaemia. *J R Coll Physicians Lond* **25**: 102–104.

18. Miller PF, Sheps DS, Bragdon EE *et al.* (1990) Aging and pain perception in ischemic heart disease. *Am Heart J* **120**: 22–30.

19. AIMS Trial Study Group (1988) Effect of intravenous APSAC on mortality after acute myocardial infarction: preliminary report of a placebo-controlled clinical trial. *Lancet* **i**: 545–549.

20. AIMS Trial Study Group (1990) Long-term effects of intravenous antistreplase in acute myocardial infarction: final report of the AIMS study. *Lancet* **335**: 427–431.

21. ISIS-2 (Second International Study of Infarct Survival Collaborative Group) (1988) Randomised trial of intravenous streptokinase, oral aspirin, both or neither among 17178 cases of suspected acute myocardial infarction. *Lancet* **ii**: 349–360.

22. Wilcox RG, Olsson CG, Skene AM *et al.* Trial of tissue plasminogen activator for mortality reduction in acute myocardial infarction: Anglo-Scandinavian Study of Early Thrombolysis (ASSET). *Lancet* **ii**: 525–530.

23. American College of Cardiology/American Heart Association Task Force (1990) Guidelines for the early management of patients with acute myocardial infarction. *Circulation* **82**: 664–707.

24. Herlitz J, Hjalmarson A, Waagstein F (1989) Treatment of pain in acute myocardial infarction. *Br Heart J* **61**: 9–13.
25. Semple T, Williams BO (1976) Coronary care for the elderly. In *Cardiology in Old Age*, Caird FI, Dall JLC, Kennedy RD (eds). Plenum, New York.
26. Davies MJ, Moore BP and Braimbridge MV (1978) The floppy mitral valve: study of incidence, pathology and complications in surgical, necropsy and forensic material. *Br Heart J* **40**: 468–481.
27. Tresch DD, Siegel R, Keelan MH Jr *et al.* (1979) Mitral valve prolapse in the elderly. *J Am Geriatr Soc* **27**: 421–424.
28. Topol EJ, Traill TA, Fortuin NJ (1985) Hypertensive hypertrophic cardiomyopathy in the elderly. *N Engl J Med* **312**: 277–283.
29. Koch JP, Maron BJ, Epstein SE, Morrow AJ (1980) Results of operation for obstructive hypertrophic cardiomyopathy in the elderly. *Am J Cardiol* **46**: 963–966.
30. Zull DN, Cydulka R (1988) Acute paraplegia: a presenting manifestation of aortic dissection. *Am J Med* **84**: 765–770.
31. Treasure T, Raphael MJ (1991) Investigation of suspected dissection of the thoracic aorta. *Lancet* **338**: 490–495.
32. DeBakey ME, Lawrie GM (1989) Cardiovascular surgery. In *Clinical Geriatric Cardiology*, Luchi RJ (ed.). Churchill Livingstone, Edinburgh, pp. 304–326.
33. Hawkins JW, Dunn MI (1990) Primary pulmonary hypertension in adults. *Clin Cardiol* **13**: 382–387.
34. Busby W, Bayer A, Pathy J (1988) Pulmonary embolism in the elderly. *Age Ageing* **17**: 205–209.
35. Castell DC (1990) Esophageal disorders in the elderly. *Gastroenterol Clin North Am* **19**: 235–254.
36. Yelland C (1991) Disorders of the upper gastrointestinal tract. *Rev Clin Gerontol* **1**: 29–42.
37. Hellemans J, Vantrappen G, Pelemans W (1984) Oesophageal problems. In *Gastrointestinal Tract Disorders in the Elderly*, Hellemans J, Vantrappen G (eds). Churchill Livingstone, Edinburgh, pp. 17–61.
38. Mayou R (1991) Medically unexplained physical symptoms. *Br Med J* **303**: 534–553.
39. American Psychiatric Association (1987) *Diagnostic and Statistical Manual of Mental Disorders DSM III*, 3rd edn. APA, Washington.
40. Katon WJ (1990) Chest pain, cardiac disease, and panic disorder, *J Clin Psychiatry* **51** (Suppl.): 27–30.

26 Dyspnoea

ANDREW J. S. COATS AND PHILIP A. POOLE-WILSON
National Heart and Lung Institute, London, UK

Dyspnoea or breathlessness is a term used to describe an unpleasant sensation of being unable to breathe or of being aware of the need to breathe. There is no clear dividing line between the sensation of being short of breath during or after exercise that a normal person would describe and the symptom of a patient with disease that leads to excessive ventilation on exertion. It is a sensation which has proved extremely difficult to quantify or evaluate (1). It is a very common complaint in many branches of medicine and becomes increasingly common in old age.

Disorders of many systems can be associated with breathlessness (Table 1). These include respiratory, cardiac, neurological, musculoskeletal, haematological and psychological conditions, as well as gross obesity or severe wasting. Thus in the evaluation of a breathless patient a full history, examination and range of diagnostic procedures may be necessary to evaluate the cause. This chapter will review the mechanisms of breathlessness and the approach to the evaluation of an elderly patient presenting with this symptom.

APPROPRIATE VERSUS INAPPROPRIATE BREATHLESSNESS

The first decision is whether the breathlessness reflects a physiologically necessary increased ventilatory effort, or whether the patient is describing a psychological sensation of needing to breathe excessively. This can be a very difficult clinical judgement. Clues such as the circumstances of the complaint may help. If there is a predictable relationship to exercise then the sensation is more likely to be appropriate. If the sensation occurs at rest or at times of emotional stress then a psychological cause may be considered. The possibility of an intermittent disorder such as a cardiac arrhythmia or asthma should, however, also be considered in this circumstance.

If the clinical history, examination and investigations find no evidence of disease, it is necessary to confirm a diagnosis of inappropriate breathlessness. This may include recognizing the associated features of psychogenic hyperventilation such as parasthaesiae, tetany and panic attacks and being able to reproduce the sensation by stressful situations. Although blood gas analysis

Geriatric Cardiology. Principles and Practice.   Edited by A. Martin and A. J. Camm
© 1994 John Wiley & Sons Ltd

Table 1. Pathophysiological basis of dyspnoea

Appropriate (organic disease)
Respiratory
  Airway obstruction: reversible or irreversible (including extrathoracic)
  Loss of alveoli: e.g. emphysema, lung resection
  Restrictive: e.g. pulmonary fibrosis, gross obesity
  Diffusion limitation: e.g. pneumonia, infiltration
  Ventilation/perfusion mismatch: e.g. pulmonary embolus

Cardiovascular
  Diffusion limitation: pulmonary oedema secondary to cardiac dysfunction
  Ventilation/perfusion mismatch: e.g. right ventricular failure
  Other unpleasant chest sensation: e.g. angina
  Unknown mechanism: e.g. pulmonary hypertension

Neurological
  Respiratory muscle weakness: myasthenic syndromes

Musculoskeletal
  Respiratory muscle weakness: e.g. respiratory muscle fatigue
  Altered muscle signalling: severe wasting, cachexia, ?chronic heart failure

Haematological
  Reduced oxygen delivery: anaemia, altered haemoglobin–oxygen affinity

Inappropriate
Psychological conditions: e.g. hyperventilation, anxiety
  Fictitious: compensation-seeking, malingering

---

demonstrating hypocapnia with normoxia during an attack of breathlessness will strengthen the diagnosis, a definitive diagnosis can only be established by the complete resolution of symptoms after psychological or relaxation therapy. In the absence of a complete cure suspicion should always be preserved that an organic cause may underlie the symptoms.

NORMAL VERSUS ABNORMAL BREATHLESSNESS

All subjects will become short of breath with sufficient exercise. There is no consensus as to whether this 'normal' shortness of breath should be described as dyspnoea (1) or, indeed, whether it is even the same sensation as disease-induced breathlessness.

What may be considered unexpected and unacceptable shortness of breath for a young adult may be considered normal for an elderly person. Thus patients' expectations (based perhaps on their past fitness and the exercise tolerance of friends and relatives of the same age) will have a strong bearing on symptom presentation. There will be a difficult clinical decision as to what degree of exertional breathlessness in an elderly person warrants further investigation.

With ageing degenerative changes occur in many organs and exercise tolerance will decline even in the absence of clinical disease. Each patient should be compared with the normal for his or her age. To what extent shortness of breath on exercise worsens with age depends on how normal ageing is defined. If elderly subjects with any subclinical disease are excluded from a population of 'the normal elderly' then exercise intolerance will decrease less steeply with age. In mild forms conditions such as reversible airway obstruction or left ventricular diastolic impairment cannot be reliably called disease and may be an integral part of the ageing process. In any case there is no clear threshold between low normality and disease for these conditions. Thus in investigating a complaint of breathlessness the patient's symptoms and exercise tolerance must be compared against very imperfect 'normal' data.

INVESTIGATION OF BREATHLESSNESS

The list of conditions which can present with breathlessness is protean and can involve disease in many organ symptoms. The history and clinical examination should be detailed to direct further attention to specific systems. The majority of cases of breathlessness will, however, have either a cardiovascular or respiratory basis. Initial investigation should include a chest X-ray, peak flow and an electrocardiogram (ECG) as these are inexpensive and can detect important diseases not readily evident from clinical examination. The full investigation of a breathless patient may occasionally be necessary and this should include the evaluation of cardiorespiratory function under maximal exercise stress. In between these two extremes lies the majority of clinical practice. Once it is established that the patient is suffering exercise-induced dyspnoea inappropriate for the age of the patient then the search for the cause should begin.

If respiratory or cardiac disease is identified the management of the patient will be guided along conventional lines. In cases where the degree of detected disease seems insufficient to explain the symptomatic limitation, second disease processes should be sought. Cardiac and respiratory diseases are common and often share similar risk factors such as smoking history, so it will be common to have two or more causes of breathlessness coexisting. Other conditions producing breathlessness may also overlap, including, for example, the effects of obesity and physical deconditioning. Other less frequently diagnosed conditions may complicate cardiorespiratory diseases such as myasthenic syndromes associated with malignancies, respiratory muscle fatigue complicating chronic heart failure and the skeletal muscle wasting and deconditioning effects associated with any chronic activity-restricting condition.

THE CLINICAL HISTORY IN A DYSPNOEIC PATIENT

History taking is the most important and productive part of the diagnostic process. Features of the patient's history will focus attention on particular systems and raise diagnostic possibilities and probabilities. Important basic questions include previous medical and family history as well as smoking status, alcohol and drug use, allergies, occupational exposure to toxins and allergens, foreign travel and the premorbid level of physical fitness.

It is important to enquire in detail into the nature of the dyspnoea. If reliably and predictably related to exercise the cause is more likely to be a disease leading to impaired cardiopulmonary reserve. If the exercise tolerance is much more unpredictable, episodic and variable conditions such as asthma or arrhythmias should be considered. The features associated with the shortness of breath will also direct further investigation. Wheeze suggests obstructive bronchial disease, although it can also be a feature of pulmonary oedema. Inspiratory stridor suggests extrapulmonary obstruction. Exertional chest pain with breathlessness suggests angina pectoris, although it is possible for heart failure-induced exertional symptoms occasionally to be reported as a 'pressure' in the chest. Cough, especially if productive or blood-stained, is much more common in lung disease. Cardiac failure can be associated with pink frothy sputum if acute and severe and with a dry cough if chronic or especially if the patient is taking an angiotensin-converting enzyme inhibitor. Gasping, air hunger, puffing and panting and a feeling of suffocation are less discriminatory descriptions but can be useful in assessing the severity of the symptom. Fatigue associated with breathlessness is described in chronic heart failure and anaemia but less frequently in respiratory disease.

What the patient does to relieve his or her symptoms can also provide helpful information. In cardiac failure it is common for a patient to stand or sit up, presumably to reduce left ventricular filling pressures. In angina they are more likely to rest. In obstructive airway disease the patient will often expire against pursed lips to provide a degree of positive airway pressure. In painful, especially pleuritic, conditions patients will usually pant with a rapid shallow respiratory pattern.

Grading the severity of breathlessness can be difficult if the patient is not used to performing physical exercise. Some elderly people do not climb stairs or go out for walks and it may be extremely difficult to get such patients to describe their exercise tolerance. The most useful approach is to ask which regular activities are associated with breathlessness and then assess the severity of the exercise involved in such a task. It is not uncommon, however, for a patient to state that he or she no longer performs tasks that induce breathlessness because they had proved difficult in the past. Exercise testing may be necessary to determine if such patients truly are limited in their exercise capacity.

CLINICAL EXAMINATION IN THE DYSPNOEIC PATIENT

The features of general clinical examination are well described in general medical textbooks. Particular features are important, however, in the patient complaining of breathlessness. Signs of physical fitness or unfitness should be elicited, such as resting heart rate, muscle bulk and body weight. These should be assessed against the fitness assessment based on the medical history. The appearance of laboured breathing, tachycardia or visible distress performing simple tasks such as undressing or getting onto the examination couch or lying flat can be helpful.

The pattern and frequency of breathing should be assessed when the patient is unaware that the physician is observing his or her breathing. The period whilst appearing to measure the pulse is useful for this purpose. Respiratory rate, regularity, use of accessory muscles of respiration, balance between thoracic and diaphragmatic movements, tracheal tug and audible wheeze or stridor can all be assessed at this time. Psychogenic breathing disorders are occasionally detected by a dramatic change in respiratory pattern when the patient thinks the physician is observing breathing.

Chest examination and cardiological examination should be performed in detail in any breathless patient, and this should include an assessment of peak expiratory flow rate.

FURTHER INVESTIGATIONS

The choice and order of these will be determined by the history and examination and the degree of inappropriate dyspnoea. Common investigations include full blood count, chest X-ray and ECG in new patients, lung function tests or exercise testing, respectively, if angina or obstructive or restrictive lung disease is suspected, and only more extensive investigation if the cause or severity is not clearly established. Individual special tests will be used when directed by clinical suspicion. These include sputum culture for infections, cytology for suspected malignancy, and echocardiography or radionuclide ventriculography for cardiac failure. Many more advanced and possibly invasive procedures exist for particular diagnostic and staging questions but should not be used routinely. These include bronchoscopy, bronchoalveolar lavage, computed tomography (CT) or other imaging of the thorax, cardiac catheterization, biopsies, etc. A discussion of their indications and uses is beyond the scope of this chapter.

CARDIORESPIRATORY FUNCTIONAL ASSESSMENT

The best assessment of the breathless patient is the evaluation of the integrated function of the cardiorespiratory system during a maximal exercise test. Exercise testing stresses the heart, lungs, blood and skeletal muscle and the integration of these components so that the system which is deficient can be identified. This requires the measurement of respiratory gas exchange during exercise. If lung function limits exercise then at peak exercise a failure of adequate respiratory function will be seen. This can manifest by arterial oxygen desaturation or, more subtly, by a need to hyperventilate and reduce arterial carbon dioxide tensions to preserve arterial oxygenation near normal. Other conditions which lead to a similar picture include right-to-left intra- or extracardiac shunting and ventila-

584

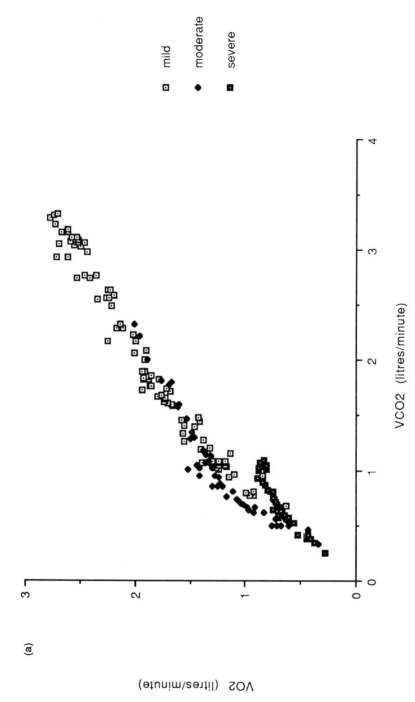

Figure 1. (a) The relationship between oxygen consumption and carbon dioxide production during incremental treadmill exercise in three patients with chronic heart failure. VO_2 = oxygen consumption in litres per minute, and VCO_2 = carbon dioxide production in litres per minute

585

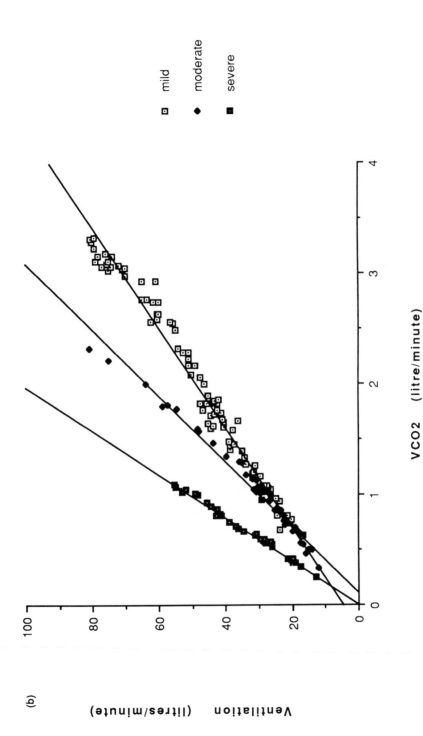

Figure 1. (b) The relationship between minute ventilation and carbon dioxide production during incremental treadmill exercise in three patients with chronic heart failure. VCO_2 = carbon dioxide production in litres per minute

tion/perfusion mismatch within the lungs. In cardiac limitation the defect is in the ability to supply the exercising muscles with enough oxygen, and hence anaerobic metabolism will occur at a low workload and become manifest by lactic acidosis and an increase in the respiratory exchange ratio. Arterial oxygen saturations do not usually fall during exercise in cardiac dysfunction unless a right-to-left shunt is present, for example, with an atrial septal defect.

In chronic heart failure cardiopulmonary functional reserve is reduced and the peak level of oxygen uptake is a good measure of the severity of the condition. During incremental exercise patients with chronic heart failure have a near-normal relationship between the rate of oxygen consumption and the rate of carbon dioxide production until the former falls off at peak exercise. In contrast there is a much steeper relationship between total minute ventilation and the rate of carbon monoxide production even at low levels of exercise (Figure 1). This increased ventilatory response is associated with an increased sensation of breathlessness, although the mechanisms of both are not fully understood.

A cardiopulmonary exercise test limited by symptoms prior to arterial oxygen desaturation or anaerobic metabolism being detected (respiratory exchange ratio exceeding unity) indicates either inadequate effort on the part of the patient or that the factor limiting exercise is neither cardiovascular nor respiratory in origin. This does not mean that the patient is not suffering exertional symptoms, merely that integrated cardiorespiratory reserve is not the limiting factor. Other unpleasant sensations such as angina, muscular fatigue, anxiety or dizziness may be expressed as shortness of breath or 'air hunger'.

Different symptoms may be produced by different forms of exercise testing. In heart failure, for example, exercise may be limited by muscle fatigue or breathlessness depending on whether a rapidly incremental exercise test or a slower protocol is used (2). This may mean that cardiorespiratory functional reserve is limiting in the fast test but not in the slower test. It is known that in chronic heart failure skeletal muscle blood flow is impaired (3) and also that intrinsic abnormalities of metabolism develop in the peripheral muscle (4), so that even where cardiac dysfunction is clearly the initiating event other changes may supervene to become the main exercise-limiting change.

MECHANISMS OF DYSPNOEA

This most fundamental of sensations is very poorly understood. It is clearly related to the control of ventilation during exercise but there is not a causal relationship between the two. Patients who are 'breathless' need not necessarily have an excessive ventilatory response to exercise, and conversely patients who exhibit hyperpnoea on exercise do not necessarily feel breathless.

There are many theories for the physiological basis of the sensation of dyspnoea, but even quantifying the sensation has proved problematical. Several excellent reviews exist on this subject to which the reader is referred (5,6). The first observation is that there is a fairly close relationship between the perception of the severity of breathless and the level of minute ventilation. It may be, therefore, that there is a perception of the respiratory effort required. In patients with respiratory disorders, however, it has been noted that with prolonged exercise this relationship is lost and breathlessness increases even during a constant workload and a constant minute ventilation. In this case the subject may be aware of a greater neural input driving ventilation with a restriction in the ability of the respiratory system to respond to the increased respiratory drive (7). Furthermore, in normals and subjects with respiratory disease, if the ventilatory response to exercise is imitated by voluntary hyperventilation then the resultant level of perceived breathlessness is reduced even if carbon dioxide gas tension is prevented from falling. It is not known if the same is true in cardiac exercise limitation. Other possible inputs to the central nervous system which may mediate the sensation of breathlessness include direct appreciation of the chemoreceptor drive and a perception of the level of respiratory stimulating factors such as arterial lactate, pH, potassium, adenosine, carbon dioxide and other unknown factors. It may be that the pattern or rhythms of these chemical signals are important rather than merely the mean blood level.

The normal mechanisms whereby ventilatory effort is matched to muscular work are imperfectly understood. From rest to peak exercise the rate of oxygen utilization and carbon dioxide can vary 20–30-fold (8). This response occurs with minor changes in arterial gas concentrations and with little time delay. Clearly there is a very effective control system. A variety of physiological approaches has led to the conclusion that there are several control systems which overlap and complement each other to match integrated cardiopulmonary function to metabolic demand. The main control systems involve the peripheral and central chemoreceptors, central command and blood-borne chemical products of exercising muscle metabolism.

In response to exercise the cardiac output increases, minute ventilation is enhanced and peripheral blood flow is directed to the exercising muscle groups. This response is rapid and appropriate to the demands placed upon the system. It requires an integrated control system. At the onset of exercise some central command signal (perhaps going in parallel with motor neurone discharge) is thought to go to putative central cardiovascular and respiratory control centres in the brain stem to increase heart rate, cardiac output and ventilation. Very soon after the onset of exercise venous return is enhanced due to the muscle pump action. This will lead to a further tachycardia and increase in cardiac output due to the combined effects of the Bainbridge reflex and Starling's law. It is not known if there is a sufficient cross-talk between the cardiac reflexes and the respiratory centre for a simultaneous increase in ventilation to accompany this change. In experiments with active and passive exercise in patients with heart or heart and lung transplantations with loss of neural connections between the heart, lungs and brain, however, there is evidence that the early respiratory response to exercise is preserved, although the mechanism of this control signal was not evaluated (9). Very quickly after the onset of exercise, blood with a reduced oxygen content and increased carbon dioxide tension could be expected to traverse the lungs and stimulate the peripheral arterial chemoreceptors and lead to a reflex increase in respiratory rate and effort. That such changes in arterial blood gases are not commonly seen at the initiation of exercise has led to the search for other respiratory stimuli (10).

When the arterial chemoreceptors are activated there is again cross-talk between cardiovascular and respiratory control mechanisms as chemoreceptor activation is thought to cause further tachycardia and reflex vasoconstriction of non-exercising muscle beds. Other more complex interactions and reflex effects also exist but with physiological roles which are far from clear.

Overall the integrated control of ventilation is sufficient to keep ventilation adequate to ensure virtually unchanged arterial blood gas concentrations throughout exercise. As no feedback loop can have infinite gain there must be a residual blood gas abnormality to maintain the increased ventilatory effort, unless other factors contribute to the maintenance of increased ventilation. Many other factors have been identified, some of which may be better substrates for the primary control mechanisms, perhaps indicating that the chemoreceptors may serve to fine-tune ventilatory responses rather than being the primary drive. These factors include arterial potassium, pH, lactate, adenosine or its meta-bolites all acting as blood-borne factors, neural messages reflecting the state of the exercising skeletal muscle (ergo- or metaboloreceptors) or respiratory muscles, or alterations in the temporal patterns of any of the above. The precise control mechanisms in this basic exercise response is very poorly understood. Our ability to understand the basis of pathophysiological conditions associated with disordered control of breathing or perceptions of breathlessness may need to await a better understanding of integrated cardiopulmonary physiology.

SUMMARY

Dyspnoea is a common but poorly understood symptom. Many diseases in the elderly and indeed the ageing process itself can lead to this symptom. The assessment of the dyspnoeic elderly patient should be thorough but realistic, and should be directed towards the identification of conditions or pathophysiological processes amenable to amelioration.

REFERENCES

1. Adams L, Guz A (1991) Dyspnea on exertion. In *Exercise: Pulmonary Physiology and Pathophysiology*. Whipp BJ, Wasserman K (eds). Marcel Dekker, New York, 449–494.
2. Lipkin DP, Canepa-Anson R, Stephens MR, Poole-Wilson PA (1986) Factors determining symptoms in heart failure: comparison of fast and slow exercise tests. *Br Heart J* **55**: 439–445.
3. Zelis R, Mason DT, Braunwald E (1968) A comparison of the effects of vasodilator stimuli on peripheral resistance vessels in normal subjects and in patients with

congestive heart failure. *J Clin Invest* **47**: 960–970.

4. Massie B, Conway M, Yonge R *et al.* (1987) Skeletal muscle metabolism in patients with congestive heart failure: relation to clinical severity and blood flow. *Circulation* **76**: 1009–1019.

5. Stark RD (1988) Dyspnoea: assessment and pharmacological manipulation. *Eur Respir J* **1**: 280–287.

6. Wasserman K, Casaburi R (1988) Dyspnea: physiological and pathological mechanisms. *Annu Rev Med* **39**: 503–515.

7. O'Neill PA, Stark RD, Allen SC, Stretton TB (1986) The relationship between breathlessness and ventilation during steady state exercise. *Clin Respir Physiol* **33**: 247–250.

8. Astrand P-O, Rodahl K (1986) *Textbook of Work Physiology: Physiological Bases of Exercise.* McGraw-Hill, New York.

9. Adams L, Guz A, Innes JA, Murphy K (1987) The early circulatory and ventilatory response to voluntary and electrically induced exercise in man. *J Physiol (Lond)* **383**: 19–30.

10. Clark A, Coats A (1992) The mechanisms underlying the increased ventilatory response to exercise in chronic stable heart failure. *Eur Heart J* (in press).

Part VI

MAJOR ELEMENTS OF
THERAPY

27 Drug Treatment

CHARLES F. GEORGE AND DEREK WALLER
University of Southampton, Southampton, UK

The past 40 years have seen a major change in the age structure of our population. In 1951 the population of England and Wales contained 4.83 million persons aged 65 or over, but by 30 years later the figure had risen to 7.57 million. By the turn of the century the figure should exceed 8 million elderly people. More important is the number of 'old elderly' persons, the number of whom has risen from 1.57 million in 1951 to more than 3 million at present. This figure is particularly important in view of the high rate of illness in the latter age category. Several studies have shown that the elderly are prescribed more medicines than younger people (1–4). Although much of the prescribing is beneficial there is concern about the high incidence of iatrogenic illness in the elderly, and much of this is avoidable (5–9).

Two recent studies have examined the nature of medicines prescribed for old people living in the community. The first from Southampton (4) assessed prescribing for a systematic 1:200 sample of the adult population by means of postal questionnaire. As anticipated, women were prescribed more medicines than men, and drug therapy was twice as common among those over the age of 55 compared to those under that age (60.8% versus 31.5%; $p < 0.001$). Overall, 42.4% (188 respondents) had been prescribed a medicine by their general practitioner during the previous month. Drugs with an action on the heart and circulation were those which were most commonly in use (Table 1). In particular, β-adrenoceptor antagonists, diuretics and vasodilator compounds were in widespread use. A larger study by Cartwright and Smith (8) used a different method of survey. A structured random sample of people aged 65 and over was drawn from the electoral registers of 10 parliamentary constituencies in England. Information was obtained for 78% (805 patients) of the 1032 included in the original sample. Sixty per cent of these people had taken one or more prescribed medicines within the preceding 24 hours. Despite the different approach, this survey confirmed that drugs for diseases of the heart and circulation were widely prescribed. Overall, diuretics formed the therapeutic category in most widespread use, followed by analgesics, hypnotics, sedatives and anxiolytics, drugs for rheumatism and gout and then β-adrenoceptor antagonists.

Geriatric Cardiology. Principles and Practice.   Edited by A. Martin and A. J. Camm
© 1994 John Wiley & Sons Ltd

Table 1. Cardiovascular drugs taken by 50 people identified in a systematic sample of Southampton residents (classified according to the *British National Formulary* system)

2.	Cardiovascular system	
2.1	Cardiac glycosides	3
2.2	Diuretics	17
2.3	Antiarrhythmic drugs	1
2.4	β-Adrenoceptor blocking drugs	18
2.5	Antihypertensive drugs	1
2.6	Vasodilators	9
2.8	Anticoagulants	1
		50

Modified from Ridout *et al.* (4).

These 50 people were drawn from a total of 188 who were prescribed a medicine during the previous month.

ADVERSE DRUG REACTIONS

An adverse drug reaction (ADR) has been defined as any noxious change in a patient's condition due to drug therapy. Most commonly ADRs represent an excessive response to the drug's primary or secondary pharmacological actions (type A) (10). Thus, most ADRs indicate the need to stop the offending drug, or reduce its dosage.

Secondly, patients who are affected by an adverse effect of one drug are more liable to develop unwanted effects from subsequent drug therapy. Finally, some unwanted effects may themselves require treatment. Several reasons have been identified as being responsible for the increased incidence of adverse drug reactions in old people (11). These are: (i) multiple drug prescribing; (ii) altered pharmacokinetics; and (iii) altered pharmacodynamics.

Multiple drug therapy

Several legitimate reasons exist for polypharmacy in the elderly. First, the prevalence of many diseases is age-related and several may coexist in the same patient: hypertension (12), osteoarthrosis (13) and prostatic hypertrophy (14), for example. Second, it may not be possible to achieve an adequate therapeutic response from the use of a single drug. Thus, a patient with asthma may require not only a bronchodilator but also an inhaled corticosteroid to suppress the inflammatory response in the bronchi (15). Similarly, some patients with angina pectoris will require a calcium channel-blocking drug as well as a β-adrenoceptor antagonist (16) to produce an adequate response. Third, a second drug may be required to counteract or minimize a type A effect. For example, potassium loss can be corrected with spironolactone, amiloride (17) or triamterene (18) in patients who are receiving either a benzothiadiazine or loop-type diuretic.

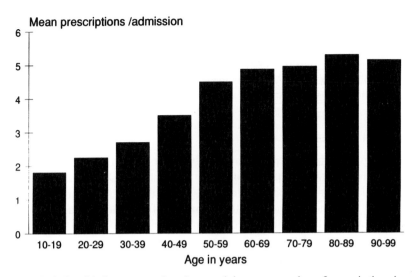

Figure 1. Relationship between patients' age and the mean number of prescriptions issued for 5284 admissions to medical wards in Southampton

However, one of the most important predictors for adverse drug reactions is the total number of drugs given simultaneously (19–21). In this context, Moir and Dingwall-Fordyce (22) found that 28% of those aged 65 years and living at home had no medication, 57% had one to three prescribed drugs and 15% received four or more. In the study by Cartwright and Smith (8) the average number of medicines prescribed per patient was 2.8. Even larger numbers of drugs are prescribed for patients in hospital (Figure 1) and the incidence of adverse drug reactions is higher. In addition, polypharmacy in the elderly can cause confusion and lead to errors in medicine taking, particularly in those over the age of 85 (23,24).

Drug–drug interactions

Another consequence of multiple prescribing for old people is the occurrence of drug–drug interactions. The latter may be defined as an alteration in either the magnitude or the duration of a drug's effects caused by the introduction or presence of a second. The chances of an adverse consequence of multiple drug therapy rise exponentially with the number given simultaneously (5,25). However, some agents are far more likely than others to give rise to such problems. Notable amongst these are agents with a narrow therapeutic index (25,26), i.e. the dose or plasma concentration of drug which is effective lies close to that which causes toxicity. Among those agents whch fall into the above category are antihypertensive drugs, cardiac glycosides and oral anticoagulants (26). Antagonism of their actions will render them ineffective, while synergism with such agents can cause profound toxicity (see below).

Altered pharmacokinetics

The term 'pharmacokinetics' applies to the processes and rates of drug absorption, distribution, metabolism and elimination. Alterations can be produced either by age *per se* or by disease processes, many of which increase in their prevalence with age.

Absorption

Most drugs are administered by mouth, both for convenience and because this route affords a greater margin of safety than others. Drugs administered by mouth will normally reach the stomach, where disintegration and dissolution occur (27). For most there is little absorption from the stomach because its surface area is small and the pH is unfavourable for this to occur (the majority of drugs are ionized at the acidic pH of gastric contents). By contrast, in the more alkaline environment of the small intestine, absorption is favoured both by pH (and the fact that the drug is less ionized) and because the surface area available for absorption is large due to the presence of the villous projections and the microvilli present on the surface of each mucosal cell (27). In practical terms, the majority of drug absorption takes place from the intestine rather than the stomach. It follows that absorption cannot occur until the stomach has emptied. Numerous studies have attempted to examine gastric emptying and its relationship to increasing age (28–31). Many such studies are difficult to interpret because of the presence of coexistent disease and drug treatment for the latter. However, any changes in motility due to age appear to be quite small. Furthermore, although achlorhydria is more common with increasing age (32), it has little effect on the absorption of the majority of drugs.

By contrast, there is evidence for impaired absorption of some drugs in the presence of cardiac failure (33–36). The best-documented examples are of metolazone, prazosin and quinidine. The precise explanation of these changes is unclear but the possibilities include oedema of the intestinal wall and the diminished blood flow (37). The latter parameter is well recognized to determine the rate and extent of drug absorption in experimental animals and from other sites of drug administration in man.

Drug distribution

In general, old people show an increased amount of adipose tissue and a reduced lean body mass (38). As a consequence, the distribution volume of lipid-soluble products may increase. However, the situation is complicated because the majority of drugs are either weak acids or weak bases. As a consequence they bind to either basic or acidic plasma proteins (39). Albumin present in the blood has an affinity for both types of molecules, particularly those which are acidic. Albumin concentrations decline only slightly in fit old people (40,41) but are reduced in those who are sick or frail (40–42). As a consequence, plasma protein binding of acidic drugs may be diminished and their distribution volumes increased. Furthermore, since it is the fraction of drug which is free in plasma water that is active (43,44), pharmacological effects may be increased. By contrast, basic molecules such as propranolol and lignocaine are bound to the acidic protein α_1-acid glycoprotein (45,46). Concentrations of this acute-phase protein are influenced by concomitant diseases (47) which tend to be more prevalent in old age. In their presence, the binding of some drugs, e.g. propranolol, can be increased and its distribution reduced (48). Alterations in protein binding can occur also with concomitant drug therapy (26). For the most part these are short lived because any displacement from protein binding tends to be compensated for by increased distribution, metabolism and elimination (25,26).

For some drugs, particularly digoxin, binding to muscle is an important determinant of its distribution within the body (49). The reduced lean body mass influences its distribution volume and the loading dose required.

Drug metabolism

Although some drugs can be eliminated unchanged via the kidneys (see below) the majority are reabsorbed and must undergo metabolism prior to their elimination from the body. Drug metabolism takes place in two phases: phase I and phase II (or both) (44,45). In phase I reactions the drug undergoes either oxidation, reduction or hydrolysis to reveal or append reactive chemical groupings which may be liable to subsequent conjugation or phase II reactions. Some examples are shown in Table 2. Most phase I reactions lead to a diminution in pharmacological activity but there are exceptions. Thus, 4-hydroxypropranolol is also an active β-adrenoceptor antagonist, and there are several active metabolites of antiarrhythmic drugs, e.g. amiodarone, encainide, procainamide and verapamil.

Drug oxidation takes place in the mixed function oxidases which are present in a variety of body tissues. However, the largest concentration and activity of these is located in the liver. Although collectively known as cytochrome P_{450} because of the fact that their maximum absorption of ultraviolet light occurs at 450 nm (51), there is, in fact, a family of isoenzymes many of which have now been sequenced and cloned (52,53). Genetic polymorphism in the activity of such enzymes has been well demonstrated (54), particularly for that which metabolizes not only debrisoquine but also a variety of β-adrenoceptor antagonists. This enzyme is now classified as cytochrome P_{450} 2D6. Between 5% and 10% of the population show impaired metabolism of debrisoquine (and 20 or so other compounds) and this deficiency is inherited in an autosomal recessive manner. Poor metabolizers of debrisoquine are more susceptible to its effects and develop postural hypotension. Other substrates include the antiarrhythmics, encainide and propafenone, and a variety of β-adrenoceptor antagonists including alprenolol,

Table 2. Pathways of drug elimination in man

Phase	Reaction	Enzyme	Examples
I	Oxidation of aliphatic and aromatic groups, etc.	Cytochrome P_{450} Flavin monooxygenases	Propranolol and other lipid-soluble β-adrenoceptor antagonists
	Reduction of azo, nitro and sulphoxide groups, etc.	Aldehyde oxidase	Sulindac
	Hydrolysis	Esterases Amidases	Procaine Lignocaine Esters
II	Glucuronide synthesis	Glucuronyl-transferase	Paracetamol Chloramphenicol
	Glycine conjugation	Transacylase	Salicylate
	Ethereal sulphate synthesis	Sulphokinase	Isoprenaline
	Methylation	Catechol-O-methyl-transferase	Isoprenaline
	Acetylation	N-Acetyl-transferase	Hydralazine
	Mercapturic acid synthesis	Glutathione-transferases	Paracetamol

bopindolol, bufuralol, metoprolol, penbutolol, propranolol and timolol. Deficient metabolism explains some adverse effects, which were previously regarded as being idiosyncratic, e.g. vomiting with bufuralol.

Besides genetic influences, drug metabolism is affected by environmental factors such as chemicals present in tobacco smoke, foodstuffs and other drugs (25,26,44). But old age itself can affect the rate and extent of drug metabolism (55,56). However, the direction and magnitude of such effects vary according to the substrate in question. Furthermore, in the past, problems have arisen because only half-lives have been used to estimate drug metabolism. Although this parameter is simple to estimate it is influenced not only by the elimination rate of the drug in question, but also by its distribution volume. Since the latter is often affected by ageing (see above) it is easy to infer that drug metabolism is reduced when it is not. In our view, clearance is a more precise measure of the rate of drug elimination and this concept can be applied either to drug metabolism or renal elimination.

Clearance is the volume of blood (or plasma) from which a drug is totally removed in unit time. It therefore has the dimensions of millilitres or litres per minute, hour or day. Further precision can be added by relating these values to the weight of the individual. Typically, clearance of a drug is then expressed in terms of millilitres per kilogram per minute (or hour).

The physiochemical characteristics of a drug are very important in determining its rate of metabolic clearance. Basic drugs such as propranolol that are bound to α_1-acid glycoprotein (45) are transported to the liver, where at least 75% of what is presented is extracted during passage through this organ (57). Liver blood flow averages 20 ml/kg per minute (58), so that propranolol's hepatic clearance can be as high as 15 ml/kg per minute. Clearly, hepatic blood flow is an important determinant of clearance for drugs (59) which, like propranolol, are subject to extensive extraction and metabolism (60). Examples include other lipid-soluble β-adrenoceptor antagonists, e.g. labetalol (61), the calcium channel-blocking drugs such as verapamil (62) and many members of the dihydropyridine group, e.g. nifedipine (63).

When such compounds are administered intravenously to an old person it is to be anticipated that their clearance from the plasma will be diminished as compared with that of young people (Figure 2). By contrast, there is little evidence to show any change in the systemic clearance of drugs such as the long-acting non-steroidal anti-inflammatory drugs, e.g. isoxicam (64). The clearance of such agents is more often affected by a balance between the intrinsic

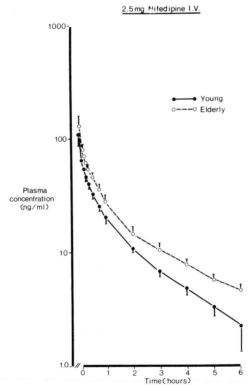

Figure 2. Plasma concentrations of nifedipine following 2.5 mg intravenously in volunteers. Clearance is delayed in the elderly, averaging 348 ± 83 ml/min compared with 519 ± 125 ml/min in the young

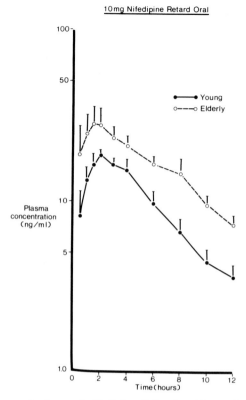

Figure 3. Plasma concentrations of nifedipine following 10 mg of a sustained release formulation given to volunteers. The data were obtained from the same individuals as those shown in Figure 2. The calculated bioavailability is 61% in the elderly compared with 46% in the young, and the area under the concentration-time curve is 281 ± 64 ng/ml hour compared with 136 ± 56 ng/ml hour

metabolic capacity of the liver and the delaying effect of binding to plasma proteins.

Changes in the pharmacokinetics of drugs which undergo extensive metabolism within the liver tend to be more obvious when they are given by the oral route (65). Following their absorption from the gastrointestinal tract (which is often complete due to their high lipid solubility) a major portion of the agent is eliminated prior to reaching the systemic circulation. Thus, the bioavailability (the proportion of the drug reaching the systemic circulation unchanged) is around 25–30% for propranolol (60) and 46% for nifedipine in young adults (63). However, higher bioavailabilities occur with ageing (Figure 3) (66). If the dynamic response is unchanged, these pharmacokinetic changes will cause an increased magnitude and duration of response.

Controversy remains as to the precise cause of the diminished presystemic metabolism seen for drugs administered to old people. Readers are referred to a recent review by Woodhouse and James (56). From this it is clear that for a majority of drugs any diminution in first-pass metabolism occurring in the elderly is chiefly the result of an age-related reduction in liver volume (67), rather than in specific enzyme activity. But for nifedipine it seems possible that some of the age-related differences could result from an alteration in intestinal metabolism.

A specific cytochrome P_{450} known as 3A is the dominant enzyme involved in the metabolism of nifedipine and the other dihydropyridines (68). This enzyme is also present in the intestinal wall at the tips of the villi and is the dominant cytochrome P_{450} present at this site (69,70).

Drug metabolism can occur also within the microorganisms of the gastrointestinal tract (71). The majority of these are located in its more distal reaches, i.e. beyond the ileocaecal valve. They are responsible for the bioactivation of sulphinpyrazone to its metabolite, sulphinpyrazone sulphide (72), which has 'antiplatelet' effects by inhibiting cyclooxygenase therein (73). Digoxin is also subject to metabolism within the colon but the extent of this reaction varies markedly from one individual to another (74). Concurrent administration of antimicrobials can profoundly affect the metabolism of both sulphinpyrazone (75,76) (reducing the formation of its active metabolite) and of digoxin, leading to intoxication (74).

Phase II reactions

Phase II reactions can occur in both the liver and intestine (44,77). In phase II reactions chemical groupings, e.g. glucuronide or sulphate, are added to the products of phase I metabolism (or for suitable substrates directly to the parent moiety). This has two effects: first, the molecule is rendered more polar and suitable for excretion by the kidneys (44,50). Second, the enhanced molecular weight of the product can facilitate its elimination in the bile (78). Many phase II reactions are not rate-limiting and therefore show little effect due to ageing. However, genetic polymorphism is apparent for some reactions, especially that carried out by N-acetyltransferase (79). This enzyme is present in both the intestinal wall and liver (80) and is responsible for the metabolism of the vasodilator compound, hydralazine (81), and the antiarrhythmic, procainamide (79). Poor metabolizers of hydralazine show a greater pharmacological response but are more liable to develop the systemic lupus erythematosus syndrome (81).

Drug elimination

The kidneys represent the major site of drug elimination for drugs which are themselves soluble in water (polar), e.g. amiloride (82), atenolol (83), digoxin (84), procainamide (85) (in part) and the aminoglycoside antibiotics (86). For the majority of compounds filtration of the fraction which is free in plasma water occurs at the glomerulus. However, there can be pH-dependent reabsorption in the tubules, e.g. of procainamide. But for a small number of compounds, especially the β-lactam antibiotics (penicillins, cephalosporins), active tubular secretion occurs. This latter process can be blocked by the co-administration of probenecid (87).

It follows that the rate of drug clearance by the kidneys depends upon blood flow to these organs. An age-related decline in glomerular filtration has been well documented (88,89) due either to nephrosclerosis (90) or a reduction in cardiac output. A further example is seen in patients with myxoedema in whom the clearance of digoxin is reduced (91). The introduction of thyroxine treatment causes glomerular filtration to return towards normal rates. Conversely, in thyrotoxicosis the clearance of digoxin is increased and this accounts in part for resistance to its effects.

Changes in renal function consequent upon ageing and disease can have major effects on the rate of elimination of water-soluble compounds (92). The administration of the usual therapeutic dose (100 mg) of atenolol can, for example, lead to its accumulation in the elderly and excessive pharmacological effects occurring (Figure 4). Similarly, the elderly are well known to be at greater risk from therapy with digoxin (90) than younger patients and as a consequence many doctors tend to protect their patients by using much smaller doses than usual. It should be remembered that even in patients who are anephric digoxin can be cleared by non-renal routes (93).

Apart from influencing the rate of elimination of polar drugs themselves, renal function can modulate the clearance of active metabolites. Thus, for acebutolol its active acetyl metabolite can accumulate in renal failure (94). Like its parent compound, the metabolite has β-adrenoceptor-blocking properties but it may be less cardioselective.

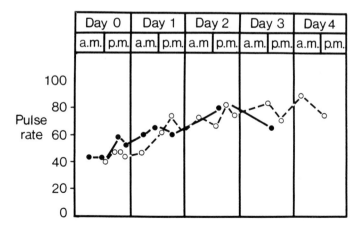

Figure 4. Pulse rates obtained in two elderly patients admitted because of syncopal attacks. Both received atenolol orally which was withdrawn on admission to hospital because of the bradycardia

Identifying and coping with changes in renal function

In our experience, doctors frequently base their assumptions of renal function on measures of blood urea or creatinine. However, blood urea is a poor guide to the glomerular filtration rate (GFR) since it varies widely with changes in diet and urine flow rate. But if the blood urea is raised in the presence of a normal blood creatinine, it can provide useful information (Table 3). Blood creatinine provides a better indicator of GFR but frequently remains within the laboratory reference range in elderly people despite compromised renal function. This is due to their loss of muscle mass and the fact that many old people consume less protein than do younger persons. The common practice of providing a single reference range for all age groups can therefore be dangerously misleading. Thus, a muscular 30-year-old man weighing 80 kg and an 80-year-old woman weighing 50 kg may have identical plasma creatinine concentrations of 120 μmol/l. In the young man, this will reflect a GFR of about 90 ml/min, compared with a value of 25 ml/min in the elderly woman. If, however, changes in both age and weight are taken into account, fairly reliable estimates of GFR can be calculated (95) (Figure 5). Such equations make assumptions about the rate of creatinine excretion in urine and produce values of GFR which are comparable to those obtained by direct measurement. They have a considerable advantage over the more widely used (measured) creatinine clearance which relies on accurate urine collections. Obtaining accurate 24-hour urine collections can require two or three attempts in the elderly, even in those who are hospitalized. Estimates may be complicated by small urine volumes, incomplete bladder emptying (due to prostatism or vaginal prolapse) or by urinary incontinence. Although shorter periods of urine collection have been proposed, the accuracy of creatinine clearance measurements is reduced when based on 2- or 4-hour collections (96).

Table 3. Relationship between blood urea and creatinine

Urea and creatinine raised to a similar extent
Chronic renal failure
Established acute renal failure

Urea disproportionately increased compared to creatinine
Salt and water depletion
Diuretic therapy
Heart failure
Gastrointestinal bleeding
High protein intake
Protein catabolism, e.g. infection, glucocorticoids

Urea disproportionately depressed compared to creatinine
Liver failure
High fluid intake
Low protein intake

$$\text{Male } C_{cr} = \frac{1.23 \times (140 - \text{age in years}) \times (\text{weight in kg})}{\text{plasma creatinine } \mu\text{mol/1}}$$

$$\text{Female } C_{cr} = \frac{1.04 \times (140 - \text{age in years}) \times (\text{weight in kg})}{\text{plasma creatinine } \mu\text{mol/1}}$$

Figure 5. Cockcroft and Gault's formula for calculating creatinine clearance based upon the knowledge of age, gender, weight and plasma creatinine

Although creatinine clearance predicted by these formulae is normally accurate, there are some situations in which their use can be misleading. One of these is gross obesity, which results in a substantial overestimate of GFR. Second, there are problems when renal function is changing rapidly and there is a lag before a change in blood creatinine concentration is seen. Third, renal tubular secretion of creatinine occurs and is important when renal function is impaired. The renal tubular excretion can be blocked by other drugs, including cimetidine, trimethoprim, triamterene, spironolactone and amiloride: all of these may elevate blood creatinine concentrations without altering GFR (97,98). Additionally, there is some evidence that the formulae are inaccurate in patients with coexisting liver disease perhaps due to reduced production of creatinine (95,99).

When an accurate knowledge of GFR is required, either for the determination of drug doses or to monitor the effects of a potentially nephrotoxic drug, there is no substitute for the use of a radioisotopic clearance method. The plasma clearance of labelled chelates, particularly ^{51}Cr-labelled ethylendiaminetetra-acetic acid (^{51}Cr-EDTA) and ^{99m}Tc-labelled diethylenetriaminepentaacetic acid (^{99m}Tc-DTPA), give values for GFR which correlate closely with those obtained using inulin, the accepted 'gold standard' (100). Reliable estimates of GFR can be obtained from one or two blood samples taken within 4 hours of the intravenous injection of either chelate and without urine collection (101). However, the additional expense and complexity involved make these methods unsuitable (and unnecessary) for most clinical situations.

When considering impaired renal function and drug handling, it is important to remember that while GFR is an important index of renal function it does not always reflect renal tubular function. In the ageing kidney, renal GFR and tubular functions appear to decline at similar rates (renal plasma flow falls between 1% and 2% per annum after the age of 20 (102) and GFR by about 0.5% per year (103). Urine-concentrating ability reflecting distal tubular function and maximum reabsorptive capacity for glucose also show a progressive decline (104,105). But superimposed on this age-related decline in renal function, intrinsic renal disease may further impair the ability to handle drugs. In this situation a decline in tubular function may not always be reflected in the GFR, particularly in the case of some forms of tubulointerstitial disease. Drug accumulation may therefore be greater than anticipated from either the serum creatinine or GFR measurement. Drugs for which tubular excretion is important include the β-lactam antibiotics and many diuretics.

For some drugs with a narrow therapeutic index, chemical or bioassay methods exist for their estimation in plasma (106). Thus, the estimation of digoxin concentrations can help dosage adjustment, particularly when renal function is changing fairly rapidly or when interactions with other drugs are possible. By contrast, when using an aminoglycoside antibiotic to treat infective endocarditis it would be negligent to do so without measuring the plasma/serum concentration at appropriate times (peak and trough values) and adjusting the dosage accordingly (107). Failure to observe this precaution increases the risk of toxicity to the hair cells within the ear and of nephrotoxicity occurring (108).

Pharmacodynamic variation with ageing

Estimation of pharmacodynamic variation with ageing is hampered by a lack of methods for quantifying the effects of drugs on the target tissue(s). But because of the simplicity of measuring pulse, blood pressure and the existence of reliable tests of coagulation, many of the best-documented examples can be found in the sphere of cardiovascular medicine. Almost certainly these represent the tip of a much larger iceberg. We have confined ourselves to some of the better-documented examples.

Anticoagulants

In most centres warfarin is regarded as the preferred anticoagulant because of its much lower incidence of type B unwanted effects, e.g. rashes.

The effects of warfarin are monitored routinely using tests such as the INR, for which a therapeutic range of 2–3 is often recommended. Several studies have shown that the elderly require less warfarin than average to bring their INR values into the therapeutic range (109). However, the mechanism underlying the age-related difference has been disputed. In a study by Shepherd and colleagues (110) an age-related difference in the sensitivity of the vitamin K_1 receptor was claimed, but this was not confirmed by other authors in a subsequent study (111). Nevertheless, whatever the mechanism involved it is clear that warfarin therapy requires careful justification if it is to be used in the elderly (112), and the dose requires modification and careful monitoring.

Antihypertensives

In recent years several studies have shown the benefits of antihypertensive therapy in elderly people (113–117) (up to the age of 80 years). However, inappropriate antihypertensive therapy can lead to syncopal attacks (118) and to fractures occurring.

Homeostatic mechanisms are impaired in this age group and postural hypotension occurs in up to one person in 10 (in the absence of drug therapy) (119). Diuretics which diminish plasma volume, and those antihypertensive

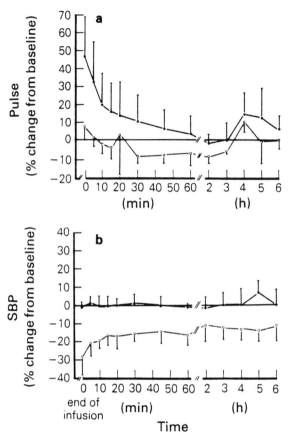

Figure 6. The effects of nifedipine 2.5 mg given intravenously to young (●) and elderly (○) volunteers. There is no change in the blood pressure of the young volunteers but a marked increase in heart rate. By contrast, in the elderly heart rate is unaffected but there is a pronounced reduction in systolic blood pressure

agents which have a predominantly postural effect on blood pressure (119), are likely to be particularly problematic.

Baroreflexes show an age-related decline (120–123): thus, the heart rate response to standing is diminished. Two explanations are possible. First, compliance of the carotid sinuses can be reduced due to atheroma. Second, there is a diminished sensitivity of β-adrenoceptors to catecholamines, both in the circulation and liberated from noradrenergic nerve endings (124). An example of the diminished cardioacceleratory response in the elderly is shown for intravenously administered nifedipine (66) (Figure 6).

Problems with postural hypotension are to some extent dose-related but are more likely to occur with the first dosage of inhibitors of the angiotensin-converting enzyme (125) or the α-adrenoceptor-blocking agent prazosin (126). Such problems tend to be magnified by concurrent diuretic therapy (127). It is also important to remember that 'non-cardiac' drugs can cause similar problems (128). Examples include L-dopa and a variety of psychotropic agents, e.g. phenothiazines, butyrophenones, tricyclic antidepressants and monoamine oxidase inhibitors.

Adrenoceptors

Several studies have shown that the density and responsiveness of β-adrenoceptors are reduced in the elderly (129–135). As a consequence there is a reduced responsiveness of the heart and bronchi to isoprenaline, and the cyclic AMP response of human lymphocytes is diminished. More recently, abnormalities in the sensitivity of the α_1 and α_2-adrenoceptors have been demonstrated (135,136).

Frusemide

The onset of the diuretic effect of intravenous frusemide tends to be delayed in old people (137). This may reflect its slower distribution into the renal tubular fluid but, in addition, the intensity of the diuretic response shows a greater variation in the elderly.

Other problems with drug therapy in the elderly

The potential problems of drug therapy for old people were well documented in a report of the Royal College of Physicians (London) published in 1984 (11). Summarized briefly and paraphrased, they include:

1. Excessive prescribing of certain categories of medicine.
2. Failure to adjust for age-related changes in the pharmacokinetics and pharmacodynamics of drugs (see above).
3. Excessive numbers of drugs given simultaneously.
4. Regimens which are too complex.
5. Inadequate supervision.

To these can be added the failure of many doctors (and pharmacists) to give patients adequate information about their medicines (4).

Excessive prescribing of drugs from certain therapeutic categories

Probably the best example of excessive use of a cardiovascular drug therapy is that of diuretics. Many old people are poorly mobile and as a consequence can develop gravitational oedema. Diuretics are not indicated for this purpose (nor for oedema associated with the use of drugs such as nifedipine). Several studies have shown that diuretics can be withdrawn quite safely (138–140)—in the absence of heart failure—thereby avoiding their undesirable metabolic effects, which include glucose intolerance (141). Second, other 'non-cardiac' drugs tend to be used to excess in the elderly (8). These include prochlorperazine (Stemetil), which is all too often prescribed for 'giddiness' (142). It is, however, a neuroleptic with a broad spectrum of pharmacological actions.

Osteoarthrosis is common in the elderly, and its identification in the knees or hips frequently leads to the prescription of non-steroidal anti-inflammatory drugs (143–145). Often, simple analgesics such as paracetamol, together with a programme of weight reduction and exercises (to strengthen the muscles and thereby stabilize joints) would be more appropriate (146). Non-steroidal anti-inflammatory drugs give rise to more gastrointestinal bleeding in this age group (147). But, in addition, they can antagonize the effects of loop diuretics (148), as well as reducing the effects of many antihypertensive agents, e.g. β-adrenoceptor antagonists (149), angiotensin-converting enzyme (ACE) inhibitors and benzothiadiazine diuretics. The combination of non-steroidal anti-inflammatory drug therapy, ACE inhibitor and diuretics (particularly potassium-conserving ones) appears to be particularly hazardous (150).

Failure to adjust for age-related changes in the pharmacokinetics and pharmacodynamics of drugs

See above and tables.

Excessive numbers of drug/complex regimens

Although many elderly people appear to cope quite well when given several medicines it is particularly in people who are over the age of 85 that problems tend to occur. Problems are most likely when more than three medicines are used simultaneously and these are given at different times of the day (one from another) (23).

Inadequate supervision

The meticulous study by Cartwright and Smith (8) led to the identification of numerous shortcomings in the supervision of medication for old people. Our own studies from Southampton confirm that when old people are commenced on drug treatment it tends to be continued for periods in excess of 6 months (4). Regular review is important, particularly for patients on potent cardiovascular drug therapy, such as digoxin (151). Finally, in recent years several studies have identified that patients want and need more information than they currently receive from their medical practitioners and pharmacists (4). A significant number of people are unaware of the fact that they should swallow medicines with either food or fluid and that failure to do so may lead to a drug sticking in the gullet (4). This can be particularly hazardous with agents such as Slow-K (152), a product which is in any event undesirable for old people.

When problems with coping exist, it is often useful to enlist the help of a relative/neighbour (or even the district nurse) in the supervision of medicine taking (153). This is particularly important if there are problems of either failing vision or intellect present.

Inadequate information

Many people seem uncertain about what to do if they forget to take a dose of their medicine. Our biggest concern is the fact that the majority of people are totally unaware of any adverse effects that can result from potent cardiovascular drug therapy, unless they have themselves experienced such a problem(s). It is clear that information leaflets can facilitate communication with patients and enhance their knowledge without necessarily influencing their behaviour (154,155). However, contrary to previous assumptions most elderly people are just as likely as younger people to want information leaflets. Furthermore, because they are more likely to be on treatment they are more likely to derive benefit.

CONCLUSIONS

The questions posed by the late James Crooks (156) are as valid today as they were when published in 1983. When considering the use of cardiovascular drugs in the elderly we would do well to ask the following:

1. Is drug therapy required?
2. If drug treatment is required, which drug is appropriate?
3. What side-effects are more likely to occur in the elderly?
4. Is there a need for continued medication?
5. Can the patient 'manage' the number of different drugs prescribed?
6. Can the patient 'manage' the dosage regimen of the individual drugs prescribed?
7. What is the most appropriate type of preparation to be prescribed in respect of tablets or capsules (size, shape and colour, liquid preparations, suppositories, etc.)?
8. Can the drug be specially packed and labelled for use by elderly patients?
9. Can the patient carry out the prescribing instructions in his or her normal environment?

Tables 4–13 give examples of special problems for cardiovascular drugs in the elderly, using the British National Formulary classification.

Table 4. Positive inotropic drugs[a]

Drug	Mode of elimination	Comments
2.1.1 Cardiac glycosides		
Digoxin	Mainly renal ($\frac{3}{4}$): reduced in the elderly	Narrow therapeutic index. Important interactions with diuretics and antiarrhythmics. Therapeutic monitoring available
Digitoxin	Metabolism and enterohepatic recirculation (EHR)	Metabolism can be induced: EHR interrupted by cholestyramine
Lanatoside C	Metabolized in the gut to digoxin	Variable plasma concentrations
2.1.2 Phosphodiesterase inhibitors		
Enoximone (fenoximone)	Hepatic metabolism	Active sulphoxide metabolite accumulates in renal failure
Milrinone	Mainly renal	Clearance is reduced by heart failure and by renal disease

[a]See also sympathomimetics (Table 9).

Table 5. Diuretics

	Drug	Method of elimination	Comments
2.2	Diuretics		
2.2.1	Thiazides and related diuretics		
	Bendrofluazide	70% metabolized 30% renal tubular excretion	Metabolic disturbance, volume depletion and renal impairment more common in elderly
	Chlorothiazide	Renal tubular secretion	Renal impairment in the elderly or in heart failure may reduce access to the site of action and decrease effectiveness as a diuretic
	Chlorthalidone	2/3 renal tubular secretion 1/3 probably biliary	Conversely higher plasma concentrations may produce a greater antihypertensive effect
	Clopamide	1/3 renal 2/3 hepatic metabolism	To avoid metabolic effects, doses should be reduced in the elderly
	Cyclopenthiazide	Renal tubular secretion	
	Hydrochlorothiazide	Renal tubular excretion	
	Hydroflumethiazide	2/3 renal tubular secretion 1/3 metabolized in liver	
	Indapamide	95% metabolized in liver 5% excreted unchanged in urine	
	Mefruside	Hepatic metabolism 2/3 metabolites excreted in urine	
	Methyclothizide	Probable renal secretion	
	Metolazone	80% renal tubular secretion	
	Polythiazide	25% renal tubular secretion 75% presumed metabolized	
	Xipamide	50% renal tubular secretion 50% hepatic conjugation	
2.2.2	Loop diuretics		
	Frusemide	50% renal tubular secretion 50% conjugation	
	Bumetanide	50% renal tubular excretion 50% hepatic conjugation	
	Ethacrynic acid	2/3 renal tubular secretion 1/3 hepatic metabolism	
2.2.3	Potassium-sparing diuretics		
	Amiloride	Glomerular filtration and renal tubular secretion	Increased risk of acidosis and hyperkalaemia in the elderly with renal impairment
	Potassium canrenoate	Liver metabolism then renal excretion	
	Spironolactone	Liver metabolism then renal excretion	
	Triamterene	Hepatic metabolism then 50% renal elimination	

Table 6. Antiarrhythmics (see also Table 5, p. 295)

Drug	Mode of elimination	Comments
2.3 Amiodarone	Slow metabolism: possible enterohepatic circulation	Active metabolite. Interacts with digoxin and warfarin
Disopyramide	Renal elimination and hepatic metabolism	Clearance reduced in renal disease. Antimuscarinic effects can precipitate urinary retention
Flecinide	Hepatic metabolism and pH-dependent renal excretion	Cimetidine inhibits metabolism
Procainamide	Hepatic metabolism and pH-dependent renal elimination	Excretion delayed in renal disease
Quinidine	Hepatic metabolism + 20% renal excretion	Active metabolite(s). Interacts with digoxin, encainide and propafenone
Bretylium tosylate	Poor absorption	Accumulates in renal failure
Lignocaine	Hepatic metabolism	Kinetics altered in heart failure
Mexiletine	Metabolism and pH-dependent renal excretion	Metabolism increased by phenytoin and rifampicin
Phenytoin	Dose-dependent hepatic metabolism	Induces metabolism of many drugs, especially dihydro-pyridine calcium antagonists
Propafenone	Hepatic metabolism. Dose-dependent kinetics	Subject to genetic polymorphism. Quinidine interacts
Tocainide	Metabolism and renal excretion (40%)	Clearance reduced by hepatic and/or renal disease

Table 7. β-Adrenoceptor-blocking drugs

Drug	Method of elimination	Comments
2.4 Propranolol	Hepatic metabolism	Diminished first-pass metabolism in the elderly
Acebutolol	Hepatic metabolism and some renal elimination	Active metabolite accumulates in renal failure
Atenolol	Renal	Accumulates in renal disease
Betaxolol	Hepatic metabolism	Caution recommended in elderly
Bisoprolol	Renal excretion and metabolism	Dosage unchanged
Carteolol	$\frac{2}{3}$ by renal elimination	Accumulates in renal disease
Metoprolol	Hepatic metabolism	Displays genetic polymorphism
Nadolol	Renal	Accumulates in renal disease
Oxprenolol	Hepatic/intestinal metabolism	Dosage unchanged
Pindolol	Hepatic metabolism and renal excretion (40%)	Dosage unchanged
Sotalol	Renal excretion (75%)	Accumulates in renal failure
Timolol	Mainly hepatic metabolism	Reduced dosage recommended

Table 8. Antihypertensives

	Drug	Route of elimination	Comments
2.5.1	Diazoxide	Mainly renal	Extensively bound to plasma proteins. Glucose intolerance with repeated use
	Hydralazine	Metabolism in gut wall and liver	Genetic polymorphism affects response and incidence of systemic lupus erythematosus
	Minoxidil	Metabolized in liver	Low starting dose advisable. Concurrent use of diuretics and β-blocker essential
	Sodium nitroprusside	Mainly renal	Reduced dosage required in the elderly
2.5.2	Clonidine	Renal + hepatic metabolism	Accumulates in renal failure. Interacts with β-blockers
	Methyldopa	Metabolism and renal excretion	Active metabolite(s). Little change with age
	Reserpine	Metabolism + faecal excretion	Risk of depression with doses exceeding 50 mg per day
2.5.3	Guanethidine	Renal + hepatic metabolism	Long half-life. Postural hypotension common
	Bethanidine	Renal	Clearance reduced in renal failure. Postural hypotension common
	Debrisoquine	Hepatic and renal	Genetic polymorphism in its metabolism. Postural hypotension
2.5.4	Doxazosin	Hepatic metabolism	No significant change with ageing but postural hypotension occurs
	Indoramin	Hepatic metabolism	Half-life prolonged in the elderly
	Phenoxybenzamine	Metabolized	Irreversible binding to α-adrenoceptors. Postural hypotension
	Phentolamine	Metabolized	Postural hypotension
	Prazosin	Hepatic metabolism	Postural hypotension especially with first dose
	Terazosin	Hepatic metabolism	Postural hypotension especially with first dose
2.5.5	Captopril	Renal and hepatic metabolism	Accumulates in renal failure
	Enalapril	Metabolized to active moiety	First dose effect
	Lisinopril	Renal	Accumulates with age
	Perindopril	After metabolic activation, elimination is renal	Prodrug of perindoprilat
	Quinapril	After activation, elimination is by renal route	Prodrug of quinaprilat
	Ramipril	After activation, undergoes metabolism	Prodrug of ramiprilat
2.5.6	Trimetaphan	Uncertain	Beware hypotension
2.5.7	Metirosine	Renal	

Table 9. Nitrates

Drug	Route of elimination	Comments
2.6 Glyceryl trinitrate	Hepatic metabolism (plasma hydrolysis)	
Isosorbide dinitrate	Hepatic metabolism	
Isosorbide 5-mononitrate	Hepatic metabolism	Probably unaffected by age or hepatic disease

Table 10. Sympathomimetics

Drug	Route of elimination	Comments
2.7 Adrenaline	Uptake into nerve endings and metabolism	Uptake delayed in elderly people but reduced receptor sensitivity
2.7.1 Dobutamine	Rapid clearance	Intravenous only
Dopamine	Renal	Intravenous only
Dopexamine	Fate unknown	
Isoprenaline	Metabolism and some renal excretion	Reduced effect in elderly
Xamoterol	Renal elimination	Clearance reduced
2.7.2 Metaraminol	Uncertain	Caution advised in elderly
Methoxamine		
Phenylephrine	Renal clearance	

Table 11. Antiplatelet drugs

Drug	Route of elimination	Comments
2.9 Aspirin	Dose-dependent metabolism and renal elimination	No change with ageing
Dipyridamole	Hepatic metabolism	No information available

Table 12. Fibrinolytics

	Drug	Route of elimination	Comments
2.10	Streptokinase	Complexing with antibodies and plasma inhibitors Proteolysis in plasma	Probably unaffected by age. Increased risk of haemorrhage may relate to low body weight. In patients under 67 kg a reduced dose may be desirable
	Alteplase	Hepatic metabolism	
	Anistreplase	Complexing with plasma inhibitors. Proteolysis in plasma	
	Urokinase	Hepatic metabolism	
2.11	Antifibrinolytic drugs and haemostatics		
	Aprotinin	Renal metabolism	
	Tranexamic acid	Renal elimination by glomerular filtration	Dose reduction only if renal impairment

Table 13. Lipid-lowering drugs

	Drug	Route of elimination	Comments
2.12	Cholestyramine	Not absorbed	
	Colelistopol	Not absorbed	
	Bezafibrate	50% liver metabolism and 50% renal elimination	Dose reduction in hepatic and renal failure
	Clofibrate	Hepatic metabolism	
	Fenofibrate		
	Gemfibrozil	50% liver metabolism 50% renal elimination	
	Acipimox		
	Nicofuranose		
	Nicotinic acid	Saturable hepatic metabolism	Avoid in liver disease
	Omega-3-marine triglycerides		
	Probucol	Biliary excretion	
	Pravastatin	Mainly renal elimination including tubular secretion. Some hepatic metabolism	Avoid in liver disease
	Simvastatin	Hepatic metabolism	Avoid in liver disease

REFERENCES

1. Dunnell K, Cartwright A (1972) *Medicine Takers, Prescribers and Hoarders.* Routledge & Kegan Paul, London.
2. Skegg, DCG, Doll R, Perry J (1977) Use of medicines in general practice. *Br Med J* i: 1561–1563.
3. Anderson RM (1980) Prescribed medicines: who takes what? *J Epidemiol Commun Health* **34**: 299–304.
4. Ridout S, Waters WE, George CF (1986) Knowledge of and attitudes to medicines in the Southampton community. *Br J Clin Pharmacol* **21**: 701–712.
5. Seidl LG, Thornton GF, Smith JW Cluff LE (1966) Studies on the epidemiology of adverse drug reactions. *Bull Johns Hopkins Hosp* **119**: 299–315.
6. Hurwitz N (1969) Predisposing factors in adverse reactions to drugs. *Br Med J* i: 536–539.
7. Williamson J, Chopin JM (1980) Adverse reactions to prescribed drugs in the elderly: a multicentre investigation. *Age Ageing* **9**: 73–80.
8. Cartwright A, Smith C (1988) *Elderly People, their Medicines and the Doctors.* Routledge, London.
9. Leape LL, Brennan TA, Laird N *et al.* (1991) The nature of adverse events in hospitalized patients. *New Engl J Med* **324**: 377–384.
10. Rawlins MD, Thompson JW (1977) Pathogenesis of adverse drug reactions. In *Textbook of Adverse Drug Reactions*, Davies DM (ed.). Oxford University Press, Oxford, p. 10.
11. Report of the Royal College of Physicians (1984) Medication for the elderly. *J R Coll Physicians Lond* **18**: 7–17.
12. Hawthorne VM, Greaves DA, Beevers DG (1974) Blood pressure in a Scottish town. *Br Med J* **3**: 600–603.
13. Lawrence JS (1977) *Rheumatism in Populations.* Heinemann, London.
14. Berry SJ, Coffey DS, Walsh PC, Ewing LL (1984) The development of human benign prostatic hyperplasia with age. *J Urol* **132**: 474–479.
15. Woolcock AJ (1987) Disorders of the airways: asthma. In *Oxford Textbook of Medicine*, 2nd edn, Weatherall DJ, Ledingham JGG, Warrell DA (eds). Oxford University Press, Oxford, pp. 15.75–82.
16. Challenor VC, Waller DG, George CF (1989) Beta-adrenoceptor antagonists plus nifedipine in the treatment of chronic stable angina pectoris. *Cardiovasc Drugs Ther* **3**: 275–285.
17. George CF, Breckenridge AM, Dollery CT (1973) Comparison of the potassium-retaining effects of amiloride and spironolactone in hypertensive patients with thiazide-induced hypokalaemia. *Lancet* ii: 1288–1290.
18. Amery A, de Schaepdryver A (1973) European Working Party on High Blood Pressure in the Elderly (EWPHE): organisation of a double-blind multicentre trial on antihypertensive therapy in elderly patients. *Clin Sci Mol Med* **45**: 71–73S.
19. Leach S, Roy SS (1986) Adverse drug reactions: an investigation of an acute geriatric ward. *Age Ageing* **15**: 241–246.
20. Bax DE, Woods HS, Christie J *et al.* (1987) Therapeutic audit on a general medical ward. *Clin Sci* **72**: (Suppl. 16): 29P.
21. Atkin P, Shenfield GN. Personal communication.
22. Moir DC, Dingwall-Fordyce I (1980) Drug taking in the elderly at home. *J Clin Exp Gerontol* **2**: 329–332.
23. Parkin DM, Henney CR, Quirk J, Crooks J (1976) Deviation from prescribed drug treatment after discharge from hospital. *Br Med J* ii: 686–688.
24. Vestal RE (1978) Drug use in the elderly: a review of problems and special

considerations. *Drug* **16**: 358–382.

25. Dollery CT, George CF, Orme ML'E (1974) Drug interactions affecting cardiovascular therapy. In *Clinical Effects of Interaction between Drugs* Cluff LE, Petrie JC (eds). Excerpta Medica, Amsterdam, pp. 117–151.

26. Orme ML'E (1977) Drug interactions of clinical importance. In *Textbook of Adverse Drug Reactions*, 4th edn, Davies DM (ed.). Oxford University Press, Oxford, pp. 788–810.

27. George CF (1976) Disease of the alimentary system: absorption, distribution and metabolism of drugs. Effects of disease of the gut. *Br Med J* **ii**: 742–744.

28. Evans MA, Broe GA, Triggs EJ *et al.* (1981) Gastric emptying rate and the systemic availability of levodopa in the elderly Parkinsonian patient. *Neurology* **31**: 1288–1294.

29. Evans MA, Triggs EJ, Cheung M *et al.* (1981) Gastric emptying rate in the elderly: implications for drug therapy. *J Am Geriatr Soc* **29**: 201–205.

30. Horowitz M, Maddern GJ, Chatterton BE *et al.* (1984) Changes in gastric emptying rates with age. *Clin Sci* **67**: 213–218.

31. Robertson DRC, Renwick AG, Macklin B *et al.* (1992) The influence of levodopa on gastric emptying in healthy elderly volunteers. *Eur J Clin Pharmacol* **42**: 409–12.

32. Bender AD (1968) Effect of age on intestinal absorption: implications for drug absorption in the elderly. *J Am Geriatr Soc* **16**: 1331–1339.

33. Benet LZ, Greither A, Meister W (1976) Gastrointestinal absorption of drugs in patients with cardiac failure. In *The Effect of Disease Status on Drug Pharmacokinetics*, Benet LZ (ed.). American Pharmaceutical Association, Washington, pp. 33–50.

34. Tilstone WJ, Dargie H, Dargie EN *et al.* (1974) Pharmacokinetics of metolazone in normal subjects and in patients with cardiac or renal failure. *Clin Pharmacol Ther* **16**: 322–329.

35. Jaillon P, Rubin P, Yee Y-G *et al.* (1979) Influence of congestive heart failure on prazosin kinetics. *Clin Pharmacol Ther* **25**: 792–794.

36. Crouthamel WG (1975) The effect of congestive heart failure on quinidine pharmacokinetics. *Am Heart J* **90**: 335–339.

37. Haass A, Lullmann H, Peters Th (1972) Absorption rates of some cardiac glycosides in portal blood flow. *Eur J Pharmacol* **19**: 366–370.

38. Greenblatt DJ, Sellers EM, Shader RI (1982) Drug disposition in old age. *N Engl J Med* **306**: 1081–1088.

39. Wallace SM, Verbeeck RK (1987) Plasma protein binding of drugs in the elderly. *Clin Pharmacokinet* **12**: 41–72.

40. Dybkaer R, Lauritzen M, Krakauer R (1981) Relative values for clinical chemical and haematological quantities in 'healthy' elderly people. *Acta Med Scand* **209**: 1–9.

41. Campion EW, deLabry LO, Glynn RJ (1988) The effect of age on serum albumin in healthy males: report from the Normative Aging Study. *J Gerontol* **43**: M18–M20.

42. Woodford-Williams E, Alvarez AS, Webster D *et al.* (1964) Serum protein patterns in normal and pathological ageing. *Gerontologia* **10**: 86–99.

43. McDevitt DG, Frisk-Holmberg M, Hollifield JW, Shand DG (1976) Plasma binding and the affinity of propranolol for the beta receptor in man. *Clin Pharmacol Ther* **20**: 152–157.

44. George CF, George RH, Howden CW (1992) The liver and response to drugs. In *Wright's Liver and Biliary Disease*, 3rd edn, Millward-Sadler GH, Wright R, Arthur M (eds). Saunders, London, Ch. 17.

45. Piafsky KM, Borga O, Odar-Cederlof I *et al.* (1978) Increased plasma protein binding of propranolol and chlorpromazine mediated by disease-induced elevations of plasma α_1-acid glycoprotein. *N Engl J Med* **299**: 1435–1439.

46. Cusack B, O'Malley K, Lavan J *et al.* Protein binding and disposition of lignocaine in the elderly. *Eur J Clin Pharmacol* **29**: 323–329.

47. Abernethy DR, Kerzner L (1984) Age effects on alpha-1-acid glycoprotein concentration and imipramine plasma protein binding. *J Am Geriatr Soc* **32**: 705–708.

48. Waller DG, Smith CL, Renwick AG, George CF (1982) Intravenous propranolol in patients with inflammation. *Br J Clin Pharmacol* **13**: 577–578.

49. Hager WD, Fenster R, Mayersohn M *et al.* (1979) Digoxin–quinidine interaction: pharmacokinetic evaluation. *N Engl J Med* **300**: 1238–1241.

50. Parke DV, Smith RL (1977) *Drug Metabolism: From Microbes to Man.* Taylor & Francis, London.

51. Estabrook RW, Cooper DY, Rosenthal O (1963) The light reversible carbon monoxide inhibition of the steroid C21-hydroxylase system of the adrenal cortex. *Biochem Z* **338**: 741–755.

52. Guengerich FP, Distlerath LM, Reilly PEB *et al.* Human liver cytochromes P-450 involved in polymorphisms of drug oxidations. *Xenobiotica* **16**: 367–378.

53. Guengerich FP, Umbenhauer DR, Churchill PF *et al.* (1987) Polymorphism of human cytochrome P-450. *Xenobiotica* **17**: 311–316.

54. Idle JR, Smith RL (1979) Polymorphisms of oxidation at carbon centers of drugs and their clinical significance. *Drug Metab Rev* **9**: 301–317.

55. O'Malley K, Crooks J, Duke E, Stevenson IH (1971) Effect of age and sex on human drug metabolism. *Br Med J* **3**: 607–609.

56. Woodhouse KW, James OFW (1990) Hepatic drug metabolism and ageing. *Br Med Bull* **46**: 22–35.

57. Weiss YA, Safar ME, Lehner JP *et al.* (1978) (+)-Propranolol clearance: an estimation of hepatic blood flow in man. *Br J Clin Pharmacol* **5**: 457–460.

58. Ohnhaus EE (1979) Methods of the assessment of the effect of drugs on liver blood flow in man. *Br J Clin Pharmacol* **7**: 223–229.

59. George CF (1979) Drug kinetics and hepatic blood flow. *Clin Pharmacokinet* **4**: 433–448.

60. Castleden CM, George CF (1979) The effect of ageing on the hepatic clearance of propranolol. *Br J Clin Pharmacol* **7**: 49–54.

61. Kelly JG, McGarry K, O'Malley K, O'Brien ET (1982) Bioavailability of labetalol increases with age. *Br J Clin Pharmacol* **14**: 304–305.

62. Abernethy DR, Schwartz JB, Todd EL *et al.* (1986) Verapamil pharmacodynamics and disposition in young and elderly hypertensive patients. *Ann Intern Med* **105**: 329–336.

63. Waller DG, Renwick AG, Gruchy BS, George CF (1984) The first pass metabolism of nifedipine in man. *Br J Clin Pharmacol* **18**: 951–954.

64. George CF, Renwick AG, Darragh AS *et al.* (1986) A comparison of isoxicam pharmacokinetics in young and elderly subjects. *Br J Clin Pharmacol* **22**: 129S–134S.

65. Wilkinson GR, Shand DG (1975) A physiological approach to hepatic drug clearance. *Clin Pharmacol Ther* **18**: 377–390.

66. Robertson DRC, Waller DG, Renwick AG, George CF (1988) Age related changes in the pharmacokinetics and pharmacodynamics of nifedipine. *Br J Clin Pharmacol* **25**: 297–305.

67. Wynne HA, Cope LH, Mutch E *et al.* (1989) The effect of age upon liver volume and apparent liver blood flow in healthy men. *Hepatology* **9**: 297–301.

68. Guengerich FP, Brian WR, Iwasaki K *et al.* (1991) Oxidation of dihydropyridine calcium channel blockers and analogues by human liver cytochrome P-450IIIA$_4$. *J Med Chem* **34**: 1838–1844.

69. Watkins PB, Wrighton SA, Schuetz EG *et al.* (1987) Identification of glucocorticoid-

inducible cytochrome P-450 in the intestinal mucosa of rats and man. *J Clin Invest* **80**: 1029–1036.

70. Peters WHM, Kremers PG (1989) Cytochromes P-450 in the intestinal mucosa of man. *Biochem Pharmacol* **38**: 1535–1538.

71. George CF, Renwick AG (1987) The role of the intestinal flora in the metabolism of xenobiotics. In *Topics in Pharmaceutical Sciences*, Breimer DD, Speiser P (eds). Elsevier, Amsterdam.

72. Strong HA, Oates J, Sembi J *et al.* (1984) Role of the gut flora in the reduction of sulfinpyrazone in humans. *J. Pharmacol Exp Ther* **230**: 726–732.

73. Kirstein Pedersen A, Jakobsen P (1979) Two new metabolites of sulphinpyrazone in the rabbit: a possible cause of the prolonged in vivo effect. *Thromb Res* **16**: 871–876.

74. Lindenbaum J, Rund DG, Butler VP *et al.* (1981) Inactivation of digoxin by the gut flora: reversal by antibiotic therapy. *N Engl J Med* **305**: 789–794.

75. Strong HA, Renwick AG, George CF (1984) The site of reduction of sulphin-pyrazone in the rabbit. *Xenobiotica* **14**: 815–826.

76. Strong HA, Angus R, Oates J *et al.* (1986) Effects of ischaemic heart disease, Crohn's disease and antimicrobial therapy on the pharmacokinetics of sulphinpyrazone. *Clin Pharmacokinet* **11**: 402–410.

77. Renwick AG (1982) First-pass metabolism within the lumen of the gastrointestinal tract. In *Presystemic Drug Elimination*, George CF, Shand DG, Renwick AG (eds). Butterworths, London, pp. 3–28.

78. Hirom PC, Milburn P, Smith RL, Williams RT (1972) Species variations in the threshold molecular-weight factor for the biliary excretion of organic amines. *Biochem J* **129**: 1071–1077.

79. Rawlins MD, Thompson JW (1991) Mechanisms of adverse drug reactions. In *Textbook of Adverse Drug Reactions*, 4th edn, Davies DM (ed.) Oxford University Press, Oxford, pp. 18–45.

80. Blondheim SH, Kunkel HG (1950) Portal blood in collateral veins of patients with cirrhosis: acetylation by the intestine. *Proc Soc Exp Biol Med* **73**: 38–41.

81. Perry HM, Sakamoto A, Tan EM (1967) Relationship of acetylating enzyme to hydralazine toxicity. *J Lab Clin Med* **70**: 1020–1021.

82. George CF (1980) Amiloride handling in renal failure. *Br J Clin Pharmacol* **9**: 94–95.

83. McAinsh J (1977) Pharmacokinetics of atenolol. *Postgrad Med J* **53**: (Suppl. 3): 74–78.

84. Smith TW (1973) Digitalis glycosides. *N Engl J Med* **288**: 719–722, 942–946.

85. Reidenberg MM, Camacho MC, Kluger J, Drayer DE (1980) Aging and renal clearance of procainamide and acetylprocainamide. *Clin Pharmacol Ther* **28**: 732–735.

86. Saltissi D, Pusey CD, Rainford D (1979) Recurrent acute renal failure due to antibiotic-induced interstitial nephritis. *Br Med J* **i**: 1182–1183.

87. Kampann J, Hansen JM, Siersbaek-Nielsen K, Laursen H (1972) Effect of some drugs on penicillin half-life in blood. *Clin Pharmacol Ther* **13**: 516–519.

88. Davies DF, Schock NW (1950) Age changes in glomerular filtration rate, effective renal plasma flow, tubular excretory capacity in adult males. *J Clin Invest* **29**: 496–507.

89. Brod J (1968) Changes in renal function with age. *Scripta Med* **41**: 223–229.

90. Cusack B, Kelly J, O'Malley K *et al.* (1979) Digoxin in the elderly: pharmacokinetic consequences of old age. *Clin Pharmacol Ther* **25**: 772–776.

91. Croxson MS, Ibbertson HK (1975) Serum digoxin in patients with thyroid disease. *Br Med J* **iii**: 566–568.

92. Molholm-Hansen J, Kampmann J, Laursen H (1970) Renal excretion of drugs in the elderly. *Lancet* **i**: 1170.

93. Caldwell JH, Caldwell PB, Murphy JW, Beachler CW (1980) Intestinal secretion of digoxin in the rat. Augmentation by feeding activated charcoal. *Naunyn-Schmiedebergs Arch Pharmacol* **312**: 271–275.

94. Smith RS, Warren DJ, Renwick AG, George CF (1983) Acebutolol pharmacokinetics in renal failure. *Br J Clin Pharmacol* **16**: 253–258.

95. Cockcroft DW, Gault MH (1976) Prediction of creatinine clearance from serum creatinine. *Nephron* **16**: 31–41.

96. Waller DG, Fleming JS, Ramsay B, Gray J (1991) The accuracy of creatinine clearance with and without urine collection as a measure of glomerular filtration rate. *Postgrad Med J* **67**: 42–46.

97. Young DS, Pestamer LC, Gibberman V (1975) Effects of drugs on clinical laboratory tests. *Clin Chem* **21**: 286–287D.

98. Payne RB (1986) Creatinine clearance: a redundant clinical investigation. *Ann Clin Biochem* **23**: 243–250.

99. Cochetto DM, Tschanz C, Bjornsson TD (1983) Decreased rate of creatinine production in patients with hepatic disease: implications for estimation of creatinine clearance. *Ther Drug Monit* **5**: 161–168.

100. Rehling M, Moller ML, Thamdrup B *et al.* (1984) Simultaneous measurement of renal clearance and plasma clearance of ^{99m}Tc DTPA, ^{51}Cr EDTA and inulin in man. *Clin Sci* **66**: 613–619.

101. Waller DG, Keast CM, Fleming JS, Ackery DM (1987) Measurement of glomerular filtration rate with Tc^{99m}-DTPA: comparison of plasma clearance techniques. *J Nucl Med* **28**: 372–377.

102. Bender AD (1965) The effect of increasing age on the distribution of peripheral blood flow in man. *J Am Geriatr Soc* **13**: 192–198.

103. Rowe JW, Andres R, Tobin JD *et al.* (1976) The effect of age on creatinine clearance in man: a cross-sectional and longitudinal study. *J Gerontol* **31**: 155–163.

104. Miller JH, McDonald RK, Shock NW (1952) Age changes in the maximal rate of renal tubular reabsorption of glucose. *J Gerontol* **7**: 196–200.

105. Rowe JW, Shock NW, De Fronzo RA (1976) The influence of age on the renal response to water deprivation in man. *Nephron* **17**: 270–278.

106. Davies DS, Prichard BNC (eds) (1973) *Biological Effects of Drugs in Relation to their Plasma Concentrations*. Macmillan, London.

107. British Medical Association and Royal Pharmaceutical Society of Great Britain (1991) *British National Formulary* **22**: 202–203.

108. Friedlander IR (1979) Ototoxic drugs and the detection of ototoxicity. *N Engl J Med* **301**: 213–214.

109. O'Malley K, Stevenson IH, Ward CA *et al.* (1977) Determinants of anticoagulant control in patients receiving warfarin. *Br J Clin Pharmacol* **4**: 309–314.

110. Shepherd AMM, Hewick DS, Moreland TA, Stevenson IH (1977) Age as a determinant of sensitivity to warfarin. *Br J Clin Pharmacol* **4**: 315–320.

111. Routledge PA, Chapman PH, Davies DM, Rawlins MD (1979) Pharmacokinetics and pharmacodynamics of warfarin at steady state. *Br J Clin Pharmacol* **8**: 243–247.

112. Gurwitz JH, Goldberg RJ, Holden A *et al.* (1988) Age-related risks of long-term oral anticoagulant therapy. *Arch Intern Med* **148**: 1733–1736.

113. Hypertension Detection and Follow-up Program Cooperative Study (1979) Five year findings of the Hypertension Detection and Follow-up Program 2: mortality by race, sex and age. *JAMA* **242**: 2572–2577.

114. Amery A, Brixko P, Birkenhager W, *et al.* (1975) Mortality and morbidity results from the European Working Party on High Blood Pressure in the Elderly Trial. *Lancet* **i**: 1349–1354.

115. Amery A, Brixko P, Birkenhager W *et al.* (1986) Efficacy of antihypertensive drug

treatment according to age, sex, blood pressure and previous cardiovascular disease in patients over the age of 60. *Lancet* **ii**: 589–592.

116. Report by The Management Committee (1981) Treatment of mild hypertension in the elderly: a study initiated and administered by the National Heart Foundation of Australia. *Med J Aust* **ii**: 398–402.

117. Dahlof B, Lindholm LH, Hansson L *et al.* (1991) Morbidity and mortality in the Swedish Trial in old patients with hypertension (STOP-Hypertension). *Lancet* **338**: 1281–1284.

118. Jackson G, Pierscianowski TA, Mahon W, Condon J (1976) Inappropriate antihypertensive therapy in the elderly. *Lancet* **ii**: 1317–1318.

119. Exton-Smith AN (1989) Hypotension and syncope. In *Clinical Geriatric Cardiology*, Luchi RJ (ed.). Churchill Livingstone, Edinburgh, pp. 79–96.

120. Reid JL, Calne DB, George CF *et al.* (1971) Cardiovascular reflexes in parkinsonism. *Clin Sci* **41**: 63–67.

121. Gribbon B, Pickering TG, Sleight P, Peto R (1971) Effect of age and high blood pressure on baroreflex sensitivity in man. *Circ Res* **29**: 424–431.

122. Caird FI, Andrews GR, Kennedy RD (1973) Effect of posture on blood pressure in the elderly. *Br Heart J* **35**: 527–530.

123. Collins KJ, Exton-Smith AN, James MH, Oliver DJ (1980) Functional changes in autonomic nervous responses with ageing. *Age Ageing* **9**: 17–24.

124. Vestal RE, Wood AJJ, Shand DG (1979) Reduced β-adrenoceptor sensitivity in the elderly. *Clin Pharmacol Ther* **26**: 181–186.

125. Cleland JGF, Dargie HJ, McAlpine H *et al.* (1985) Severe hypotension after first dose of enalapril in heart failure. *Br Med J* **291**: 1309–1312.

126. Bendall MJ, Baloch KH, Wilson PR (1975) Side effects due to treatment of hypertension with prazosin. *Br Med J* **ii**: 727–728.

127. Inman WHW, Rawson NSB, Wilton LV *et al.* (1988) Postmarketing surveillance of enalapril. I. Results of prescription event monitoring. *Br Med J* **297**: 826–829.

128. George CF, Challenor VF, Swift CG (1989) Effect of commonly used non-cardiac drugs on the heart and circulation. In *Clinical Geriatric Cardiology*, Luchi RJJ (ed.). Churchill Livingstone, Edinburgh, pp. 362–390.

129. Schocken D, Roth G (1977) Reduced beta-adrenergic receptor concentrations in aging man. *Nature* **267**: 856–858.

130. Dillon N, Chung S, Kelly J, O'Malley K (1980) Age and beta adrenoceptor-mediated function. *Clin Pharmacol Ther* **27**: 769–772.

131. Ullah MI, Newman GB, Saunders KB (1981) Influence of age on response to ipratropium and salbutamol in asthma. *Thorax* **36**: 523–529.

132. Kendall MJ, Woods KL, Wilkins MR, Worthington DJ (1982) Responsiveness to β-adrenergic receptor stimulation: the effects of age are cardioselective. *Br J Clin Pharmacol* **14**: 821–826.

133. Pan HYM, Hoffman BB, Pershe RA, Blaschke TF (1986) Decline in beta-adrenergic receptor-mediated vascular relaxation with aging in man. *J Pharmacol Exp Ther* **239**: 802–807.

134. Scarpace PJ (1986) Decreased β-adrenergic responsiveness during senescence. *Fed Proc* **45**: 51–54.

135. Montamat SC, Davies AO (1989) Physiological response to isoproterenol and coupling of beta-adrenergic receptors in young and elderly human subjects. *J Gerontol* **44**: M100–105.

136. Buckley C, Curtin D, Walsh T, O'Malley K (1986) Ageing and platelet α_2-adrenoceptors. *Br J Clin Pharmacol* **21**: 721–722.

137. Andreasen F, Hansen U, Husted SE *et al.* (1984) The influence of age on renal and extrarenal effects of frusemide. *Br J Clin Pharmacol* **18**: 65–74.

138. Burr ML, King S, Davies HEF, Pathy MS (1977) The effect of discontinuing long term diuretic therapy in the elderly. *Age Ageing* **6**: 38–45.
139. Abrams J, Andrews K (1984) The influence of hospital admission on long-term medication of elderly patients. *J R Coll Physicians Lond* **18**: 225–227.
140. Pearson MW (1985) Prescribing for the elderly: an audit. *Practitioner* **229**: 85–86.
141. Amery A, Berthaux P, Bulpitt C *et al.* (1978) Glucose intolerance during diuretic therapy. *Lancet* **i**: 681–683.
142. Stephen PJ, Williamson J (1984) Drug-induced Parkinsonism in the elderly. *Lancet* **ii**: 1082–1083.
143. Baum C, Kennedy DL, Forbes MB (1985) Utilization of nonsteroidal antiinflammatory drugs. *Arthritis Rheum* **28**: 686–692.
144. Fox JS, Taggart AJ, Harron DWG (1988) Prescribing of non-steroidal anti-inflammatory drugs in Northern Ireland (1978–1986). *Int Pharm J* **2**: 171–174.
145. Blackburn SCF, Ellis RM, George CF, Kirwan J (in preparation).
146. Dieppe PA, Doherty M, MacFarlane D, Maddison P (1985) *Rheumatological Medicine*. Churchill Livingstone, Edinburgh.
147. Griffin MR, Ray WA, Schaffner W (1988) Nonsteroidal anti-inflammatory drug use and death from peptic ulcer in elderly persons. *Ann Intern Med* **109**: 359–363.
148. Watkins J, Abbot EC, Hensby CN *et al.* (1980) Attenuation of hypotensive effects of propranolol and thiazide diuretics by indomethacin. *Br Med J* **281**: 702–705.
149. Wing LMH, Bune AJC, Chalmers JP *et al.* (1981) The effects of indomethacin in treated hypertensive patients. *Clin Exp Pharmacol Physiol* **8**: 537–541.
150. Speirs CJ, Dollery CT, Inman WHW *et al.* (1988) Postmarketing surveillance of enalapril II. Investigation of the potential role of enalapril in deaths with renal failure. *Br Med J* **297**: 830–832.
151. Shaw SM, Opit LJ (1976) Need for supervision in the elderly receiving long term prescribed medication. *Br Med J* **i**: 505–507.
152. Al-Dujaili M, Salole EG, Florence AJ (1983) Drug formulation and oesophageal injury. *Adv Drug React Acute Poisoning Rev* **2**: 235–256.
153. Cartwright A (1990) Medicine taking by people aged 65 or more. *Br Med Bull* **46**: 63–76.
154. Gibbs S, Waters WE, George CF (1989) The benefits of prescription information leaflets (1). *Br J Clin Pharmacol* **27**: 727–739.
155. Gibbs S, Waters WE, George CF (1990) Prescription information leaflets: a national survey. *J R Soc Med* **83**: 292–297.
156. Crooks J (1983) Rational therapeutics in the elderly. *J Chronic Dis* **36**: 59–65.

28 Surgery

DAVID J.WHEATLEY[a] AND DAVID TAGGART[b]
[a] *University of Glasgow, and Royal Infirmary,Glasgow, UK*
[b] *Royal Brompton and National Heart and Lung Hospital, London, UK*

Cardiac surgery in the 65 and over age group is now well established and, indeed, forms an increasing proportion of cardiac surgical practice in most Western countries where the commonest pathology amenable to surgery is coronary artery disease, the prevalence of which increases with age. This, together with the growing number of elderly people in the general population, accounts in large measure for the expansion of cardiac surgery in older people, although other factors such as changing referral policies, patient expectations, and wider selection criteria for surgical candidates have also had an influence.

While the disease processes are no different from those seen in younger patients, the severity of cardiac disease (such as ventricular dysfunction or extent of coronary atheroma) is generally greater in the older age groups, and the presence of concomitant pathology more frequent. Physiological reserves, particularly pulmonary and renal, are reduced, and the ability to withstand major surgery is diminished.

Selection of patients for surgery is less straightforward in the elderly. The demarcation between those 'able to withstand' surgery and those too frail is often difficult to distinguish, and limitations imposed on recovery by diminished physiological reserves are not easy to predict. Selection of suitable surgical candidates in an elderly population must therefore take account of factors which are seldom a problem in younger patients. Preoperative investigations may need to be more extensive to better define physiological functions or concomitant pathology.

The elderly are not a homogeneous group: there are marked differences in outcome between 65-year-olds and 75-year-olds, and octogenarians are emerging as a substantial subset of the elderly population undergoing cardiac surgery in the USA.

Surgical procedures differ little from those in younger age groups, although there may well be the need for more extensive coronary surgery, and age may influence such decisions as the surgeon's choice of prosthetic valve. Elderly patients often react differently to many of the drugs used in the operative period and postoperatively run an increased risk of complications and generally have a slower recovery.

Geriatric Cardiology. Principles and Practice.   Edited by A. Martin and A. J. Camm
© 1994 John Wiley & Sons Ltd

Higher hospital mortality has been reported in the elderly age group, but many centres are now reporting only minimal increase. The long-term outcome appears at least as good, indeed in the experience of some, even better, than for the younger age groups, both symptomatically and prognostically. Although the observation that chronological and physiological age are not synonymous is something of a cliché, this may well have a bearing on the wide variation in outcome reported in different series and emphasizes the role of selection in achieving satisfactory results in the elderly.

This chapter discusses particular aspects of the surgical management of elderly patients with cardiac disease, and reviews selection criteria, experience and outcome.

GENERAL CONSIDERATIONS

Assessment for surgery at any age requires consideration of history, physical findings, and results of specialized investigations. Presentation of most cardiac disease is no different in the elderly and today limitation of activity is no more acceptable to the elderly retired than it is to the younger wage-earner. Restriction of therapy to younger, economically productive age groups in many fields of medicine has sometimes been made not only on grounds of cost, but because of misconceptions about the risks and potential benefit of interventions in the elderly (1–3).

The elderly have a higher incidence of concomitant disease and a higher likelihood of previous serious illness which may influence future prognosis as well as ability to withstand surgical intervention. Recent experience indicates that the major problem with cardiac surgery in the elderly is that of 'getting the patient through surgery'; given survival, results are as good, or better, than in younger counterparts. Increased perioperative risks in the elderly are due to a combination of natural decline in physiological reserves and an increased prevalence of other pathological processes. It is has been estimated that there is a progressive physiological deterioration in most organ systems with advancing age, with a rate of functional loss of 1–1.5% annually (4), and most of the diseases that create perioperative problems are age-related.

Among the major concerns that arise in elderly patients under consideration for cardiac surgery are impaired respiratory reserves (age-related physiological changes, chronic obstructive airways disease, emphysema), renal insufficiency, cardiovascular disease (not only the presenting problem but 'non-surgical' conditions such as hypertension), cerebrovascular disease (previous stroke, transient ischaemic episodes, carotid bruits), peripheral vascular disease, general frailty, osteoporosis, and previous or coexistent malignant disease (5).

In patients undergoing cardiac surgery, the damaging effects of cardiopulmonary bypass as a consequence of systemic activation of inflammatory mediators (6), changes in systemic blood flow, pressure and temperature (7), and microemboli in the extracorporeal circuit (8,9) must be considered in addition to the effects of conventional surgical injury. Of particular concern to the cardiac surgeon are pre-existing impairment of cardiac, respiratory, renal and neurological status, as these systems appear most clinically susceptible to the damaging effects of cardiopulmonary bypass.

With advancing age, cardiac output is preserved at rest at a level appropriate to skeletal muscle mass (5,10) but may fail to increase, or may even decrease, under stress (11). This is largely due to an inability to increase heart rate, so that increased cardiac output is achieved by increasing stroke volume as witnessed by an increased end-diastolic volume (12), but predisposing the elderly patient to congestive heart failure when given fluid loads.

Deterioration in physiological reserves is even more obvious in pulmonary function. There is a marked decline in lung volumes and ventilatory flow rates with advancing age, accompanied by an increase in physiological shunting (4,5,13). These changes increase the susceptibility of elderly patients to all postoperative pulmonary complications and, in particular, to chest infection and hypoxia.

Renal function also declines with advancing age: by the eighth decade the glomerular filtration rate may have fallen by almost 50% (5,14) despite an apparently normal serum creatinine. Serum creatinine reflects the ratio between creatinine production and clearance and, because of a significant decrease in muscle bulk in the elderly, serum creatinine may be considerably reduced. Serum creatinine is therefore a poor indicator of renal function in the elderly and explains the occasional apparent dramatic deterioration in renal function in the elderly even after minor surgical procedures. This decline in renal function must also be considered when prescribing potent drugs whose main route of elimination is by renal excretion.

More difficult to measure is the decline in cerebral function with advancing age which results from a loss of functional neurones as well as a diminution in cerebral blood flow and metabolic and neurotransmitter activity (5). Cerebrovascular disease becomes increasingly common with advancing age and, while there is still controversy over management of asymptomatic carotid disease, symptomatic disease should be investigated prior to cardiac surgery (15).

Obesity is common in patients with ischaemic heart disease but malnutrition is also common in the elderly, may be difficult to detect, and has an adverse effect on postoperative recovery (16). Malnutrition contributes to the risks of postoperative infection, as does immune senescence—the decline in both cell-mediated and humoral-mediated immunity which accompanies increased age (17).

The practical implications for the surgeon considering an elderly patient require that he seeks information on previous cardiovascular events such as transient ischaemic episodes or stroke, exercise tolerance and breathlessness, drug therapy, previous illness and, where indicated, initiate appropriate additional investigations. Most commonly this will require ventilatory function tests, tests of renal function, evaluation of the extracranial cerebral circulation and, for those in whom coronary artery disease is not the presenting problem, coronary angiography.

INTRAOPERATIVE CONSIDERATIONS

Elderly patients are more susceptible to hypothermia and decubitus ulceration in the operating room, and are less tolerant of fluctuations in fluid requirements because of impaired haemodynamic and renal reserves (5). The anaesthetist takes into consideration the reduced metabolism and excretion of all pharmacological agents in the elderly as well as a generally reduced metabolic rate. As a consequence of decreased concentrations of circulating transport proteins such as albumin in the elderly, a larger proportion of intravenous drugs remains unbound and therefore active. With advancing age, a reduction in lean body mass accompanied by an increase in adipose tissue results in increased sequestration of lipid-soluble anaesthetic agents and prolonged recovery from anaesthesia. The practical implication for the anaesthetist is the need to reduce drug dosage, allow for prolonged circulatory times, and monitor cardiovascular status in more detail—an indwelling pulmonary artery catheter is frequently a wise precaution.

Of the potential complications of cardiopulmonary bypass, one of the most important is stroke. The risk of perioperative stroke is higher in elderly patients (18), partly because of their increased prevalence of pre-existing cerebrovascular disease, as well as the greater likelihood of atheroma in the proximal aorta and arch vessels. Calcification of the ascending aorta is more common in the elderly and is easily detected by palpation, but atheromatous lesions may be less readily apparent. Any such area is avoided during cannulation, aortic clamping, and siting of proximal anastomoses, to minimize the risk of generating calcific or atheromatous emboli. Many surgeons adopt a policy of running higher perfusion pressures (> 75 mmHg) during cardiopulmonary bypass and most would avoid pressures below 50 mmHg to reduce the risk of cerebral hypoperfusion, although there is no conclusive proof that this is advantageous.

POSTOPERATIVE CONSIDERATIONS

The damaging effects of cardiopulmonary bypass (6) are characterized by increased capillary permeability, multi-organ dysfunction and a bleeding diathesis. In younger patients these adverse effects are often mild and self-limiting, producing only subtle clinical or biochemical signs of organ dysfunction and not materially influencing convalescence. In the elderly, however, physiological reserves are already diminished and consequently the damaging effects of cardiopulmonary bypass may be more obvious. Elderly patients are thus more prone to cardiac, respiratory and neurological complications (19–23).

Cardiac dysfunction

The incidence of perioperative myocardial infarction after open heart surgery is usually estimated at around 2–4%. Acinapura and colleagues reported a higher incidence of perioperative myocardial infarction (7.9% versus 2.2%), increased requirements for postoperative inotropic support (19% versus 8%), and postoperative intra-aortic balloon pumping (3.9% versus 1.4%) in their experience with 685 patients 70 years or over and 3142 patients under 70 years (22). They attribute this difference to the greater severity of disease and poorer ventricular function in the older age group. In contrast, Loop and colleagues found that perioperative myocardial infarction, defined as the appearance of new Q waves, occurred with about the same incidence regardless of age (19).

The most common cardiac complication following open heart surgery is the development of atrial fibrillation in approximately 20–30% of patients. Loop's group documented the incidence of postoperative atrial fibrillation at 18% in men aged less than 65 years, 34% in men aged 65–74 years, and 46% in men aged over 75 years (19). Atrial fibrillation commonly appears between the second and fourth postoperative days and usually responds to digitalization. In the small proportion of patients who are haemodynamically compromised, cardioversion may be required.

Respiratory dysfunction

Cardiac surgery results in some degree of respiratory impairment in all patients but particularly in the elderly, whose respiratory reserves are already diminished. Most elective patients are extubated within 12 hours of surgery and approximately 2–5% will require prolonged ventilation. Cosgrove and colleagues documented morbidity due to respiratory insufficiency in 1.2% of coronary patients aged 40–49, 1.2% aged 50–59, 2.4% aged 60–69 and 4.8% in those over 70 (18). In a recent Veterans Administration study of over 10 000 patients (mean age 61 years) undergoing cardiac surgery, the most frequent complication was the need for mechanical ventilation for at least 48 hours occurring in 8% of the 8569 coronary surgery patients and in 15% of 1912 patients undergoing valve and other cardiac surgery (24). This complication was associated with high mortality (24–25%) and increasing age was a relative risk factor in its occurrence. In the study reported by Acinapura and colleagues (22), prolonged ventilatory support was required in 10% of patients aged over 70 years, compared to 3% of those less than 70 years. Salomon and colleagues (25) reported the need for prolonged ventilatory support in 16% of patients aged over 75 years undergoing coronary surgery, compared to 4% in those aged less than 75 years.

Neurological complications

Major focal neurological abnormalities occur in 1–2% of patients following coronary revascularization and in up to 5% of patients undergoing valve replacement (24,26,27). The likelihood of a cerebrovascular accident following cardiac surgery increases with advancing age (22,25,26). Cosgrove and colleagues documented the risk of postoperative stroke for coronary patients at

0.7%, 1.2%, 2.6% and 4.5% for patients aged 40–49, 50–59, 60–69 and >70 years, respectively (18).

More recently, attention has focused on the much more common occurrence of neuropsychological abnormalities following cardiopulmonary bypass. These abnormalities can be identified in 30–50% of patients, are subtle, and usually detected only with detailed neuropsychological testing (28). They may also occur after non-cardiac surgery and, although their long-term consequence remains to be determined, it appears the majority resolve within a few months of surgery.

Renal dysfunction

The overall incidence of acute renal failure following open heart surgery is less than 1%, although biochemical indices suggesting some degree of renal dysfunction are present in up to one-third of patients. Severe postoperative oliguria has been reported in up to 11% of elderly patients (25), and in the experience of Acinapura's group dialysis was required in 3.1% of those 70 or over, compared to 0.6% in younger patients (22).

CORONARY ARTERY SURGERY

Magnitude of the problem

The volume of coronary artery bypass grafting (CABG) undertaken in Western countries has increased considerably over the last decade. This increase has been most dramatic in the USA, where it is striking that over half of CABG surgery is undertaken in patients aged 65 years or over. The estimates produced by the National Hospital Discharge Survey (NHSD)—a survey of discharges from short-stay non-Federal hospitals (military and veterans' hospitals excluded) categorized by disease or procedure undertaken during hospital admission, show a rise in the number of patients undergoing CABG from 114 000 in 1979 to 262 000 in 1990. Particularly noteworthy has been the increase in the number of elderly patients undergoing these procedures: 23% of patients having CABG in 1979 were 65 years of age or older, compared with 54.5% in 1990. A higher proportion of females (64.9%) than males (50.53%) undergoing CABG in 1990 were 65 or over (29–32).

The UK has also seen an increase in the overall volume of CABG. The UK Cardiac Surgical Register returns for the period 1977–1989 show a growth in the number of procedures involving CABG from 2881 in 1977 to 13 990 in 1989. Procedures involving coronary grafting (either as isolated CABG or combined with valve replacement, aneurysmectomy, etc.) account for an increasing percentage of total cardiac surgical workload, from 29% in 1977 to 64% in 1989 (33).

The UK Register contains no information on the age of the patient population. The Scottish Cardiac Surgical Register (34) shows that the practice

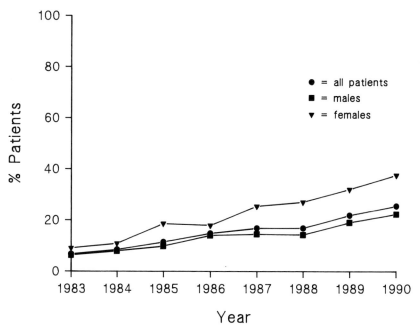

Figure 1. Percentage of patients aged >65 years undergoing isolated CABG: Scottish Cardiac Surgical Register

of isolated CABG in Scotland increased from 851 in 1983 to 1605 in 1990, and the percentage of patients 65 or over rose from 6.7% in 1983 to 25.5% in 1990. As in the USA, a higher proportion of females are in the 65 and over age group (the proportion rising from 9.0% in 1983 to 37.6% in 1990) compared with males (6.3% in 1983 rising to 22.3% in 1990) (Figure 1).

Indications for surgery

In the 1990s, indications for coronary surgery in the elderly do not differ from those in younger patients. Severe angina with unsatisfactory response to medical therapy is the commonest indication for investigation with a view to intervention. Demonstration of readily provoked myocardial ischaemia (from the history or on exercise testing) adds urgency to consideration of intervention. The finding of extensive or critically located coronary lesions (especially left main stenosis and proximal anterior descending disease), and impaired left ventricular function suggest a poor prognosis if left without effective intervention. Data from randomized studies of coronary surgery are based on trials of management which are now somewhat dated, and indeed included few or no patients over 65. However, the common finding of these trials was that prognosis was favourably influenced by surgical intervention in those with more extensive coronary disease, particularly three-vessel disease (35–37). Subsequent non-randomized studies have further emphasized the poor prognostic implications of severe symptoms, extensive coronary disease and impaired left ventricular function, and the prognostic advantages of surgical intervention in patients with these features have been shown (38–42). In the elderly it is well recognized that coronary disease is usually more extensive and that left ventricular function is more likely to be impaired—the very features associated with better prognosis if treated surgically.

In making decisions about surgery for coronary disease, it is now increasingly accepted that prognostic considerations are as valid in the 65 + age group as in the younger population. In the USA, life expectancy at 65 years of age for a man is about 15 years, for a woman about 19 years; at 75 years for a man it is just over 9 years and for a woman just over 12 years (43). Figures for Scotland indicate a life expectancy of 12.8 years for 65-year-old men and 16.5 years for women; for England and Wales the corresponding figures are 13.7 and 17.6 years (44). It is not surprising, therefore, that patient expectations are a powerful factor in the increasing population of 'elderly' cardiac surgical patients.

Alternative interventions

The increasing numbers of patients in the elderly group warranting surgery on medical grounds threaten to overwhelm resources even in the best-endowed health systems. There is inevitably pressure to limit expensive coronary surgery in the elderly, and percutaneous transluminal coronary angioplasty (PTCA) has some appeal. However, costs are still considerable and savings may not be as dramatic as is often believed. Hospital charges for PTCA and surgery have been compared in a number of studies from the USA (45–48), which have reported the initial hospital cost of PTCA to be approximately 60% of surgery. In determining the true cost-effectiveness of any intervention, however, long-term results must be considered in addition to initial hospital costs. Thus, while angioplasty may initially appear less costly than surgical revascularization, it is increasingly recognized that the initial savings may be offset by a much greater likelihood of need for subsequent reintervention in the angioplasty group. Furthermore, Hlatky and colleagues have recently demonstrated that although PTCA is less expensive than surgery, at least initially, the saving may only be in the region of 20% when the true costs of the procedure as opposed to the hospital charges are considered (48). More importantly, the generally more extensive nature of coronary disease in the elderly makes it less likely that angioplasty will be a suitable alternative to coronary surgery on technical grounds (49).

Operative procedures

In the elderly, coronary surgery is more likely to be complicated by the presence of atheroma in the ascending aorta. This can create particular problems in siting the proximal anastomoses of vein grafts. It may be necessary to resort to alternative surgical manoeuvres to deal with the problem. These may include a single aorta-to-vein anastomosis, with other vein grafts being inserted onto the vein attached to the aorta, or the choice of less diseased aortic sites made with the cross-clamped aorta being opened for viewing from the inside (50).

There has sometimes in the past been the perception that, in the elderly, surgical intervention should be kept to the minimum necessary to achieve operative survival and correction of the most critical lesions, possibly using fewer bypass grafts and omitting grafts to smaller vessels or those with relatively minor obstructions. Experience has shown, however, that elderly patients require just as many, if not more, grafts than younger patients (20,21,25) in view of the more extensive nature of coronary disease, and that complete revascularization in this group is reflected in better outcome. Our own policy is to apply the same strategy in the elderly as for any age group—that of achieving maximum revascularization. Review of practice in Glasgow Royal Infirmary during the period 1986–1991 (Figure 2) indicates that the proportion of patients having one to five or more grafts is similar in the elderly and younger age groups.

Internal mammary artery (IMA) grafts have been consistently shown to have significantly better long-term patency than saphenous vein grafts and to be associated with improved long-term survival and freedom from cardiac events or the need for reoperation (51–53). At 10 years angiographic follow-up, 25–50% of vein grafts are occluded or have significant disease, whereas 95% of IMA grafts

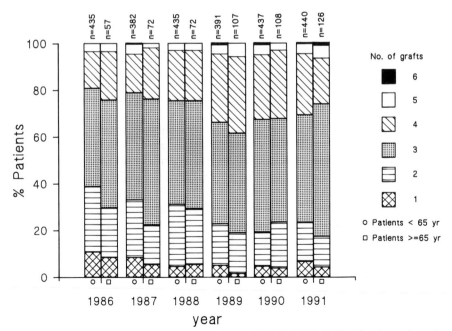

Figure 2. Glasgow Royal Infirmary: isolated CABG 1986–1991. Number of grafts inserted (%)

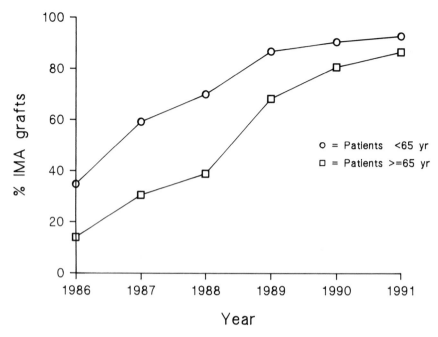

Figure 3. Glasgow Royal Infirmary: isolated CABG 1986–1991. Percentage of CABG surgery using IMA for one or more grafts

remain disease-free. This is due, at least in part, to the resistance of the IMA to the development of atherosclerosis even in patients with widespread vascular and coronary artery disease (54).

Concern has been expressed in the past about the use of the IMA in elderly patients, partly because of an anticipated increased surgical risk but also because the rationale in favour of using the IMA for its prognostic benefits was considered less relevant in the elderly. Experience has largely refuted these reservations. Review of our own practice over the period 1986–1991 shows that the proportion of patients receiving internal mammary grafts has increased in all patients, rising from 32% in 1986 to 91% in 1991 (Figure 3); initially we, like others, were more cautious with the use of the IMA in the elderly, but would now advocate no different criteria in the elderly with regard to IMA use.

Use of an IMA graft generally leads to increased mediastinal bleeding because of the additional dissection of the chest wall, but there is no consistent evidence that its use increases wound infection rates. Wareing and colleagues compared the use of a single IMA graft in 341 patients over 65 years with its use in 445 patients aged younger than 65 years and found no difference in mortality or morbidity, including sternal wound infection, perioperative infarction, or re-exploration for bleeding (55). Gardner and colleagues (56) reported similar findings in their series of more than 450 patients aged over 70 years who received an IMA graft and emphasized improved survival at 4 years in the IMA group compared to those receiving only saphenous vein grafts. There is evidence that the use of both IMAs may contribute to increased blood loss (57). Kouchoukos and colleagues reported a 6.9% incidence of wound infection with use of both IMAs compared to 1.9% with a single IMA (58). Use of both IMAs has been reported to improve long-term survival over single IMA use but at the cost of a higher operative mortality (59). While the use of a single IMA graft is therefore appropriate in the elderly (60), the increased mortality and morbidity associated with use of both IMAs, particularly in the obese and diabetics, cautions against routine use of both IMAs.

Outcome

Hospital mortality

Although elderly patients may be less attractive surgical candidates for reasons previously discussed, coronary surgery can still be performed with a relatively modest increase in mortality. Reported mortality rates are by no means uniform, reflecting variation in the size of the experience, the age distribution of the patients within the elderly group, whether surgery was undertaken on an elective or urgent basis, and the selection criteria applied to surgical candidates. However, the consensus of experience from leading centres reporting sizeable numbers of patients indicates that coronary artery bypass can be undertaken in elderly patients, particularly in the under-75-year-olds, with only a slightly elevated hospital mortality.

Loop and colleagues in comparing the postoperative course of 5070 patients aged 65 years or over with that of almost 18 000 patients aged less than 65 years undergoing coronary revascularization from 1976 to 1986 reported hospital mortality of 0.7% in patients aged less than 65 years, 2.0% in 4603 patients aged 65–74 years, and 4.7% in 467 patients aged 75 years or over (19). Carey's group reviewing 20 years experience of 2479 patients having myocardial revascularization found that hospital mortality was not higher in older patients undergoing CABG only—being 4% for the 300 patients aged 49 or younger, and 3.5% for the 230 patients 70 years or older (20). Our own experience of isolated CABG in Glasgow Royal Infirmary over the period 1986–1991 shows that age 65 or more did not increase hospital mortality; for 2520 patients aged under 65, hospital mortality was 2.4%; for the 542 patients aged 65 years and over, it was 1.7%. The claim that coronary surgery can be undertaken in the elderly with little or no increase in hospital mortality can therefore be supported by our own experience, although for Scotland as a whole for the period 1983–1990 mortality in the under-65 group (8632 patients) was 2.2%, compared with 4.1% in the 1677 patients over 65 years or over (34).

Within the 'elderly' population (over 65), experience shows that there is a distinct incremental risk with advancing age, which to a large extent explains disparity in reports of mortality and morbidity rates in the elderly in the literature. In the Scottish experience, only 4.7% of the elderly (or 0.7% of total CABG patients) were 75 years or over (34); in our own centre, the majority of elderly patients fell within the 65–70-year age range, only 18% of the group being over 70 and 3% over 75 years. Horneffer and colleagues reported a considerably higher hospital mortality of 9.3% in 228 patients aged over 70 compared with 2.2% in 228 patients aged 55–69 years (21). Acinapura and colleagues (22) reported hospital mortality of 2% in 3142 patients under 70 years (range 30–69, mean 58.5), compared with 7% in 685 patients 70 and over (range 70–85, mean 74.2).

The mortality of surgery rises significantly in octogenarians. Edmunds and colleagues reported the 90-day mortality of 41 octogenarians having isolated CABG at 24% (61). Montague's group (23) document an overall mortality of 2.7% for 597 patients aged 70 or over, compared with 0.4% in 4125 patients under 70. The mortality in the 70 and over age group was further subdivided to show that in the under 80-year-olds it was 2.4% compared with 12.5% in the ⩾80-year-olds. Other recent reports quote mortality rates varying from 0 to 10.7% in octogenarians, and it would appear that in selected elective patients a mortality of the order of 6–10% may be anticipated in octogenarians (62–66). Most reports emphasize the need to be particularly selective in this age group; most authors comment on the greater incidence of concomitant pathology which adds to risk, and nearly all confirm the greater number of patients with left main disease, three-vessel disease and poor left ventricular function in this age group.

Many groups highlight the greatly increased mortality incurred when surgery is carried out on an urgent or emergency basis; Horvath's group (67) noted a 10-told increase in mortality when emergency CABG was undertaken: an overall mortality of 10.8% was reported in their group of 222 patients ⩾75 years; when surgery was undertaken electively (in 111 patients), mortality was 3.6%; when carried out urgently (in 94 patients) it was 14.9%, and when on an emergency basis (in 17 patients), mortality rose to 35.3%.

Many reports document non-cardiac causes for the increased mortality and morbidity in older age groups—the presence of age-related concomitant disease and age-related decline in function of major systems showing their effects (19,68).

Morbidity

Reports indicate a longer postoperative stay (19,69) and prolonged ventilation times for patients aged 65 or over. Postoperative morbidity is also higher in elderly patients (19,20,39,69). In the oldest of the three age groups (< 65, 67–74, ⩾75 years) described by Loop and colleagues (19), there were statistically significant, but clinically modest, increases in reoperation for bleeding (3.5%, 4.8%, 6.4%, respectively), respiratory distress (1%, 2.6%, 4.3%, respectively), stroke (1%, 2.7%, 2.4%, respectively) and renal failure (0.2%, 0.9%, 1.7%, respectively). There was, however, no significant difference in myocardial infarction (around 1%) or wound complication (around 1%) in the three groups. Postoperative complications were also higher in older patients in Horneffer's series (21), where the outcome was compared for three groups each comprising 228 patients: <55 years, 55–69 years and ≥70 years. The frequency of reoperation for bleeding was, respectively, 0.9%, 4.0% and 7.1%, prolonged ventilation was required in 2.2%, 4.0% and 8.4%, stroke occurred in 0%, 3.1% and 7.5%, renal dialysis was needed in 0%, 1.3% and 3.1%, and wound infection was seen in 3.5%, 4.4% and 13%.

Long-term outcome

The Cleveland Clinic group's 10-year survival data for 1439 64–74-year-olds following CABG performed between 1976 and 1980 is reported as 64.2%, and compares well with the age and gender-matched US population (61.7%). Their 75 and over group (84 patients) showed favourable 8-year actuarial survival of 53.3% compared with 48.6% for the age- and gender-matched US population (19). This group also reported relief of angina at 8 years to be significantly better in patients aged 75 years (81%) than in those aged 65–74 years (77%) and those less than 65 years (73%).

Rahimtoola and colleagues (69) report actuarial survival data in three groups of patients following CABG surgery defined by age: 55–64 years, 65–74 years and 75–84 years. Five-year survival, respectively, was 91%, 83% and 73%; 10-year survival was 77% and 66% in the first two age groups, and 7-year survival of 65% is reported in the oldest age group. For all groups, survival data compared favourably with expected mortality for the relevant general population.

Gardner and colleagues report a significantly improved 4-year survival in patients 70 years or older who had received an IMA graft compared to those without (86% versus 77%) (56).

Carey and colleagues (20) noted that reoperation rate was less in patients over 60 than in those under 60, that improvement lasted longer, and that quality of life (as measured by health index status) was better. Horneffer (21) reports no differences in completeness of rehabilitation or in duration of convalescence in all three age groups in his study (<55 years, 55–69 years and ≥70 years), all groups showing substantial improvement in activity level following CABG. A survival advantage was demonstrated after year 3 in elderly patients compared with the age-, race- and sex-matched peers in the general population (from 91% in year 1 to 101% and 107% in years 4 and 5), while relative survival in younger patients similarly matched remained stable at 95%.

Even in octogenarians, coronary surgery in appropriately selected patients can achieve very good longer-term results. Mullany's group (63) reporting results in 159 octogenarians showed 1- and 5-year survival of 84% and 71%, respectively (comparing favourably with age- and gender-matched populations), with 79% angina-free at mean follow-up of 29 months.

Redo surgery

There is recurrence of angina at a rate of 5% yearly following successful coronary surgery due to appearance of disease in the bypass conduits or progression of disease in native vessels (70). There is some evidence, however, that the risk of requiring redo surgery is less when surgery is performed in patients in the sixth and seventh decades and followed for a comparable time to younger patients (20,71). Approximately 20% of patients receiving only vein grafts will subsequently require reoperation for recurrence of symptoms within 10 years of the initial operation, compared to 10% of patients where one IMA graft was used in addition to vein grafts (72). Reoperations are associated with increasing mortality and morbidity in all patients, and particularly in the elderly. At the Cleveland Clinic the overall mortality for 1500 redo coronary operations increased with advancing age, but was still only 4% for 47 patients aged over 70 years in 1982–1984 (72). Morbidity was also increased in the reoperation group, especially from perioperative myocardial infarction, stroke, reoperation for bleeding, respiratory distress, wound complications and renal impairment (72). Salomon and colleagues reported the mortality of redo surgery at 12.5% in 16 patients with a mean age of 78 years, compared to 6.8% in patients with a mean age of 59 years, and emphasized the increased hospital costs and complications in the elderly (25).

In summary, therefore, the elderly group can be seen to be heterogeneous. The increased likelihood of age-related concomitant illness and the natural age-related decline in physiological function of many of the body's systems makes it important to exercise care and clinical acumen in selection for coronary surgery. Operative mortality and morbidity rise little, if at all, in the first few years beyond 65. By 70 years, there is a discernible increase in operative mortality and morbidity which becomes more marked in the next 5–10 years, but even in octogenarians coronary surgery can be accomplished with acceptable mortality and morbidity. Given survival, the symptomatic and survival status of the elderly following CABG is at least as good and possibly better than for younger groups.

Surgery for complications of coronary artery disease

Left ventricular aneurysm

Left ventricular aneurysm may complicate myocardial infarction, and when left heart failure becomes a significant clinical problem there is a role for surgical intervention with resection. As with coronary disease generally, there has been a rise in the age of the surgical population undergoing left ventricular aneurysm resection. The risk factors for this form of surgery are little different from those in CABG surgery. Cosgrove's group (73) reported recent practice with left ventricular aneurysm resection in 212 patients, 31.6% of whom were over 65 years of age. Hospital mortality was 8%. Advancing age, although identified as a risk factor, did not appear to play a major role. McGovern's group (74) reporting surgical results in 197 patients with a mean age of 58 (range of 29–76 years) showed an overall hospital mortality rate of 9.6%; age over 65 did not influence hospital mortality or length of survival.

Postinfarction ventricular septal defect

Surgery for rupture of the ventricular septum following myocardial infarction carries a very high mortality at any age; mortality without intervention is even higher. Hill and Stiles recently reviewed the literature and found only five reports in which survival data could be distinguished for age. There was an operative survival rate of 52% for 27 patients aged over 65 and 45% for 22 patients under 65 (no significant difference) (75).

VALVULAR HEART SURGERY

In the past few decades, there has been a change in the nature of valvular heart disease in most Western countries. The prevalence of rheumatic heart disease has declined and the elderly are forming an increasing proportion of the population, resulting in a growing volume of surgery for aortic valve degenerative disease. Aortic stenosis in the elderly is now most frequently due to calcification in a congenitally bicuspid aortic valve, or in the very elderly to degenerative valvular calcification. There has been a decrease in the frequency of mitral stenosis, mitral valve disease in the elderly being increasingly a consequence of degenerative and ischaemic pathologies (76).

The age of patients undergoing valve surgery generally has risen, and there has been an increase in the number of operations in which coronary artery bypass grafting and valve surgery are combined. In the UK in 1989, 37% of patients undergoing valve surgery were over the age of 65 (77). In Scotland the percentage of patients aged 65 or over undergoing valve surgery rose from 17% to 37% over the period 1983–1990 (34). During the period 1975–1987, 41.4% of 2717 patients undergoing valve replacement in Jamieson's centre in Vancouver were 65 years or older (78). Important issues in surgery for valvular heart disease in the elderly include consideration of valve repair or balloon valvuloplasty rather than replacement, the choice of valve prosthesis, and the need for concomitant coronary artery bypass grafting.

Alternatives to replacement

Balloon valvuloplasty

The heavily calcified aortic valves which are usually encountered in the elderly are rarely suitable for conservative procedures. Attempts to decalcify such valves (79) have been disappointing. For the moribund or very frail elderly patient with calcific aortic stenosis, the possibility of a less invasive form of intervention is attractive. However, the initial promise of percutaneous balloon valvuloplasty for aortic and mitral valve stenosis as an alternative to surgery seems to have faded as 'long-term' results become available. The hospital mortality of aortic balloon valvuloplasty has been reported at around 3.5%, and the increase in the mean aortic orifice area at less than 0.5 cm² (80,81). Much of the initial benefit may be lost within 8 days (82) with evidence of residual benefit in only 50% of patients at 6 months, and no improvement in survival at 1 year compared to untreated patients has been shown in at least one study (83). The temporary nature of any improvement with balloon aortic valvuloplasty has been confirmed by other workers (84), who reported that event-free survival was only 18% amongst 205 patients at a mean of 2 years' follow-up, and that the best improvements occurred in those who would have been expected to have had excellent long-term results after aortic valve replacement.

There is considerably less experience with percutaneous balloon valvotomy for mitral stenosis, but preliminary results for fused, pliable and non-calcified leaflets have been modestly encouraging in young patients (85). Such leaflets are, however, rarely seen in the elderly where calcified, shrunken leaflets and a fused subvalvar apparatus are much more common.

Surgical repair

Procedures which conserve the native valve are most often applicable to the mitral and tricuspid valves and require pliable valve leaflets and a non-calcified, non-fused subvalvar apparatus. The advantages of repair rather than replacement are well established (86). Although much of the pioneering work with the Carpentier techniques of mitral valve reconstruction was undertaken in younger patients frequently with rheumatic disease, it is apparent that the same techniques can be applied in suitable patients well into the elderly age group. Spencer's group (87) have made a plea for widening indications for reconstruction to almost all patients with mitral regurgitation regardless of age or aetiology, and their own patient group ranged in age from 2 to 77 years. Cosgrove's group (88) report a series of 117 patients with mitral valve reconstruction with a mean age of 60; 35 of these patients were more than 70 years of age.

The mortality for repair of the mitral valve is higher in the elderly (the overall mortality in Cosgrove's group of 4.3% was incurred in those aged over 65 with severe symptoms) (88). Fremes and colleagues (89) reported similar mortality rates of 15% and 16%, respectively, for repair and replacement procedures in patients aged over 70 years, compared to 2% and 7%, respectively, in younger patients, and speculated that the less favourable results of repair procedures in the elderly might be due to poorer tissue viability.

Choice of prosthesis

Increasing awareness of the limited durability of bioprosthetic valves in young patients has largely led to their abandonment in patients less than 65 years old, except in circumstances where there is a strong contraindication to the use of warfarin. The choice of bioprosthetic or mechanical valve in the elderly, however, remains controversial. Proponents of bioprosthetic valves point to the virtual lack of mechanical failure of porcine valves in patients aged over 70 years at 10–12 years' follow-up (78) and the possibility, therefore, of minimizing thromboembolic and haemorrhagic complications associated with mechanical valves and anticoagulants (78,90–92). Nevertheless, some groups have advocated the use of mechanical valves in the elderly on the basis that anticoagulant-related problems are no more common in patients aged over 65 years than in a younger population (93). Indeed, it has been reported that thromboembolic events are less common with mechanical valves and adequately controlled anticoagulation than with bioprosthetic valves without anticoagulation (92,93). However, the advantages of independence from anticoagulation are significant, and in patients older than 70 years it would be our practice to use a bioprosthetic valve for the aortic position—a policy also favoured by other groups (78,89,94,95).

Concomitant coronary disease

Elderly patients undergoing valve replacement are much more likely to have poorer left ventricular function and significant coronary artery disease than a younger population (89,96,97). In view of the increased operative risks of combined valvular surgery and coronary revascularization in the early era of cardiac surgery (98–100), some groups advocated isolated valve replacement even in the presence of significant (> 50% stenosis) coronary artery disease (102). Although there was no increase in operative mortality with this approach, there was an earlier recurrence of angina in the patients who did not undergo revascularization. Failure to deal with associated coronary artery disease is increasingly recognized to be a cause of early and late mortality following otherwise successful valve replacement (89,102), and coronary arteriography is now an essential part of investigation in the elderly under consideration for valve replacement. Significant coronary obstructions are bypassed at the time of valve replacement.

Outcome

The increased likelihood of age-related disease and decline in physiological reserves results in an increasing mortality for valve replacement with advancing age, together with a greater risk of postoperative complications and delayed recovery. Apart from advanced age, the main factors which influence mortality are the presence of coronary artery disease and the urgency of surgery. In general, aortic valve replacement has a lower risk than mitral valve replacement—probably the consequence of impairment of pulmonary function and pulmonary vascular changes which are more common with mitral valve disease.

There are now many reports in the literature of experience of valve replacement in elderly populations, and mortality ranging from 0% (103,104) to as high as 36% has been documented for subgroups identified by such parameters as procedure performed, lesion, priority of operation, advanced age or preoperative risk factors. The influence of such variables is well shown by Azariades and colleagues (105), who report an overall hospital mortality of 16% in a group of 88 patients over 80 years undergoing aortic valve replacement: the mortality for 52 patients in whom surgery was performed electively was 6% but rose to 36% in 14 patients where emergency operation was necessary.

For patients below the age of 70 years, the operative risk of aortic valve replacement is little different from that in younger patients. Risk is significantly higher after age 70, although for elective operation the increase need not be dramatic. In the Cleveland Clinic's more recent experience, aortic valve replacement for aortic stenosis incurred an overall hospital mortality of 1.5%; in the subgroup of 88 patients aged 70 or over mortality was 2.3% (106). In a large experience in Toronto (96), elective aortic valve surgery at age 40–60 carried a mortality of 2.5% and at age 60–70 mortality was 2.4%; in those over 70 it rose to 6.5%.

Jamieson's report (78) of valve replacement surgery in 1127 patients 65 years and over confirms the incremental risk which accompanies advancing age: the 65–69-year-olds (465 patients) had a hospital mortality of 7.3%, the 70–79-year-olds (618 patients) 10.7% and the 80 and over (52 patients) 15.4%. In this experience, mortality for aortic valve replacement was 6.3% for the entire group.

Simultaneous CABG may increase the risk of aortic valve replacement in the elderly (89,91). The 2.7% operative mortality for aortic valve replacement in patients aged 70 years and over in the Toronto group's experience rose to 8% when coronary surgery was combined with aortic valve replacement; those patients with coronary disease who did not have concomitant CABG, however, incurred the highest operative risk (10%) (89). This increased mortality for concomitant CABG has not been universal experience. Indeed, there are reports of lower mortality in elderly patients having combined aortic valve replacement and CABG compared to those having only aortic valve replacement (104,105). Azariades' overall 16% operative mortality in 88 patients aged ⩾ 80 years having aortic valve replacement was reduced to 8% in the 38 who underwent concomitant CABG (105), in Arom's series mortality for aortic valve replacement alone was 9.8% in 41 patients aged 70 or over; there was no mortality in the 43 patients having aortic valve replacement combined with coronary grafting (104).

Although, inevitably, there are exceptions (93), reports of valve surgery in the elderly suggest that mitral valve replacement carries a higher operative mortality than replacement of the aortic valve (78,89,104). More important, however, is the degree to which the risk is increased in the elderly compared with the younger population in the same experience. Such comparative studies as are available show a higher risk for mitral valve replacement in the older population. Thus,

Fremes and colleagues (89) in comparing results for patients 70 and over with those under 70 show operative mortality of 8.6% versus 3.2%, and Arom and colleagues (104) report operative mortality of 8.3% versus 4.5% in the same age groups. In both reports, the addition of coronary surgery increased mortality—to 19.6% in Fremes' series and to 12.5% in Arom's series. Fremes, however, noted the highest mortality (33.3%) in those with coronary disease in whom additional CABG was not undertaken.

When replacement of both mitral and aortic valves is required, mortality ranging from 14% to over 30% has been reported (78,89,93,104).

In summary, elective aortic valve replacement in the elderly can be accomplished with a mortality of 5–10%; the need for concomitant coronary surgery may increase the mortality. Elective mitral valve replacement in the elderly has a higher mortality, probably 8–15%; associated coronary disease makes mitral valve replacement more risky. Urgent or emergency surgery adds considerably to the mortality for aortic or mitral valve surgery.

The longer-term outcome after aortic valve replacement in the elderly is generally good, with loss of symptoms, return of activity, improvement in both quality of life and life expectancy, with late survival not greatly different from, or even better than, age- and gender-matched populations (89,103,105,107,108). Although there are fewer reports in the literature of late outcome for mitral valve replacement in the elderly, it seems likely that these patients do not differ unduly from aortic valve patients (78).

Endocarditis

The diagnosis of endocarditis is often delayed in the elderly because of atypical presentation and/or confusion with other pathological processes and consequently results in a higher overall mortality. Staphylococci and streptococci are now the most common causative organisms of endocarditis in all age groups, with staphylococci also being the predominant organism in prosthetic valve endocarditis. Absolute indications for surgical intervention in endocarditis are the same in all age groups: progressive haemodynamic instability refractory to medical therapy, or uncontrollable infection. Relative indications include systemic embolization, the appearance of conduction defects and the nature of the causative organism; for example, infection with *Staphylococcus aureus* or coagulase-negative staphylococci, particularly on prosthetic valves, is likely to require surgery.

OTHER CONDITIONS

Aneurysm or dissection of the ascending aorta

Atherosclerosis and hypertension are the most important aetiological factors in the development of aortic aneurysms and dissections, which are increasingly prevalent in the elderly population. Aneurysm and dissection of the ascending aorta presenting in the elderly require consideration for surgery in the same way as in younger patients. However, a much greater likelihood of concomitant disease, and the decline in physiological reserves in the elderly, combine to make the surgical risk higher for this age group. Associated coronary disease is a particular risk, and coronary angiography is required in the routine investigation for surgery. In a large series reported by Crawford (109) the median age of his 717 patients was 61 and the oldest 88. Increasing age was one of the predictors of early death. Mortality increased from 5% in patients less than 50 years to 9% in those aged 50–74 years and 22% in those aged over 75.

Congenital heart disease in the elderly

Apart from congenital bicuspid aortic valve, which presents in the elderly as a calcified stenotic valve, and prolapsing mitral valve, few haemodynamically important congenital defects are seen in the elderly. Atrial septal defect is one condition which can escape earlier detection and treatment, and when it presents in the older patient with progressive ventricular dysfunction, dysrhythmias or pulmonary infection and embolism, closure of such defects is feasible provided that the shunting is still predominantly left to right. In one series of 66 patients aged over 60 years the operative mortality of atrial septal defect closure was 6% and was related to performance of an additional procedure (110). Late cardiac failure, stroke and atrial fibrillation were noted to be more frequent in the older patient.

CONCLUSION

Not only is it possible to undertake virtually the full range of cardiac surgical procedures in the elderly, but in many countries this is already established practice. Surgery is a valid therapeutic option for clinical heart disease in the elderly as it is in younger patients. Apart from the important economic implications, there are additional risk factors attached to surgery in this age group. A successful outcome is more likely if surgery is undertaken timeously and electively. With careful selection and appropriate intervention, surgery can offer relief of symptoms, improved quality of life and restoration of life expectancy.

REFERENCES

1. Wetle T (1987) Age as a risk factor for inadequate treatment. JAMA **258**: 516.
2. Yusuf S, Furberg CDE (1991) Are we biased in our approach to treating elderly patients with heart disease? *Am J Cardiol* **68**: 954–956.
3. Report of a Working Group of the Royal College of Physicians (1991) *Cardiological Intervention in Elderly Patients.* Royal College of Physicians of London.
4. Evans TI (1973) The physiological basis of geriatric general anaesthesia. *Anaesth Intens Care* **1**: 319–322.

5. Muravchick S (1990) Anesthesia for the elderly. In *Anesthesia*, 3rd edn, Miller RD (ed.). Churchill Livingstone, Edinburgh, pp. 1969–1983.

6. Kirklin JK, Westaby S, Blackstone EH *et al.* (1983) Complement and the damaging effects of cardiopulmonary bypass. *J. Thorac Cardiovasc Surg* **86**: 845–847.

7. Fox LS, Blackstone EH, Kirklin JW *et al.* (1992) Relationship of whole body oxygen consumption to perfusion flow rate during hypothermic cardiopulmonary bypass. *J Thorac Cardiovasc Surg* **83**: 239–248.

8. Aris A, Solanes H, Camara ML *et al.* (1986) Arterial line filtration during cardiopulmonary bypass: neurologic, neurophysiologic, and hematologic studies. *J Thorac Cardiovasc Surg* **91**: 526–533.

9. Blauth C, Smith P, Newman S *et al.* (1989) Retinal microembolism and neuro-psychological deficit following clinical cardiopulmonary bypass: comparison of a membrane and a bubble oxygenator. *Eur J Cardiothorac Surg* 135–139.

10. Gerstenblith G, Lakatta EG, Leisfeldt ML (1976) Age changes in myocardial function and exercise response. *Prog Cardiovasc Dis* **XIX**: 1–21.

11. Craig DB, McLeskey CH, Mitkeno PA *et al.* (1987) Geriatric anaesthesia. *Can J Anaesth* **34**: 156–167.

12. Rodeheffer RJ, Gerstenblith G, Becker LC *et al.* (1984) Exercise cardiac output is maintained with advancing age in healthy human subjects: cardiac dilatation and increased stroke volume compensate for a diminished heart rate. *Circulation* **69**: 203–213.

13. Wahba WM (1983) Influence of aging on lung function: clinical significance of changes from age twenty. *Anesth Analg* **62**: 764–776.

14. Lindeman RD, Tobin J, Shock NW (1985) Longitudinal studies on the rate of decline in renal function with age. *J Am Geriatr Soc* **33**: 278–285.

15. Newman DC, Hicks RG (1988) Combined carotid and coronary artery surgery: a review of the literature. *Ann Thorac Surg* **45**: 574–581.

16. Warnold I, Lundholm KO (1983) Clinical significance of preoperative nutritional status in 215 noncancer patients. *Ann Surg* **199**: 299–305.

17. Weksler ME (1981) The senescence of the immune system. *Hosp Pract* **16**: 53–64.

18. Cosgrove DM, Loop FD, Lytle BW *et al.* Primary myocardial revascularisation: trends in surgical mortality. *J Thorac Cardiovasc Surg* **88**: 673–684.

19. Loop FD, Lytle BW, Cosgrove DM *et al.* (1988) Coronary artery bypass graft surgery in the elderly: indications and outcome. *Cleve Clin J Med* **55**: 23–34.

20. Carey JS, Cukingnan RA, Singer LKM (1992) Quality of life after myocardial revascularization: effect of increasing age. *J Thorac Cardiovasc Surg* **103**: 108–151.

21. Horneffer PJ, Gardner TJ, Manolio *et al.* (1987) The effects of age on outcome after coronary bypass surgery. *Circulation* **76** (Suppl. V): V-6–V-12.

22. Acinapura AJ, Rose DM, Cunningham JN Jr *et al.* (1988) Coronary artery bypass in septuagenarians: analysis of mortality and morbidity. *Circulation* **78** (Suppl. I): I-179–I-184.

23. Montague NT, Kouchoukos NT, Wilson TAS *et al.* (1985) Morbidity and mortality of coronary bypass grafting in patients 70 years of age and older. *Ann Thorac Surg* **39**: 552–557.

24. Hammermeister KD, Burchfiel C, Johnson R, Grover FL (1990) Identification of patients at greatest risk for developing major complications at cardiac surgery. *Circulation* **82** (Suppl. IV): IV-380–IV-389.

25. Salomon NW, Page US, Bigelow JC *et al.* (1991) Coronary artery bypass grafting in elderly patients: comparative results in a consecutive series of 469 patients older than 75 years. *J Thorac Cardiovasc Surg* **101**: 209–218.

26. Furlan AJ, Bruer AC (1984) Central nervous system complications of open heart surgery. *Stroke* **15**: 912–915.

27. Taggart DP, Reece IJ, Wheatley DJ (1987) Cerebral deficit after elective cardiac surgery. *Lancet* **i**: 47.
28. Anonymous (1989) Brain damage and open heart surgery. *Lancet* **ii**: 364–366.
29. Feinleib M, Havlik RJ, Gillum RF *et al.* (1989) Coronary heart disease and related procedures: National Hospital Discharge Survey data. *Circulation* **79**: (Suppl. I): I-13–I-18.
30. Graves EJ (1991) 1989 Summary: National Hospital Discharge Survey. Advance data from vital and health statistics; no. 199. National Center for Health Statistics, Hyattsville, MD.
31. Graves EJ (1992) 1990 Summary: National Hospital Discharge Survey. Advance data from vital and health statistics; no. 210. National Center for Health Statistics, Hyattsville, MD.
32. Pokras R (1992) Personal communication. Chief, Hospital Care Statistics Branch, Division of Health Care Statistics, National Center for Health Statistics, Hyattsville, MD.
33. UK Cardiac Surgical Register (1989).
34. Scottish Cardiac Surgical Register (1983–1990).
35. Varnauskas E and the European Coronary Surgery Study Group (1988) Twelve-year follow-up of survival in the randomized European Coronary Surgery Study. *N Engl J Med* **319**: 332–337.
36. Veterans Administration Coronary Artery Bypass Surgery Cooperative Study Group (1984) Eleven-year survival in the Veterans Administration randomized trial of coronary bypass surgery for stable angina. *N Engl J Med* **311**: 1333–1339.
37. CASS Principal Investigators and their associates (1983) Coronary Artery Surgery Study (CASS) a randomized trial of coronary artery bypass surgery. Quality of life in patients randomly assigned to treatment groups. *Circulation* **68**: 951–960.
38. Kaiser GC, Davis KB, Fisher *et al.* (1985) Survival following coronary artery bypass grafting in patients with severe angina pectoris (CASS): an observational study. *J Thorac Cardiovasc Surg.* **89**: 513–524.
39. Gersh BJ, Kronmal RA, Schaff HV *et al.* and the participants in the Coronary Artery Surgery Study (1985) Comparison of coronary artery bypass surgery and medical therapy in patients 65 years of age or older: a nonrandomized study from the Coronary Artery Surgery Study (CASS) Registry. *N Engl J Med* **313**: 217–224.
40. Loop FD (1985) CASS continued. *Circulation* **72** (Suppl. II): II-1–II-6.
41. Alderman EL, Bourassa MG, Cohen LS *et al.* for the CASS Investigators (1990) Ten-year follow-up of survival and myocardial infarction in the Randomized Coronary Artery Surgery Study. *Circulation* **82**: 1629–1946.
42. Kaiser GC, Schaff HB, Killip T (1989) Myocardial revascularization for unstable angina pectoris. *Circulation* **79** (Suppl. I): I-60–I-67.
43. US Bureau of the Census (1989) Current population reports, series P-25, no. 1018, *Projections of the Population of the United States, by Age, Sex, and Race: 1988 to 2080.* US Government Printing Office, Washington, DC.
44. *Scottish Health Statistics* (1990) Common Services Agency/Crown Copyright, Scottish Health Service, Edinburgh.
45. Weinstein MC, Stason WB (1982) Cost-effectiveness of coronary artery bypass surgery. *Circulation* **66** (Suppl. III): III-56–III-66.
46. Kelly ME, Taylor GJ, Moses HW *et al.* (1985) Comparative cost of myocardial revascularization: percutaneous transluminal angioplasty and coronary artery bypass surgery. *J Am Coll Cardiol* **5**:16–20.
47. Wilson JM, Dunn EJ, Wright CB *et al.* (1986) The cost of simultaneous surgical standby for percutaneous transluminal coronary angioplasty. *J Thorac Cardiovasc Surg* **91**: 362–370.

48. Hlatky MA, Lipscomb J, Nelson C *et al.* (1990) Resource use and initial cost of coronary revascularisation: coronary angioplasty versus coronary bypass surgery. *Circulation* **82** (Suppl. IV): IV-208–IV-213.

49. Kowalchuk GJ, Siu SC, Lewis SM (1990) Coronary artery disease in the octogenarian: angiographic spectrum and suitability for revascularisation. *Am J Cardiol* **66**: 1319–1323.

50. Landymore R, Spencer F, Colvin S *et al.* (1982) Management of the calcified aorta during myocardial revascularisation. *J Thorac Cardiovasc Surg* **84**: 455–456.

51. Loop FD, Lytle BW, Cosgrove DM *et al.* (1986) Influence of the internal-mammary-artery graft on 10-year survival and other cardiac events. *N Engl J Med* **314**: 1–6.

52. Cameron A, Davis KB, Green GE *et al.* (1988) Clinical implications of internal mammary artery bypass grafts: the Coronary Artery Surgery Study experience. *Circulation* **77**: 815–819.

53. Cosgrove DM, Loop FD, Lytle BW *et al.* (1985) Determinants of 10-year survival after primary myocardial revascularization. *Ann Surg* **202**: 480–490.

54. Sims FH (1983) A comparison of coronary and internal mammary arteries and implications of the results in the etiology of arteriosclerosis. *Am Heart J* **105**: 560–566.

55. Wareing TH, Saffitz JE, Kouchoukos NT (1990) Use of single internal mammary artery grafts in older patients. *Circulation* **82** (Suppl. IV): IV-224–IV-228.

56. Gardner TJ, Greene PS, Rykiel MF *et al.* (1990) Routine use of the left internal mammary artery graft in the elderly. *Ann Thorac Surg* **49**: 188–194.

57. Cosgrove DM, Lytle BW, Loop FD *et al.* (1988) Does bilateral internal mammary artery grafting increase surgical risk? *J Thorac Cardiovasc Surg* **95**: 850–856.

58. Kouchoukos NT, Wareing TH, Murphy SF *et al.* (1990) Risks of bilateral internal mammary artery bypass grafting. *Ann Thorac Surg* **49**: 210–219.

59. Fiore AC, Naunheim KS, Dean P *et al.* (1990) Results of internal thoracic artery grafting over 15 years: single versus double grafts. *Ann Thorac Surg* **49**: 202–209.

60. Azariades M, Fessler CL, Floten HS, Starr A (1990) Five-year results of coronary bypass grafting for patients older than 70 years: role of internal mammary artery. *Ann Thorac Surg* **50**: 840–845.

61. Edmunds LH Jr, Stephenson LW, Edie RN, Ratcliffe MB (1988) Open-heart surgery in octogenarians. *N Engl J Med* **319**: 131–136.

62. Utley JR, Leyland SA (1991) Coronary artery bypass grafting in the octogenarian. *J Thorac Cardiovasc Surg* **101**: 866–870.

63. Mullany CJ, Darling GE, Pluth JR *et al.* (1990) Early and late results after isolated coronary artery bypass surgery in 159 patients aged 80 years and older. *Circulation* **82** (Suppl. IV): IV-229–IV-236.

64. Weintraub WS, Clements SD, Ware J *et al.* (1991) Coronary artery surgery in octogenarians. *Am J Cardiol* **68**: 1530–1534.

65. Mick MJ, Simpfendorfer C, Arnold AZ *et al.* (1991) Early and late results of coronary angioplasty and bypass in octogenarians. *Am J Cardiol* **68**: 1316–1320.

66. Tsai T-P, Nessim S, Kass R *et al.* (1991) Morbidity and mortality after coronary artery bypass in octogenarians. *Ann Thorac Surg* **51**: 983–986.

67. Horvath KA, DiSesa VJ, Peigh PS *et al.* Favorable results of coronary artery bypass grafting in patients older than 75 years. *J Thorac Cardiovasc Surg* **99**: 92–96.

68. Rich MW, Keller AJ, Schechtman KB *et al.* (1988) Morbidity and mortality of coronary bypass surgery in patients 75 years of age or older. *Ann Thorac Surg* **46**: 638–644.

69. Rahimtoola SH, Grunkemeier GL, Starr MD (1986) Ten year survival after coronary artery bypass surgery for angina in patients aged 65 years and older.

Circulation **74**: 509–517.

70. Grondin CM (1986) Graft disease in patients with coronary bypass grafting. Why does it start? Where do we stop? *J Thorac Cardiovasc Surg* **92**: 323–329.

71. Rogers WB, Von Dohlen TW, Frank MJ (1991) Management of coronary heart disease in the elderly. *Clin Cardiol* **14**: 635–642.

72. Lytle BW, Loop FD, Cosgrove DM *et al.* (1987) Fifteen hundred coronary reoperations: results and determinants of early and late survival. *J Thorac Cardiovasc Surg* **93**: 847–859.

73. Cosgrove DM, Lytle BW, Taylor PC *et al.* (1989) Ventricular aneurysm resection: trends in surgical risk. *Circulation* **79** (Suppl. I): I-97–I-101.

74. Magovern GJ, Sakert T, Simpson K *et al.* (1989) Surgical therapy for left ventricular aneurysms: a ten-year experience. *Circulation* **79** (Suppl. I): I-102–I-107.

75. Hill JD, Stiles QR (1989) Acute ischemic ventricular septal defect. *Circulation* **79** (Suppl. I): I-112–I-115.

76. Seltzer A (1987) Changing aspects of the natural history of valvular aortic stenosis. *N Engl J Med* **317**: 91–98.

77. Taylor KM (1991) Heart valve surgery in the United Kingdom: present practice and future trends. *Br Heart J* **66**: 335–336.

78. Jamieson WRE, Burr LH, Munro AI *et al.* (1989) Cardiac valve replacement in the elderly: clinical performance of biological prostheses. *Ann Thorac Surg* **48**: 173–185.

79. King MR, Pluth JR, Giuliani ER, Piehler JM (1986) Mechanical decalcification of the aortic valve. *Ann Thorac Surg* **42**: 269–272.

80. Cribier A, Savin T, Berland J *et al.* (1987) Percutaneous transluminal balloon valvuloplasty of adult aortic stenosis: report of 92 cases. *J Am Coll Cardiol* **9**: 381–386.

81. Safian RD, Berman AD, Diver DJ *et al.* (1988) Balloon aortic valvuloplasty in 170 consecutive patients. *N Engl J Med* **319**: 125–130.

82. Commeau P, Grollier G, Lamy *et al.* (1988) Percutaneous balloon dilatation of calcific aortic valve stenosis: anatomical and haemodynamic evaluation. *Br Heart J* **59**: 227–238.

83. Sprigings DC, Jackson G, Chambers JB *et al.* (1988) Balloon dilatation of the aortic valve for inoperable aortic stenosis. *Br Med J* **297**: 1007–1011.

84. Kuntz RE, Tosteson, AN, Berman AD (1991) Predictors of event-free survival after balloon aortic valvuloplasty. *N Engl J Med* **325**: 17–23.

85. Casale PN, Stewart WJ, Whitlow PL (1991) Percutaneous balloon valvotomy for patients with mitral stenosis: initial and follow-up results. *Am Heart J* **121**: 476–479.

86. Taggart DP, Wheatley DJ (1990) Mitral valve surgery: to repair or replace? *Br Heart J* **64**: 234–235.

87. Spencer FC, Colvin SB, Culliford AT, Isom OW (1985) Experiences with the Carpentier techniques of mitral valve reconstruction in 103 patients. *J Thorac Cardiovasc Surg* **90**: 341–350.

88. Cosgrove DM, Chavez AM, Lytle BW *et al.* (1986) Results of mitral valve reconstruction. *Circulation* **74** (Suppl. I): I-82–I-87.

89. Fremes SE, Goldman BS, Ivanov J *et al.* and the Cardiovascular Surgeons at the University of Toronto (1989) Valvular surgery in the elderly. *Circulation* **80** (Suppl. I): I-77–I-90.

90. Fiore AC, Naunheim KS, Barner HB *et al.* (1989) Valve replacement in the octogenarian. *Ann Thorac Surg* **48**: 104–108.

91. Galloway AC, Colvin SB, Grossie *et al.* (1990) Ten-year experience with aortic valve replacement in 482 patients 70 years of age or older: operative risk and long-term results. *Ann Thorac Surg* **49**: 84–93.

92. McGrath LB, Adkins MS, Chen C *et al.* (1991) Actuarial survival and other events

following valve surgery in octogenarians: comparison with an age-, sex-, and race-matched population. *Eur J Cardiothorac Surg* **5**: 319–325.

93. Antunes MJ (1989) Valve replacement in the elderly: is the mechanical valve a good alternative? *J Thorac Cardiovasc Surg* **98**: 485–491.
94. Borkon AM, Soule LM, Baughman KL *et al.* (1988) Aortic valve selection in the elderly patient. *Ann Thorac Surg* **46**: 270–277.
95. Blakeman BM, Pifarre R, Sullivan HJ *et al.* (1987) Aortic valve replacement in patients 75 years and older. *Ann Thorac Surg* **44**: 637–639.
96. Christakis GT, Weisel RD, David TE *et al.* and the Cardiovascular Surgeons at the University of Toronto (1988) Predictors of operative survival after valve replacement. *Circulation* **78** (Suppl. I): I-25–I-34.
97. Jameison WR, Dooner J, Munro AI *et al.* (1981) Cardiac valve replacement in the elderly: a review of 320 consecutive cases. *Circulation* **64**: (Suppl. II): II-177–I-183.
98. Berndt TB, Hancock EW, Shumway NE, Harrison DC (1974) Aortic valve replacement with and without coronary artery bypass surgery. *Circulation* **50**: 967–971.
99. Rossiter SJ, Hultgren HN, Kosec JC *et al.* (1974) Ischemic myocardial injury with aortic valve replacement and coronary bypass. *Arch Surg* **109**: 652–657.
100. Miller DC, Stinson EB, Rossiter SJ *et al.* (1978) Impact of simultaneous myocardial revascularization on operative risk, functional result and survival following mitral valve replacement. *Surgery* **84**: 848–856.
101. Bonow RO, Kent KM, Rosing DR *et al.* (1981) Aortic valve replacement without myocardial revascularization in patients with combined aortic valvular and coronary artery disease. *Circulation* **63**: 243–251.
102. Lytle BW (1988) Combined surgery for valve and coronary artery disease. *Cleve Clin J Med* **55**: 79–87.
103. Hochberg MS, Morrow AG, Michaelis LL *et al.* (1977) Aortic valve replacement in the elderly: encouraging postoperative clinical and hemodynamic results. *Arch Surg* **112**: 1475–1480.
104. Arom KV, Nicoloff DM, Lindsay WG *et al.* (1984) Should valve replacement and related procedures be performed in elderly patients? *Ann Thorac Surg* **38**: 466–472.
105. Azariades M, Fessler CL, Ahmad A, Starr A (1991) Aortic valve replacement in patients over 80 years of age: a comparative standard for balloon valvuloplasty. *Eur J Cardiothorac Surg* **5**: 373–377.
106. Lytle BW, Cosgrove DM, Taylor PC *et al.* (1989) Primary isolated aortic valve replacement: early and late results. *J Thorac Cardiovasc Surg* **97**: 675–694.
107. Deleuze Ph, Loisance DY, Besnainou F *et al.* (1990) Severe aortic stenosis in octogenarians: is operation an acceptable alternative? *Ann Thorac Surg* **50**: 226–229.
108. Levinson JR, Akins CW, Buckley MJ *et al.* (1989) Octogenarians with aortic stenosis: outcome after aortic valve replacement. *Circulation* **80** (Suppl. I): I-49–I-56.
109. Crawford ES, Svensson LG, Coselli JS *et al.* (1989) Surgical treatment of aneurysm and/or dissection of the ascending aorta, transverse aortic arch, and ascending aorta and transverse aortic arch: factors influencing survival in 717 patients. *J Thorac Cardiovasc Surg* **98**: 659–674.
110. St John Sutton MG, Tajik AJ, McGoon DC (1981) Atrial septal defect in patients aged 60 years or older: operative results and long-term postoperative follow-up. *Circulation* **64**: 402–409.

29 Cardiac Pacing: General Overview and Specific Considerations for Pacing in the Elderly

DAVID L. HAYES

Mayo Clinic and Mayo Foundation, and Mayo Medical School, Rochester, Minnesota, USA

Although permanent pacemakers are implanted in patients of all ages, cardiac pacing is often thought of strictly in terms of the elderly. In the 1989 Survey of Cardiac Pacing Practices in the United States (1), the age for primary or initial permanent pacemaker implantation was 61–80 years for 69% of pacemakers implanted and greater than 80 years for 17% of pacemakers implanted. Given these figures, it is understandable why cardiac pacing is an important aspect of cardiac disease in the elderly.

There is some physiological explanation for the higher incidence of symptomatic bradyarrhythmias in the elderly (2). The number of pacemaker cells in the sinoatrial node has been shown to decrease with age. After age 75, the total number of pacemaker cells may be less than 10% of the normal number. In addition, there may be a significant decrease in fibres from the fascicles of the left bundle branch beginning at age 60 and some replacement of distal conduction system fibres with fibrous tissue. (3).

EVOLUTION OF CARDIAC PACING

The first cardiac pacemaker was implanted in Sweden in 1958 (4). In the ensuing three decades, remarkable progress occurred (5). The first decade of cardiac pacing saw the development of mercury–zinc oxide batteries as a power source, the first transvenous pacing system, and rapid improvement in pacemaker lead technology. Between 1968 and 1977, improvements included development and institution of inhibited, or demand-mode, pacing; improved reliability by hermetic sealing of the pulse generator; significant reduction in size of the pulse generator through the use of hybrid technology; inclusion of defibrillation protection in the pacemaker to prevent pacemaker damage from power surges such as defibrillation; and inclusion of circuitry to prevent rapid, life-threatening

Geriatric Cardiology. Principles and Practice. Edited by A. Martin and A. J. Camm
© 1994 John Wiley & Sons Ltd

pacing rates. Pacemaker longevity also was increased significantly with the introduction of lithium battery technology. During the third decade of cardiac pacing, programmability and telemetric functions were made possible by microprocessor-based circuitry without serious compromise of size or battery longevity. Advances in lead technology and transvenous implantation technique also evolved rapidly. DDD pacing was introduced early in the decade, and during the latter portion of the decade single-chamber rate-adaptive pacing was introduced. Dual-chamber rate-adaptive pacing followed in the first years of the fourth decade of cardiac pacing.

PACEMAKER NOMENCLATURE

A universal code representing various pacing systems has been developed, and understanding this code is essential to any discussion of permanent pacemakers. A three-letter code describing the basic function of the pacing systems was first proposed in 1974 by a combined task force from the American Heart Association and the American College of Cardiology. Since that time, responsibility for periodically updating the code has been assumed by a committee consisting of members of the North American Society of Pacing and Electrophysiology Group (NASPE) and the British Pacing and Electrophysiology Group (BPEG) (6). The code now has five positions, but the first three are the most frequently used (Table 1).

The first position reflects the chamber or chambers in which stimulation

Table 1. The NASPE/BPEG[a] Generic (NBG) Pacemaker Code

I	II	III	IV
Chamber(s) paced	Chamber(s) sensed	Response to sensing	Programmability, rate modulation
O = None	O = None	O = None	O = None
A = Atrium	A = Atrium	T = Triggered	P = Simple programmable
V = Ventricle	V = Ventricle	I = Inhibited	M = Multiprogrammable
D = Dual	D = Dual	D = Dual	C = Communicating
(A + V)	(A + V)	(T + I)	R = Rate modulation

Modified from Bernstein *et al.* (6).
A, atrial application, e.g. an A in the first position denotes the capability of atrial pacing; V, ventricular application, e.g. a V in the second position denotes the capability to sense events arising in the ventricle; D, atrial and ventricular, or 'dual', application, e.g. a D in the first position denotes pacing capability in both chambers; O, absence of a particular function, e.g. in the DOO mode the pacemaker is capable of pacing in both chambers but incapable of sensing any events or responding to any sensed events; I, inhibition of the pacemaker by an intrinsic cardiac event, e.g. in a VVI pacemaker only ventricular activity is sensed and any sensed ventricular event will inhibit pacemaker output; T, triggering of a pacemaker output will occur when an intrinsic cardiac event occurs, e.g. in the AAT mode of pacing only atrial activity is sensed and any sensed atrial event will result in a pacemaker output; P, simple programmability or capability of only one or two programmable features, most commonly rate or output programming only; M, capability of programmability for more than two programmable functions; C, telemetric capability; R, rate-adaptive capability of the pacemaker, which is determined by measurement of some variable other than the sinus rate, e.g. mechanical vibration or respiration.
[a]North American Society of Pacing and Electrophysiology and British Pacing and Electrophysiology group.

occurs. 'A' refers to the atrium, 'V' indicates the ventricle, and 'D' means dual-chamber, or both atrium and ventricle. There can also be an 'O' in the first position when the device is capable of antitachycardia pacing or defibrillation but has no bradycardia support function.

The second position refers to the chamber or chambers in which sensing occurs. The letters are the same as those for the first position. Manufacturers are also allowed to use 'S' in both the first and the second positions to indicate that the device is capable of pacing by a single cardiac chamber. Once the device is implanted and connected to a lead in either the atrium or the ventricle, 'S' should be changed to either an 'A' or a 'V' in the clinical record to reflect the chamber in which pacing and sensing are occurring.

The third position refers to the mode of sensing, or how the pacemaker responds to a sensed event. 'I' means that a sensed event inhibits the output pulse and causes the pacemaker to recycle for one or more timing cycles. 'T' means that an output pulse is triggered in response to a sensed event. 'D', in a manner similar to that in the first two positions, means that there are dual modes of response. This designation is restricted to dual-chamber systems. An event sensed in the atrium inhibits the atrial output but triggers a ventricular output. Unlike the single-chamber triggered mode, in which an output pulse is triggered immediately on sensing, the dual mode features a delay between the sensed atrial event and the triggered ventricular output to mimic the normal P–R interval. If a native ventricular signal or R wave is sensed, it will inhibit the ventricular output and possibly even the atrial output, depending on where sensing occurs.

The fourth position of the code reflects both programmability and rate modulation. 'O' indicates that none of the settings of the pacing system can be non-invasively altered. 'P' is simple programmability; one or two variables can be changed, but this code does not specify which ones. 'M' is multiparameter programmability, which means that three or more variables can be changed. 'C' reflects the ability of the pacemaker to communicate with the programmer; namely, it has telemetry. By convention, it also means that the pacemaker has multiparameter programmability. An 'R' in the fourth position indicates that the pacemaker has a special sensor to control the rate independently of endogenous electrical activity of the heart. Virtually all pacemakers with a sensor also have extensive telemetric and programmable capabilities. The type of sensor being utilized is not indicated in the code.

The fifth position is restricted to antitachycardia capabilities but does not specify the regimen or stimulation sequence. Antitachycardia pacing, used relatively infrequently in the elderly population, will not be discussed in this chapter.

INDICATIONS FOR PERMANENT PACING

The indications for permanent pacing vary considerably among countries. In some areas of the world, limited resources allow pacing only in patients with lethal bradycardias. Generally agreed upon guidelines for permanent pacing

Table 2. Indications for permanent pacemaker[a]

Acquired atrioventricular (AV) block (AVB)

I.
1. Complete heart block (CHB), permanent or intermittent associated with any symptomatic bradycardia, congestive heart failure, asystolic pauses > 3 s, or rates < 40 beats/min
2. Second-degree AVB with symptomatic bradycardia
3. Atrial fibrillation with AVB and symptomatic bradycardia

II.
1. Asymptomatic CHB
2. Asymptomatic Mobitz II second-degree AVB
3. Asymptomatic Mobitz I second-degree AVB at intra-His or infra-His level

III.
1. First-degree AVB
2. Asymptomatic Mobitz I second-degree AVB at the supra-His (AV nodal) level

AVB after myocardial infarction

I.
1. Persistent high-grade AVB with block in the His–Purkinje system
2. Transient high-grade AVB and associated bundle branch block

II.
1. Persistent first-degree AVB and new bundle branch block
2. Persistent high-grade AVB at AV nodal level

III.
1. Transient AV condition disturbances without intraventricular conduction defects
2. Transient AVB with isolated left anterior hemiblock
3. New left anterior hemiblock without AVB

Bifascicular (BiB) and trifascicular block (TriB)

I.
1. BiB with intermittent CHB with symptomatic bradycardia
2. BiB or TriB with intermittent Mobitz II second-degree AVB

II.
1. BiB or TriB with syncope and no other identifiable cause
2. Pacing-induced infra-His block
3. Markedly prolonged HV interval

III.
1. Fascicular block without AVB or symptoms
2. Fascicular block and first-degree AVB without symptoms

Table 2. (*continued*)

Sinus node dysfunction (SND)

I
1. SND with symptomatic bradycardia

II.
1. SND with heart rates <40 beats/min even if clear correlation between symptoms and bradycardia is not documented
2. Syncope with associated bradycardia induced by tilt-table testing (syncope prevented with temporary pacing on second attempt)

III.
1. SND in asymptomatic patients
2. SND when symptoms are clearly not associated with bradycardia

Carotid sinus hypersensitivity

I.
1. Recurrent syncope with clear, spontaneous events provocable by carotid sinus massage

II.
1. Recurrent syncope without clear provocative events but with asystole >3 s with carotid sinus massage

III.
1. Abnormal response to carotid sinus massage in absence of symptoms
2. Abnormal response to carotid sinus massage in patient with vague symptoms, e.g. dizziness

---

Data from ACC/AHA Task Force (8).
[a] I, conditions for which there is general agreement that pacemaker is indicated; II, conditions for which pacemaker is generally used but some controversy exists; III, conditions for which there is general agreement that pacemaker is not indicated.

exist among the USA, Europe and the Pacific rim nations. Because of changes in diagnosis and therapy as well as continued technological developments, some degree of constant change affects absolute indications for permanent pacing. A joint committee of the American College of Cardiology and the American Heart Association has developed guidelines for permanent pacemaker implantation. The original guidelines, published in 1984 (7), were updated in 1991 (8). These guidelines are summarized in Table 2.

SPECIAL CONSIDERATIONS FOR PACING IN THE ELDERLY

Pacemaker selection criteria should be applicable to all patients regardless of age (9). Previous studies have shown that even in the very elderly, a permanent pacemaker, when indicated, significantly prolongs life and improves quality of life with minimal associated morbidity and mortality (2,10,11). In an excellent editorial, Spielman and Segal (12) stressed that before a pacemaker is implanted in an elderly patient, three factors should be given specific attention. First, they cautioned that cerebral symptoms, such as dizziness, syncope and seizures, should be fully evaluated before it is assumed that the cause is bradycardia. Second, a pacemaker is generally not indicated for a patient with chronic bifascicular block who does not have cerebral symptoms. Third, sinus bradycardia, which is not uncommon in the elderly patient, should not require permanent pacing unless the patient has cerebral symptoms that can be correlated with the bradycardia.

This final point is controversial with current state-of-the-art rate-adaptive pacemakers. It is not uncommon to see elderly patients with vague cerebral symptoms, such as dizziness, fatigue and demonstrable chronotropic incompetence. A rate-adaptive pacemaker could correct the chronotropic incompetence and, potentially, the patient's vague symptoms. However, some implanters do not agree that chronotropic incompetence alone is a justifiable reason for permanent pacing. Such symptoms unarguably deserve a cardiac evaluation and ambulatory or transtelephonic monitoring, if necessary, to correlate the patient's cardiac rhythm with the symptoms. In a study by Martin et al. (13), a significant number of symptomatic bradyarrhythmias in the elderly were diagnosed when long-term ambulatory monitoring was made more available to the clinician.

Other specific issues have been raised about pacing in the elderly, including cost and associated irreversible debilitating or life-threatening illnesses. In the otherwise healthy, active elderly patient, we have avoided using cost as a factor in choosing the best pacemaker for the patient; for example, if the patient appears to be best served by a dual-chamber pacemaker, a dual-chamber pacemaker rather than a less costly single-chamber pacemaker is implanted. This philosophy has also been voiced by others (9,14). Rising medical costs may soon alter this approach, but at present we are not restricted from using the best pacemaker for the patient as long as the need can be documented clinically.

A more difficult decision arises if the patient has associated irreversible debilitating or life-threatening illnesses other than the conduction system disease. In such circumstances, one could argue that it may be in the patient's best interest not to pace. If it is determined that pacing is warranted despite the associated problems, it is reasonable to use a simple VVI system. A VVI pacing system should prevent symptomatic bradycardias while limiting costs. (If the patient will be pacemaker-dependent and ventricular pacing provokes symptoms—see 'pacemaker syndrome' below—consideration should be given to an alternative pacing mode.)

SELECTION OF THE APPROPRIATE PACING MODE

Once it is established that the elderly patient has a conduction disorder that warrants permanent pacing, one must determine which pacemaker to prescribe. The patient's overall physical condition, associated medical problems, exercise

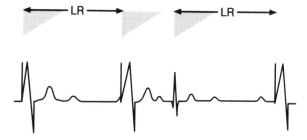

Figure 1. The VVI timing cycle consists of a defined lower rate limit (LR) and a ventricular refractory period (VRP), represented by the triangle. When the LR timer is complete, a pacing artefact is delivered in the absence of a sensed intrinsic ventricular event. If an intrinsic QRS occurs, the LR timer is started from that point. A VRP begins with any sensed or paced ventricular activity. From Hayes and Levine (110), by permission of Blackwell Scientific Publications Inc.

capacity, and chronotropic response to exercise must be considered along with the underlying rhythm disturbance.

VVI pacing remains the most commonly used pacing mode (Figure 1). Although VVI pacing protects the patient from lethal bradycardias, this mode has significant limitations. Pacemaker syndrome with VVI pacing is well documented.

The earliest indication for cardiac pacing was high-grade or complete heart block with recurrent Stokes–Adams attacks. In patients with this disorder, establishing a stable ventricular rhythm was life-saving and prevented catastrophic asystole. This fact alone overshadowed the observation that although ventricular pacing improved cardiac output or symptoms (or both), it did not re-establish normal function. In addition, some patients with intermittent heart block experienced symptomatic haemodynamic deterioration with ventricular pacing (Figure 2).

Adverse haemodynamics associated with a normally functioning pacing system resulting in overt symptoms or limiting the patient's ability to achieve optimal functional status is referred to as 'pacemaker syndrome' (15,16). Pacemaker syndrome is the result of ventriculoatrial (VA) conduction or contraction of the atria against a closed atrioventricular (AV) valve that occurs when AV synchrony is lost. VA conduction may result in AV valve insufficiency and abnormal venous pulsations that may produce symptoms. VA conduction can result in activation of stretch mechanoreceptors in the walls of the atria and pulmonary veins. Vagal afferents transmit these impulses centrally, and the result is reflex peripheral vasodilation, which may cause dizziness, near-syncope or syncope. Pacemaker syndrome may therefore be manifested by a variety of symptoms, including weakness, near-syncope, syncope, fatigue, lassitude, cough, chest pain, hypotension, congestive heart failure, shortness of breath, apprehension, jugular venous pulsations and abdominal pulsations. Physical findings in pacemaker syndrome may include cannon A waves, decrease in blood pressure during ventricular pacing from that during normal sinus rhythm, and cyclic

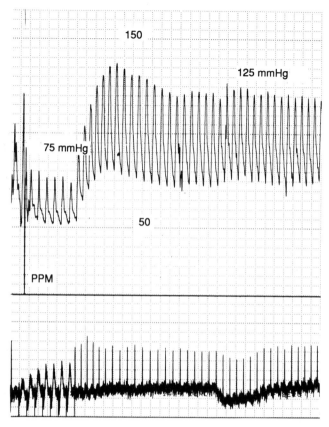

Figure 2. Simultaneous electrocardiogram (bottom) and arterial pressure tracing (top). During the initial portion of the tracing, ventricular pacing is accompanied by a significantly lower arterial pressure than that with normal sinus rhythm in the latter portion of the tracing

variation in cardiac output, arterial pressure and peripheral vascular resistance during haemodynamic monitoring. Pacemaker syndrome was initially recognized with ventricular (VVI) pacing. However, pacemaker syndrome may occur any time there is AV dissociation. It has also been described with AAI and DDI pacing modes (17,18).

The incidence of pacemaker syndrome is difficult to determine and depends on how one defines pacemaker syndrome. If the definition is limited to clinical limitations in patients, during any pacing mode that results in AV dissociation, the incidence is probably in the range of 7–10% of patients with VVI pacing, as estimated in a review by Ausubel and Furman (16). However, in a recent study by Heldman *et al.* (19), patients with DDD pacemakers were randomized to DDD or VVI pacing mode for 1 week, subsequently had their devices programmed to the alternative mode, and were asked to complete questionnaires comparing 16

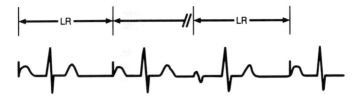

Figure 3. The AAI timing cycle consists of a defined lower rate limit (LR) and an atrial refractory period (ARP). When the LR timer is complete, a pacing artefact is delivered in the atrium in the absence of a sensed atrial event. If an intrinsic P wave occurs, the LR timer is started from that point. An ARP begins with any sensed or paced atrial activity. From Hayes and Levine (110), by permission of Blackwell Scientific Publications Inc.

different symptoms during each pacing mode. With this approach, pacemaker syndrome was thought to be present in 83% of the patients studied. The most common symptoms reported were shortness of breath, dizziness, fatigue, pulsations in the neck or abdomen, cough and apprehension. The authors concluded that if patients with VVI pacing have some basis for comparison, they may be more aware of symptoms with VVI pacing. Although these symptoms may be severe at times, as in the 7%–10% of patients described by Ausubel and Furman, some awareness of symptoms can be elicited in a much higher proportion of patients if symptoms are carefully sought.

AAI pacing is appropriate for patients with sinus node dysfunction but is infrequently used in most countries (Figure 3). The obvious disadvantage of atrial pacing is lack of ventricular support should AV block occur. If the patient with sinus node dysfunction is assessed carefully for AV node disease at the time of pacemaker implantation, the occurrence of clinically significant AV nodal disease is 2–3% a year (20,21). This assessment should include incremental atrial pacing at the time of pacemaker implantation. The patient should be capable of 1:1 conduction through the AV node to rates of 120–140 beats/min (the criteria vary among implanters and institutions) (20).

DVI pacemakers, at one time implanted in large numbers, performed adequately in many patients (Figure 4). However, DVI pacing is limited by the lack of atrial sensing, which prevents the restoration of rate responsiveness in the chronotropically competent patient. In addition, lack of atrial sensing may lead to competitive atrial pacing and initiation of atrial rhythm disturbances. For these reasons, DVI pacing is rarely used as the mode of choice at the time of implantation. It is a programmable option in most DDD pacemakers and may be used in the patient with a DDD pacemaker and in whom atrial failure to sense develops.

The competitive atrial pacing with DVI pacing can be avoided by use of the DDI pacing mode. In this pacing mode, atrial sensing and pacing are present but the pacemaker is incapable of tracking intrinsic atrial activity. Therefore, only a single rate is programmed, and the paced ventricular rate never exceeds the programmed rate (Figure 5). This mode may be advantageous in the patient with

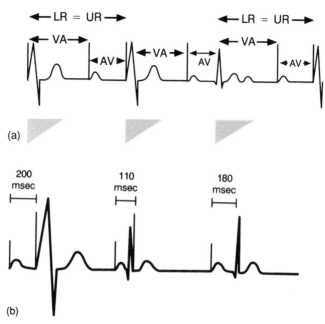

Figure 4. DVI. (a) In the non-committed version of DVI pacing, components of the timing cycle include a lower rate limit (LR), an atrioventricular (AV) interval, and a ventricular refractory period (VRP). The VRP is initiated with any sensed or paced ventricular activity. If ventricular activity is sensed after the atrial pacing artefact, ventricular output will be inhibited, i.e. the ventricular pacing artefact is not committed to the previous atrial pacing artefact. UR, upper rate limit; VA, ventriculoatrial; VV, ventricular event to ventricular event. Triangles represent the postventricular atrial refractory period. (b) In modified or partially committed DVI, ventricular events sensed within the non-physiological AV interval do not inhibit ventricular output, and a ventricular pacing stimulus will occur at the end of the interval. Ventricular events occurring within the physiological AV interval inhibit pacemaker function. In this example, the first paced atrial and ventricular events represent normal DVI pacing. The second paced atrial and intrinsic ventricular complex demonstrates a spontaneous ventricular event occurring within the non-physiological AV interval, resulting in a ventricular pacing stimulus. In the third event shown, after an atrial paced event, a spontaneous ventricular event falls within the physiological AV interval, resulting in inhibition of ventricular pacing function. From Hayes and Levine (110), by permission of Blackwell Scientific Publications Inc.

paroxysmal supraventricular tachycardias that could result in rapid ventricular pacing if the device were programmed to the DDD mode.

'Stand-alone' VDD pacemakers had largely been supplanted by DDD pacemakers (Figure 6). Most DDD pacemakers can be programmed to the VDD mode. If the patient's sinus node function is normal, a DDD pacemaker in effect

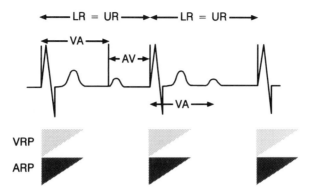

Figure 5. The DDI timing cycle consists of a lower rate limit (LR), an atrioventricular (AV) interval, a ventricular refractory period (VRP) and an atrial refractory period (ARP). The VRP is initiated by any sensed or paced ventricular activity, and the ARP is initiated by any sensed or paced atrial activity. DDI can be conceptualized as DDD pacing without the capability of P wave tracking or DVI without the potential for atrial competition by virtue of atrial sensing. The LR cannot be violated even if the sinus rate is occurring at a faster rate. For example, the LR is 1000 ms, 60 ppm, and the AV interval 200 ms. If a P wave occurs 500 ms after a paced ventricular complex, the AV interval is initiated, but at the end of the AV interval, 700 ms from the previous paced ventricular activity, a ventricular pacing artefact cannot be delivered because it would violate the LR. UR, upper rate limit; VA, ventriculoatrial. From Hayes and Levine (110), by permission of Blackwell Scientific Publications Inc.

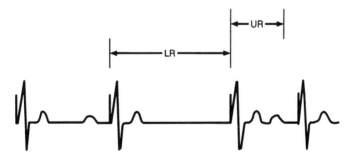

Figure 6. The VDD timing cycle consists of a lower rate limit (LR), atrioventricular (AV) interval, ventricular refractory period, postventricular atrial refractory period (PVARP) and an upper rate limit (UR). A sensed P wave initiates the AV interval (during this interval, the atrial sensing channel is refractory). At the termination of the AV interval, a ventricular pacing artefact is delivered if no intrinsic ventricular activity has been sensed, i.e. P wave tracking. Ventricular activity, paced or sensed, initiates the PVARP and the ventriculoatrial interval (the LR interval minus the AV interval). If no P wave activity occurs, the pacemaker will escape with a ventricular pacing artefact at the LR. From Hayes and Levine (110), by permission of Blackwell Scientific Publications Inc.

operates as a P-synchronous device. More recently, however, several manufacturers have introduced a single-lead pacing system capable of VDD pacing, and this may increase the use of 'stand-alone' VDD pacemakers.

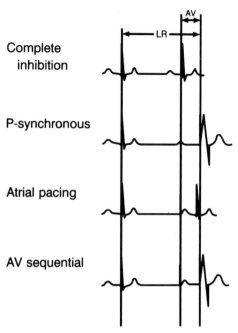

Figure 7. The DDD timing cycle consists of a lower rate limit (LR), atrioventricular (AV) interval, ventricular refractory period, postventricular atrial refractory period and upper rate limit. There are four variations of the DDD timing cycle. If intrinsic atrial activity and ventricular activity occur before the LR times out, both channels will be inhibited and no pacing occurs (top panel). If a P wave is sensed before the ventriculoatrial (VA) interval is completed (the LR minus the AV interval), output from the atrial channel will be inhibited. The AV interval is initiated, and if no ventricular activity is sensed before the AV interval terminates, a ventricular pacing artefact is delivered, i.e. P-synchronous pacing (middle top panel). If no atrial activity is sensed before the VA interval is completed, an atrial pacing artefact is delivered, which initiates the AV interval. If intrinsic ventricular activity occurs before the termination of the AV interval, ventricular output from the pacemaker is inhibited, i.e. atrial pacing (middle bottom panel). If no intrinsic ventricular activity occurs before the termination of the AV interval, a ventricular pacing artefact is delivered, i.e. AV-sequential pacing (bottom panel). From Hayes and Levine (110), by permission of Blackwell Scientific Publications Inc.

The DDD pacing system combines ventricular, atrial, AV sequential and atrial synchronous functions (Figure 7). As the letter code implies, pacing and sensing occur in both atrium and ventricle. The atrium is stimulated if sinus bradycardia exists. Both atrium and ventricle are stimulated if bradycardia exists independently in both chambers. If heart block exists with normal sinus function, the ventricle is paced in synchrony with the atrium, and if sinus rhythm exists, the pacemaker is totally inhibited. Therefore, four different rhythms can be seen as a result of normal pacemaker function: (i) normal sinus rhythm; (ii) atrial pacing; (iii) AV sequential pacing; and (iv) P-synchronous pacing.

Upper and lower rate limits must be set for atrial tracking or P-synchronous pacing. If the atrial rate falls below the lower rate limit, AV sequential pacing

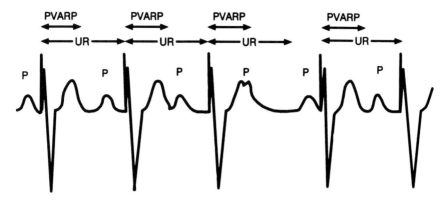

Figure 8. In the DDD pacing mode, the programmed upper rate limit (UR) cannot be violated regardless of the sinus rate. Several mechanisms exist to limit the UR, the most commonly used being pseudo-Wenckebach block. When a P wave is sensed after the postventricular atrial refractory period (PVARP), the atrioventricular (AV) interval is initiated. If, however, delivering a ventricular spacing artefact at the end of the AV interval would violate the UR, the ventricular pacing artefact cannot be delivered. The pacemaker would wait until completion of the UR and then deliver the ventricular pacing artefact. This action would result in a prolonged AV interval, or pseudo-Wenckebach effect. From Hayes and Levine (110), by permission of Blackwell Scientific Publications Inc.

occurs. If the atrial rate exceeds the upper limit, some form of pacemaker-induced heart block occurs. This pacemaker-induced heart block is most commonly a pseudo-Wenckebach type of block, although other upper rate behaviour occurs in some pacemakers (Figure 8).

The DDD pacing mode is most successful for patients with normal sinus node function and AV block. DDD pacing is considered by some to be the mode of choice in carotid sinus hypersensitivity with symptomatic cardioinhibition.

DDD pacing is not the 'universal' pacing mode it was first purported to represent. It was apparent from the outset that DDD, or P-synchronous, pacing had definite limitations in some patients. P-synchronous pacing is not possible in patients with chronic atrial fibrillation or a paralysed or non-excitable atrium. A limitation not well appreciated until more recently is chronotropic incompetence—inability to appropriately increase the atrial rate with exercise. Patients in sinus rhythm but chronotropically incompetent do not realize the full benefit of P-synchronous pacing.

The first single-chamber rate-adaptive pacemaker was made commercially available in the USA in 1986 (22,23), and the first dual-chamber device was commercially released in 1989. At this time, three types of sensors—activity, minute volume and temperature—are commercially available in the USA (24–27). Additional sensors are available in Europe, including a QT interval sensor, which has been used in large numbers (28,29). Multiple physiological sensors are undergoing evaluation (30–34) (Table 3). Pacemakers that incorporate dual sensors are also in evaluation (35).

Table 3. Rate-adaptive sensors: market-released or undergoing clinical investigation

---

Activity (motion-sensing)
Minute volume
Temperature
Q–T (evoked response)
Pre-ejection interval and stroke volume
Paced depolarization interval
dP/dt
O_2 saturation
Respiratory rate

INDICATIONS FOR RATE-ADAPTIVE PACEMAKERS

Current indications for rate-adaptive pacemakers are listed in Table 2 (36). VVIR pacing, like VVI, is contraindicated if ventricular pacing results in retrograde (VA) conduction or a decrease in blood pressure (see 'pacemaker syndrome', above). VVIR pacing should not be used as an excuse to forgo attempts at placing an atrial lead in a patient who is undergoing pacemaker implantation, has normal sinus node function, and would benefit from rate-adaptive pacing. If the sinus node is intact, P-synchronous pacing should still be considered the optimal rate-adaptive variable and be used when possible.

AAIR pacing could be considered in the patient with sinus node dysfunction and normal AV node function, because this mode restores rate responsiveness and maintains AV synchrony. If AAIR pacing is contemplated, normal AV node conduction must first be determined, as previously discussed for AAI pacing.

The ideal patient for DDDR pacing is one with combined sinus nodal and AV nodal dysfunction in whom DDDR pacing would restore rate responsiveness and AV synchrony (Figure 9). In a patient with paroxysmal atrial rhythm disturbances, programming the pacemaker to the DDIR mode allows rate modulation and AV synchrony but not tracking of any rapid pathological atrial rhythms (DVIR can be used when DDIR is not available, but DVIR is less ideal because atrial competition can occur) (37).

HAEMODYNAMIC INFLUENCE ON MORBIDITY AND MORTALITY

When all factors that influence haemodynamics and long-term improvement with permanent pacing are considered, the ideal pacing system maintains AV synchrony and allows or provides rate responsiveness. Several investigators have compared morbidity and mortality after DDD or AAI pacing with those after VVI pacing (38–43). Most of this information has been collected retrospectively, but some definite conclusions can be drawn. In patients with sinus node

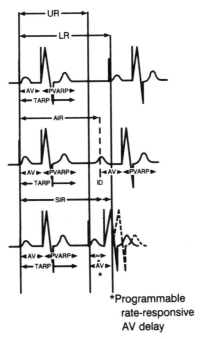

*Programmable
rate-responsive
AV delay

Figure 9. DDDR pacemakers are capable of all pacing variations previously described for DDD pacemakers (Figure 8). When the device is functioning above the programmed lower rate limit (LR), it may increase the heart rate on the basis of the atrial indicted rate (AIR) (middle panel) or the sensor-indicated rate (SIR) (bottom panel). In current DDR pacemakers, the postventricular atrial refractory period (PVARP) remains fixed regardless of cycle length. A programmable feature in one DDDR pacemaker allows the length of the atrioventricular (AV) interval to vary with the SIR, i.e. as the SIR increases, the AV interval shortens. Incorporation of a rate-responsive AV delay, even though the PVARP does not change at faster rates, may result in shortening of the total atrial refractory period (TARP) because of the changing AV interval (bottom panel). ID, intrinsic deflection. From Hayes and Levine (110), by permission of Blackwell Scientific Publications Inc.

dysfunction, incidences of atrial fibrillation and embolic events are significantly higher after VVI pacing than after DDD or AAI pacing. Rosenqvist *et al.* (38) demonstrated that in patients with sinus node dysfunction, survival was significantly better with AAI pacing than with VVI pacing. Alpert *et al.* (39,40) demonstrated that 5-year survival rates for both sinus node dysfunction and AV block in patients with congestive heart failure were improved when paced in a dual-chamber mode. Table 4 summarizes studies comparing morbidity and mortality of VVI pacing with those of DDD or AAI pacing. Although the validity of any retrospective data can be questioned, it is impressive that findings are similar among these studies. In addition, designing a randomized prospective study would be difficult without recruiting a significantly biased study population.

Table 4. Comparison of morbidity and mortality between VVI pacing and DDD or AAI pacing

Ref.	No. of pts	Pacing modality (no. of pts)			Atrial fibrillation (%)				Mortality (%)				Thromboembolic events (%)				Congestive heart failure (%)			
		AAI	DDD	VVI	AAI	DDD	VVI	p_a	AAI	DDD	VVI	p_a	AAI	DDD	VVI	p_a	AAI	DDD	VVI	p_a
(38)	168	89		79	6.7		47	<0.0005	8		23	<0.05	2				15		37	<0.005
(44)	339	135	79	125	4	13	47	<0.001	13	16	30	<0.001		2.5	8	NS				
(45)	110	53		57	3.8		17.5	0.025	9.4		17.5	NS	0		7		1.9		5.3	
(46)	222	110		112	6		19		17		27	b								
(40)	128		49[c]	79						22[d]	26	NS[e]								
										25[f]	43	<0.03[e]								
(42)	49	12	12	25	0	0	36	<0.01		7	15	j	0	0	20	<0.05	4.2[g]		28	NS[h]
(47)	220		110[i]	110		8	18	<0.05										27	26	NS
(41)	90[k]	45[g]		45	8.8[l]		24.4	<0.05[h]	15.4[g]		22.1	NS[h]	0	0	6.6					
(43)	1092[k]		649	443		5.5	9.2	<0.03[m]		15	29	<0.003[m]								
(39)	180[n]		48[o]	132						30[d]	27	NS[e]								
										31[f]	53	<0.02[e]								

[a] For difference between VVI and AAI unless otherwise noted.
[b] Cumulative survival not statistically significant when overall groups compared. For subgroups with coronary disease, survival in AAI > VVI, $p < 0.02$. For subgroups without underlying heart diseases, survival in AAI > VVI, $p < 0.05$.
[c] DDD, 11; DVI, 38.
[d] Without congestive heart failure.
[e] For difference between VVI and DDD + DVI.
[f] With congestive heart failure.
[g] Value is for AAI and DDD together.
[h] For difference between VVI and AAI + DDD.
[i] DDD or DDI.
[j] Not analysed.
[k] Mixed conduction disturbances requiring pacing, not just sinus node dysfunction.
[l] Classified as overall occurrence of atrial arrhythmias, not just atrial fibrillation.
[m] For difference between VVI and DDD.
[n] Patients with atrioventricular block.
[o] DDD, 12; DVI, 36.

IMPLANTATION TECHNIQUE

A detailed explanation of pacemaker implantation technique is not appropriate for a text concentrating on the broad issues of cardiac disease in the elderly. For such a description, the reader is referred to one of several texts that provide this information (48, 49).

Pacemaker implantation technique need not be altered for even the very elderly. If the subclavian puncture technique is used, it must be remembered that altered anatomy in the elderly patient, e.g. marked kyphosis, may alter the usual landmarks for subclavian puncture. If intravenous sedation is routinely used in addition to a local anaesthetic at the time of pacemaker implantation, smaller amounts of intravenous sedatives may be necessary in the very elderly to avoid over-sedation and respiratory depression. When the pacemaker pocket is created, it must be of optimal size, because the elderly asthenic patient may be predisposed to pacemaker erosion if the pocket is too tight. Conversely, too large a pocket may predispose the elderly patient with loose connective tissues to pacemaker migration or 'twiddler's syndrome' (see below).

PROGRAMMABILITY

Programmability refers to the ability to alter a pacemaker setting non-invasively. If a pacemaker is capable of 'simple' programmability, only one or two functions, most commonly rate or output, are programmable. Multiprogrammability refers to two or more programmable parameters (Table 5). Programmability is accomplished via a radiofrequency link between the pacemaker and the designated programmer. Pacemaker programmers contain software that makes them pacemaker-specific. Although there has been enthusiasm in the physician community to develop a 'universal programmer', i.e. a single programmer that would be capable of programming some or all functions of all pacemakers, this goal has not been achieved. In the USA, all pacemakers implanted are capable of some degree of programmability. However, non-programmable pacemakers are commonly used in other countries because they remain less expensive than programmable devices.

Programmability can be of paramount importance in any patient but may be especially helpful in the elderly patient. In the patient with a non-programmable pacemaker, any pacing malfunction, e.g. failure to capture or sensing abnormalities, may require another invasive procedure to restore normal pacing. In the patient with a programmable pacemaker, many pacing problems can be corrected non-invasively, obviating another invasive procedure and its associated morbidity and mortality (50–54).

Programming today's pacemakers can at times be very complex. For the purposes of this chapter, only the most commonly programmed parameters will be considered.

Table 5. Potential programmable options in current pacemakers

Mode
Lower rate limit
Maximum pacing rate[a,b]
Hysteresis
Atrioventricular delay[a]
Adaptive atrioventricular delay[a]
Atrial refractory period
Postventricular atrial refractory period[a]
Ventricular refractory period
Pulse width (atrial or ventricular, or both)
Pulse amplitude (atrial or ventricular, or both)
Sensitivity (atrial or ventricular, or both)
Blanking period[a]
Polarity
Rate adaptation (on or off)[c]
Rate-adaptive sensor variables[d]

[a]Applicable to dual-chamber pacemakers only.
[b]In dual-chamber rate-adaptive pacemakers, the maximum pacing rate may be a single programmable value, or maximum P-tracking rate and maximum sensor-driven rate may be independently programmable.
[c]Rate adaptation may be a function of the programmed mode, e.g. the pacemaker may have DDDR as a programmable option, or rate adaptation may require programming 'on' in conjunction with the desired pacing mode, e.g. programming the mode to DDD and rate adaptation 'on' will deliver DDDR pacing.
[d]Rate-adaptive sensor variables are not listed separately because they vary significantly from sensor to sensor.

Rate

Pacemaker rate is the most commonly programmed feature (55). The major use of programming is to allow a patient to remain in sinus rhythm rather than in paced rhythm when associated symptomatic bradycardia is present only intermittently. Programming the rate to 60 beats/min, or even as low as 40–50 beats/min, might allow the patient's intrinsic rhythm to exist most of the time but still protect the patient from symptomatic bradycardia. Lower pacing rates may also be helpful in the patient with pacemaker syndrome by minimizing ventricular pacing and subsequent VA conduction. Faster pacing rates, i.e. greater than 70 beats/min, are most commonly used in paediatric patients to increase cardiac output for any reason, transiently or permanently, and are occasionally used to prevent other rhythm disturbances (overdrive pacing) (55).

Output

Probably the most important programmable feature is the energy output (pulse width or voltage amplitude, or both). For patients with high pacing thresholds and failure to capture, increasing the output may restore effective pacing (52) (Figure 10). Conversely, reduction of energy output is safe for many patients and

VVI–70PPM; PW.03

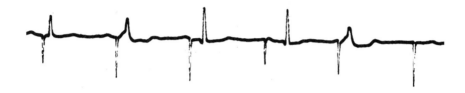

VVI–70PPM; PW.05

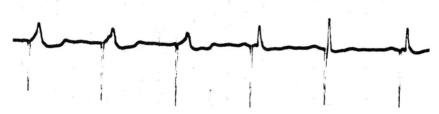

Figure 10. Failure to capture demonstrated during threshold determination in a patient with a VVI pacemaker programmed to a voltage output of 2.5 V and rate of 70 ppm. In the top panel, the pulse width (PW) was reduced to 0.03 ms and intermittent failure to capture is noted at the third, fourth and sixth pacing artefacts. In the bottom panel, the pulse width is reprogrammed to 0.05 ms and there is consistent capture

translates into prolonged longevity of the pulse generator. With good implantation technique and newer low-threshold lead designs, voltage output is commonly programmed to 2.5 V rather than the previously used 5 V. By programming the output at an efficient but safe level, one can theoretically increase the projected battery life by 30–50% (51). A decrease in energy output can be used not only to increase pulse generator longevity but also to eliminate phrenic or diaphragmatic stimulation and to eliminate local pectoral muscle stimulation (56).

Sensitivity

Terminology for sensitivity can be very confusing. When the pacemaker fails to sense intrinsic activity, sensitivity is increased, i.e. the device is made more sensitive. The numerical values are opposite to the terminology. For example, if a VVI pacemaker is programmed to a sensitivity of 2.5 mV (Figure 11) and under-sensing occurs, the problem is corrected by increasing the sensitivity to 1.25 mV. Doing so actually decreases the amplitude of the signal required to trigger the pacemaker. Sensitivity programmability can obviate additional

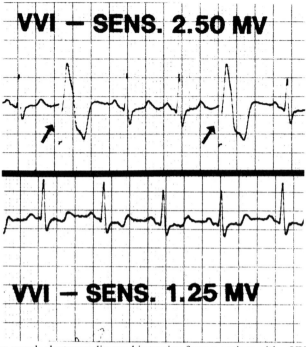

Figure 11. Top panel: electrocardiographic tracing from a patient with a VVI pacemaker programmed to a rate of 70 ppm and sensitivity of 2.5 mV. Inappropriate pacing after the first and third intrinsic QRS complexes demonstrates intermittent failure to sense (arrows). Bottom panel: sensitivity has been increased to 1.25 mV, and sensing is normal. Reproduced from Holmes *et al.* (48) by permission of The Mayo Foundation for Medical Education and Research

operative procedures (50,51,53,54). Under-sensing or failure to sense is the most common abnormality requiring sensitivity programming. Increased sensitivity is also useful when atrial sensing is required, because these signals are usually far smaller than those during ventricular stimulation (57). Decreasing sensitivity is useful in eliminating over-sensing of non-physiological electromagnetic interference signals or such physiological signals as pectoral muscle artifacts (56,58).

Hysteresis

Hysteresis permits prolongation of the first escape interval, i.e. the first interval after an intrinsic beat (Figure 12). For example, the pacemaker programmed at a rate of 60 beats/min, 1000 ms cycle length, and at a hysteresis of 50 beats/min, 1200 ms, will pace at 1200 ms after an intrinsic beat. Unless an intrinsic beat occurs within the following 1000 ms, the pacemaker will continue to pace at 1000 ms intervals, or 60 beats/min. Hysteresis allows maintenance of the patient's intrinsic rhythm as much as possible (59). By minimizing VA conduction, it is especially helpful in the patient with pacemaker syndrome.

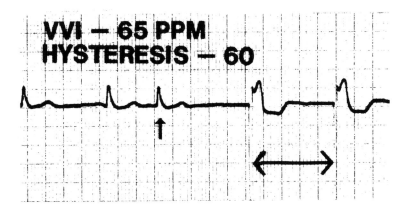

Figure 12. Normal function in a patient with a VVI pacemaker programmed to a rate of 65 ppm and hysteresis at 60 ppm (1000 ms). After the third intrinsic QRS complex (arrow), no paced activity for 1000 ms indicates the hysteresis escape interval. The subsequent pacing interval is 923 ms or 65 ppm—the programmed rate (double-headed arrow)

Refractory period

The refractory period is that portion of the pacemaker's timing cycle after a paced or sensed event during which the pacemaker is insensitive. In a single-chamber pacemaker, refractory period programmability may be helpful in several specific situations. Premature ventricular contractions occurring shortly after a paced ventricular event during VVI pacing are not sensed if they occur during the refractory period. Shortening the refractory period allows sensing of the premature events. Occasionally, the T wave is of sufficient amplitude to be sensed by the pacemaker and therefore to lengthen the paced cycle length by resetting the pacemaker's timing cycle. Lengthening the refractory period of a VVI pacemaker so that the T wave occurs during the refractory period prevents further T wave sensing. During AAI pacing, a refractory period long enough to include the intrinsic QRS complex prevents sensing of the QRS on the atrial sensing circuit and resetting of the pacemaker's timing cycle (Figure 13).

Refractory period operation in dual-chamber pacemakers is much more complex (Figure 14). The refractory period for the ventricular channel behaves as it would for single-chamber pacing. The operation of the atrial channel refractory period is much different. After an event is sensed on the atrial sensing circuit, the atrial sensing amplifier becomes refractory for the duration of the AV interval. When a ventricular event occurs, the atrial sensing amplifier becomes refractory for the programmed postventricular atrial refractory period (PVARP). (The combination of the AV interval and the PVARP is the total atrial refractory period.) The PVARP is critical for the prevention of endless-loop tachycardia (see below).

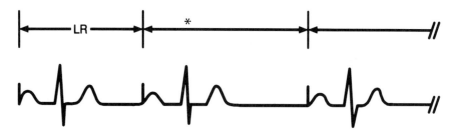

Figure 13. In this example of AAI pacing, the AA interval is 1000 ms (60 ppm). The interval between the second and third paced atrial events is > 1000 ms. The interval from the second QRS complex to the subsequent atrial pacing artefact is 1000 ms. This difference occurs because the second QRS complex (*) has been sensed on the atrial lead (far-field sensing) and has inappropriately reset the timing cycle. LR, lower rate limit. From Hayes and Levine (110), by permission of Blackwell Scientific Publications Inc.

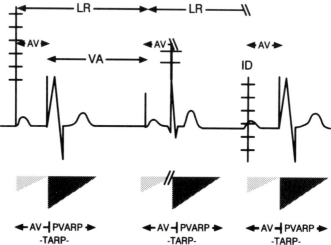

Figure 14. In the DDD pacing mode, the atrial sensing circuit of the pacemaker is refractory throughout the atrioventricular (AV) interval and during the postventricular atrial refractory period (PVARP). The combination of these two intervals represents the total atrial refractory period (TARP). The AV interval begins with either a sensed or a paced atrial event, and the PVARP begins with either a sensed or a paced ventricular event. ID, intrinsic deflection; LR, lower rate limit; VA, ventriculoatrial. From Hayes and Levine (110), by permission of Blackwell Scientific Publications Inc.

Polarity

Programmability of polarity allows the pacemaker to operate in either the unipolar or the bipolar configuration (60,61). (A bipolar lead must be in place to allow bipolar operation.) Polarity programmability may be helpful for the patient whose device is in the unipolar configuration and in whom over-sensing of myopotentials or other electromagnetic signals develops. Reprogramming to the bipolar configuration may prevent further over-sensing of these signals.

Phantom programming

When programming is inadvertent, phantom programming is said to occur. This most commonly takes place when there is human failure to record a programming change or accidental programming of one or more parameters when another change is being made. Pacemakers can occasionally be reprogrammed by external electrical signals, such as those produced by electrocautery (62,63).

PACEMAKER MALFUNCTION

Pacemaker malfunction may be caused by a primary problem with the pacing system (either the pulse generator or the pacing lead or leads) or be secondary to environmental influences. The problem may manifest itself as abnormal pacing or sensing, extracardiac stimulation, or their combination. The few 'true' pacemaker emergencies that can occur with contemporary pacemakers are most likely to affect pacemaker-dependent patients, for whom transient sensing or pacing abnormalities may be catastrophic. The same malfunction may be without consequence in the non-pacemaker-dependent patient. Several series have reviewed the incidence and types of pacemaker problems identified during follow-up (53,64–67) (Table 6). Battery depletion is not considered a malfunction, because it is an expected phenomenon except when it occurs prematurely or in an unpredictable fashion (68). With current lithium-powered pacemakers, the battery life ranges from 4 years to more than 12 years, depending on the current drain, which is determined by the degree of the patient's dependency, thresholds, single- or dual-chamber pacing, and presence of a rate-modulating sensor or other feature that requires additional current drain. Lithium iodine, currently the most commonly used battery, has shown predictable battery depletion, i.e. end-of-life (EOL) characteristics (69). Once initial EOL changes occur, usually a period of months elapses before the battery reaches a critically low voltage and the pacemaker fails.

A clear distinction in terminology must be made between failure to output, i.e. a pacemaker stimulus is not emitted, and failure to capture, i.e. a pacemaker stimulus is ineffective. Failure to output from the pacemaker system can be catastrophic for the pacemaker-dependent patient. Failure to pace can result from rare random component failure and total battery depletion, which is avoidable if routine pacemaker follow-up has been adequate and non-urgent battery replacement is planned when EOL limits are reached. Lead fracture and disconnection of the lead from the pacemaker can also result in failure to pace. Pacemaker lead fracture has become less common as lead technology has improved but must be considered as a possible cause of sudden failure to output. Disconnection of the lead from the pacemaker occurs only when the lead is not adequately secured within the connector block at the time of implantation. Disconnection requires surgical intervention to secure the lead in the connector block of the pacemaker.

Table 6. Type and number of pacemaker problems in recent studies

| Ref. | Year | Pacemaker evaluated | No. of pts | No. of instances | | | |
				Failure to capture	Sensing abnormality	Capture and sensing abnormality	Failure to output
(64)	1986	S & D	2934[a]	67	93	35	3
(53)	1986	S & D	1065	11	35	4	—
(65)	1986	D	345	15	10	—	3[b]
(66)	1987	S & D	100	10	23	—	12
(67)	1990	D	67	6[c]	24	—	—[c]

D, dual-chamber; S, single-chamber.

[a]Total study population, 25919. Malfunctions given specifically for 2934 pacemakers: single-chamber, 2414; dual-chamber, 520.

[b]Described as 'component failure' without further specification.

[c]Data given as 'ventricular pacing' abnormalities and not defined as capture or output.

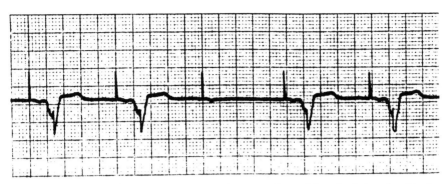

Figure 15. Electrocardiographic recording from a patient with a dual-chamber bipolar pacing system. Of five atrial pacing artefacts, four (the first, second, fourth and fifth) are followed by paced ventricular activity. (Very small pacing artefacts, such as those preceding the ventricular events in this example, are at times a function of a bipolar pacing system and at other times due to the equipment used to record the electrocardiographic signals. This recording was made in a pacemaker-dependent patient who would have had asystole without ventricular pacing.) The absence of paced ventricular activity after the third paced atrial beat occurred because of cross-talk. Cross-talk occurs when activity in one cardiac chamber is sensed by the sensing circuit in the other cardiac chamber. In this example, the ventricular sensing circuit sensed the atrial activity and the ventricular pacing artefact was inhibited

Although not a true malfunction of the pacing system, 'cross-talk', i.e. far-field sensing or, in a dual-chamber pacemaker, sensing in one chamber of a pacemaker stimulus in the other chamber, may cause failure of output (70). If an atrial depolarization is sensed on the ventricular lead, ventricular output may be inhibited (Figure 15). For the pacemaker-dependent patient, inhibition could result in ventricular asystole. Most pacemakers protect against this by incorporating ventricular 'safety pacing', whereby any event sensed on the ventricular sensing circuit within a defined early portion of the AV delay initiates the delivery of a ventricular pacing stimulus (Figure 16). This interval, the time from the atrial sensed event to ventricular safety pacing, is usually in the range of 100–120 ms. If the event sensed by the ventricular sensing circuit is intrinsic ventricular activity, the delivered ventricular pacing stimulus most likely will fall within the intrinsic QRS complex, i.e. a non-vulnerable portion of the cardiac cycle. Conversely, if the event sensed by the ventricular sensing circuit is indeed cross-talk from the atrium, asystole is prevented.

Failure to capture is most commonly due to dislodgement of the pacemaker lead from the endocardial surface and usually occurs in the early postimplantation period. With newer designs of active and passive fixation leads, the incidence of dislodgement has decreased strikingly (71). (Although the absolute acceptable rates for lead dislodgement are difficult to define, they should be less than 2% for ventricular leads and well below 5% for atrial leads (72).)

Failure to capture can also occur when a break in the insulation of the pacemaker catheter allows some of the current from the electrode to escape into

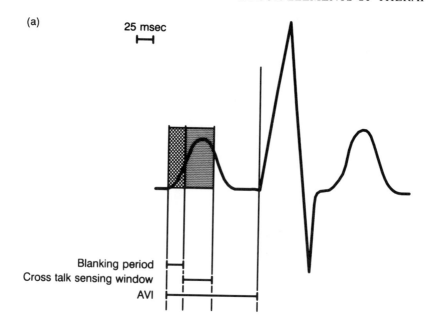

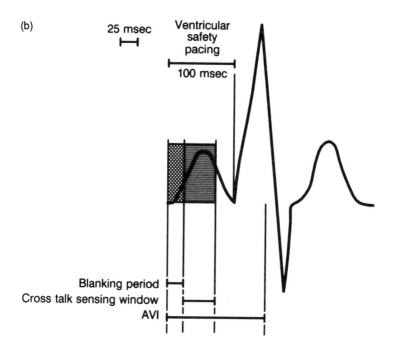

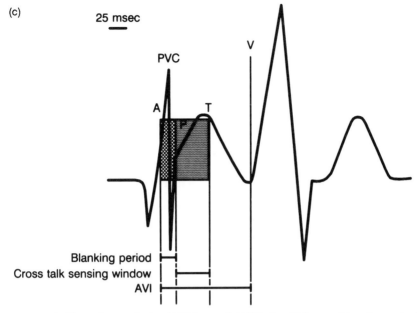

Figure 16. (a) The atrioventricular (AV) interval (AVI) should be considered as a single interval with two subportions. The entire AVI corresponds to the programmed value, i.e. the interval after a paced or sensed atrial beat allowed before a ventricular pacing artefact is delivered. The initial portion of the AVI is the blanking period. This interval is followed by the cross-talk sensing window. (b) If the ventricular sensing circuit sensed activity during the cross-talk sensing window, a ventricular pacing artefact is delivered early, usually at 100–110 ms after the atrial event. This has been referred to as 'ventricular safety pacing', '110 ms phenomenon' and 'non-physiological AV delay'. (c) The initial portion of the AVI in most dual-chamber pacemakers is designated as the blanking period. During this portion of the AVI, sensing is suspended. The primary purpose of this interval is to prevent ventricular sensing of the leading edge of the atrial pacing artefact. Any event that occurs during the blanking period, even if it is an intrinsic ventricular event, as shown in this figure, is not sensed. In this example, the ventricular premature beat that is not sensed is followed by a ventricular pacing artefact delivered at the programmed AVI and occurring in the terminal portion of the T wave. PVC, premature ventricular contraction. From Hayes and Levine (110), by permission of Blackwell Scientific Publications Inc.

the surrounding tissues. If the current leakage is sufficient, complete or intermittent failure of myocardial capture results.

High pacing thresholds may lead to intermittent or total failure to capture and early battery depletion. High thresholds are usually due to poor lead position but in a minority of patients are due to exit-block. Exit-block refers to high pacing thresholds without radiographic evidence of dislodgement and possibly is related to excessive fibrosis at the attachment of the electrode to the myocardium. In a patient with exit-block, recurrence can usually be prevented with the use of a steroid-eluting lead (73).

Failure to capture may also be caused by marked metabolic abnormalities, e.g.

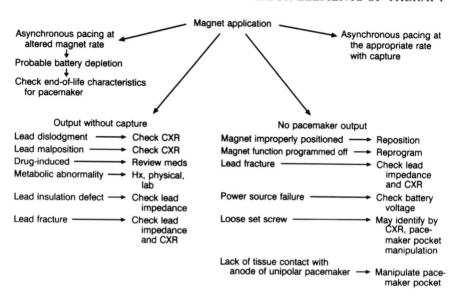

Figure 17. Algorithm for evaluating failure of output or capture, or both, by magnet application. If the magnet function of the pacemaker is rendered inactive for any reason, this algorithm would not apply. Although the chest radiograph (CXR) may be helpful, normal radiographic appearance does not exclude an abnormality of the pacing system. Many factors, such as patient position and CXR penetration, may prevent radiographic identification of a malfunction

hyperkalaemia, and some cardioactive drugs, e.g. flecainide, which alter the myocardium at the cellular level (74). Figure 17 provides an algorithm for determining the cause of failure to output and failure to capture.

Inappropriately rapid pacing rates

There are several causes for inappropriately rapid pacing rates, but few are due to true malfunction of the pacing system. One true malfunction that may be lethal for pacemaker-dependent and non-pacemaker-dependent patients alike is 'runaway pacemaker'. Runaway pacemaker occurs so infrequently with current pulse generators that it can be argued that it does not warrant discussion (75,76). When runaway pacemaker does occur, it is a true emergency. Inappropriate very rapid pacing rates are usually associated with haemodynamic instability and can result from battery failure, random component failure, or component failure induced by therapeutic radiation (77,78). Treatment must be initiated promptly if haemodynamic compromise is present (75,76).

Sensing abnormalities may also result in inappropriately rapid pacing rates, either by ventricular tracking of atrial tachyarrhythmias in a dual-chamber pacing system or by induction of tachydysrhythmias due to under-sensing and

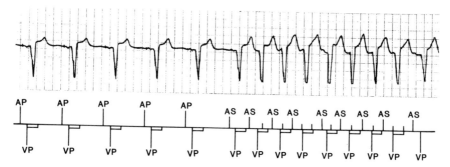

Figure 18. Resting electrocardiogram, demonstrating atrioventricular sequential pacing at base rate (55 ppm) followed by paroxysmal atrial flutter with ventricular tracking at maximum tracking rate (110 ppm). Marker channel-like diagram (Medronic, Inc.) shows atrial paced events (AP), atrial sensed events (AS), and ventricular paced events (AP) with their postventricular atrial refractory periods. Short unlabelled ticks represent unsensed atrial activity occurring in atrioventricular interval or postventricular atrial refractory period. Reproduced from Higano *et al.* (37) by permission of The Mayo Foundation for Medical Education and Research

competitive pacing (see 'Sensing malfunction', below). So that the intermittent rapidly paced ventricular rates that could occur during paroxysms of supraventricular tachycardia can be avoided, tracking of atrial fibrillatory or flutter waves may require that the pacemaker be programmed to some mode that does not allow atrial tracking (Figure 18). In the past, this meant sacrificing rate responsiveness. With current DDDR pacemakers, however, several other options are available (37). If the pacemaker is programmed to the DDIR mode, rate responsiveness is still possible via the sensor but tracking is disabled. Another DDDR device is capable of reversion to VVIR pacing if the patient has a rhythm that meets the pacemaker's criteria for pathological atrial rhythm disturbance (79). When these criteria are no longer met, the device reverts back to the DDDR pacing mode.

Endless-loop tachycardia (ELT) occurs when sensing of retrograde atrial depolarization initiates ventricular pacing, which in turn causes retrograde conduction (80,81) (Figure 19). Several methods have been used to prevent ELT. Programmable PVARPS have had the greatest impact in preventing ELT. Unfortunately, lengthening the PVARP may significantly limit the upper rate limit. A number of algorithms have been incorporated in DDD pacemakers to recognize and terminate ELT (82,83). The increased programmable flexibility of current pacemakers and ELT-terminating algorithms have made ELT relatively easy to correct in most patients.

Extracardiac stimulation

Extracardiac stimulation usually involves the diaphragm or pectoral muscle. Diaphragmatic stimulation may be due to direct stimulation of the diaphragm

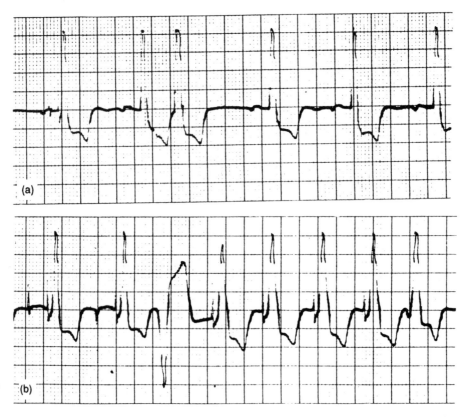

Figure 19. (a) Endless loop tachycardia (ELT) in a patient with a DDD pacemaker. In this example, a premature ventricular contribution occurs with subsequent tachycardia at the programmed upper rate limit of the pacemaker. (b) Same patient again has a premature ventricular contraction but without subsequent ELT. After the first detected episode of ELT, the postventricular atrial refractory period had been prolonged in an effort to prevent recurrent episodes of ELT. Bottom panel reproduced from Holmes *et al.* (48) by permission of The Mayo Foundation for Medical Education and Research. (b) From Hayes and Levine (110), by permission of Blackwell Scientific Publications Inc.

(usually stimulation of the left hemidiaphragm) or stimulation of the phrenic nerve (usually stimulation of the right hemidiaphragm). The potential for diaphragmatic stimulation should be tested at the time of implantation. If any stimulation is noted with 10 V of stimulation, the pacing lead should be repositioned. Diaphragmatic stimulation occurring during the early postimplantation period can be due to either microdislodgement or macrodislodgement of the pacing lead. (Although perforation of the myocardium by the pacing lead may result in diaphragmatic pacing, perforation occurs uncommonly.) Stimulation may be diminished or alleviated by decreasing the voltage output or the pulse width, or both. (An adequate pacing margin of safety must still be maintained after the output parameters have been decreased.)

Local muscle stimulation occurs much more frequently with unipolar than with bipolar pacemakers and is usually noted in the early postimplantation period. Pectoral muscle stimulation may be due to an insulation defect of the pacing lead, current leakage from the connector or sealing plugs, erosion of the pacemaker's protective coating (84), or rapid high-amplitude atrial output in a unipolar dual-chamber pacemaker (85). If the problem is due to an insulation defect on either the unipolar pacemaker or the pacemaker lead, the stimulation may be minimized by decreasing the voltage output or the pulse width, but it may be necessary to replace the defective portion of the system. (If an activity-sensing rate-adaptive pacemaker is in place, muscle stimulation could theoretically result in sensor activation and inappropriately rapid pacing rates for a given level of activity.)

Sensing malfunction

Under-sensing

Failure to sense (under-sensing), be it intermittent or total, is rarely an urgent problem (Figure 11). Lack of sensing of intrinsic cardiac activity—a relatively common abnormality—results in pacemaker output that is undesirably competitive with the intrinsic rhythm. Although competitive pacing can result in an unwanted rhythm, e.g. atrial fibrillation if there is competitive pacing in the atrium or ventricular tachycardia or fibrillation if pacing is in the ventricle, such rhythms are actually uncommon. Under-sensing may be the result of magnet application that renders the pacemaker asynchronous or, rarely, a defect in the reed switch (the switch that closes with magnet application to produce asynchronous pacing). Under-sensing is more likely due to lead dislodgement, poor lead position at the time of implantation, or interruption in the insulation of the pacing catheter. (An insulation defect may be manifested as under-sensing or over-sensing, or both.) Under-sensing may also be the result of delivery of a poor cardiac electrical signal to a normally functioning pacing system. The size of the electrical signal can be determined only from the intracardiac electrogram (ECG). Many factors may influence the size of the signal from the intracardiac ECG, e.g. concomitant drug therapy, myocardial infarction and cardiomyopathic process, such that an initially acceptable R or P wave amplitude may be diminished to a level that cannot be sensed by the pulse generator. Also, the size of the atrial signal may diminish with exercise (86). Under-sensing can frequently be corrected by reprogramming the sensitivity of the pacemaker.

In dual-chamber pacemakers, the initial portion of the AV delay is known as the blanking period. During this interval the ventricular channel of the pacemaker is insensitive to avoid sensing the atrial stimulus and depolarization. Any intrinsic ventricular event that occurs during the blanking period will give the appearance of under-sensing (87,88). Ths can often be corrected by reprogramming the blanking period.

An approach to the evaluation of sensing abnormalities is shown in Figure 20.

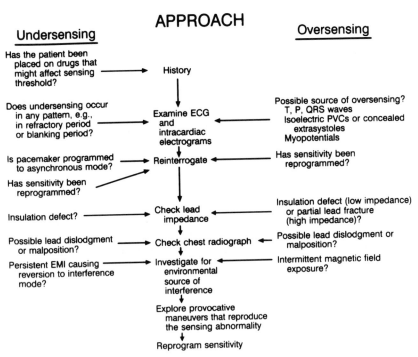

Figure 20. Approach to the evaluation of sensing abnormalities. Normal radiographic appearance does not exclude minimal lead displacement, i.e. microdislodgment. ECG, electrocardiogram; EMI, electromagnetic interference; PVC, premature ventricular contraction

Over-sensing

Over-sensing is associated with the unexpected sensing of an intracardiac or extracardiac signal (89). It may be intermittent, resulting in irregularly delayed pacemaker stimulation, or it may be permanent, leading to a decreased pacing rate or total inhibition of pacemaker output. Electrical signals that may cause over-sensing are myopotential interference, T waves, delayed afterpotentials, P waves and isoelectric extrasystoles. (Over-sensing of myopotentials in a single-chamber pacemaker may result in pauses, whereas over-sensing of myopotentials by the atrial sensing circuit of a dual-chamber pacemaker may result in rapid paced rhythms. The myopotentials are interpreted as atrial activity, and the pacemaker 'tracks' the signals with ventricular pacing.)

Over-sensing can be corrected frequently by reprogramming the sensitivity or at times by reprogramming the refractory period of the pacemaker so that the event being inappropriately sensed occurs in the refractory period and therefore does not alter the timing cycle of the pacemaker. Over-sensing of extracardiac events occurs much less commonly with bipolar sensing (90).

Pacemaker lead malfunction

Lead malfunction can be summarized simply as a fracture or insulation defect. Lead fracture, common in the early years of cardiac pacing, has become less common as lead technology has evolved. Most often, lead fractures occur adjacent to the pulse generator or near the site of venous access (91), i.e. at a stress point (92,93), although fracture of more distal portions of the pacing lead has also been reported (94). Although uncommon, direct trauma may result in damage to the pacing lead (95).

Both polyurethane and silicone are used as insulating materials for most permanent pacing leads. In the early 1980s, concern arose about the long-term performance of the polyurethane lead because of the early failure of several specific polyurethane leads (96,97). In these specific leads, difficulties in manufacturing were identified that appear to have been limited to those leads and are not indicative of overall experience with polyurethane. Insulation defects of polyurethane leads have also been described at stress points, specifically at the costoclavicular space when placement is via the subclavian puncture technique (98).

Twiddler's syndrome

'Twiddler's syndrome' refers to dislodgement or fracture of a transvenous pacing electrode by repeated manipulation and turning of the pulse generator in the subcutaneous pocket (Figure 21). Twiddling can result in retraction of the electrode into the right atrium or superior vena cava. This cause of lead dislodgement is uncommon. Although no one has reported a large collection of such cases, twiddler's syndrome seems to be most common in elderly women. Predisposing factors include large, loose pulse generator pockets and pendulous breasts that may actually contribute to pacemaker movement. It has been said in the past that such patients tend to be neurotic and repetitively turn the pacemaker as a nervous habit, but this association has never been clearly shown. Most patients with this problem adamantly deny manipulating the pacemaker.

This problem may be prevented by (i) avoiding the creation of an excessively large pocket, (ii) placing the pacemaker in a Parsonnet pouch, which is a snugly fitting Dacron pouch that reduces migration and torsion of the pacing system by promoting tissue ingrowth and stabilization of the pacemaker, (iii) fixing the pulse generator by an anchoring suture, or (iv) anchoring the lead to the prepectoral fascia by a sleeve.

Environmental causes of pacemaker malfunction

Numerous environmental factors can induce pacemaker malfunction. The most important of these are in the hospital environment. Electrocautery is the most common piece of medical equipment to affect pacemaker function. Most

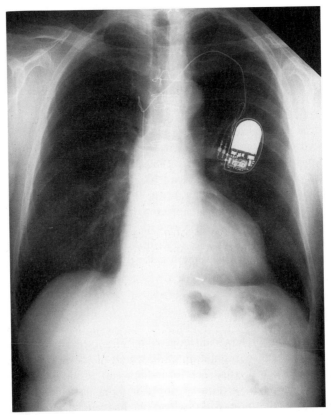

Figure 21. Posteroanterior chest radiograph in a patient with a single-chamber ventricular pacing system. The pacing lead is twisted in the superior vena cava because of twiddler's syndrome, i.e. patient manipulation of the pulse generator resulted in twisting of the pacing lead

commonly, it reprograms the pacemaker, although it can result in permanent alteration of the pacemaker circuitry (99). After electrocautery is used in a patient with a permanent pacemaker, the pacemaker should be checked to confirm proper function and expected programmed parameters.

Magnetic resonance imaging (MRI) remains questionable for pacemaker patients. In animal studies, MRI resulted in unpredictable rapid pacing and haemodynamic instability (100). In non-pacemaker-dependent patients, MRI has been performed after the pacemaker was disabled by programming to the OOO mode (101). In general, however, MRI examinations should still be avoided in patients with pacemakers.

Therapeutic radiation may cause pacemaker malfunction by damaging the complementary metal oxide semiconductors used in the integrated circuits of pacemakers (102). Sudden loss of output or runaway may occur. Because the damage to the circuit is random and the radiation dose cumulative, no specific prediction about the dose can be made.

Transthoracic defibrillation may result in permanent or transient electrical damage to the pulse generator; onset may be delayed for several days. The effects on the pacing system may be due to myocardial thermal damage secondary to transmission of defibrillation discharge to the heart via the lead or leads (resulting in myocardial infarction or ventricular fibrillation, or both), inappropriate reprogramming of programmable pulse generators, or damage to the pacemaker circuitry (103). The potential for such damage is minimized by the incorporation of a circuit (Zener diode) into the pacemaker to shunt excess energy away from the pacemaker (103). Further steps can be taken clinically to minimize the chance of pacemaker malfunction with defibrillation by positioning the defibrillation paddles anteroposteriorly and as far from the pacemaker or subcutaneous lead as possible.

Extracorporeal shock wave lithotripsy can be used in patients with dual-chamber pacemakers, but reprogramming to a different pacing mode may be required beforehand to ensure patient safety (104,105). The use of trans-cutaneous electrical nerve stimulation in paced patients remains somewhat controversial. Although one study demonstrated no pacing abnormalities in 51 patients in whom 20 different pacemakers were evaluated (106), individual case reports have shown pacemaker inhibition by such stimulation (107). At this time, it is advisable to monitor pacemaker-dependent patients during initial trans-cutaneous electrical nerve stimulation and to avoid application directly to the pacemaker in all paced patients.

Environmental influences outside the hospital are unlikely to cause permanent malfunction of a pacemaker. However, any high-energy transient, e.g. arc welding or electrical shock, coupled into the patient could potentially result in asynchronous pacing or reversion of the pacemaker to the manufacturer's preset parameters.

Prevention of pacing system malfunctions requires not only that the pacemaker and pacing lead be reliable but also that the implanter of the system be knowledgeable and have expertise in pacemaker implantation. In a survey conducted by Parsonnet *et al.* (108), the number of complications was inversely proportional to the implanter's experience.

PACEMAKER FOLLOW-UP

After pacemaker implantation, the patient must be seen regularly to ensure normal pacemaker function (109). Pacemaker follow-up requires periodic evaluations in the physician's surgery or hospital. If transtelephonic monitoring is part of the follow-up, office visits may be less frequent. At the election of the physician implanting the pacemaker, transtelephonic monitoring may be done at the implanter's institution or through a commercial pacemaker follow-up centre.

However, transtelephonic pacemaker monitoring is common only in the USA. In most parts of the world, regular office visits are the mainstay of follow-up.

The most important reason for careful pacemaker follow-up still is to identify pacemaker failure before it occurs. The incidence of catastrophic pacemaker failure continues to decline with advances in pacemaker technology. With current lithium batteries, failure usually occurs very slowly, i.e. over a period of months, giving the physician ample time to detect the impending failure and electively replace the pulse generator. Other important reasons for periodic follow-up are lowering of pacemaker output (voltage amplitude and pulse width), when possible, to maximize battery longevity and correction of other detected abnormalities, such as under-sensing or over-sensing and ELT. Patients with rate-adaptive pacemakers may also require alteration of rate-response parameters to optimize rate response. Their rate-response requirements may increase or decrease over time, depending on their level of conditioning and associated medical problems. This is especially true in the elderly population, because cardiac, neurological or orthopaedic problems may significantly alter rate-response requirements.

REFERENCES

1. Bernstein AD, Parsonnet V (1992) Survey of cardiac pacing in the United States in 1989. *Am J Cardiol* **69**: 331–338.
2. Berman ND, Mitchell JM, Dickson SE (1983) Pacemaker therapy in the seventies: interaction of patient age, time of implant, and indications for pacing. *PACE* **6**: 247–252.
3. Davies MJ (1976) Pathology of the conduction system. In *Cardiology in Old Age*, Caird FI, Dall JLC, Kennedy RD (eds). Plenum Press, New York, pp. 57–80.
4. Elmqvist R, Senning A (1960) An implantable pacemaker for the heart. In *International Conference on Medical Electronics*, 2nd edn, Smyth CN (ed.). Iliffe, Paris, pp. 253–254.
5. Sutton R, Bourgeois I (1991) *The Foundations of Cardiac Pacing, Part 1: An Illustrated Practical Guide to Basic Pacing*. Futura, Mount Kisco, NY, pp. 319–324.
6. Bernstein AD, Camm AJ, Fletcher RD *et al.* (1987) The NASPE/BPEG generic pacemaker code for antibradyarrhythmia and adaptive-rate pacing and antitachyarrhythmia devices. *PACE* **10**: 794–799.
7. A Report of the Joint American College of Cardiology/American Heart Association Task Force on Assessment of Cardiovascular Procedures (Subcommittee on Pacemaker Implantation) (1984) Guidelines for permanent cardiac pacemaker implantation, May 1984. *J Am Coll Cardiol* **4**: 434–442.
8. ACC/AHA Task Force (1991) Guidelines for implantation of cardiac pacemaker and antiarrhythmia devices: a report of the American College of Cardiology/American Heart Association Task Force on assessment of diagnostic and therapeutic cardiovascular procedures (committee on pacemaker implantation). *J Am Coll Cardiol* **18**: 1–13.
9. Jordaens L, De Backer G, Clement DL (1988) Physiologic pacing in the elderly: effects on exercise capacity and exercise-induced arrhythmias. *Jpn Heart J* **29**: 35–44.
10. Amikam S, Lemer J, Roguin N *et al.* (1976) Long-term survival of elderly patients after pacemaker implantation. *Am Heart J* **91**: 445–449.

11. Strauss HD, Berman ND (1978) Permanent pacing in the elderly. *PACE* **1**: 458–464.
12. Spielman SR, Segal BL (1986) Pacemakers in the elderly: new knowledge, new choices (Editorial). *Geriatrics* **41** (2): 13–14.
13. Martin A, Nathan AW, Camm AJ (1985) Cardiac pacing in an elderly population with a satellite clinic in a district general hospital. *Age Ageing* **14**: 333–338.
14. Galassi A, Dottore E (1989) Cost effectiveness of today's cardiac pacing. *Cardiologia* **34**: 113–116.
15. Levine PA, Mace RC (1983) Pacemaker syndrome. *Pacing Therapy: A Guide to Cardiac Pacing for Optimum Hemodynamic Benefit*, Levine PA, Mace RC (eds). Futura, Mount Kisco, NY, pp. 3–18.
16. Ausubel K, Furman S (1985) The pacemaker syndrome. *Ann Intern Med* **103**: 420–429.
17. Den Dulk K, Lindemans FW, Brugada P *et al.* (1988) Pacemaker syndrome with AAI rate variable pacing: importance of atrioventricular conduction properties, medication, and pacemaker programmability. *PACE* **11**: 1226–1233.
18. Cunningham TM (1988) Pacemaker syndrome due to retrograde conduction in a DDI pacemaker. *Am Heart J* **115**: 478–479.
19. Heldman D, Mulvhill D, Nguyen H *et al.* (1990) True incidence of pacemaker syndrome. *PACE* **13**: 1742–1750.
20. Hayes DL, Furman S (1984) Stability of AV conduction in sick sinus node syndrome patients with implanted atrial pacemakers. *Am Heart J* **107**: 644–647.
21. Rosenqvist M (1990) Atrial pacing for sick sinus syndrome. *Clin Cardiol* **13**: 43–47.
22. Benditt DG, Milstein S, Buetikofer J *et al.* (1987) Sensor-triggered, rate-variable cardiac pacing: current technologies and clinical implications. *Ann Intern Med* **107**: 714–724.
23. Fearnot NE, Smith HJ (1986) Trends in pacemakers which physiologically increase rate: DDD and rate responsive. *PACE* **9**: 939–947.
24. Hayes DL, Christiansen JR, Vlietstra RE, Osborn MJ (1989) Follow-up of an activity-sensing, rate-modulated pacing device, including transtelephonic exercise assessment. *Mayo Clin Proc* **64**: 503–508.
25. Mond H, Strathmore N, Kertes P *et al.* (1988) Rate responsive pacing using a minute ventilation sensor. *PACE* **11:** 1866–1874.
26. Sellers TD, Fearnot N (1988) Kelvin 500 Investigator Group: a multicenter experience with a temperature based rate modulating pacemaker (Kelvin 500) (Abstract). *PACE* **11**: 486.
27. Lau C-P, Wonk C-K, Leung W-H *et al.* (1989) A comparative evaluation of a minute ventilation sensing and activity sensing adaptive-rate pacemakers during daily activities. *PACE* **12**: 1514–1521.
28. Rickards AF, Norman J (1981) Relation between QT interval and heart rate: new design of physiologically adaptive cardiac pacemaker. *Br Heart J* **45**: 56–61.
29. Boute W, Derrien Y, Wittkampf FHM (1986) Reliability of evoked endocardial T-wave sensing in 1,500 pacemaker patients. *PACE* **9**: 948–953.
30. McGoon MD, Olive A, Salo R *et al.* (1988) Pre-ejection interval as a determinant of physiologic pacing rate (Abstract). *Pace* **11**: 499.
31. Olson WH, Bennett TD, Beck RD *et al.* (1985) Stroke volume controlled rate responsive pacing in exercising heart-blocked canines (Abstract). *Circulation Suppl* **72** (Suppl. 3): III-432.
32. Sharma AD, Bennett T, Sutton R *et al.* (1988) The effect of variable pacing rate on maximum positive right ventricular DP/DT: implications for a new rate responsive pacing system (Abstract). *J Am Coll Cardiol* **11**: 165A.
33. Snell J, Cohen D, Hedberg SE *et al.* (1988) In-vivo performance of a hemo-reflective type oxygen sensor for rate responsive pacing (Abstract). *PACE* **11**: 504.

34. Callaghan F, Camerlo J, Tarjan P (1987) The ventricular depolarization gradient: exercise performance of a closed-loop rate responsive pacemaker (Abstract). *PACE* **10**: 1212.
35. Landman MAJ, Senden PJ, Van Rooijen H, Van Hemel NM (1990) Initial clinical experience with rate adaptive cardiac pacing using two sensors simultaneously. *PACE* **13**: 1615–1622.
36. Hayes DL (1989) Rate-modulating pacemakers. *Cardiovasc Rev Rep* **10**: 20–26.
37. Higano ST, Hayes DL, Eisinger G (1989) Advantage of discrepant upper rate limits in a DDDR pacemaker. *Mayo Clin Proc* **64**: 932–939.
38. Rosenqvist M, Brandt J, Schuller H (1988) Long-term pacing in sinus node disease: effects of stimulation mode on cardiovascular morbidity and mortality. *Am Heart J* **116**: 16–22.
39. Alpert MA, Curtis JJ, Sanfelippo JF *et al.* (1986) Comparative survival after permanent ventricular and dual chamber pacing for patients with chronic high degree atrioventricular block with and without preexistent congestive heart failure. *J Am Coll Cardiol* **7**: 925–932.
40. Alpert MA, Curtis JJ, Sanfelippo JF *et al.* (1987) Comparative survival following permanent ventricular and dual-chamber pacing for patients with chronic symptomatic sinus node dysfunction with and without congestive heart failure. *Am Heart J* **113**: 958–965.
41. Ebagosti A, Gueunoun M, Saadjian A *et al.* (1988) Long-term follow-up of patients treated with VVI pacing and sequential pacing with special reference to VA retrograde conduction. *PACE* **11**: 1929–1934.
42. Sasaki Y, Shimotori M, Akahane K *et al.* (1988) Long-term follow-up of patients with sick sinus syndrome: a comparison of clinical aspects among unpaced, ventricular inhibited paced, and physiologically paced groups. *PACE* **11**: 1575–1583.
43. Hayes DL, Neubauer SA (1990) Incidence of atrial fibrillation after DDD pacing (Abstract). *PACE* **13**: 501.
44. Santini M, Alexidou G, Ansalone G *et al.* (1990) Relation of prognosis in sick sinus syndrome to age, conduction defects and modes of permanent cardiac pacing. *Am J Cardiol* **65**: 729–735.
45. Zanini R, Facchinetti AI, Gallo G *et al.* (1990) Morbidity and mortality of patients with sinus node disease: comparative effects of atrial and ventricular pacing. *PACE* **13**: 2076–2079.
46. Stangl K, Seitz A, Wirtzfeld A *et al.* (1990) Differences between atrial single chamber pacing (AAI) and ventricular single chamber pacing (VVI) with respect to prognosis and antiarrhythmic effect in patients with sick sinus syndrome. *PACE* **13**: 2080–2085.
47. Feuer JM, Shandling AH, Messenger JC, with the technical assistance of Castellanet CD, Thomas LA (1989) Influence of cardiac pacing mode on the long-term development of atrial fibrillation. *Am J Cardiol* **64**: 1376–1379.
48. Holmes DR Jr, Hayes DL, Furman S (1989) Permanent pacemaker implantation. In *A Practice of Cardiac Pacing*, 2nd edn, Furman S, Hayes DL, Holmes DR Jr (eds). Futura, Mount Kisco, NY, pp. 239–287.
49. Sutton R, Bourgeois I (1991) *The Foundations of Cardiac Pacing, Part 1: An Illustrated Practical Guide to Basic Pacing.* Futura, Mount Kisco, NY, pp. 177–234.
50. O'Keefe JH Jr, Hayes DL, Holmes DR Jr, Vlietstra RE (1983) Clinical use of multiparameter programmability in the early and late follow-up periods (Abstract). *PACE* **6**: A-102.
51. Hauser RG (1983) Multiprogrammable cardiac pacemakers: applications, results and follow-up. *Am J Surg* **145**: 740–745.

52. Furman S, Pannizzo F (1981) Output programmability and reduction of secondary intervention after pacemaker implantation. *J Thorac Cardiovasc Surg* **81**: 713–717.
53. Griffin JC, Schuenemeyer TD, Hess KR *et al.* (1986) Pacemaker follow-up: its role in the detection and correction of pacemaker system malfunction. *PACE* **9**: 387–391.
54. Pless P, Simonsen E, Arnsbo P, Fabricius J (1986) Superiority of multiprogrammable to nonprogrammable VVI pacing: a comparative study with special reference to management of pacing system malfunction. *PACE* **9**: 739–744.
55. Hayes DL (1989) Programmability. In *A Practice of Cardiac Pacing*, 2nd edn, Furman S, Hayes DL, Holmes DR Jr (eds). Futura, Mount Kisco, NY, pp. 563–596.
56. Hauser RG (1982) Bipolar leads for cardiac pacing in the 1980s: a reappraisal provoked by skeletal muscle interference. *PACE* **5**: 34–37.
57. Klementowicz PT, Furman S (1985) Stability of atrial sensing and pacing after dual chamber pulse generator implantation. *J Am Coll Cardiol* **6**: 1338–1341.
58. Gould L, Reddy CVR, Singh BK, Zen B (1979) Inappropriate slowing of the pacemaker rate with programmable demand pacemaker. *PACE* **2**: 370–372.
59. Rosenqvist M, Vallin HO, Edhag KO (1984) Rate hysteresis pacing: how valuable is it? A comparison of the stimulation rates of 70 and 50 beats per minute and rate hysteresis in patients with sinus node disease. *PACE* **7**: 332–340.
60. Smyth NPD, Sager D (1983) A multiprogrammable pacemaker with unipolar or bipolar option. *Am Heart J* **106**: 412–414.
61. Nielsen AP, Cashion WR, Spencer WH *et al.* (1985) Long-term assessment of unipolar and bipolar stimulation and sensing thresholds using a lead configuration programmable pacemaker. *J Am Coll Cardiol* **5**: 1198–1204.
62. Fieldman A, Dobrow RJ (1978) Phantom pacemaker programming. *PACE* **1**: 166–171.
63. Sinnaeve A, Piret J, Stroobandt R (1980) Potential causes of spurious programming: report of a case. *PACE* **3**: 541–547.
64. Dreifus LS, Zinberg A, Hurzeler P *et al.* (1986) Transtelephonic monitoring of 25,919 implanted pacemakers. *PACE* **9**: 371–378.
65. Markewitz A, Hemmer W, Weinhold C (1986) Complications in dual chamber pacing: a six-year experience. *PACE* **9**: 1014–1018.
66. Janosik DL, Redd RM, Buckingham TA *et al.* (1987) Utility of ambulatory electrocardiography in detecting pacemaker dysfunction in the early postimplantation period. *Am J Cardiol* **60**: 1030–1035.
67. Heinz M, Zitzmann E, Coenen M, Alt E (1990) Malfunctioning of DDD pacemakers despite correct functioning of routine pacemaker controls (Abstract). *PACE* **13**: 560.
68. Collins DWK, Black JL, Sinclair IN (1985) Predicted early failure of cardiac pacemakers. *PACE* **8**: 544–548.
69. Hauser RG, Wimer EA, Timmis GC *et al.* (1986) Twelve years of clinical experience with lithium pulse generators. *PACE* **9**: 1277–1281.
70. Sweesy MW, Batey RL, Forney RC (1988) Crosstalk during bipolar pacing. *PACE* **11**: 1512–1516.
71. Mugica J, Ripart A (1984) Twelve years experience with cardiac pacing leads: clinical conclusions for 8,004 cases. *Clin Prog Pacing Electrophysiol* **2**: 513–532.
72. Hayes DL (1989) Pacemaker complications. In *A Practice of Cardiac Pacing*, Hayes DL (ed.). Futura, Mount Kisco, NY, p. 497.
73. Hayes DL, Broadbent JC, Holmes DR Jr *et al.* (1985) Steroid-tipped leads: 1-year follow-up. In *Pacemaker Leads. (Proceedings of the International Symposium on Pacemaker Leads, Leuven, Belgium, September 5–7, 1984)*, Aubert AE, Ector H (eds). Elsevier, Amsterdam, pp. 317–322.
74. Reiffel JA, Coromilas J, Zimmerman JM, Spotnitz HM (1985) Drug–device

interactions: clinical considerations. *PACE* **8**: 369–373.

75. Campo A, Nowak R, Magilligan D, Tomlanovich M (1983) Runaway pacemaker. *Ann Emerg Med* **12**: 32–34.

76. Mickley H, Andersen C, Nielsen LH (1989) Runaway pacemaker: a still existing complication and therapeutic guidelines. *Clin Cardiol* **12**: 412–414.

77. Lee RW, Huang SK, Mechling E, Bazgan I (1986) Runaway atrioventricular sequential pacemaker after radiation therapy. *Am J Med* **81**: 883–886.

78. Katzenberg CA, Marcus FI, Heusinkveld RS, Mammana RB (1982) Pacemaker failure due to radiation therapy. *PACE* **5**: 156–159.

79. Ilvento J, Fee JA, Shewmaker S (1990) Automatic mode switching from DDDR to VVIR: a management algorithm for atrial arrhythmias in patients with dual chamber pacemakers (Abstract). *PACE* **13**: 1199.

80. Furman SF, Fisher JD (1982) Endless loop tachycardia in an AV universal (DDD) pacemaker. *PACE* **5**: 486–489.

81. Akhtar M, Gilbert C, Rehan M *et al.* (1985) Pacemaker-mediated tachycardia: underlying mechanisms, relationship to ventriculoatrial conduction characteristics, and management. *Clin. Prog. Electrophysiol. Pacing* **3**: 90–104.

82. Hayes DL (1988) Endless-loop tachycardia: the problem has been solved? In *New Perspectives in Cardiac Pacing*, Barold SS, Mugica J (eds). Futura, Mount Kisco, NY, pp. 375–386.

83. Nitzsché R, Gueunoun M, Lamaison D *et al.* (1990) Endless-loop tachycardias: description and first clinical results of a new fully automatic protection algorithm. *PACE* **13**: 1711–1718.

84. Chauvin M, Brechenmacher C (1987) Muscle stimulation caused by a pacemaker current leakage: the role of the insulation failure of a polyurethane coating. *J Electrophysiol* **1**: 326–329.

85. Stroobandt R, Willems R, Depuydt P *et al.* (1989) The superfast atrial recharge pulse: a cause of pectoral muscle stimulation in patients equipped with a unipolar DDD pacemaker. *PACE* **12**: 451–455.

86. Fröhlig G, Schwerdt H, Schieffer H, Bette L (1988) Atrial signal variations and pacemaker malsensing during exercise: a study in the time and frequency domain. *J Am Coll Cardiol* **11**: 806–813.

87. Berman ND, George CA, Duxbury GB (1987) Apparent pacemaker malfunction due to ventricular blanking. *Can J Cardiol* **3**: 63–65.

88. Bertuso J, Kapoor AS, Schafer J (1986) A case of ventricular undersensing in the DDI mode: cause and correction. *PACE* **9**: 685–689.

89. Barold SS, Falkoff MD, Ong LS, Heinle RA (1985) Oversensing by single-chamber pacemakers: mechanisms, diagnosis, and treatment. *Cardiol Clin* **3**: 565–585.

90. Gabry MD, Behrens M, Andrews C *et al.* (1987) Comparison of myopotential interference in unipolar–bipolar programmable DDD pacemakers. *PACE* **10**: 1322–1330.

91. Alt E, Völker R, Blömer H (1987) Lead fracture in pacemaker patients. *Thorac Cardiovasc Surg* **35**: 101–104.

92. Suzuki Ym Fujimori S, Sakai M *et al.* (1988) A case of pacemaker lead fracture associated with thoracic outlet syndrome. *PACE* **11**: 326–330.

93. Conklin EF, Giannelli S Jr, Nealon TF Jr (1975) Four hundred consecutive patients with permanent transvenous pacemakers. *J Thorac Cardiovasc Surg* **69**: 1–7.

94. Clarke B, Jones S, Gray HH, Rowland E (1989) The tricuspid valve: an unusual site of endocardial pacemaker lead fracture. *PACE* **12**: 1077–1079.

95. Grieco JG, Scanlon PJ, Pifarré R (1989) Pacing lead fracture after a deceleration injury. *Ann Thorac Surg* **47**: 453–454.

96. Phillips R, Frey M, Martin RO (1986) Long-term performance of polyurethane

pacing leads: mechanisms of design-related failures. *PACE* **9**: 1166–1172.

97. Stokes KB, Church T (1986) Ten-year experience with implanted polyurethane lead insulation. *PACE* **9**: 1160–1165.

98. Fyke FE III (1988) Simultaneous insulation deterioration associated with side-by-side subclavian placement of two polyurethane leads. *PACE* **11**: 1571–1574.

99. Levine PA, Balady GJ, Lazar HL *et al.* (1986) Electrocautery and pacemakers: management of the paced patient subject to electrocautery. *Ann Thorac Surg* **41**: 313–317.

100. Hayes DL, Holmes DR Jr, Gray JE (1987) Effect of 1.5 tesla nuclear magnetic resonance imaging scanner on implanted permanent pacemakers. *J Am Coll Cardiol* **10**: 782–786.

101. Alagona P Jr, Toole JC, Maniscalo BS *et al.* (1989) Nuclear magnetic resonance imaging in a patient with a DDD pacemaker (Letter to the editor). *PACE* **12**: 619.

102. Adamec R, Haefliger JM, Killisch JP *et al.* (1982) Damaging effect of therapeutic radiation on programmable pacemakers. *PACE* **5**: 146–150.

103. Aylward P, Blood R, Tonkin A (1979) Complications of defibrillation with permanent pacemaker in situ. *PACE* **2**: 462–464.

104. Cooper D, Wilkoff B, Masterson M *et al.* (1988) Effects of extracorporeal shock wave lithotripsy on cardiac pacemakers and its safety in patients with implanted cardiac pacemakers. *PACE* **11**: 1607–1616.

105. Fetter J, Patterson D, Aram G, Hayes DL (1989) Effects of extracorporeal shock wave lithotripsy on single chamber rate response and dual chamber pacemakers. *PACE* **12**: 1494–1501.

106. Rasmussen MJ, Hayes DL, Vlietstra RE, Thorsteinsson G (1988) Can transcutaneous electrical nerve stimulation be safely used in patients with permanent cardiac pacemakers? *Mayo Clin Proc* **63**: 443–445.

107. Chen D, Philip M, Philip PA, Monga TN (1990) Cardiac pacemaker inhibition by transcutaneous electrical nerve stimulation. *Arch Phys Med Rehabil* **71**: 27–30.

108. Parsonnet V, Bernstein AD, Lindsay B (1989) Pacemaker-implantation complication rates: an analysis of some contributing factors. *J Am Coll Cardiol* **13**: 917–921.

109. Furman S (1989) Pacemaker follow-up. In *A Practice of Cardiac Pacing*, 2nd edn, Furman S, Hayes DL, Holmes DR Jr (eds). Futura, Mount Kisco, NY, pp. 511–544.

110. Hayes DL, Levine PA (1992) Pacemaker timing cycles. In *Cardiac Pacing*, Ellenbogen KA (ed). Blackwell Scientific Publishers, Cambridge, MA, pp. 263–308.

30 Interventional Techniques

ANGUS TURNER AND DAVID WARD
St George's Hospital, London, UK

The field of interventional cardiology has rapidly expanded in recent years. The techniques employed allow patients to be managed in a relatively conservative manner and make it feasible to offer active treatment for some individuals who are considered to be unsuitable for surgery. On top of this, the nature of the procedure, as well as the reduced time spent in hospital, make interventional techniques an economically attractive proposition.

These features are becoming increasingly relevant with respect to the expanding elderly population with heart disease. In this chapter, consideration will mainly be given to percutaneous transluminal coronary angioplasty (PTCA) and valvuloplasty.

ANGIOPLASTY

Introduction

The first PTCA was carried out in 1977 by Gruntzig. This was a revolutionary step and since then the technique has gained wide acceptance as an alternative to coronary artery bypass surgery for treatment of angina pectoris in patients with suitable coronary anatomy.

In considering PTCA for elderly patients, i.e. over the age of 65 years, account must be taken of the increased risk with respect to younger patients (1) as well as coexistent medical conditions and the unsuitability, or otherwise, of the patient for coronary artery bypass surgery.

Mechanism of percutaneous transluminal coronary angioplasty

By inflating a balloon across an atheromatous lesion, PTCA causes disruption of both an atherosclerotic plaque and the associated vessel wall to bring about restoration of the affected arterial segment's lumen to a more normal dimension.

During effective PTCA, the atherosclerotic plaque is split at its weakest point. This split involves the intima and media, and as the balloon expands further the media and adventitia expand to accommodate the angioplasty balloon. During

Geriatric Cardiology. Principles and Practice. Edited by A. Martin and A.J. Camm
© 1994 John Wiley & Sons Ltd

the procedure, the outer layers of the vessel become distorted and slightly aneurysmal. This controlled 'injury' is the basis of angioplasty (2).

The coronary complications of PTCA are often caused by the traumatic nature of the procedure and, given the greater fragility of older arteries, may be expected to be more common in the elderly. The exposure of the atheromatous plaque and arterial collagen leads to platelet deposition and activation and thrombus formation, which in turn would lead to acute occlusion. This is the basis behind giving antiplatelet treatment prior to an anticoagulant and intravenous nitrate therapy during and immediately after the procedure. Damage to the media commonly causes a localized dissection of the coronary artery, which can be a major determinant in vessel occlusion.

Practical aspects of percutaneous transluminal coronary angioplasty

The fasted patient is consented for the procedure and the possible complications are explained. If the patient is not already on aspirin therapy, this is commenced 24 hours prior to the procedure. Premedication is often given in the form of a benzodiazepine derivative or as an opiate when the patient is in the laboratory; also a low-dose intravenous nitrate infusion may be commenced 10 minutes before starting the procedure. In view of the possible acute complications which might arise, it is imperative that there is access to surgical assistance in the event of bypass grafting being required.

The procedure is usually carried out from the right femoral artery approach, but the brachial approach may also be used. An 8–9 French sheath is inserted into the right femoral artery using the Seldinger technique, and at this stage 10 000 units of heparin is administered intravenously. A guiding catheter, usually of the Judkins type, is advanced retrogradely up the aorta to the coronary ostea. The guide wire is removed and a set of diagnostic angiograms is performed to confirm the location of the target lesion and to assess any possible disease progression if there has been a significant interval since the last cardiac catheterization.

The balloon catheter is then advanced up the guiding catheter, with the balloon fully deflated. Nearly all balloon catheters are of the steerable type, i.e. there is a lumen present which allows passage of a floppy tipped, high-torque radio-opaque guide wire of 0.010–0.018 inch diameter. The guide wires vary in stiffness and configuration to allow differing degrees of support and flexibility as the situation demands.

With the balloon catheter in the distal part of the guiding catheter, the guide wire is advanced and manipulated across the lesion. The position is checked with a contrast injection, for instance to confirm that the distal end of the wire is not in a side branch of the artery. The balloon catheter is then advanced over the guide wire and across the lesion. Difficulty may be experienced at this stage due to disengagement of the guiding catheter or inappropriate balloon profiles. The position of the balloon is visualized by radio-opaque markers in the catheter and confirmed by contrast injection (Figure 1).

The balloon can now be inflated across the lesion. Balloons are made of polyvinyl chloride or polyethylene, both of which have a high tensile strength. The standard length of a balloon is 2.0 cm and the inflated diameter varies between 1.5 and 4.2 mm. Balloon rupture is a risk at inflation pressures of 8 atmospheres or greater. The duration and number of inflations vary between operators and patients. Two to four inflations of 60–120 seconds each are often made. The results of the dilatations can be checked by contrast injection with the balloon catheter withdrawn, but the guide wire still *in situ* across the lesion. Angina and ST segment changes often occur with balloon insufflation but these usually resolve with deflation.

After the procedure, the patient should be closely observed on a high-dependency unit with facilities for continuous cardiac monitoring. The intra-venous nitrates are reduced and stopped over the next 12 hours and the patient continues on intravenous heparin until 16–24 hours after the procedure. During this time the atrial sheath is left *in situ*, both to prevent bleeding complications in the anticoagulated patient and to allow access in case of the need for repeat PTCA. Six-hourly electrocardiograms (ECGs) and cardiac enzymes are checked to enable early detection of myocardial ischaemia and infarction. Successful PTCA might be defined as the reduction of the target coronary lesion or lesions by greater than 50% with no complications.

Complications of percutaneous transluminal coronary angioplasty in the elderly

Local complications may occur at the site of insertion of the femoral cannula, such as bleeding or distal embolization (see Chapter 10). The risk of aortic trauma and trauma to the coronary arteries with the guiding catheter is the same as in routine angiography. Disturbances in cardiac rhythm may also occur as does chest pain, but these are usually easily reversible.

The most important complications arise from vessel occlusion at the site of balloon dilatation and consist of myocardial infarction and death. Vessel occlusion can result as a consequence of coronary artery dissection, spasm or from thromboembolism, and usually results in emergency coronary bypass. Occlusion usually occurs within the first 1–2 hours of the procedure, and rarely occurs after 6 hours (3).

Dissection

A limited or controlled dissection is part of the mechanism of a successful angioplasty. However, approximately half the cases of acute occlusion occur as a result of more extensive dissection, resulting in compromise to coronary blood flow. It commonly arises as a direct result of balloon inflation, but can be caused by manipulation of the guide wire or balloon. An obvious dissection (on arteriography) occurs with compromise to flow, and careful observation is required for 10–20 minutes, followed by repeat contrast injection. A degree of

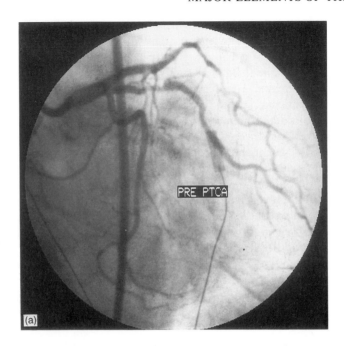

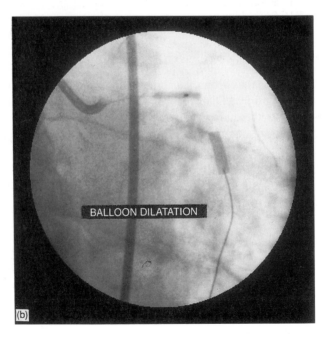

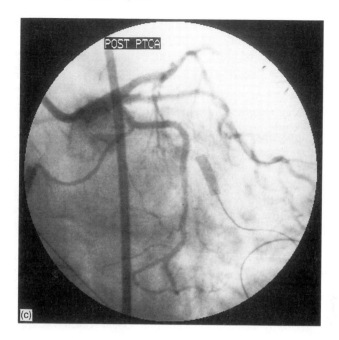

Figure 1. Stenotic lesion of an intermediate branch of the left coronary artery: (a) (opposite) pre-PTCA; (b) (opposite) during balloon inflation; (c) post-PTCA

obstruction can be reversed by repeat balloon inflation, but if further compromise is evident or complete occlusion occurs, emergency bypass grafting should be considered.

Coronary artery spasm

Coronary artery spasm may be a cause of complete occlusion in its own right or be a significant contributing factor in conjunction with dissection. Spasm may be due to the interaction of vasoactive factors released by platelets and the exposed arterial media. The situation may be promptly relieved by intracoronary injection of glyceryl trinitrate at a dose of 100–400 μg.

Occlusion secondary to thromboembolism

Thromboembolic occlusion is usually the result of poor PTCA technique combined with inadequate anticoagulation. For this reason, it is suggested that additional heparinization is given if the procedure is to last longer than 1 hour. Conscientious flushing of all catheters and cleaning of guide wires is essential to avoid these complications.

The occurrence of complications of PTCA in the elderly has been recorded at 3.2%, with a 1.4% incidence of Q wave myocardial infarction and a 0.8%

incidence of emergency bypass procedures (4). Complication rates occurring within the catheter laboratory are not significantly different between patients over and under the age of 65 years. However, patients over the age of 65 years are more likely to require emergency bypass grafting (1).

Indications for percutaneous transluminal coronary angioplasty in the elderly

Patients presenting with either chronic stable angina or unstable angina, which is proving refractory to standard medical therapy and has amenable disease shown on the cardiac catheterization, are suitable candidates for consideration of PTCA. When the procedure was first introduced, it was uncommon to attempt PTCA in patients over 65 years of age, the mean age of one of the first studies being 49 years (5). However, with improved methods, there is a body of evidence to suggest that age should not be a contraindication.

Angiographic criteria

The angiographic criteria are an important factor for considering PTCA in the elderly, as it is in younger patients. Lesions of less than 60% of the luminal diameter are generally not considered good target lesions as their doubtful haemodynamic significance does not outweigh the risk of complications—which is the same as in more severe lesions.

Ideally an atherosclerotic stenosis should be in a proximal position, be discrete and not involve any major side branches. As the sophistication of PTCA develops, increasingly more difficult lesions, e.g. those distally placed, eccentric in nature or involving arterial branches, are being attempted with success. Complete occlusions are also suitable for PTCA if viable myocardium has been demonstrated in the area supplied by the affected vessel. The elderly population have a high incidence of multivessel disease. In this situation PTCA is usually attempted on the stenosis considered to be most symptomatic, rather than aiming for complete revascularization, which would put the patient at increased risk.

However, multivessel PTCA is becoming more widespread and is often carried out as a staged procedure over more than 1 day. Obviously the risk of complications is increased in this setting.

Lesions which are highly likely to cause a significant amount of haemodynamic compromise are obviously best approached with caution. Such a situation would be a stenosis of one major vessel which also supplies a significant collateral flow to one or other major branches. Unprotected left main stem stenosis is also a contraindication to PTCA.

In the elderly population it is commoner to find cardiac anatomy which is more suitable for coronary bypass grafting than for PTCA (6). Obviously any coexistent medical condition, such as diabetes, respiratory disease or malignancy, must be taken into consideration.

Efficacy, mortality and survival of percutaneous transluminal coronary angioplasty in the elderly

The success rate for PTCA of coronary lesions in the elderly is high, with figures of 82% in patients aged 65–74 years and 92.8% in patients 75 years and older (7). In a study of octogenarians only, immediate angiographic success was demonstrated in 91% of lesions dilated (8).

Long-term efficacy of PTCA in the elderly is encouraging, with less than 25% of patients over 65 years reporting any residual angina at 2 years (1). However, patients over 65 with residual pain at 2 years required more severe therapy to control their symptoms than those under 65 years, and a greater proportion of these patients required repeat PTCA (38% versus 6%) coronary artery bypass grafts (26% versus 10%) or both (5% versus 4%) (1).

Restenosis is one of the most significant aspects of PTCA. The true incidence is difficult to ascertain due to lack of routine follow-up angiographic data. However, one study managed to acquire routine angiography 6 months post PTCA in 62% of a population of octogenarians who underwent the procedure. Restenosis (defined as the recurrence of greater than 50% luminal narrowing in the previously dilated vessel) was seen in 31% (8). This compares well with similar studies performed on a population with a wider range of age groups (9).

The mortality and survival figures of PTCA in the elderly compare well with those of coronary artery bypass grafting. The reported in-hospital mortality for PTCA varies from 1.6% to 6.8% (4,7) with patients over 75 years contributing most to the higher end of the spectrum. The comparable perioperative mortality for coronary artery bypass grafts has been noted as 4.6% in patients aged 65–69 years, 6.6% in those aged 70–74 years and 9.5% in people aged 75 years and older (10).

With respect to longer-term follow-up, patient populations aged over 65 having undergone successful PTCA have shown surivival figures of 92% at 1 year, 86% at 3 years and 75% at 5 years (4). Other studies have confirmed these encouraging statistics (1,7,8). These figures are comparable with long-term survival following coronary bypass surgery.

When compared with patients under the age of 65 years, elderly patients have a greater incidence of multivessel disease, left main coronary artery disease and low left ventricular ejection fractions (less than 50%), as well as a history of hypertension and a higher proportion of women. These are all factors which increase the risk of PTCA, and when these are taken into account the relative risk of PTCA in patients over the age of 65 is reduced, when compared with patients under the age of 65, but still remains significant (1).

PERCUTANEOUS BALLOON VALVULOPLASTY

Percutaneous balloon valvuloplasty is the method of treating stenotic valve lesions whereby a balloon, introduced on the end of a catheter, is inflated across the affected valve, resulting in an increase in the orifice dimensions and the relief of the stenosis.

Mitral valvuloplasty

Mitral valvuloplasty was first reported by Inoue in 1984 (11). Since that time, percutaneous mitral balloon valvuloplasty has become an accepted technique which has success and mortality rates comparable with surgical valvulotomy in selected patients. The mechanism of this procedure centres around commissural splitting of the stenotic valve leaflets and, if present, fracturing of any nodular calcium deposits, although the latter mechanism is much less important (12).

Practical considerations

The most commonly used method for a percutaneous mitral balloon valvulo-plasty is the anterograde approach. Here, the femoral vein is cannulated and a guide wire inserted into the left atrium via a trans-septal route. The balloon catheter is then advanced over the guide wire and into the left atrium. At this point, heparin 100 units/kg is given intravenously. A pigtail catheter is then advanced from the femoral artery retrogradely into the left ventricle and the mitral valve gradient is measured. The balloon is then manipulated across the mitral valve orifice and the distal half inflated and gently withdrawn until some resistance is felt from the ventricular side of the stenotic mitral valve. The proximal portion of the balloon is then inflated quickly across the stenotic valve. The inflation time is usually of the order of 3 seconds (11,13).

The balloon catheter is then withdrawn across the atrial septum and left ventricular angiography performed through the pigtail catheter to assess the degree of resultant mitral regurgitation; oximetry measurements are then carried out to detect any left–right shunt across the atrial septum. The size of the balloon varies from 3 to 5 cm in length and from 18 to 25 mm inflated diameter. Single and double balloon techniques have been used (Figure 2).

Complications and outcome

Complications include embolic phenomena (including air embolus from balloon rupture), the creation of mitral regurgitation, transient conduction disturbances, the creation of an intra-atrial septal defect and pericardial effusion and tamponade secondary to cardiac perforation (11,12,24). Local complications of catheter insertions into the femoral artery and vein also occur.

The initial success rate of the procedure is high, with significant increase in mitral valve area (Figure 3), reduction of left atrial pressure and valve gradients, and increase in cardiac output seen in 85–95% of patients of all ages (14,15). The procedural mortality rate is low, and the incidence of restenosis is likely to be similar of that with surgical commissurotomy, e.g. with approximately 10% of patients requiring a repeat procedure in 5 years and 60% within 20 years (16).

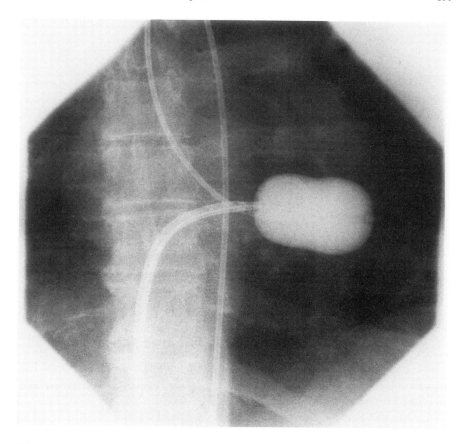

Figure 2. Mitral valvuloplasty balloon inflated across the mitral valve

Application to the elderly population

None of the present studies in percutaneous mitral balloon valvuloplasty have concentrated on the elderly population. In view of the relatively conservative nature of the procedure and the good success rates, mitral valvuloplasty would appear to be an excellent method of treating this condition; however, note must be taken of factors which have been known to influence the success of valvuloplasty as well as contraindications.

Suboptimal results (e.g. post-procedure mitral valve gradient of 10 mmHg or more) have been noted to occur in patients with severe mitral valve thickening, valvular calcification, involvement of the subvalvular mechanism and atrial fibrillation. Definite contraindications include left atrial thrombus and severe mitral regurgitation. It seems likely that these factors will be more prevalent in the older population in view of the fact that the disease has been present for a greater length of time and the condition is progressive.

This technique would therefore seem to be most applicable for patients with

(a)

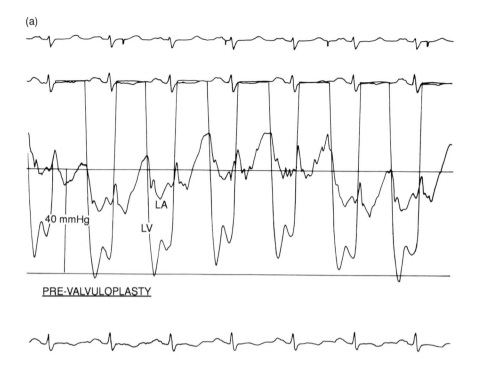

PRE-VALVULOPLASTY

Figure 3. Measurements of mitral valve gradient in a case of mitral stenosis: (a) pre- and (b) (opposite) post-balloon valvuloplasty

pliable non-calcified valve leaflets and no left atrial thrombus, or for those individuals with less than ideal valvular criteria, but whose general physical state makes them poor candidates for surgical treatment.

AORTIC BALLOON VALVULOPLASTY

This technique was first performed by Cribier in 1985. The indications for its use are still controversial. A major point of discussion is the application of aortic balloon valvuloplasty in the elderly population who are symptomatic but are considered unfit for open heart surgery due to cardiac or non-cardiac factors.

Method, mechanisms and considerations

The balloon is inserted across the aortic valve retrogradely, usually from the femoral artery (Figure 4). During the procedure, the balloon is inflated one to three times and the peak-to-peak aortic valve gradient monitored (calculated by the Gorlin continuity equation or the simpler Hakki equation). The mechanism

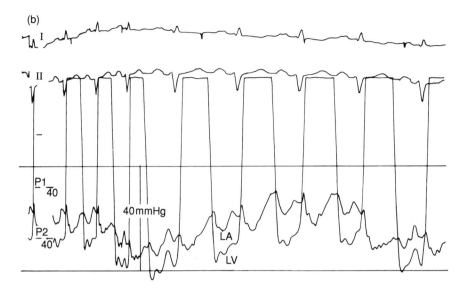

(b)

POST-VALVULOPLASTY

behind the procedure is thought to be due to the stretching of the aortic valve ring and fracturing of the calcified skeleton of the valve (17). This is in marked contrast to the predominant commissural stretching of mitral valvuloplasty.

Analysis of the initial reduction and aortic valve gradient (Figure 5) and increasing orifice diameters is encouraging (18,19), with corresponding improvement in ejection fraction and NYHA status (19,26). The in-hospital procedural mortality is significant, as is the occurrence of rapid restenosis; in one study of 44 patients (mean age 77.8 years), 10 had died and 15 had undergone aortic valve replacement for worsening NYHA status within 15.5 months after the procedure (19). Another study done with follow-up catheterization found that most of the benefit of valvuloplasty had been lost within 8 days (20). The longer-term mortality data also helped to put the procedure in perspective, with 28% mortality at 6 months and 65% mortality at 1 year in one series (21).

The mechanism behind valvular restenosis after aortic balloon valvuloplasty is not known, but it is likely to be determined by the intrinsic architecture of the stenotic valve (27). This is supported by the observation that more frequent complications occur when valvuloplasty is performed on a bicuspid valve (28–30) than when aortic stenosis is due to commissural fusion (31).

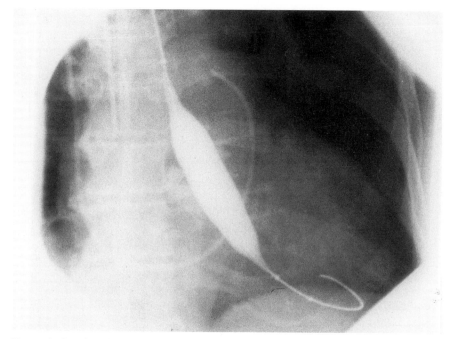

Figure 4. Aortic valvuloplasty balloon inflated across the aortic valve

Application of percutaneous aortic balloon valvuloplasty in the elderly

In view of the early deterioration of benefit shown in elderly patients after aortic balloon valvuloplasty, the procedure cannot be looked upon as a viable long-term treatment for aortic stenosis in this group, although there is still discussion about this point (22). Aortic valvuloplasty has been used in patients with severe aortic stenosis as a method of relieving the gradient to enable general anaesthesia for emergency non-cardiac surgery (23,24) or as a 'bridging' procedure in a compromised patient awaiting definitive treatment for aortic stenosis, i.e. aortic valve replacement.

ECONOMIC FACTORS IN INTERVENTIONAL TECHNIQUES

The economic considerations for interventional procedures at first appear to be attractive. The techniques require less time in hospital, generally only local anaesthesic and less hospital staff than the corresponding surgical treatment. However, against this must be considered the possibility of emergency surgery in the event of serious complications occurring as well as the cost of repeat procedures due to recurrence of the original condition, which is an important feature of both PTCA and percutaneous valvuloplasty.

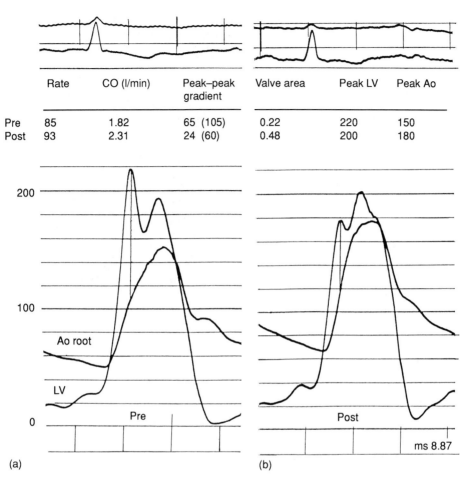

	Rate	CO (l/min)	Peak–peak gradient	Valve area	Peak LV	Peak Ao
Pre	85	1.82	65 (105)	0.22	220	150
Post	93	2.31	24 (60)	0.48	200	180

(a) (b)

Figure 5. Measurements of aortic valve gradients in a case of aortic stenosis: (a) pre- and (b) post-balloon valvuloplasty

Patients over the age of 65 years with cardiac disease are considered to have a poor prognosis with respect to outcome from interventional techniques when compared with patients under 65 years. Comparison of patients over 65 years treated with interventional methods against age-matched patients treated more conservatively for similar conditions may reveal a more striking survival benefit amongst the elderly patients managed aggressively.

Approximately one-fifth of health care costs in the elderly are incurred in the last 6 months of an individual's life. Any method which might prevent the complications of disease, e.g. PTCA relieving myocardial ischaemia and preventing myocardial infarction and heart failure, could be seen as economically as well as symptomatically beneficial (25).

Until further trials are performed using a greater number of elderly patients, there is little clear data to act as guidance. In the meantime, indications for the applications of interventional techniques must rely upon clinical assessment as to the relevance of these methods, rather than predicted economic advantages.

REFERENCES

1. Kelsey S, Miller D, Holubkov R et al. (1990) Results of percutaneous transluminal angioplasty in patients 65 years of age (from the 1985 to 1986 National Heart, Lung and Blood Institute's Coronary Angioplasty Registry). Am J Cardiol 66: 1033–1038.
2. Block P (1984) Mechanism of transluminal angioplasty. Am J Cardiol 53: 69C–71C.
3. Shiu M (1989) Interventional cardiac catheterisation: transluminal angioplasty. In Diseases of the Heart, Julian DG, Camm AJ, Fox KM, Hall R, Poole-Wilson PA (eds). Ballière Tindall, London, pp. 403–404.
4. Bedotto J, Rutherford B, McConahay DK et al. (1991) Result of multivessel percutaneous transluminal coronary angioplasty in persons aged 65 years and older. Am J Cardiol 67: 1051–1055.
5. Gruntzig A (1978) Transluminal dilatation of coronary artery stenosis. Lancet i: 263.
6. Kowalchuk G, Siu S, Lewis S (1990) Coronary artery disease in the octogenarian: angiographic spectrum and suitability for revascularization. Am J Cardiol 66: 1319–1323.
7. Thompson R, Holmes D, Gesh E et al. (1991) Percutaneous transluminal coronary angioplasty in the elderly: early and long-term results. J Am Coll Cardiol 17: 1245–1250.
8. Jackman J, Avetta F, Smith J et al. (1991) Percutaneous transluminal coronary angioplasty in octogenarians as an effective therapy for angina pectoris. Am J Cardiol 68: 116–119.
9. Leimgruber P, Roubin G, Anderson H et al. (1985) Influence of intimal dissection on restenosis after successful coronary angioplasty. Circulation 72: 530–535.
10. Gersh B, Kronmal R, Frye R et al. (1983) Coronary arteriography and coronary artery bypass surgery: morbidity and mortality in patients aged 65 years and older. Circulation 67: 483–491.
11. Inoue K, Owaki T, Nakamua T et al. (1984) Clinical application of transvenous mitral commissurotomy by a new balloon catheter. J Thorac Cardiovasc Surg 87: 394–402.
12. McKay R, Lock J, Safian R et al. (1987) Balloon dilation of mitral stenosis in adult patients: postmortem and percutaneous mitral valvuloplasty studies. J Am Coll Cardiol 9: 723–731.
13. Strauss B (1990) Percutaneous valvuloplasty as a treatment for aortic and mitral valve disease. Am Heart J 119: 1184–1192.
14. Levine M, Berman A, Safian R et al. (1988) Palliation of valvular aortic stenosis by balloon valvuloplasty as preoperative preparation for noncardiac surgery. Am J Cardiol 62: 1309–1310.
15. Palacios I, Block P, Wilkins G, Weymon A (1989) Follow up of patients undergoing percutaneous mitral balloon valvotomy: analysis of factors determining re-stenosis. Circulation 79: 573–579.
16. Ellis L, Singh J, Morales D, Harken D (1973) Fifteen to twenty five year study of one thousand patients undergoing closed mitral valvuloplasty. Circulation 48: 357–364.
17. Beatt K (1989) Balloon dilatation of the aortic valve in adults: a physician's view. Br Heart J 63: 207–208.
18. Letac B, Cribier A, Koning R, Lefebvre E (1989) Aortic stenosis in elderly patients aged 80 years or older: treatment by percutaneous balloon valvuloplasty in a series of

92 cases. *Circulation* **80**: 1514–1520.

19. Rodriguez A, Kleiman N, Minor S *et al.* (1990) Factors influencing the outcome of balloon aortic valvuloplasty in the elderly. *Am Heart J* **120**: 373–380.
20. Commeau P, Grollier G, Lamy E *et al.* (1988) Percutaneous balloon dilatation of calcified aortic valve stenosis: anatomical and haemodynamic evaluation. *Br Heart J* **59**: 227–238.
21. Sherman W, Hershman R, Lazzam C *et al.* (1989) Balloon valvuloplasty in adult aortic stenosis: determinants of clinical outcome. *Ann Intern Med* **110**: 421–425.
22. Cheitlin M (1989) Severe aortic stenosis in the sick octogenarian: a clear indicator for balloon valvuloplasty as the initial procedure. *Circulation* **80**: 1906–1908.
23. Roth R, Palacios I, Block P (1989) Percutaneous aortic balloon valvuloplasty: its role in the management of patients with aortic stenosis requiring major non-cardiac surgery. *J Am Coll Cardiol* **13**: 1039–1041.
24. Bassand JP, Schiele F, Bernard Y *et al.* (1991) The double balloon and Inoue techniques in percutaneous mitral valvuloplasty: comparative results in a series of 232 cases. *J Am Coll Cardiol* **18**: 982–989.
25. Yusuf S, Furberg C (1991) Are we biased in our approach to treating elderly patients with heart disease? *Am J Cardiol* **68**: 954–956.
26. Safian RD, Berman AD, Diver DJ *et al.* (1988) Balloon aortic valvuloplasty in 170 consecutive patients. *N Engl J Med* **319**: 125–130.
27. Bashore TM, Davidson DF (1991) Follow-up recatheterisation after balloon aortic valvuloplasty. *J Am Coll Cardiol* **17**: 1188–1195.
28. Kennedy KD, Hauck AF, Edwards WD *et al.* (1988) Mechanism of reduction of aortic valvular stenosis by percutaneous transluminal balloon valvuloplasty: report of five cases and review of literature. *Mayo Clin Proc* **63**: 769–776.
29. Davidson CT, Skelton TN, Kisslo KB *et al.* (1988) The risk for systemic embolisation associated with percutaneous balloon valvuloplasty in adults: a prospective comprehensive evaluation. *Ann Intern Med* **108**: 557–560.
30. Isner JM, Salem DN, Desnoyners MR *et al.* (1989) Treatment of calcific aortic stenosis by balloon valvuloplasty. *Am J Cardiol* **59**: 313–317.
31. Medina A, Bethencourt A, Coello I *et al.* (1989) Combined percutaneous mitral and aortic balloon valvuloplasty. *Am J Cardiol* **64**: 620–624.

31 Fitness for Anaesthesia and Surgery in the Elderly Cardiac Patient

MICHAEL W. PLATT AND R. M. JONES
St Mary's Hospital Medical School, London, UK

As the general age of the population increases, the proportion of the surgical population aged over 65 years is expanding (1). In this age group only some 15% can be described as 'physiologically normal' with respect to haemodynamic, respiratory and renal function (2). The increase in perioperative mortality and morbidity in the elderly reflects the importance of these age-related physiological changes as well as the increased incidence of coexisting medical disease and associated drug therapy. In the UK in 1986, a combined surgical and anaesthetic working party examined all deaths occurring within 30 days of operation in three regional health authorities (3). The overall mortality was 0.7%, in some half million operations. Three-quarters of deaths were in patients over 70 years of age who made up only 22% of the surgical population in England and Wales in 1986. The majority of deaths occurred within 2 weeks of operation. Twenty-one per cent of deaths occurred following emergency (immediate) surgery and 40% occurred following urgent surgery (within 24 hours).

A recent multi-centre study of general anaesthesia in the USA attempted to identify and quantify independent predictors of severe perioperative adverse outcomes (4). Significant predictors of any severe outcome as well as death included the following: a history of myocardial infarction or cardiac failure within the previous year; ASA (American Society of Anesthesiologists) physical status 3 or 4 (Table 1) (5,6); age more than 50 years; cardiovascular, thoracic or neurological surgery; and type of anaesthetic used. Significant predictors for severe cardiovascular outcomes included: history of ventricular arrhythmia; hypertension; cardiac failure; myocardial ischaemia; myocardial infarction within the previous year; myocardial infarction more than 1 year previously plus smoking; ASA physical status; age; type of surgery; and type of anaesthetic.

These observations reinforce the conclusion that patients who are both elderly and with a significant history of cardiac disease present an appreciably increased risk during surgery.

Geriatric Cardiology. Principles and Practice. Edited by A. Martin and A. J. Camm
© 1994 John Wiley & Sons Ltd

Table 1. The American Society of Anesthesiologists classification of preoperative status

ASA I:	Healthy patient
ASA II:	Mild systemic disease with no functional limitation
ASA III:	Severe systemic disease with functional limitation
ASA IV:	Systemic disease that is a constant threat to life
ASA V:	Moribund patient not expected to survive more than 24 hours

It is not age alone which results in a higher morbidity and mortality, but the effects of ageing on the physiological processes of different organ systems, and how these depleted processes react to surgery and anaesthesia (7). The respiratory and cardiovascular systems are the most important systems in this regard, particularly in the immediate perioperative period. It is probable that 25–50% of all perioperative deaths (involving non-cardiac surgery), independent of age group, are directly related to the cardiovascular system (8). In the USA approximately 25% of patients aged over 65 have profound functional abnormalities of the cardiac or respiratory system, refractory to treatment, which may result in perioperative death (2). It is probable that some 5% of perioperative deaths in the elderly are as a result of advanced neoplasia and not to complications of surgery and anaesthesia (9). Pringle (10) looked at the outcome in a prospective study of 505 elderly patients admitted to a general surgical unit. He suggests that a new system of audit should be used to account for 'potentially viable' and 'non-viable' patients in this age group. When this system was applied to the study there was a significant decrease in the overall mortality from 14.5% to 3.6%; from 12% to 5.8% for major operations; from 6.1% to 0% for minor operations; and from 24.3% to 2.0% for those who had no surgery. It is clear from these figures that the mortality and morbidity from anaesthesia and surgery in the elderly patient with cardiac disease depend very much on the general physiological status of the patient.

PHYSIOLOGICAL EFFECTS OF AGEING, RELATED TO ANAESTHESIA AND SURGERY

Surgery and anaesthesia set a major burden on the performance of organ systems in the body. The physiological infrastructure must be capable of dealing with the stress of trauma and surgery, making use of its reserve capacity, this being greater in the younger than the older patient. As a general guide it has been estimated that over the age of 30 many physiological functions deteriorate at the rate of about 1% per year, but because of innate differences in reserve capacity some organ systems will fare worse than others.

The elderly patient, with a cardiac output capable of coping with a low skeletal muscle mass and low basal metabolic rate, may not have sufficient reserve capacity to cope with the stress response of surgery, or the complications of hypovolaemia, drug-induced hypotension, hypertension or hypoxia. A number of factors combine to cause a decrease in cardiovascular fitness (7): arteriosclerosis causes a decrease in arterial elasticity; increasing peripheral vascular resistance may result in ventricular hypertrophy, contributing to myocardial ischaemia and decreased ventricular compliance; fibrosis of the myocardium and conducting system occurs, together with calcification of valves and atherosclerosis of the coronary arteries; and, along with reductions of heart rate and cardiac output, the sympathetic nervous system response may be blunted, probably due to a reduction in adrenergic receptor density and some element of general autonomic dysfunction. Patients with a combined decrease in cardiovascular and respiratory reserve are at particular risk.

In the lungs, anatomical modifications occur with loss of lung elastin and a reduction of alveolar membrane surface area. A decline in chest wall and lung compliance also occurs, contributing to effects on the rate and depth of ventilation. All these changes lead to an increase in residual and closing volumes of the lung, as well as reduced vital capacity and functional residual capacity. These changes are particularly relevant to anaesthesia, as both general and regional anaesthesia tend to cause a further decline in functional residual capacity and an increase in closing volume. In either event the net effect is a widening of the alveolar–arterial oxygen difference and a decrease in oxygenation. The energy component of the work of breathing also tends to increase in the elderly, causing a rise in oxygen consumption. The combination of lung and cardiovascular changes exaggerates ventilation–perfusion inequalities, contributing further to diminished oxygen content of arterial blood—a factor of special significance to the anaesthetist. With these pre-existing conditions, little is required to precipitate major physiological decompensation, for example an acute chest infection. Any such intercurrent chest disease must be adequately treated preoperatively—and lung function optimized before surgery.

Reduced renal blood flow and diminished renal function are reflected in an impaired ability of the kidneys to handle water and sodium loads, and their decreased efficiency at clearing drugs and metabolites from plasma. There is progressive reduction in renal plasma flow, renal tubular function and glomerular filtration rate as age increases. Perioperative renal insufficiency is commonly seen after major aortic and cardiac surgery, or associated with hepatic failure, septicaemia and multiple organ failure. Renal protection (in the form of adequate hydration, osmotic diuretics and dopaminergic agonists such as dopamine or dopexamine) is usually started preoperatively or intraoperatively in order to minimize postoperative deterioration of renal function in high-risk cases. In addition, the use of nephrotoxic drugs, such as aminoglycoside antibiotics, should be avoided if possible.

Gastrointestinal function in this age group can be compromised by intercurrent disease. Peritonitis is more likely to occur (2.6% of general surgical patients), and is likely to be silent (11). The commonest causes are mesenteric infarction and viscus perforation secondary to gastric or duodenal ulceration, or to diverticulosis. The patient should be stabilized and resuscitated as a matter of urgency before any surgery or anaesthetic intervention.

Hepatic microsomal and non-microsomal enzyme function in the elderly is usually not compromised. However, liver function may be affected due to reduced hepatic mass and blood flow. This may affect drug metabolism and excretion, so drug dosage and frequency of administration need to be regularly monitored. Drugs used in anaesthesia, such as non-depolarizing muscle relaxants and opioids, may be particularly affected.

The half-life of lipid-soluble drugs is affected in the elderly, mainly as a result of changes in the body habitus. There is an increase in the lipid fraction, with a reduction in skeletal muscle mass; plasma proteins such as albumin are reduced; and there is reduced bone density due to osteoporosis. A diminished metabolic rate and reduced oxygen consumption, in addition to the above changes, result in thermoregulation being adversely affected. Attempts should be made to minimize heat loss perioperatively with the use of insulating and heat-reflective blankets, as well as a warming mattress, warming coils for intravenous infusions, and warming and humidification of inspired gases while anaesthetized. Loss of heat during surgery can decrease the core body temperature to levels at which ventricular fibrillation is more likely to occur. In addition, drug action may be potentiated by cold, for example the non-depolarizing muscle relaxants.

Reduced immunological and endocrinological system function leads to an increased incidence of perioperative infection and a decreased ability to mount a stress response to the surgery, which may influence the healing process (especially with respect to release of interleukins, inflammatory mediators and tissue growth factors). Anaesthesia reversibly downgrades immune function, and can ablate the stress response, aggravating the preoperative immune status of the patient.

Cerebral disease, acute or chronic, is a relatively common problem in this age group. Underlying causes of acute confusional states and delirium should be treated as a matter of urgency before surgery. Some of the commoner causes include sepsis, acid–base imbalance, metabolic upset, drugs and hypoxia. Atrophic changes with age tend to cause a reduction in brain size and weight, and sensitivity to noxious stimuli tends to decrease with age. Stroke occurs more commonly in general surgical patients of this age group. The incidence is difficult to assess, because there is commonly no obvious neurological deficit, except to fine neurobehavioural testing. Perioperative stroke tends to present within the first 2 weeks of operation. Factors predisposing to stroke in the elderly include hypertension, arteriosclerosis and peripheral vascular disease (especially carotid artery occlusion), and cervical spondylosis. The perioperative avoidance of extremes of blood pressure changes, careful positioning of the patient during surgery and care with the head and neck during laryngoscopy will help to minimize the effects of surgery and anaesthesia on brain blood flow. Parkinson's disease tends to worsen following anaesthesia and surgery, and adequate control should be maintained up to the time of operation. Postoperatively, the patient should be carefully monitored and drug therapy altered as necessary to control the disease.

Even minor changes in patterns of regional blood flow through different organs, as a result of the stress of surgery and anaesthesia, can be significant. For example, transiently reduced renal blood flow may precipitate renal failure in an elderly patient with diminished renal function. A significant decrease in cerebral or coronary blood flow may cause severe morbidity and obviously is more likely to be fatal. Generally, anaesthesia and surgery tend to adversely affect all elderly organ systems, and test their reserve capacities.

PREOPERATIVE ASSESSMENT AND PREPARATION OF THE ELDERLY PATIENT WITH CARDIAC DISEASE AND SOME SPECIFIC CONSIDERATIONS

Generally, the elderly cardiac patient should undergo anaesthesia and surgery in the most optimal physiological state. Unless surgery needs to be performed immediately to be life-saving (even here, adequate resuscitation measures should be performed first), it should be delayed where possible for appropriate treatment of intercurrent illness. Examples include acute respiratory infection, uncontrolled cardiac failure, untreated hypertension and uncontrolled diabetes mellitus.

History

In addition to basic information such as anaesthetic, family and relevant past medical history, a detailed review of the patient's history should include indications of organ function relating especially to cardiac, respiratory, renal, cerebral and hepatic performance.

Factors relating specifically to the elderly patient with cardiac disease include the following:

1. An assessment of cardiac function and associated disease state. For example, the adequacy of control of arrhythmias and cardiac failure.
2. History of recent myocardial infarction; an infarction in the 6 months before surgery carries a particularly high risk.
3. History of angina, including any worsening of symptoms, particularly unstable angina.
4. Exercise tolerance—especially cardiac-related limitations.
5. Many of these patients are also hypertensive, usually with essential hypertension which is often associated with significant arteriosclerosis (especially with systolic hypertension), but sometimes secondary to renal disease. Antihypertensive treatment should be maintained (or commenced and continued) up to surgery to minimize the effects of anaesthesia and surgery on blood pressure lability.

6. A full history of medication requirements should be obtained. Drug therapy needs to be reviewed before surgery and maintained throughout the period of operation, particularly if it is to control cardiac arrhythmias or hypertension. Anticoagulant therapy should be reviewed, and adjusted prior to surgery. Oral anticoagulants should be stopped at least 3 days before surgery, and if continued anticoagulation is essential heparin therapy should be instituted; anticoagulation can be promptly reversed with protamine if this becomes necessary. Aspirin, because of its irreversible effect on platelet function, should probably be stopped 10 days before major surgery if the bleeding time is significantly prolonged, to allow the growth of normal platelets and the development of a normal bleeding time. However, evidence is mounting that aprotinin, a protease inhibitor, can reverse these effects of aspirin.

Specialized investigations

Elderly cardiac patients in particular need a thorough preoperative assessment which will include certain specialized investigations. Chest X-ray, electrocardiogram (ECG), baseline biochemistry and haematology values should be available. Many elderly patients, particularly cardiac patients, take diuretic drugs, emphasizing the importance of basic biochemical tests—especially plasma potassium and magnesium concentrations. Anaemia can be insidious in onset, and haemoglobin estimation is important. A haemoglobin concentration of less than 8 g/dl may mean a doubling of cardiac output to maintain an adequate tissue oxygen delivery, resulting in an increase in myocardial work.

More specialized investigations may be indicated in this group of patients. Exercise stress testing, now refined to improve interpretation, may be a useful non-invasive diagnostic test for patients with atypical angina, but is obviously contraindicated in the presence of suspected myocardial infarction or unstable angina.

Echocardiography is now easily done by the bedside and is non-invasive. Echocardiography can visualize ventricular and atrial function, including estimation of ejection fraction. Gradients across narrowed valves and outlets can also be assessed. Knowledge of left ventricular performance is particularly useful in patients with a poor cardiac history.

Coronary angiography is commonly performed to assess patients for coronary bypass surgery. It gives more definitive information on coronary flow, obstruction and collateral flow. Some patients may present for non-cardiac surgery prior to having coronary artery bypass surgery, for example for carotid endarterectomy. In these cases it is important to fully assess cardiac function and its limitations in terms of withstanding surgery and anaesthesia.

Arrhythmias

Perioperatively, haemodynamic, fluid, electrolyte and acid–base disorders all contribute to myocardial irritability. To contain risk, pre-existing arrhythmias

Table 2. Vaughan Williams' classification of antiarrhythmic drugs

Class Ia:	Quinidine, procainamide, diisopyramide
Class Ib:	Lignocaine, mexilitine, tocainide
Class Ic:	Flecainide
Class II:	β-Adrenergic antagonists
Class III:	Amiodarone, sotalol, bretilium
Class IV:	Calcium antagonists

should be controlled before the imposition of surgical and anaesthetic stress.

Sinus bradycardia or tachycardia (less than 50 beats/min or greater than 120 beats/min) should be treated appropriately, according to probable cause. Sinus node disease ('sick sinus syndrome', 'tachycardia–bradycardia syndrome') should be treated by implantation of a demand pacemaker—especially if major surgery is proposed. Tachyarrhythmias may need to be controlled with appropriate drug therapy. These patients are often anticoagulated to control potential thromboembolism, and may need to be changed to heparin for surgery.

Atrial fibrillation or flutter is a relatively common supraventricular arrhythmia. Prophylaxis may be required with the use of Vaughan Williams' class Ia, Ic or class III antiarrhythmic drugs (see Table 2). If cardioversion fails, the ventricular rate should be controlled with the use of atrioventricular (AV) nodal blocking drugs such as digoxin. Anticoagulant therapy will again need to be adjusted for surgery, and probably changed to heparin.

Paroxysmal atrial tachycardia, atrial tachycardia with AV conduction block, or chronic atrial tachycardia should be controlled and prevented with class Ia, Ic or III drugs.

First- and second-degree AV block usually require no specific treatment, as long as the anaesthetist is aware and prepared to treat possible complications intraoperatively. Patients with third-degree block should always have a pacemaker inserted before any form of surgery.

Junctional tachycardia can be a difficult problem for the anaesthetist. There are two types of re-entrant junctional tachycardia: intra-AV nodal, in which the re-entrant circuit is entirely in the AV node and its surrounding myocardium; and AV, in which the circuit is large, encompassing the AV node and the bundle of His, with the ventricle and the atrium connected by an abnormal connection. Both may be controlled and prevented with the use of drugs that impair AV nodal conduction (classes II and IV and digoxin), impair abnormal conduction (classes Ia and III), or suppress initiation of the arrhythmia by suppressing abnormal beats (drugs from classes I, II and III). These types of arrhythmias should be controlled prophylactically preoperatively.

Patients with Wolff–Parkinson–White syndrome, a re-entrant tachycardia caused by an abnormal connection between atrium and ventricle (bundle of Kent), should be given appropriate prophylactic therapy as above before surgery.

Intraventricular conduction disturbances such as His bundle delay, bundle branch conduction delay and bundle branch block cause few problems during surgery. However, it is often recommended that for His bundle conduction block (producing AV block) and bifascicular block a pacemaker is inserted prior to surgery. Notwithstanding this, most studies suggest that the prophylactic insertion of a transvenous pacemaker in an asymptomatic patient with combined right bundle branch block and left anterior hemiblock is not necessary (10).

Of the four main types of ventricular tachyarrhythmias, only ventricular premature beats are likely to be present in a patient presenting for surgery. Ventricular tachycardia, fibrillation and *torsades des pointes* are usually associated with patients who are unlikely to present for surgery untreated. Frequent ventricular premature beats (more than five per minute on the preoperative ECG), those that occur on preceding 'R' waves ('R-on-T'), runs of two or more beats, and bigeminal or multifocal premature beats are more serious than occasional ectopic beats. In the presence of myocardial ischaemia, ventricular premature beats are also sinister. Before surgery, prophylaxis and control should be achieved with drugs from classes I, II or III.

Ventricle and valve function

It is vitally important that ventricular function is optimized prior to surgery. Disordered left ventricular function is strongly implicated in the poor prognosis of patients with ischaemic heart disease (14). Patients with evidence of ventricular impairment should be treated without delay. A combination of rest, removal of precipitating factors (such as infection, infarction, arrhythmias, anaemia and fluid overload) and drug therapy as appropriate should be instigated, provided the time is available. If urgent surgery is necessary, control of cardiac failure should be achieved as much as possible with intravenous drug therapy prior to anaesthesia.

For those patients with evidence of coronary insufficiency, nitrates should be commenced, if not already being administered. These can be administered topically by dermal patches, intravenously or sublingually.

Patients with valvular heart disease exposed to anaesthesia and surgery are at high risk of cardiac failure, arrhythmias, infective endocarditis and embolic phenomena (8). As with ventricular disease, which usually accompanies severe valve disease, patients with serious impairment of cardiac reserve will tolerate surgery poorly. Patients with significant aortic or mitral stenosis are particularly prone to sudden death or acute left ventricular failure during the perioperative period. Those patients with severe stenotic or regurgitant valve disease should probably undergo valve surgery before an elective operation. Significant aortic valve disease may encompass the coronary sinuses, and coronary insufficiency can be aggravated.

All patients with valve or other mechanical disease of the heart should have prophylactic antibiotic cover prior to surgery, especially dental, genitourinary or intestinal surgery.

The cardiomyopathies present a particularly difficult problem for the anaesthetist. There are three types: hypertrophic (including hypertrophic obstructive, HOCM), dilated (formerly known as congestive), and restrictive/obliterative cardiomyopathy. In the UK the two commoner types are dilated and hypertrophic (usually presenting as HOCM). Patients known to have a cardiomyopathy should be aggressively monitored perioperatively, and ventricular filling pressures optimized to reduce risks of haemodynamic decompensation. Those with hypertrophic cardiomyopathy with a ventricle of low compliance are intolerant of hypovolaemia (or peripheral vasodilation), which results in a reduction of the high preload necessary to maintain ventricular filling. In those patients with HOCM, sudden increases in ventricular contractility may cause increasing outlet obstruction, requiring the administration of a β-receptor antagonist. Dilated cardiomyopathy, if aggravated, may respond to treatment with inotropic agents. The cardiomyopathies carry a grave prognosis, and represent a rare cause of sudden death perioperatively.

Assessment of perioperative risk

The assessment of fitness for surgery is a complex consideration and should include not only a thorough history, examination and investigation, but also the application of risk probability based on known data. The simplest qualitative system, developed specifically for surgery, is the ASA's physical status (5,6) rating scale shown in Table 1. This index is a measure of the physiological state of the patient according to the degree of illness and whether the surgery is an emergency. If the operation is an emergency, the letter 'E' is placed after the status number. This classification takes no account of any specific preoperative factors such as age, specific disease states or type of operation. It is not intended to be a predictor of outcome, but has been used as a crude measure of preoperative physical status for over 50 years.

Perioperative risk can also be assessed with the use of predictors to calculate overall risk. The best known quantitative example of the latter is Goldman's risk evaluation for perioperative cardiac complications (12,13). Goldman and colleagues (12,13), found nine specific factors that were successfully used to predict operation outcome. Seven of the nine factors relate to cardiac function and fitness of the patient, the other two being related to the type of operation. Each factor is weighted with a number of points, according to its weight as a predictor of adverse outcome:

1. Gallop rhythm (S3), or evidence of raised central venous pressure, during preoperative visit.   11 points
2. Myocardial infarction within 6 months.   10 points
3. Arrhythmias on preoperative ECG (not sinus or premature atrial contractions).   7 points
4. More than five ventricular premature beats per minute documented at any time preoperatively.   7 points
5. Age over 70 years.   5 points

6. Aortic stenosis.   3 points
7. Any of the following, suggesting poor organ function:
   $PaO_2 < 8\,kPa$, or $PaCO_2 > 6.7\,kPa$*
   serum bicarbonate $< 20\,mmol/l$
   serum urea $> 18\,mmol/l$
   serum creatinine $> 265\,\mu mol/l$
   signs of chronic liver disease
   bedridden from any cause.   3 points
8. Intraperitoneal, intrathoracic or aortic operations.   3 points
9. Emergency operations.   4 points

The points are added, producing a cardiac risk index for each patient. Goldman's group recognized four categories of patient:

   Class 1: score 0–5   lowest risk
   Class 2: score 6–12
   Class 3: score 13–25
   Class 4: score > 26   highest risk†

The risk of perioperative reinfarction decreases with time following a previous myocardial infarction. The best-known study is Tarhan *et al.* (15), who studied the risks of reinfarction during the first postoperative week. If operation is performed within 3 months of infarction, some 37% of patients will reinfarct. If the operation occurs within 6 months, but more than 3 months, 16% of patients will tend to reinfarct. Over 1 year, the risk decreases to less than 1%. The mortality of perioperative reinfarction was 54%, with 80% of deaths occurring within 48 hours of the myocardial infarction. This study was performed in a mixed age group patient population and the risks in the elderly can be expected to be greater.

Rao *et al.* (16) and Wells and Kaplan (17) showed that if high-risk patients are aggressively managed perioperative mortality decreases significantly. Their patients were admitted to intensive care units prior to surgery and invasive monitoring was instigated, especially pulmonary artery flow-directed catheterization. Haemodynamic variables were controlled within tight limits, and cardiac output and oxygen delivery optimized. Both stress the importance of all patients remaining in intensive care with full invasive monitoring for at least 3 days postoperatively, this being the most likely time interval for serious postoperative complications (15).

General preparation and premedication of the patient

With myocardial factors under adequate control, other organ systems should also be optimized during the preoperative preparation of the patient. Ventilation

---

* PaO_2, arterial oxygen tension; $PcCO_2$, arterial carbon dioxide tension.
† Three-quarters of these patients suffered life-threatening cardiac complications postoperatively, (half these dying). Of the above factors, several are avoidable or treatable.

and gas exchange should be the best possible for the patient (bearing in mind that many of these patients have coexisting chest disease). As mentioned above, the patient should be well hydrated and nourished, with optimal renal and hepatic function.

Premedication will include those drugs required to maintain cardiac function and control blood pressure and symptoms of angina pectoris. For example, in addition to sedation, a nitrate for cutaneous administration may be prescribed to help maintain coronary perfusion. Drugs such as warfarin or aspirin should be stopped, or substituted for reversible agents as discussed, in time for function to be restored, if possible.

Patients at very high risk of perioperative mortality are often admitted to intensive care preoperatively. Here, they can be invasively monitored and cardiac preload and afterload tightly controlled. They can then be monitored post-operatively, in the same controlled conditions. This has been shown to improve mortality, but is expensive (15,16).

INTRAOPERATIVE MANAGEMENT

Patients may have general or local anaesthesia depending on the surgical procedure. In the majority of cases, those with cardiac problems are better managed under general anaesthesia. Under general anaesthesia, response to stress is better controlled, airway and oxygenation are optimized, and the patient, being unconscious, has no anxiety. Regional procedures carry the risk of hypotension associated with sympathetic blockade and the presence of any anxiety will tend to increase systemic arterial blood pressure and thus increase myocardial oxygen demand. Combined regional and general anaesthesia may be employed, having the advantage of providing optimum postoperative anal-gesia—especially administering opioids by epidural catheter after appropriate procedures.

General anaesthesia for elderly patients with cardiac disease will generally consist of those agents shown to have minimal effects on cardiac function. Since most anaesthetic agents depress myocardial function, they are given sparingly and titrated carefully against patient response. Sodium thiopentone is still the most commonly used agent for induction of anaesthesia, although etomidate is sometimes used as it better maintains cardiac output. However, it is not used routinely as it can cause pain on injection. Of the non-depolarizing muscle relaxants, vecuronium has least effect on the cardiovascular system. Pan-curonium is a chronotropic agent, and may increase blood pressure by its effect of releasing nonadrenaline from sympathetic nerve endings. Its use is relatively contraindicated in patients with ischaemic heart disease. Atracurium, although it causes some histamine release, is especially easy to reverse at the end of surgery and thus is widely used, as significant residual paralysis is a major cause of postoperative morbidity. For maintenance, the volatile agent of choice is generally held to be isoflurane, as it causes the least myocardial depression, has the least effect on splanchnic blood flow, and has minimal effects on cardiac rhythm. A background of nitrous oxide gas is often administered to aid anaesthesia and provide additional analgesia. Opioid supplementation is often used to reduce volatile agent requirements and to blunt the stress response, especially for laryngoscopy, but postoperative recovery may be delayed, depending on drug-handling ability.

Minimal standards of monitoring, which include blood pressure, ECG, pulse oximetry and end-tidal carbon dioxide, will generally be used. Depending on the type of surgery, and the state of the patient, more invasive monitoring, including an indwelling arterial cannula (for blood gas analysis as well as real-time measurement of arterial blood pressure), central venous pressure monitoring, and perhaps pulmonary artery pressure, wedge pressure, cardiac output and mixed venous oxygen saturation, may be used. Heat loss is a common problem in the elderly, and core temperature should be monitored, ideally by way of a tympanic membrane probe. As mentioned earlier, heat loss can be minimized with the use of blankets, heat-reflective sheets and warming mattresses, together with warming and humidification of inspired gases and warming of intravenous infusions.

Inotropic, chronotropic and antihypertensive drugs will be used as necessary to maintain cardiac output and blood pressure within acceptable limits. Prophylactic or regular antibiotics will be given as prescribed, particularly during surgery involving the genitourinary system, gut, dental procedures, or infective disease such as abscess drainage. As described above, this is particularly important for those patients with cardiac valve disease or who otherwise need prophylaxis for infective endocarditis.

POSTOPERATIVE RECOVERY

Postoperatively, patients are more likely to die within the first week, particularly in this age group (3). The likely contributing factors (apart from terminal disease for which surgery was unsuccessful), discussed at length above, include hypoxia, myocardial infarction and cardiac arrhythmias.

Adequate postoperative monitoring of cardiac and general physiological status, during the ensuing postoperative days, will give early warning of the onset of complications and help to decrease the morbidity and mortality of patients. The use of pulse oximetry on surgical wards postoperatively could help to identify those at risk of hypoxia—especially during sleep and the onset of sleep apnoea, which is common in this age group. Ideally, ECG and blood pressure should be monitored for at least 5 days postoperatively, but this is often impracticable on understaffed, under-equipped wards, although admission to coronary care may be appropriate in cases with cardiac instability.

CONCLUSION

The elderly cardiac patient is at an increased risk when undergoing even minor surgery, and efforts should be made to ensure that adequate preoperative preparation, perioperative management, and postoperative observation and treatment are all to high standards. Admission to coronary or intensive care may be appropriate both pre- and postoperatively, in the especially high-risk patient.

* PaO$_2$, arterial oxygen tension; PcCO$_2$, arterial carbon dioxide tension.
† Three-quarters of these patients suffered life-threatening cardiac complications postoperatively, half of these dying). Of the above factors, several are avoidable or treatable.

REFERENCES

1. Muravchick S (1981) Anaesthesia for the elderly. In *Anesthesia*, Vol. 2, Miller RD (ed.). Churchill Livingstone, Edinburgh, p. 1969.
2. Del Guercio, LRM, Cohn JD (1980) Monitoring operative risk in the elderly. *JAMA* **243**: 1350–1355.
3. Buck N, Devlin HB, Lunn JN (1987) *The Report of a Confidential Enquiry into Perioperative Deaths*. Nuffield Provincial Hospitals Trust and King's Fund Publishing Office, London.
4. Forrest JB, Rehder K, Cahalan MK, Goldsmith CH (1992) Multicenter Study of General Anesthesia: III. Predictors of severe perioperative adverse outcomes. *Anesthesiology* **76**: 3–15.
5. Saklad M (1941) Grading of patients for surgical procedures. *Anesthesiology* **2**: 281–284.
6. Dripps RD, Lamont A, Eckenhoff JE (1961) The role of anesthesia in surgical mortality. *JAMA* **178**: 261–266.
7. Desmeules H, Fournier L, Tremblay P-R (1985) Systemic changes in the elderly patient and their anaesthetic implications. *Can Anaesth Soc J* **32**: 184–187.
8. Wolf MA, Braunwald MD (1984) General anesthesia and noncardiac surgery in patients with heart disease. In *Heart Disease: A Textbook of Cardiovascular Medicine*, 2nd edn, Braunwald MD (ed.). Saunders, Philadelphia, p. 1820.
9. Seymour DG, Pringle R (1983) Post-operative complications in the elderly surgical patient. *Gerontology* **29**: 262–270.
10. Pringle R (1991) Safety of surgery in elderly. *Ann Acad Med Singapore* **20**: 260–264.
11. Wroblewski M, Mikulowski P (1991) Peritonitis in geriatric patients. *Age Ageing* **20**: 90–94.
12. Goldman L, Caldera DL, Nussbaum SR *et al.* (1977) Multifactorial index of cardiac risk in noncardiac surgical procedures. *N Engl J Med* **297**: 845–850.
13. Goldman L (1983) Cardiac risks and complications of noncardiac surgery. *Ann Intern Med* **98**: 504–513.
14. Burggraf GW, Parker JO (1975) Prognosis in coronary artery disease: angiographic, hemodynamic, and clinical factors. *Circulation* **51**: 146–156.
15. Tarhan S, Moffitt EA, Taylor WF, Giuliani ER (1972) Myocardial infarction after general anaesthesia. *JAMA* **220**: 1451–1454.
16. Rao TL, Jacobs KH, El-Etr AA (1983) Reinfarction following anesthesia in patients with myocardial infarction. *Anesthiology* **59**: 499–505.
17. Wells PH, Kaplan JA (1981) Optimal management of patients with ischaemic heart disease for noncardiac surgery by complementary anesthesiologist and cardiologist interaction. *Am Heart J* **102**: 1029–1037.

32 Quality of Life: Its Relevance and Applicability to Elderly Patients with Cardiac Illness

NANETTE K. WENGER
Emory University School of Medicine, and Grady Memorial Hospital, Atlanta, Georgia, USA

DEMOGRAPHIC ISSUES: ELDERLY PATIENTS WITH CARDIAC ILLNESS

The almost doubling of life expectancy at birth, from 40 to about 80 years (1), that has occurred since the mid-nineteenth century has engendered the need to care for an exponentially expanding elderly population—currently 12% of the US population and projected to increase to 21% by the year 2030. The size of the 'oldest old' subset of this population continues to increase, and favourable health-related behavioural changes may further accentuate this trend. The challenge to the medical care system in an era of upwardly spiralling health care costs is to provide an increased duration of active life expectancy, rather than an expanded period of frailty and dependency (2).

Currently four of five persons in the USA older than age 65 have at least one chronic illness, and many have multiple chronic illnesses. Based on reports of a decade ago, 39% of elderly persons in the USA have hypertension and 26% have some type of heart disease. Because of this increased likelihood of comorbidity and of potentially complicating therapies, the 'noise' generated by these features may make the 'signal' of the cardiac disorder in elderly patients more difficult to detect as the aetiology of alterations in the patient's quality of life.

Much of the medical care of elderly patients involves the management of chronic disease, where the therapeutic goal is to limit the consequences of the illness and to optimize life quality, since elimination or cure of an illness defined as chronic is not possible. Issues that mandate evaluation when a treatment is undertaken relate to the alleviation or limitation of the patient's symptoms; maintenance of a sense of well-being; restoration or preservation of physical and mental functional abilities that permit relative self-sufficiency and independence; and retardation of the progression of the underlying disease if feasible (3).

The heterogeneity of the elderly population poses major challenges, in that the

Geriatric Cardiology. Principles and Practice. Edited by A. Martin and A. J. Camm
© 1994 John Wiley & Sons Ltd

variance of any variable is likely to increase with increasing age. This is of particular concern in the very elderly, age 85 years and older, often designated the 'oldest old', and currently the fastest-growing population segment in many industrialized nations. Among the important factors contributing to this heterogeneity are the variable changes of ageing in multiple organ systems, varying concomitant disease states, multiple drug therapies that increase not only the potential for drug toxicity but for drug interactions, and the varying social settings in which an illness occurs. There may be major variability between custodial and independent living settings and with differing degrees of social support. The women in the 'oldest old' age group are likely to be widowed, with frequent resultant lowered socio-economic status, decreased social support and less access to medical care. Although stereotypes of elderly patients with cardiac illness have often characterized them as having increasing disability and dependency, many contemporary elderly cardiac patients appear and behave younger than their chronological age and anticipate an extended and active retirement.

Current improvements in cardiac care appear to have postponed mortality; it remains uncertain whether there has been comparable delay in the onset of morbidity and disability. The concerns of care should focus on limiting the frailty of elderly patients with chronic cardiac illness, i.e. lessening the adverse effects of non-fatal but highly disabling conditions. Quality-of-life assessments tap this domain, addressing those interventions likely to contribute to the amelioration of non-fatal chronic diseases of ageing. Stated otherwise, quality-of-life attributes are important outcome measures to determine the preservation and improvement of health status in the elderly, which should be the focus of therapeutic interventions, rather than simply a prolongation of life in a dependent and non-functional state (2).

QUALITY OF LIFE: ITS DOMAINS IN THE MEDICAL CARE CONTEXT AND ITS RELEVANCE TO MEDICAL CARE OF ELDERLY CARDIAC PATIENTS

Quality of life, in the medical care setting, denotes a wide range of capabilities, limitations, symptoms and psychosocial characteristics that describe an individual's ability to function and to derive satisfaction from a variety of roles (4). This is a measurable and quantifiable concept that considers a patient's total well-being, both physical and psychological, and describes the ways a patient's life is affected by an illness and by its care. Alterations of life quality in elderly patients with cardiac illness may result from the physiological characteristics and consequences of the specific disease, from its therapy, or from a concurrent illness and its management. Treatments that decrease symptoms are likely to enhance the patient's functional effectiveness and sense of well-being; treatments that cause new symptoms or side-effects exert a deleterious effect on life quality because of the diminished sense of well-being and decreased ability to function.

Although traditional medical care has characteristically focused on the relief of symptoms, there has been little consideration of a number of more subtle aspects of a patient's well-being: life satisfaction, hopefulness, self-confidence, social functioning, etc.

Health-related quality of life, described by Spitzer as addressing 'clinically relevant human attributes' (5), is characteristically defined in terms of the major components that contribute to it: functional capacity, perceptions, and symptoms and their consequences. *Functional capacity*, which addresses the activities of personal and social living, has five subcomponents: the ability to perform activities of daily life (including mobility, independence, the energy to carry out self-care, the possibility to obtain adequate sleep and rest, and the ability to participate in occupational or leisure activities); social function, which encompasses informal activities with friends, community interactions, family relationships and marital satisfaction; intellectual function (including memory, alertness, the ability to communicate, confidence in making decisions and judgement); emotional function (mood changes, sick role behaviours, satisfactions, expectations, fears and concerns about the future); and the ability to maintain a satisfactory economic status or standard of living (income, insurance eligibility, employment or retirement, etc.). *Perceptions* are an individual's subjective assessment of his or her situation; they constitute a personal value judgement or perspective about general health status, current level of well-being and satisfaction with the current ability to engage in valued activities. Personal potential and goals are also considered. These inherently individual and personal perceptions and judgements often differ from objective measures of the sphere being evaluated, but both must be considered as valid. The final component of life quality involves *symptoms*: the severity of those due to the cardiac illness and the resultant degree of functional impairment, the amount of medication required to alleviate symptoms, and those symptoms induced by treatments or by a concomitant illness. Symptoms are likely to influence the two other components, functional capacity and perceptions, and vice versa.

As noted, symptoms and functional ability, as perceived by the patient, do not always parallel physiological outcome measures; since symptomatic status and functional ability appear more salient to patients than do laboratory or other objective measurements, it appears prudent to directly measure the domains of an individual's subjective quality of life than to infer them from measurable, objective attributes. The challenge is to select assessment measures that are applicable to the issues important in an elderly population and responsive to the small changes in clinical status that are typical of this population. This highlights the importance of quality-of-life information in enhancing our ability to assess the effectiveness of care as perceived by the patient and to compare benefits of alternative management strategies that reflect the patient's values of outcomes of treatment. As such, quality-of-life outcomes become relevant to determining health-related public policy—a concept currently undergoing evaluation in the USA in the Medical Outcomes Study (6).

What quality-of-life measures can and should be used? Global or generic quality-of-life measures such as the Sickness Impact Profile (7), Nottingham Health Profile (8) and Quality of Well-Being Scale (9) address a variety of dimensions of quality of life and can aid in identifying both anticipated and unanticipated benefits and adverse effects of interventions. Whereas disease-specific quality-of-life measures (10–12) have been suggested to more effectively examine selected quality-of-life issues unique to a disease, even within a particular disease or disease category there may be marked differences in measures appropriate for examining life quality in young versus elderly patients. Further, the clinical setting of the illness, as well as its severity, may determine the spectrum of questions appropriate for quality-of-life ascertainment as well. The quality-of-life measures of function and of social relationships appropriate for a younger active population may have limited applicability to older and more impaired patients; important outcomes related to independence and small variations in function may not be discernible by the instruments used for younger populations. Further, disease-specific measures may fail to ascertain interre-lationships among quality-of-life dimensions, i.e. an increase in physical symptoms and functional limitation resulting in depression or other emotional dysfunction; or depression or emotional dysfunction inducing a limitation of physical function. Combinations of global and disease-specific measures often provide optimal information about quality of life.

A number of measures of health-related quality of life have been validated in elderly populations (13,14) with a variety of chronic illnesses. Many of these measurement strategies are designed to focus more on activities of daily living, on cognitive functioning, on use of medical services, and on requirements for social support than do comparable instruments for younger populations. Important is that elderly patients often rate their functional status higher than do their family members or nurses, suggesting first biasing effects of using different data sources to assess life quality and, even more salient, the importance of determining the patient's viewpoint whenever feasible.

In terms of quality years of life resulting from a cardiac intervention, and variation in patient preferences for different health states, we must learn why some elderly patients who incur major intrusions on their health-related quality of life continue to value living. We must learn about health status and health preferences and their variations at differing points from the probable end of lifespan (15).

GOALS OF THERAPY OF CARDIAC ILLNESS IN ELDERLY PATIENTS

The goal of most therapies for elderly patients is, or should be, the restoration, maintenance and extension of a reasonably independent and active life, with preservation and possibly even improvement of life quality. As more people live to older age, they have greater needs for and increasing use of medical services;

and elderly patients have become more sophisticated consumers of medical care, educated to query the anticipated benefits of recommended therapies. Quality-of-life endpoints may be equally or more important to patients than mortality outcomes; however, morbidity outcomes may substantially influence life quality. Alterations in quality of life assume major importance in selecting these medical interventions and services appropriate for the growing elderly population of most countries.

Is preventive therapy, using coronary heart disease as an example, appropriate for elderly persons? Despite the substantial decline in coronary heart disease mortality in persons of all ages in the USA during the 1970s, coronary disease remains the major cause of death in the US population older than age 65. The continued reduction of mortality from coronary heart disease at younger age will significantly increase the prevalence of this problem in the elderly population. The current life expectancy of a US male aged 65 is almost 15 years, and that of a US female aged 65 almost 19 years. Given the high prevalence of traditional coronary risk factors in elderly populations, coronary risk reduction in elderly persons with and without clinical evidence of coronary heart disease, in addition to decreasing disability and societal dependency, may increase survival as well. However, in undertaking preventive therapies, a wide spectrum of benefit: harm ratios must be addressed. Patient perceptions assume major importance, because these influence adherence to preventive therapies, which in turn influence outcome. We must ascertain the effect of recommended lifestyle modifications on an elderly patient's desired lifestyle, versus the importance of coronary risk reduction to the individual patient. The requirement is that components of risk modification should be reasonable, individualized, designed to maintain functional status, and compatible with the patient's desired life quality, i.e. alterations in perceived health status or well-being must be appropriate for the benefit anticipated. Quality-of-life considerations are included in current recommendations for the management of hypertension (16) and are cited as concerns in recommendations for preventive therapies of the British Cardiac Society and the European Atherosclerosis Society (17,18).

Elderly patients are major consumers of cardiovascular care. In ascertaining the cost-effectiveness of this care, the cost and survival data are readily obtainable. Given the considerable cost of contemporary high-technology cardiovascular interventions, what is required is the determination of the resultant functional state of the patients. What are the resources that must be expended relative to the health benefits obtained? Currently over one-third of all diagnostic and therapeutic cardiovascular procedures performed in the USA are applied to patients older than age 65 (19). Return to remunerative work, often used as a surrogate measure for quality of life, is an inappropriate expectation for many elderly patients; the focus, rather, should be on their resultant independence and life satisfaction—both quality-of-life attributes.

The outcomes warranting consideration in ascertaining the quality of care for chronic illness include limiting the disabling consequences of the cardiac problem, i.e. the total consequences of the disease and of its therapies. Mosteller elegantly cites the interdependencies of chronic illness and life quality:

> Public impression to the contrary, the bulk of medical and surgical treatment is not life-saving, but is aimed at improving the state or quality of life. Most disease is not dramatically fatal but chips away at confidence and happiness. At the same time, treatments for life-threatening diseases often have different impacts on patient comfort. To the extent that we are unable to measure and compare the effects of treatments on the quality of the patient's life, we are unable to document the advantages of the treatments as well as their defects (20).

INFLUENCE OF THE SEVERITY OF THE CARDIAC ILLNESS: SYMPTOMATIC AND FUNCTIONAL LIMITATIONS

Quality-of-life concerns vary as a function of the severity and symptomatic and other physiological limitations of a cardiovascular problem. Thus the evaluative measures used must be tailored to the disease. Although physical capacity, mental capacity and freedom from pain are targeted as critical life quality attributes in the setting of severe or terminal cardiac illness (21), other aspects may be more relevant with stable, less disabling cardiac problems: level of function and adjustment, quality of interpersonal relationships, mobility, residential considerations, recreation, organizational involvement, financial adequacy, life satisfaction (22–25). Even within the care of a particular disease, the severity of illness and setting of care may be more important than the actual aetiological problem in determining the quality-of-life areas that should be examined to determine the effects of the illness and the interventions. Different aspects assume importance in a custodial care setting such as a nursing home, among independently living elderly patients, and among the subset of independent elderly patients who pursue an active lifestyle. Using coronary heart disease as a example, different life quality attributes must be considered in ambulatory elderly patients with chronic stable angina pectoris cared for in a surgery setting or a clinic; elderly patients hospitalized for acute myocardial infarction in an intensive care unit versus those receiving usual hospital care; patients with complications of coronary heart disease, particularly chronic congestive heart failure, whose care is primarily delivered in an ambulatory setting, but who have frequent intermittent hospitalizations; or elderly patients hospitalized for invasive procedures such as coronary arteriography, coronary angioplasty or coronary bypass surgery; even different issues are important for elderly coronary patients participating in exercise rehabilitation.

Hypertension, by contrast, is an asymptomatic illness, with therapy undertaken for the lifelong prevention of late complications, i.e. progression of the disease or deterioration of function. Because elderly patients with hypertension have no overt manifestations of illness, interference with any component of functional capability by a therapy raises practical and ethical considerations. In a symptomless patient, therapies can only engender symptoms that may adversely alter the patient's functional status. Thus a wide spectrum of benefit: harm ratios must be examined. There should be no resultant symptoms, limitation of physical function, decrease in energy or well-being, or unfavourable alteration of self-image. Because hypertension has a favourble short-term prognosis and a low incidence of early complications, morbidity and mortality outcome are insensitive measures for characterizing the impact of a therapy; particularly for elderly patients, there may be little effect on life expectancy. Quality-of-life alterations can effectively compare the benefits and harms of interventions as to demands of medication taking or diet on daily routines, requirements for clinical or laboratory surveillance, impairment of alertness or intellective function, depression, irritability, activity intolerance, sexual dysfunction, sleep disturbances, coping behaviour and life satisfaction. Adverse effects of therapy that impair any of these functional spheres are likely to lessen adherence to the therapy and thereby limit the potential benefits of blood pressure control that are dependent on adherence to diet, medications and the like. Application of quality-of-life information regarding a therapy may help to individualize management and optimize outcome. Comparable issues are raised in the decision for and evaluation of treatments of asymptomatic hypercholesterolaemia in elderly patients.

A large number of categories of antihypertensive medications may have equal efficacy in lowering blood pressure in elderly patients; those therapies with the most favourable long-term effect on life quality attributes, those perceived to interfere least with the elderly patients' desired lifestyle, seem the desirable choices. Several medications tested in clinical trials of antihypertensive therapy for elderly patients fulfil these requirements. For example, in an Italian Multicenter Trial (26), quality-of-life aspects showed improvement in the treated group; these included feeling fit, improved well-being, normal mood and increased sexual desire. A randomized study comparing atenolol, enalapril and diltiazem for blood pressure control in elderly women (27) showed that all three treatment regimens effectively lowered blood pressure, and that there were no significant differences in adverse effects or deleterious effects on life quality.

The Systolic Hypertension in the Elderly Program (SHEP) (28) demonstrated substantial benefit from the control of this problem. However, in the initial design of the trial there was concern that no harm should result from the management of this common asymptomatic problem in an elderly population. Recognizing the multidimensional aspects of life quality, a wide variety of potential adverse effects on personal lifestyle and enjoyment were carefully examined. In the Pilot Study, levels of depression fell in both the treatment and placebo groups; increases in symptoms or side-effects attributed to therapy were also comparable in both groups (29).

In contrast to patients with hypertension, where there is concern that any adverse effect of therapy may impair the health-related well-being of an asymptomatic patient, with more symptomatic illnesses such as angina pectoris and advanced heart failure, therapy is likely to improve symptomatic status and activity level. Particularly in the patient treated for heart failure, an improvement in the activities that can be performed and a reduction of symptoms may improve the patient's perception of health status and enable the performance of increased leisure and occupational activities. As with other cardiovascular problems, the aspects of life quality to be assessed in judging the efficacy of management of heart failure include the symptomatic well-being, the activity level and the psychological status. Entry into a study often makes patients feel better, so that their quality of life may improve, as do other aspects of clinical trial data, even when treated with a placebo; thus placebo therapy values must be compared with those related to the intervention (30,31).

At the other extreme of the symptomatic spectrum from hypertension is advanced congestive heart failure, the end result of a variety of cardiac disorder and the most common hospital discharge diagnosis in elderly patients. In addition to having a poor prognosis, these patients are highly symptomatic, have significant limitation of activity, with dietary restrictions, requirements for multiple medications, at times have associated dementia or cognitive or memory disorders related to diminished cerebral blood flow, and have frequent hospitalizations for exacerbations of the severity of the heart failure. Because advanced heart failure is a highly symptomatic disorder with a grave prognosis, morbidity and mortality data are insensitive measures for comparing outcomes. Only recently have selected vasodilator drugs been shown to prolong survival (32,33); nevertheless, the major thrust of therapy remains improvement in symptoms of dyspnoea or fatigue, in activity intolerance, in the ability to obtain adequate sleep and rest, and in mood and emotional stability; with resulting enhancement of autonomy, comfort, expectations, coping behaviour and life satisfaction. Ascertainment of these life quality outcomes can help gauge the efficacy of an intervention in ameliorating or relieving symptoms for the remaining duration of life and in maintaining the limited functional capacity. Because maintenance of independence is so precarious among these elderly patients, any adverse effect of therapy may challenge this valued status. Some of the newer therapies for advanced heart failure require hospitalization, often in an intensive care setting; others may markedly improve symptoms but have substantial toxicity, including the risk of sudden arrhythmic death. Patient preferences and expectations assume major importance in selecting options for treatment, i.e. the value of quality versus quantity of life, the negative impact of loss of control during hospitalizations, the personal value of maintenance of functional independence. Physicians are charged to act in the best interests of their patients; clinicians must appreciate the elderly patient's personal value systems, health beliefs, and their desired outcomes of cardiovascular interventions in delineating treatment options and in making recommendations among them. There may be prominent discordance between objective measures of improvement and favourable changes in symptomatic status (32). As an example, in patients with heart failure there is little relationship between indices of ventricular function and symptomatic status or objectively determined physical work capacity (34,35); and their interrelationships with life quality characteristics have not been ascertained. Nevertheless, a favourable outcome (as perceived by the patient) must include an improved functional status and life quality profile, not solely an improvement in the physiological parameters of heart failure. Patients' satisfaction with their care—a component of the evaluation of the effectiveness of any intervention—often reflects the meeting of their perceived needs, resultant comfort and self-sufficiency.

Patients with coronary heart disease who present with chest pain symptoms value the outcome (by medical or surgical therapy) of alleviation of the pain and a consequent improvement in functional status. The substantial survival advantage offered by acute thrombolysis or acute angioplasty to elderly patients at least to age 75 (36) in the setting of acute myocardial infarction is judged by most patients to counterbalance the potential risk of cerebrovascular or other bleeding complication, with possible resultant major deterioration of life quality. We currently lack data to advise elderly patients older than 75 years of their benefit: harm ratio from these dramatic revascularization procedures, owing to the extreme heterogeneity of coronary patients beyond age 75. However, physicians today face an added challenge: to guide the elderly coronary patient in limiting the progression or potentially inducing regression of the underlying atherosclerosis. We must then determine the impact of preventive interventions on a patient's resultant quality of life. Many elderly (as well as younger) patients perceive as unacceptable alterations in their diet, physical activity levels, smoking behaviour or alcohol use. Clinicians must also address some of the adverse psychological consequences of illness; in a number of studies of coronary patients, psychological problems entail more invalidism than does physiological impairment. We must determine the psychological consequences of illness that lead to unwarranted invalidism, defining the characteristics of those elderly patients who fail to return to normal functioning after a coronary event, despite satisfactory physiological status.

Quality-of-life data were reported for 10 years of follow-up in the Coronary Artery Surgery Study (CASS), which compared medical and surgical treatments of patients with asymptomatic coronary heart disease (37). Measures of recreational status, employment status, frequency of heart failure and hospitalizations were similar for both medically and surgically assigned groups throughout follow-up. Indexes of life quality such as angina relief, increased physical activity and decreased antianginal medication use were initially superior in the group randomized to surgical therapy; by 10 years, these advantages were greatly attenuated, predominantly due to the referral to late surgery of a large proportion of medically assigned patients, with this therapy rendering them asymptomatic. These data relate to patients over a wide age range. Consistent observations have been reported from the Veterans Administration Cooperative Study of Coronary Artery Surgery (38) and the European Coronary Surgery Study (39).

Although traditional morbidity and mortality data are comparable for some subsets of coronary patients who receive medical versus surgical therapies, and appear similar in others treated with coronary bypass surgery or percutaneous transluminal coronary angioplasty (40–42), other determinants than morbidity and mortality are also important to elderly coronary patients. Some interventions entail multiples of cost, of days in the hospital away from family and friends. Many require lifelong adherence to diet and medications, with the latter often costly in the long term. Two clinical trials currently in progress, sponsored by the US National Heart, Lung and Blood Institute, are designed to compare morbidity and mortality outcomes in patients randomly allocated to coronary angioplasty or coronary artery bypass surgery (CABG); elderly patients are included in the study populations. If survival and morbidity are comparable, a spectrum of quality-of-life outcomes will assume major importance in subsequent clinical decision making. How do patients view the life quality intrusions of the perioperative period following CABG versus the fear and anxiety regarding the potential for late angioplasty failure? Are there subtle alterations in memory, motor coordination, reasoning and other neuropsychological functions related to the cardiopulmonary bypass procedure needed for open heart surgery (41), and how are these impairments viewed by patients? Are they more frequent or extensive in elderly patients?

THE ROLE OF PATIENT EXPECTATIONS OF OUTCOMES OF TESTS AND TREATMENTS

In this heterogeneous population, age-related issues reflect, in addition to the cardiac disease under question, the degree of independence and activities before, during and following an acute cardiac problem; prior disabilities unrelated to the cardiac disease or disorder being addressed, i.e. the impact of comorbidity on life quality; and particularly patient expectations. It is important to examine whether the patient's expectations are merely for survival and recovery, with little concern for subsequent life quality; whether the patient hopes to feel better or even to be completely well, but does not consider issues of independence; or whether an elderly patient anticipates resumption of an active lifestyle (and even a return to work, which may constitute a reasonable expectation for some). With increasingly severe symptoms and resulting activity restrictions, patient expectations as to the degree of improvement that can be attained are likely to lessen. This considerable spectrum of outcome expectations demands that different components of what gives quality to a patient's life be explored.

An individual patient's perceptions are important constituents of his or her quality of life that require assessment, but these perceptions can be substantially influenced by the patient's expectations. Although altered expectations of outcome have been described in elderly patients, it remains unsure whether these reflect age *per se* or whether they are related to medical care systems in specific countries, where options for medical care available to elderly patients differ from those for a younger population. Stated another way, if access to and availability of health care differ for elderly patients, these factors may adversely affect their expectations of the outcome of a cardiac illness and thereby alter their perceptions of the impact of therapy on life quality. In a health care delivery system where age influences health policy, elderly patients may have different expectations of the outcomes of the management of an illness.

Elderly cardiac patients' perceptions of their quality of life have been shown to correlate significantly with their physical health status (determined by restriction of activities and by the number of visits to physicians), as well as level of discomfort. Perceptions of health status also correlate well with the mortality risk of elderly patients (43). In one study (44), physicians rated their patients' life quality more negatively than did their geriatric patients, based on physical health and discomfort, emotional status, and cognitive and physical activity impairments (compared to other individuals of same age and gender). These findings, among others, suggest the need for physicians to incorporate the values of what gives quality to their elderly patients' lives into decisions about cardiac care; different values of treatment outcomes likely underlie the patient–physician lack of congruence in assessing life quality (45). Of interest is the substantial number of women evaluated in the study cited (54%) and the 30-year average younger age of the physicians than the patients.

QUALITY-OF-LIFE DATA FROM CLINICAL TRIALS: EXTRAPOLATION TO CLINICAL CARE

Extrapolation of clinical trial data about therapies to the clinical care of elderly patients, including issues of quality-of-life assessment, presents a major challenge. The population currently selected for most clinical trials only minimally reflects the total population likely to receive a therapy, and these differences are magnified in elderly as compared with younger cardiac patients. Screening for participation in most clinical trials initially involves assessment of the patient's competence to agree to participate, the multiple features involved in the actual ability to participate, and the typically lesser comorbidity required so that there can be precise assessment of the problem addressed by the clinical trial. Thus the application of results to the total elderly population likely to have the disease and receive the therapy is limited. These exclusions from randomized trials can seriously affect the validity of conclusions—different patients face different probabilities because of their different comorbidities and severities. As quality-of-life outcome measures are addressed in clinical trials, for this information to be applicable to clinical care of elderly patients attention is required to those quality-of-life variables that are either unique to an elderly population or that are more specifically or frequently applicable in the elderly.

ROLE OF LIFE QUALITY OUTCOMES IN CLINICAL DECISION MAKING: SHOULD TESTS OR TREATMENTS BE UNDERTAKEN?

A current trend in medical care, particularly in the USA, is that of 'informed consumerism', such that patients as consumers of health care actively seek information from their physicians about their cardiac illness and about the options available to them for treatment of specific cardiovascular problems; this information enables them to participate in decisions as to the choice of management. Their queries relate both to the traditional morbidity and mortality (biomedical) outcomes and to psychosocial (life quality) outcomes. These concerns are equally applicable to elderly patients; particularly for elderly patients, where the survival benefit of an intervention may be limited and may not always be the patient's priority, quality-of-life issues are reflected in questions raised about the diagnostic procedures and therapies recommended for a cardiac problem under consideration. The compelling issue is typically whether postponement of severe or debilitating disease is likely to occur as a result of the intervention.

Satisfaction of elderly patients with their medical care in a number of surveys has shown that their preferred outcomes included the resultant comfort and sense of well-being; the degree to which they could maintain reasonable physical, emotional and intellective function; and their ability to continue to participate in valued activities in the family, occasionally at work, and in the community. With the proliferation of comparably effective therapies (in regard to morbidity and mortality) for a variety of cardiovascular illnesses, their positive and negative influences on the patient's quality of life should help in selection of the optimal therapy.

Daniel Callahan, director of the Hastings Center (46), has challenged medicine to 'give up its relentless drive to extend the life of the aged, turning its attention to the relief of their suffering and an improvement in their physical and mental quality of life'. He emphasizes the importance of relief of suffering and improvement of the physical and mental life quality of elderly patients, rather than simply the forestalling of their death. Callahan identifies as the three pivotal quality-of-life criteria the capacity to think, to feel and to interact with others. He suggests that therapies should be addressed towards relieving any severe pain or suffering or effects of medications or therapies that thwart this capacity to think, to feel and to interact with others. The same outcomes that are used to decide among interventions for a particular cardiac illness should also be used to address whether an intervention should be undertaken in a seriously ill elderly cardiac patient. Many diagnostic and therapeutic cardiovascular procedures are feasible to perform in octogenarians and nonagenarians; anticipated quality-of-life outcomes, favourable and unfavourable, may help in the decision about whether they should be performed. For example, coronary bypass surgery or cardiac valve replacement in elderly patients entails an excess of morbidity and periprocedural mortality, with less potential to prolong survival than in younger populations; the critical issue appears to be whether an increase in meaningful long-term survival can be effected.

SUMMARY

To ascertain the total impact of a diagnostic or therapeutic intervention in elderly patients with cardiovascular illness, quality-of-life attributes must be examined, in addition to the traditional measures of morbidity and mortality. Quality-of-life domains tap areas of function and performance that are valued by elderly patients as result of treatment, most prominent of which are their resultant comfort and well-being.

Knowledge of these life quality outcomes, added to standard morbidity and mortality data, can help in decisions as to whether an intervention is appropriate in an elderly patient with cardiovascular illness, as well as to select among several potential approaches the one likely to best meet the elderly cardiac patient's desires and expectations of therapy.

Acknowledgements

With appreciation to Jeanette Zahler and Julia Wright for assistance in the preparation of this manuscript.

REFERENCES

1. Dublin LI, Lotka AI, Spiegelman M (1949) *Length of Life*. Ronald, New York, pp. 26–43.
2. Olshansky SJ, Carnes BA, Cassel C (1990) In search of Methuselah: estimating the upper limits of human longevity. *Science* **250**: 634–640.
3. Deyo RA (1991) The quality of life, research, and care. *Ann Intern Med* **114**: 695–697.
4. Wenger NK, Mattson ME, Furberg CD, Elinson J (eds) (1984) *Assessment of Quality of Life in Clinical Trials of Cardiovascular Therapies*. LeJacq, New York.
5. Spitzer WO (1987) Keynote address. State of science 1986: quality of life and functional status as target variables for research. *J Chronic Dis* **40**: 465–471.
6. Tarlov AR, Ware JE Jr, Greenfield S *et al.* (1989) The Medical Outcome Study: an application of methods for monitoring the results of medical care. *JAMA* **262**: 925–930.
7. Bergner M, Bobbitt RA, Carter WB *et al.* (1981) The Sickness Impact Profile: development and final revision of a health status measure. *Med Care* **19**: 787–805.
8. Hunt SM, McKenna SP, McEwen J (1985) A quantitative approach to perceived health. *J Epidemiol Community Health* **34**: 281–295.
9. Bush JW (1984) General health policy model/quality of well-being (QWB) scale. In *Assessment of Quality of Life in Clinical Trials of Cardiovascular Therapies*, Wenger NK, Mattson ME, Furberg CD, Elinson J (eds). LeJacq, New York, pp. 189–199.
10. Goldman L, Hashimoto B, Cook EF, Loscalzo A (1981) Comparative reproducibility and validity of systems for assessing cardiovascular functional class: advantages of a new Specific Activity Scale. *Circulation* **64**: 1227–1234.
11. Rose GA, Blackburn H (1986) *Cardiovascular Survey Methods*. World Health

Organization, Geneva, No. 56, pp. 1–188.

12. Mahler DA, Weinberg DM, Wells CK, Feinstein AR (1984) The measurement of dyspnoea: content, interobserver agreement and physiologic correlates of two new clinical indexes. *Chest* **85**: 751–758.

13. Erickson P (1986) Measuring health-related quality of life among the elderly. *Qual Life Cardiovasc Care* **2**: 182–185.

14. Erickson P (1986) Measures and determinants of health-related quality of life among the elderly. *Qual Life Cardiovasc Care* **2**: 235–237.

15. Lawton MP (in press) A multidimensional view of quality of life in frail elders. In *The Concept and Measurement of Quality of Life*, Birren JE, Lubben JE, Rowe JC, Deutchman DE (eds). Academic Press, New York.

16. 1988 Joint National Committee (1988) The 1988 Report of the Joint National Committee on Detection, Evaluation, and Treatment of High Blood Pressure. *Arch Intern Med* **148**: 1023–1038.

17. Shultz NR Jr, Dineen JT, Elias MF *et al.* (1979) W.A.I.S. performance for different age groups of hypertensive and control subjects during administration of a diuretic. *J Gerontol* **34**: 246–253.

18. Bulpitt CJ, Fletcher AE (1985) Quality of life in hypertensive patients on different antihypertensive treatments: rationale for methods employed in a multicentre randomized controlled trial. *J Cardiovasc Pharmacol* **7**: S137–S145.

19. Wenger NK, Marcus FI, O'Rourke RA (eds) (1987) 18th Bethesda Conference: Cardiovascular Disease in the Elderly. *J Am Coll Cardiol* **10** (Suppl. A).

20. Mosteller F, Gilbert JP, McPeek B (1980) Reporting standards and research strategies for controlled trials. *Controlled Clin Trials* **1**: 37–58.

21. Bayles MD (1978) Euthanasia and the quality of life. In *Medical Treatment of the Dying: Moral Issues*, Bayles MD, High DM (eds). Schenkman, Cambridge, MA, pp. 143–152.

22. Deniston OL, Jette A (1980) A functional status assessment instrument: validation in an elderly population. *Health Serv Res* Spring: 21–34.

23. Campbell A, Converse PE, Rodgers WL (1976) *The Quality of American Life Perceptions, Evaluations and Satisfactions*. Russel Sage, New York.

24. Stock WA, Okun MA (1982) The construct validity of life satisfaction among the elderly. *J Gerontol* **37**: 625–627.

25. Spreitzer E, Snyder E (1979) The relative effects of health and income on life satisfaction. *Int J Aging Hum Dev* **10**: 283–288.

26. Ambrosio GB, Zamboni S, Botta G for The Study Group on Captopril in the Elderly (1988) Captopril in elderly hypertensive patients: results from a Multicenter Italian Trial. *Am J Med 84* (Suppl. 3A): 152–154.

27. Applegate WB, Phillips HL, Schnaper H *et al.* (1991) A randomized controlled trial of the effects of three antihypertensive agents on blood pressure control and quality of life in older women. *Arch Intern Med* **151**: 1817–1823.

28. SHEP Cooperative Research Group (1991) Prevention of stroke by antihypertensive drug treatment in older persons with isolated systolic hypertension: final results of the Systolic Hypertension in the Elderly Program (SHEP). *JAMA* **265**: 3255–3264.

29. Gurland BJ, Teresi J, Smith WM *et al.* (1988) Effect of treatment for isolated systolic hypertension on cognitive status and depression in the elderly. *J Am Geriatr Soc* **36**: 1015–1022.

30. Mann AH (1984) Hypertension: psychological aspects and diagnostic impact in the clinical trial. *Psychol Med.* Monograph Suppl. 5.

31. Bulpitt CJ, Fletcher AE (1988) Measurement of the quality of life in congestive heart failure: influence of drug therapy. *Cardiovasc Drugs Ther* **2**: 419–424.

32. Cohn JN, Archibald DG, Ziesche S *et al.* (1986) Effect of vasodilator therapy on

mortality in chronic congestive heart failure: results of a Veterans Administration Cooperative Study. *N Engl J Med* **314**: 1547–1552.

33. The CONSENSUS Trial Study Group (1987) Effects of enalapril on mortality in severe congestive heart failure: results of the Cooperative North Scandinavian Enalapril Survival Study (Concensus). *N Engl J Med* **316**: 1429–1435.

34. Guyatt GH (1985) Methodologic problems in clinical trials in heart failure. *J Chronic Dis* **38**: 353–363.

35. Franciosa JA (1986) Epidemiologic patterns, clinical evaluation, and long-term prognosis in chronic congestive heart failure. *Am J Med* **80** (Suppl. 2B): 14–21.

36. Tanaka T, Wenger NK (1991) Acute myocardial infarction in the elderly: diagnosis, management, prognosis. *Mod Med* **59**: 48–65.

37. Rogers WJ, Coggin CJ, Gersh BJ *et al.* for the CASS Investigators (1990) Ten-year follow-up of quality of life in patients randomized to receive medical therapy or coronary artery bypass graft surgery: the Coronary Artery Surgery Study (CASS). *Circulation* **82**: 1647–1658.

38. Peduzzi P, Hultgren NH (1979) Effect of medical vs surgical treatment on symptoms in stable angina pectoris: the Veterans Administration Cooperative Study of Surgery for Coronary Arterial Occlusion Disease. *Circulation* **60**: 888–900.

39. European Coronary Surgery Study Group (1982) Long-term results of prospective randomised study of coronary artery bypass surgery in stable angina pectoris. *Lancet* **ii**: 1173–1180.

40. Olsson G, Lubsen J, van Es GA, Rehnqvist N (1986) Quality of life after myocardial infarction: effect of long-term metoprolol on mortality and morbidity. *Br Med J* **292**: 1491–1493.

41. Shaw PJ, Bates D, Cartlidge NEF *et al.* (1987) Neurologic and neuropsychological morbidity following major surgery: comparison of coronary artery bypass and peripheral vascular surgery. *Stroke* **18**: 700–707.

42. Allen JK, Fitzgerald ST, Swank RT, Becker DM (1990) Functional status after coronary artery bypass grafting and percutaneous transluminal coronary angioplasty. *Am J Cardiol* **65**: 921–925.

43. Mossey JM, Shapiro E (1982) Self-rated health: a predictor of mortality among the elderly. *Am J Public Health* **72**: 800–808.

44. Pearlman RA, Uhlmann RF (1986) Perceptions of quality of life in elderly patients with cardiovascular disease. *Qual Life Cardiovasc Care* **2**: 149–158.

45. LaRue A, Bank L, Jarvik L, Hetland M (1979) Health in old age: how do physicians' rating and self-ratings compare? *J Gerontol* **34**: 687–691.

46. Callahan D (1988) *Setting Limits: Medical Goals in an Aging Society.* Simon & Schuster, New York, pp. 256.

Part VII

RESEARCH INTO HEART DISEASE IN OLD AGE

33 A North American Perspective

EDWARD G. LAKATTA[a] **AND BERNARD J. GERSH**[b]

[a] *National Institute on Aging, Johns Hopkins School of Medicine, and University of Maryland School of Medicine, Baltimore, Maryland, USA*
[b] *Mayo Clinic, and Mayo Medical School, Rochester, Minnesota; present address Georgetown University School of Medicine, Washington D.C., USA*

At present, approximately 12.05% of the US population is 65 years or older. By the year 2000, this group will constitute over 14% of the population—an increase from 26 to 36 million people. Furthermore, the major increase among the elderly will be among patients aged 75 years or older, and recent estimates predict a 30% increase in their numbers over the next 10 years (1,2) (Figure 1). Octogenarians are already the fastest-growing group in our society (4).

Although old age and cardiac disease are not synonymous, the prevalence of heart disease, particularly symptomatic coronary artery disease, increases strikingly with age (5,6). Moreover, as the incidence of cardiovascular disease declines among those of middle age and the median age of the population increases, it is likely that the prevalence of symptomatic cardiovascular disease among people of advanced age will increase further, and this comes at a time when the costs of medical care are undergoing increasing scrutiny. Cardiovascular disease accounts for about one-sixth of overall health care expenditures (Figure 2) and somewhat more among patients over the age of 65 years (7). Overall health care costs for patients of extreme age (aged 85 years and above) are projected to escalate inexorably (3). Further advances in the prevention and treatment of cardiovascular disease in elderly individuals will require a more aggressive attitude of society with respect to both basic and clinical research directed at the ageing issues. The basic research required includes an evaluation of how ageing *per se* affects cardiovascular structure and function at the cellular and molecular levels as well as at the organ system levels. Clinical research issues include more sensitive detection of vascular disease and application of gene therapies as these become available. The judicious utilization of currently available cardiovascular procedures in the elderly will require a multicentre database that does not presently exist.

The population of the USA is growing older, and with it come a growing awareness of the demographic and sociological implications of a large and rapidly expanding elderly segment of our society (Figure 1) (2,3). In 1986, at a National Heart, Lung and Blood Institute (NHLBI) conference on the

Geriatric Cardiology. Principles and Practice.   Edited by A. Martin and A. J. Camm
© 1994 John Wiley & Sons Ltd

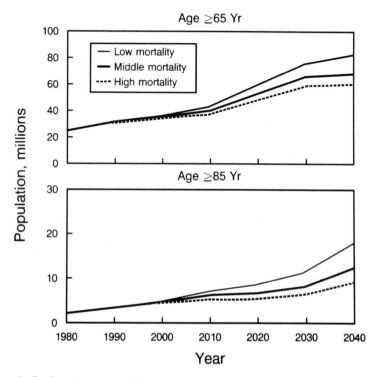

Figure 1. Projected growth of the population age 65 years and above and 85 years and above. Projections are based on low, middle and high mortality assumptions from the US Bureau of the Census (2). Modified from Schneider and Guralnik (3), *Journal of the American Medical Association*, **263**, 2335–2340. Copyright 1990, American Medical Association

Recognition and Management of Coronary Heart Disease, it was clearly stated that there was a lack of basic information regarding the prevention, diagnosis and treatment of coronary heart disease among the elderly (8). Additional issues raised at this conference questioned whether traditional risk factors for stroke and coronary artery disease were of similar predictive power for the old. The role of diet and exercise in risk factor reduction among the elderly was also discussed and the relative lack of knowledge in these areas was noted.

At the eighteenth Bethesda Conference Report of the American College of Cardiology (9), Dr Dustan highlighted the potential clash of societal and individual issues which may arise when physicians attempt to balance their obligations to their patients against their obligations to society. If the conservation of limited resources becomes a legitimate objective of society, then the extent to which society is obligated to meet all the health care needs of the elderly will be a substantive issue and the object of intense investigation and debate during this and the next decade (10).

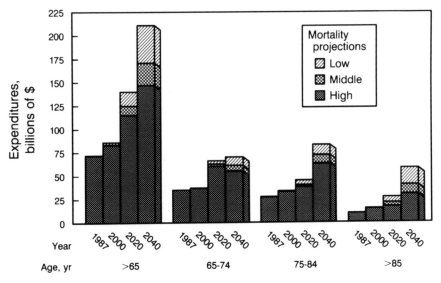

Figure 2. Actual (1987) and projected Medicare expenses in 1987 dollars by age group. Average Medicare expenses per person were obtained from data from the Health Care Financing Administration (29). Cost projects are based on low, middle and high mortality assumptions from the US Bureau of the Census (2). Adapted from Schneider and Guralnik (3), *Journal of the American Medical Association*, **263**, 2335–2340. Copyright 1990, American Medical Association

INTERPRETATION OF OUR PRESENT DATABASE REGARDING HOW AGEING AFFECTS CARDIOVASCULAR STRUCTURE AND FUNCTION

The definition of whether and how advancing age affects cardiovascular structure and function is among the most formidable research endeavours because other factors that covary with age, e.g. lifestyle and disease, each have substantial impact on cardiovascular measurements. Thus, while there is a large literature suggesting that cardiovascular function in older individuals differs from that in younger individuals, confusion arises in the interpretation of these data because of failure to acknowledge and control for *interactions* among age, disease and lifestyle, e.g. physical conditioning status. The effect of disease on cardiovascular function can go unnoticed, particularly in the case of the occult form of coronary artery disease; while 60% of male individuals aged 60 plus who died from all causes have 75–100% narrowing of at least one major coronary artery disease, only 10–15% manifest symptoms (11). Although more recent studies have employed more rigorous screening to exclude individuals with occult disease, still no 'perfect study', i.e. one that controls for both disease and lifestyle variations, has emerged.

The strategy as to which ages to compare in order to determine an effect of age has differed among studies, depending on the population available and the interest of the investigator(s). The term ageing is non-specific and has been used to indicate changes that occur with time, over those periods referred to as fetal, postpartum, neonatal, maturational, adult and senescent. Alterations in the cardiovascular regulatory mechanisms occurring over portions of this age spectrum may be the same as or opposite in direction to those occurring over other parts of the spectrum; conversely some variables may change progressively across the entire age span. Furthermore, cellular mechanisms underlying the altered function at one age may not be the same as those at another period of the life cycle. As a result, statements regarding the 'effect of age' on a given parameter, without strict qualification as to the specific age range investigated, have tended to confuse the literature on ageing. If a sufficiently broad adult age range is not investigated, erroneous conclusions, interpretations or generalizations regarding an age effect may be reached. For example, comparing cardiovascular performance in individuals ranged 20–50 may not provide the same perspective as studies comparing individuals aged 20–80 years of age. Conversely, extension of the interpretation regarding age to ages older than those studies is not warranted. In this regard very little data regarding cardiovascular regulatory mechanisms in individuals greater than 80 years of age who are healthy and retain a reasonable level of physical activity are available. Another pitfall is to generalize arbitrarily dichotomized studies, e.g. comparison of humans older and younger than 60 years of age.

Study design is another factor that complicates the interpretation of measurements seeking to address the issue of how age impacts upon the cardiovascular mechanism. Cross-sectional studies, i.e. different individuals of varying age are compared rather than the same individual at a varying age, neither quantify nor control for life-long habits of variables like nutrition and exercise or other birth cohort effects. While a longitudinal study design, i.e. repeated measurements made within an individual during his or her lifetime, intuitively appears to be superior to the cross-sectional approach, the advantage is more often apparent than real. The development of occult disease and changes in lifestyle occurring within an individual still confound the longitudinal characterization of a pure age effect. Additionally, changes in methodology or investigators over long periods of time, and substitution of new technology that enable more meaningful measurements, seriously hamper the longitudinal approach. The combination of cross-sectional and longitudinal approaches has proven fruitful in some areas of study, but these have generally been lacking with respect to cardiovascular measurements.

Because the cardiovascular system at rest functions at only a fraction of its capacity, measures at rest do not adequately characterize the system. Subtle signs of age-associated changes in cardiovascular function, in particular, become manifest during stress, e.g. during acute exercise. Non-cardiovascular factors often limit the stress response. It has long been known that most older individuals have less aerobic capacity than most younger ones. It is less often considered that the amount of work performed dictates the level of cardiovascular performance and not usually vice versa. Thus, even subtle age-associated differences in motivation to continue exercise, orthopaedic limitations, changes in body composition, changes in muscle mass and strength or in the threshold for neuromuscular fatigue can interact to limit aerobic performance in elderly individuals. In these instances the maximum measures of cardiovascular performance will be reduced, but may still be appropriate for the work performed (12). Whether age-associated differences, non-cardiac factors or cardiac factors, that may limit aerobic work capacity, are due to ageing or to the sedentary lifestyle that accompanies ageing cannot be sorted out statistically, as age and physical conditioning status are interdependent covariants and often cannot be independently statistically analysed.

Animal models provide an opportunity for mechanistic studies not available in man. Although the extrapolation from findings in animals to man introduces an additional variable, nonetheless this constraint is relatively minor as studies that address the nature of ageing, in any model, regardless of direct applicability to man, have merit in their own right. The rat is by far the most popular animal model used for ageing studies. While the problem of coronary artery disease is obviated in the species, the major issue of physical conditioning status of rats may be even more severe than in humans, and renal disease may complicate the interpretation of certain rodent measurements.

MECHANISTIC STUDIES TO CHARACTERIZE CARDIAC MYOCYTE STRUCTURE, FUNCTION AND ADAPTIVE CAPACITY WITH AGEING

Acute and chronic disease states and changes in cardiac cell function occur and permit the myocardium to adapt. When these adaptations fail, clinical signs of heart failure emerge. The incidence and prevalence of heart failure increase exponentially with older (> 60 years) age. One possible explanation for this is that with ageing there is an increased exposure time to contract specific cardiac diseases; another possibility is that most cardiac diseases increase in severity with time and thus with age. According to these two hypotheses the age association is nothing more than a time effect. An alternative hypothesis is that the substrate upon which a specific disease is superimposed becomes altered with age. According to this hypothesis, cardiac biochemistry and physiology change with age and this results in a lesser ability of the hearts of older individuals to adapt to disease states.

Cardiovascular ageing mimics hypertension

The heart and vasculature of ageing individuals whose arterial pressure is within clinically defined normal range mimics that of hypertensive patients at any age

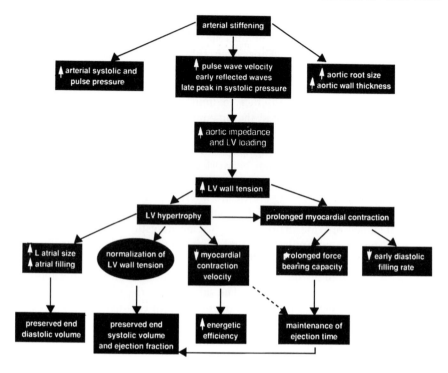

Figure 3. The interplay of vascular and adaptive cardiac changes that occur to varying degrees with ageing in otherwise healthy individuals. Adapted from *The Merck Manual of Geriatrics*, p. 318, edited by William B. Abrams and Robert Berkow. Copyright 1990 Merck & Co., Inc. Used with permission

(Figure 3). Cardiovascular changes include left ventricular hypertrophy, a diminution in resting left ventricular early diastolic filling rate, increased vascular stiffness and aortic impedance. However, an increase in peripheral vascular resistance in normotensives with ageing is not usually observed. Cardiac muscle changes with ageing in animal models also mimic those following experimental hypertension in younger animals (see below).

Hypertension and the heart

A major cardiac disease associated with the development of cases of congestive heart failure (CHF) in older patients is arterial hypertension. Cardiac cell enlargement is a major myocardial adaptive response to chronic hypertension. In animal models this results in an increase in cardiac mass due to enlargement of a relatively constant number of cardiac myocytes and reflects global activation of cardiac genes at the translational and post-translational level.

These molecular adaptations result in adaptive changes in cellular excitation–contraction mechanisms (Figure 4). The transmembrane action potential is prolonged in all models of compensated hypertension in which it has been

FUNCTIONAL MEASURE	EXPERIMENTAL LV PRESSURE LOADING	NORMOTENSIVE AGING
Contraction Duration	↑	↑
Contraction Velocity	↓	↓
Myosin Isozyme Composition	↓V_1, ↑V_3	↓V_1, ↑V_3
Sarcoplasmic Reticulum Ca^{2+} Pumping Rate	↓	↓
Cytosolic Ca^{2+} Transient Duration	↑ (Ferret)	↑
Myofilament Ca^{2+} Sensitivity	↔	↔
Action Potential Repolarization Time	↑	↑
β-Adrenergic Inotropic Response	↓	↓
Cardiac Glycoside Response	↓	↓

Figure 4. The phenotypic pattern of experimental pressure loading in young animals bears a striking resemblance to that of adult ageing and suggests that the molecular mechanisms may be similar in both cases. Adapted from Lakatta (14)

examined (15). The transient increase in cytosolic calcium concentration elicited by excitation, while not reduced in amplitude, is prolonged in duration. The rate of CA^{2+} uptake and formation of Ca^{2+}-dependent phospho-enzyme by the sarcoplasmic reticulum (SR) Ca^{2+} pump are decreased and the density of the SR Ca^{2+} pump protein (ATPase)—measured via specific monoclonal antibody—is reduced. This likely results from a decreased expression of the gene coding for the SR pump protein (16). Although the isometric force and rate of force development in rodent hypertension models are preserved, the isotonic shorten-ing velocity is decreased and contraction and relaxation times are prolonged. A decrease in the rate of ATP hydrolysis has been observed in various contractile protein preparations isolated from the myocardium of pressure-hypertrophied animals. In conjunction with this, the myosin heavy-chain isoenzyme profile in rodents shifts from the predominantly V_1 to the predominantly V_3 isoform. This shift is due, in part at least, to a selective increase in the expression of β-myosin heavy chain mRNA, as noted above. The reduction in the isotonic shortening velocity in pressure-overloaded rodent cardiac muscle is often ascribed to this shift in myosin isoforms.

Prolonged relaxation is a common feature of all experimental hypertension-loaded models. Relaxation is regulated by multiple mechanisms, which include the rate of Ca^{2+} dissociation from the myofilaments, and the duration of the cytosolic Ca^{2+} transient, which is in turn dependent upon the duration of the sarcolemmal depolarization (action potential) that initiates the increase in cytosolic [Ca], and rate of Ca^{2+} pumping into the SR or extrusion from the cell. In addition to Ca^{2+}-dependent factors, non-Ca^{2+}-dependent mechanical factors confer a load dependence to relaxation and this can modulate the contraction duration. In experimental hypertension models these relaxation 'abnormalities' can be construed as adaptive in nature as they permit prolonged force-bearing capacity required to eject blood into a stiff arterial system which, due to early reflected pulse waves, would otherwise tend to abbreviate the ejection time, increase end-systolic volume and reduce ejection fraction.

Cardiac changes with ageing

With advancing adult age in normotensive rodents, ventricular myocytes enlarge and changes in many aspects of cardiac muscle excitation–contraction coupling mechanisms occur and are strikingly similar to those in the rodent hypertensive hearts (Figure 4). Specifically, in an isometric contraction, the transmembrane action potential, the cytosolic Ca^{2+} transient and the resultant contraction are longer in duration in cardiac muscle isolated from senescent versus younger adult rats. The rate at which the SR pumps Ca^{2+} decreases with ageing and may be related to a reduction in the expression of the gene coding for the SR Ca^{2+} ATPase protein. The myosin isoenzyme composition shifts to predominantly V_3 and the myosin ATPase increases with senescence. These shifts are due to a switching of the gene coding for the β-myosin heavy chain and a switching off of the gene for the α-myosin heavy chain. In isotonic contractions, a reduction in the speed and extent of shortening occurs in muscle from senescent in contrast to that from younger adult rats. It is tempting to speculate that since the same general pattern of changes in cell mechanisms occurs in both experimental pressure overload and ageing, this pattern is a result of 'logic' within the genome that regulates the expression or multiple genes in order for cellular adaptation to occur. This adaptation allows for an energy-efficient and prolonged contraction. Still further refinement of the characterization of phenotypic cardiac changes that occur with ageing is required, as are studies to define the molecular changes of these adaptations and in particular of the transduction mechanisms involved.

The adaptive capacity of the senescent heart may be reduced

Evidence has accumulated to suggest that with ageing the extent and nature of the adaptive response of the heart to increased haemodynamic load becomes reduced (11). In human populations this may be evidenced by an exponential rise, with advancing age, in mortality following myocardial infarction. Evidence from animal studies indicates that with ageing there is a diminished capacity for adaptation to haemodynamic overload, in terms of both the hypertrophic growth response and its functional adaptations in response to mechanical stresses, e.g. pressure or volume overload that evokes substantial myocardial hypertrophy. The hypertrophic response to chronic atrioventricular block decreases with age and is also accompanied by a reduced contractile adaptation. In general, the extent to which myosin isoform ATPase activity, and action potential and contraction duration, adapt to the pressure overload correlates with the extent of hypertrophy regardless of age. A relative reduction in the extent of cardiac hypertrophy in response to a given increment on arterial pressure could also indicate an age-associated reduction in the efficiency of global activation of genes or post-transcriptional processes that result in a new increase in protein synthesis. It has also been noted that with ageing, although myocyte size increases even in the absence of experimental mechanical overload, the number of myocytes in the left ventricle significantly declines. This and a diminution in the hypertrophic response could be in part related to cell death when cell size becomes limiting, due to ischaemia or inadequacy of cell ionic or energy homeostasis for other reasons.

In summary, cardiac failure increases exponentially with advanced adult age and is essentially a 'disease' or condition of the elderly. Studies that elucidate biophysical, biochemical and molecular mechanisms of how cardiac cells age and adapt to chronic overload conditions, such as those due to specific pathological entities, are of critical importance to the development of more effective prevention and treatment modalities for heart failure in the elderly population. It is hypothesized that a relative failure of cardiac adaptive mechanisms with ageing leads to the greater incidence of clinical manifestations of heart failure in older individuals with cardiac disease. The following experimental approach is proposed.

Research strategies

Basic studies of individual freshly isolated cardiac myocytes could be utilized to define myocyte structure and function with respect to age, i.e. to characterize age-associated changes in the myocardial cell functional and biochemical phenotype, using state-of-the-art methods. Studies of molecular mechanisms that underlie the changes in myocardial cellular phenotype with age could examine specific growth factor responses to perturbations thought to transduce the cardiac cell growth response and functional cellular changes, e.g. growth factors, oncogene induction, stretch and hormones. General gene regulation mechanisms that govern protein synthesis and degradation, and specific gene-switching mechanisms that regulate the type and density of functionally important cell organelles, e.g. ion channels, pumps, carriers and myofilaments, ought to be studied. The foregoing studies could be implemented with and without the imposition of acute or chronic stress, e.g. hypertension. Novel models of pressure overloaded heart failure now render these studies feasible. Studies to define which cellular changes underlie the transition of the chronically adapted heart stage to the failing heart at different ages will also be required.

VASCULAR DISEASE AND AGEING: THE 'ULTRA-CHALLENGE' TO BIOMEDICAL RESEARCH AND CLINICAL MEDICINE

Importance of vascular disease in elderly individuals

Cardiovascular disease is acknowledged to be the leading cause of mortality in elderly individuals; the specific causes are by and large vascular in origin, i.e. coronary, cerebral and peripheral vascular atherosclerosis and essential hypertension. The major deterioration of myocardial function with ageing, in fact, results in large part from cardiac pathophysiology due to coronary artery occlusive disease and/or hypertension. These vascular disorders as a single cause occupy the leading position on lists of hospital morbidity and health care costs. Given the crucial role of vascular disease in the health problems of the elderly it might be expected that highly focused and robust research programmes on these issues would be in progress. Paradoxically, however, most studies of vascular function and pathophysiology have, in essence, excluded age as a variable.

Age-associated alterations probably occur within the vasculature and affect the prevalence, severity and prognosis of atherosclerosis and hypertension. A better understanding of vascular ageing, and its interaction with the pathophysiology of occlusive vascular disease, is urgently needed. The goals of a mechanistic vascular ageing research would be: (a) to define age-associated changes in vascular structure and intracellular mechanisms that regulate function at the biochemical, biophysical and molecular levels; and (b) to elucidate the interaction of specific vascular disease states on the age-altered vascular substrate. A general plan of the type of studies that may be considered is as follows.

A general research plan for basic vascular ageing studies

These studies could be implemented in (a) freshly isolated cells, when possible in human species from transplant donors, (b) isolated cell cultures, (c) *in situ* (wound-healing experiments), and (d) transgenic animals. Properties of cell types and matrix factors in the vascular wall as a function of age (smooth muscle cells, endothelial cells, matrix molecules) could be characterized. Biophysical measurements in vascular smooth muscle cells include: (a) intrinsic excitation–contraction mechanisms (Ca^{2+}, pH, membrane potential); (b) receptor-mediated signal transduction mechanisms; and (c) studies to measure the response of vascular smooth muscle to growth factors of importance to measure include (i) chemotaxis, (ii) invasiveness, (iii) growth and proliferation, and (iv) secretion. In endothelial cells the following studies would probably prove fruitful: signal transduction mechanisms for (a) receptor-mediated agonists (muscarinic type I and II receptors, bradykinin, histamine, ATP, 5-hydroxytryptamine (5-HT), angiotensin II, vascular permeability factor), and (b) other factors (platelet factors, thromboxane, ADP, plasmin, sheer stress, stretch, anoxia). Endothelial cell product release also requires characterization and includes the response to growth factors, e.g. fibroblast growth factor, platelet-derived growth factors and others, e.g. EDRF, EDCF, endothelin, prostacyclin, thromboxane. The response to growth factors, e.g. changes in shape, alignment or permeability (endothelial cells), proliferative capacity or angiogenesis needs to be assessed. Additionally, basement membrane changes with age, and age-associated changes of circulating blood cells (macrophages, platelets) and properties (i.e. signal transduction and production secretion after various stimuli) require characterization as do cell–cell interactions with ageing, e.g. blood cell–endothelium and endothelium–vascular smooth muscle interactions. Finally, matrix molecule–cell interactions ought to be characterized, i.e. immune type II (delayed hypersensitivity) response to induced wounds and experimental atherosclerosis (lipid and immune models). In addition the effect of altered glucose homeostatis with ageing ought to be addressed in these studies.

The constellation of research described above would allow answers as to why arteries become stiff and more prone to atherosclerotic disease with advancing age. This information could lead to the development of 'age-adjusted' therapy for hypertension and atherosclerosis.

Clinical studies

Early detection and treatment of vascular disease in humans

Can we develop or refine our current measures to stratify populations by the level of risk of individual for vascular castastrophes such as myocardial infarction or stroke? If so, this would permit the targeting of interventions to individuals most likely to respond.

Example: if we had a sensitive instrument to image an individual's vasculature non-invasively we could stratify a large number of individuals with regard to the severity of their vascular lesions rather than with regard to a plasma lipid level or blood pressure. In intervention trials we could utilize the instrument to monitor changes in the vascular lesions rather than secondary and more indirect clinical sequelae, e.g. ischaemia or infarction, of the lesions as endpoints.

Without question, on the clinical level, the greatest impediment to solving vascular problems of the elderly relates to the difficulty of non-invasively measuring vascular endpoints with existing technology. Specifically, we do not presently have sensitive instruments which permit serial and non-invasive measurements of the various subcomponents of the vascular wall and of vascular lesions in large numbers of individuals. The lack of this technology has relegated direct and quantitative studies of the progressive changes in vasculature of elderly to a 'second-rate' status and has also likely impaired clinical trials relating to risk factors for atherosclerotic disease.

Consider for the moment the results of some of our nation's largest clinical trials. Over a 10-year period the NHLBI has spent 60% of its $494 million clinical trials budget on two efforts to determine whether cholesterol is proven to be the culprit in coronary heart disease. The first of these is MRFIT (the Multiple Risk Factor Intervention Trial). This 10-year $115 million research trial selected 12 866 men out of 361 662 to obtain a sample who were at high risk for CHD from multiple factors. The sample was randomly divided into usual care and the special intervention group. The special intervention group drastically altered their eating habits by cutting cholesterol intake by 42% saturated-fat by 28% and total calories by 21% and sustained the alteration over 7 years. Almost half the smokers quit. Eighty-seven per cent of the men were treated successfully for high blood pressure and two-thirds reached their specific blood pressure goal in the normal range. Researchers expected a 25% reduction in heart disease in the special intervention group. However, no significant difference in the overall number of deaths could be found between the two groups. In addition, those treated for hypertension had a rise in blood cholesterol by 7%.

A second study, the Coronary Primary Prevention Trial, attempted to demonstrate that CHD could be prevented by intervention with the drug cholestyramine. Drug intervention gave the experiment a biochemical purity that was absent from MRFIT's broad assault on statistical risk factors. This was a double-blind placebo study, involving 3810 men selected out of a sample of 480 000. It was expected that blood cholesterol levels would be reduced by an average of 28% in the treatment group. Seven years and $142 million later the cholesterol levels in the treatment group were only 6.7% lower than those of the control group.

After examining the results of these two studies one might become wary of a mass prevention project such as we are now undertaking in the USA. *Would the outcome of these and other similar studies have differed had we been able to assess vascular endpoints rather than using clinical events as endpoints?* We need to consider whether our biomedical research ensemble can develop or refine the presently available instruments to stratify study populations by the level of risk of individuals for vascular catastrophes such as myocardial infarction or stroke by providing a 'snapshot' of their vasculature. This should permit the targeting of interventions to individuals most likely to respond. If we had sensitive instruments to image an individual's vascualture non-invasively we could indeed stratify a large number of individuals with regard to the severity of their vascular lesions rather than with regard to a plasma lipid level or blood pressure. In intervention trials we could utilize this instrumentation to monitor changes in the vasculature lesions rather than the secondary and more indirect clinical sequelae, e.g. ischaemia or infarction, of these lesions as endpoints. Adding information about an individual's blood coagulation status together with their non-invasive vascular 'snapshot' would likely permit a definition of the predictive accuracy of an intervention (e.g. diet, drug, exercise) with respect to that individual rather than with respect to population trends. The results could be black and white, rather than grey, and would result in a greater compliance of individuals to change lifestyle habits or to take medication. Millions of individuals could be assured that they do not need to change their lifestyle or take drugs—or worry about atherosclerosis. Others could be assured that they indeed are a high risk. Health care costs would be dramatically reduced; life and health care costs would be dramatically reduced; life and health insurance of older individuals could be selectively adjusted.

A concerted effort on the part of the public and private funding sector is needed to catalyse the required innovative breakthroughs in biomedical technology that would lead to the development of instrumentation capable of providing 'vascular snapshots'. Specifically required is a concerted effort of individuals (a) in academia who utilize existing imaging techniques, (b) in industry, who have provided the present instrumentation and who have ongoing research to develop more sensitive instruments, (c) in NASA and the Department of Defense (because classified technology used for imaging by these oranizations ought to be made available to the biomedical research community), and (d) in organizations such as the American Heart Association and National Institutes of Health who are research policy makers, as well as leading vascular 'pathophysiologists', *basic* as well as clinical and epidemiologist types.

UTILIZATION OF PRESENTLY AVAILABLE CARDIOVASCULAR THERAPEUTIC PROCEDURES

The utilization and potential conservation of health care resources among patients of advanced age is a critical issue which must be addressed by the medical profession and society in general.

National statistical databases point to an inescapable trend that the utilization of invasive cardiovascular procedures among the elderly is high and continues to increase rapidly. In 1983, of 188 000 coronary artery bypass operations (CABG), 35% were performed in patients aged 65 years and older, and by 1987, of 245 000 CABG procedures, almost half (48%) were among patients aged 65 years or older (17). In some large institutions, the median age for CABG is now over the age of 65 years (18) (Figure 5), and this is probably higher among patients undergoing valve replacement. Increasing numbers of recent reports deal with CABG and septuagenarians and octogenarians, and raise the issue of the 'young old' and the 'old' within the general definition of the elderly (19–22). The

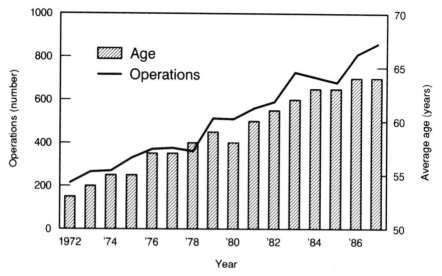

Figure 5. Isolated coronary bypass surgery at the Mayo clinic from 1972 to 1987. The scale on the left represents the number of operations, and the scale on the right the average age per year. Reproduced with permission from Dr H. V. Schaff

burgeoning rate of CABG among the elderly is not simply the result of demographic trends, but reflects to some extent the improvements in surgical techniques and outcome, which have led to an expansion of the procedure's application into a 'sicker' patient population, including the 'frail' elderly (23,24). Moreover, although the large randomized trials of CABG versus medical therapy specifically *excluded* patients over the age of 65 years, several recent reports dealing with non-randomized patients suggest that subsets of older patients might derive a *particular* benefit from CABG over medical therapy (25,26).

The utilization of other cardiovascular procedures among the elderly has undergone substantial growth. Cardiac catheterization in patients aged 65 years of age or older increased from 138 000 in 1983 to 328 000 in 1987 (a 238% increase) (17). Although the increase in pacemaker procedures has been less dramatic, this has gone from 150 000 in 1983 to 174 000 in 1987 (16% increase). Recent preliminary reports on the use of automatic implantable cardioverter–defibrillators would suggest that a substantial proportion of the patients receiving these devices in some institutions are elderly (27).

The attraction of percutaneous transluminal coronary angioplasty (PTCA) as an alternative form of coronary revascularization in elderly people is understandable, although randomized comparative trials of PTCA and CABG are still in progress (28). At the Mayo Clinic in 1980, only 10.1% of patients undergoing PTCA were aged 65 years or over, but in 1988 the elderly comprised 53.6% of the PTCA population. Moreover, among the elderly undergoing PTCA at the Mayo

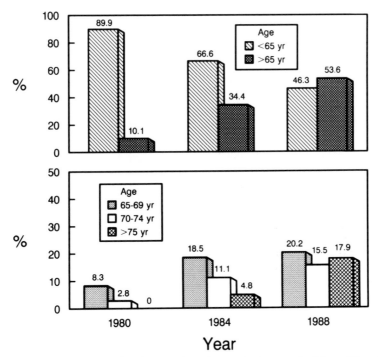

Figure 6. Percentage by age of patients undergoing angioplasty at the Mayo Clinic for the years 1980, 1984 and 1988. Top: patients <65 or ≥65 years old. Bottom: subgroup of patients over the age of 65. Reproduced from Thompson *et al.* (28) with permission from the *Journal of the American College of Cardiology*

Clinic, 20.2% were aged 65–79 years, 15.5% aged 70–74 years, and 17.9% aged 75 years or older (Figure 6). These recently published data from one institution mirror national trends (28).

Coronary artery bypass surgery

Operative morbidity and mortality increase with advancing age (23), and although the long-term survival is shorter than in younger patients, symptom relief appears to be similar (30,31). The powerful adverse impact of peripheral vascular disease and other comorbid medical conditions upon late outcome, however, needs emphasis. One of the most consistent lessons emanating from the randomized trials of CABG versus medical therapy was the demonstration that the 'sicker the patient', the greater was the survival benefit from CABG in comparison with medical therapy (24–26). In this regard, the elderly are, in many respects, 'sicker' than their younger counterparts on the basis of left ventricular dysfunction, the extent and severity of coronary disease, and the severity of symptoms and ischaemia (23). Not surprisingly, there is evidence to suggest that CABG is superior to medial therapy among particular subsets of elderly patients—the majority of whom were in the group aged 65–75 years (26,27). Moreover, the perception that the elderly are frequently intolerant of medical therapy, coupled to the comparative studies of surgery and medical therapy for symptomatic coronary disease in the elderly, have fuelled the explosion of CABG in this age group.

Among the 'old', the feasibility and efficacy of CABG are well documented (19–22), and careful patient selection to avoid the 'frail' elderly is the key to success. Nonetheless, there is a paucity of long-term follow-up data, and published series to date reflect the experience of individual centres. The results to date would suggest that operation should not be denied to patients because of age alone, but in the face of extreme age and the presence of multiple comorbid diseases, the benefits and appropriateness of CABG remain unestablished.

Percutaneous transluminal coronary angioplasty

The technical success rate of PTCA in the current era in the elderly is comparable to that achieved in younger patients (28), although in the early PTCA experience primary success rates were less (32). However, periprocedural mortality appears to be increased among the elderly, and this is a reflection, in part, of other risk factors such as extensive coronary disease, unstable angina and pre-existing heart failure in the elderly (28). The early results are also influenced by decisions made in advance not to proceed with emergency CABG in the event of PTCA failure, particularly in elderly patients with serious comorbid diseases (28).

Preliminary reports suggest that late survival is high and the subsequent incidence of non-fatal myocardial infarction or coronary bypass surgery in the elderly is low. Nonetheless, the recurrence of angina appears to be substantially greater among patients over the age of 75 years—probably the result of more extensive disease and more limited procedures leading to a greater frequency of incomplete revascularization (28).

THE ISSUES

The widespread application of invasive cardiovascular procedures in the elderly is now upon us. Ideally, cost should not be the overriding concern of the medical profession, and in the USA, by comparison with other countries, the question of cost has perhaps been underemphasized. Nonetheless, as we attempt to come to grips with the soaring cost of health care in the 1990s and a realization that resources are limited and will have to be carefully allocated in the future, the cost of cardiovascular disease and its treatment among the elderly will undergo increasing scrutiny.

Age, *per se*, should not be a contraindication to the implementation of a procedure, but the risks and costs versus benefit need to be determined among subgroups of patients. The elderly are a very heterogeneous group who differ both in chronological and 'physiological' age. Their quality of life, aspirations and motivations are more deeply rooted in their economic and sociologic well-being than in their more youthful counterparts. Whereas the potential for invasive cardiovascular procedures to prolong life in patients aged 65–80 years is well established, the long-term outcome among patients over the age of 80 or 85 years is less well known. Since maximum longevity has never increased in our species and relatively few individuals live past 100, it is clear that there must be an upper age limit at which 'meaningful' long-term survival cannot be significantly enhanced by any form of therapy. Even among the 65- to 74-year-old cohort, there are those with extensive comorbid conditions, e.g. peripheral vascular disease and renal disease, in whom it is also unlikely that a cardiovascular procedure could exert any major impact upon survival. Moreover, with advancing age, the less tangible function of the 'quality of life' becomes as important, if not more so, than survival alone. Among this diverse group of elderly patients with symptomatic coronary disease are those whose prognosis will be substantially improved by invasive therapy, and there are those in whom it will not be altered. Our ability to make these distinctions is, at this stage, limited by an inadequate database, although review of published series would suggest that clinical judgement has led to careful patient selection.

Nonetheless, society is faced with a number of difficult social, ethical and economic issues which are the direct consequence of increased survivorship and advances in medical technology. Before the decision regarding the allocation of health care resources can be made, and in order for these to be comprehensively addressed, the relevant information must be available. In this regard, it should be emphasized that a present there are insufficient data with which to formulate sound judgement. Publication of individual series which document the success or other outcomes of a procedure in highly selected subsets of patients is insufficient. What is required is a large multicentre database (prospectively entered) which will document the outcomes of different invasive cardiovascular procedures applied to patients of advanced age. Endpoints would include periprocedural morbidity and mortality, cost, long-term survival, 'quality of life' and the maintenance of functional and social independence. Only with this information will it be possible to address adequately the disquieting issue of the limits of a procedure's applicability to some segments of our society.

DESIGN OF A DATABASE

A randomized trial of invasive versus conservative therapy in the elderly would be the ideal theoretical approach to the problem. Indeed, current trials comparing PTCA versus CABG are including patients up to the age of 80 years. Nonetheless, trials of medical therapy compared to coronary revascularization in the elderly would be difficult to justify and probably impractical to implement, given the markedly symptomatic and unstable status of many elderly patients, in association with the known frequency of severe multivessel disease and left ventricular dysfunction in this age group.

An alternative approach is to establish a multicentre registry of cardiovascular procedures which would reflect the demographic and socio-economic diversity of our population. This would include (a) patients undergoing coronary angiography, (b) CABG, (c) PTCA, (d) cardiac valve surgery, (e) balloon valvuloplasty, (f) implantation of automatic antitachycardia and defibrillator devices, (g) catheterization ablation for arrhythmias; (h) patients undergoing vascular surgical procedures (all of which are strongly associated with coronary artery disease) and, more specifically, abdominal aortic aneurysm repair, carotid endarterectomy, and surgical procedures for dissecting thoracic aneurysms should likewise be included. For the purposes of a registry, the elderly could be defined as age 70 and above, with patients aged 60–69 years serving as younger controls, since it is well established that the results of many invasive procedures in patients in their 60s are not substantially different from younger patients. It is difficult to define age groups precisely within the elderly, and although chronological age is a poor predictor of functional status, 'physiological' age, while conceptually attractive, is not quantifiable. An important adjunct to a registry of patients undergoing procedures should include a sample of patients who either decline or were not offered an invasive procedure. Inclusion of these subgroups would help in identifying the impact of referral bias (10).

The period of follow-up should be sufficiently long (e.g. 10 years), so as to allow the evaluation of sufficient numbers of outliers, which would help to categorize the subset of patients with a particularly good or a particularly poor prognosis. In addition to late mortality in symptom relief, it would be necessary to prospectively define and evaluate some of the less tangible, but equally important objectives, e.g. the quality of life, functional independence and cost-effectiveness.

CONCLUSIONS

The demographics are undeniable, and our society is beginning to address the implications of the expanding elderly population upon our health care system. If physicians are to play an important role in future decision-making processes, it is imperative to construct an accurate database which will then be subjected to rigorous analysis. As a first step, it should be understood that the data we need (at least in the population over the age of 75 years) are currently unavailable, and a prospective registry might provide the framework for rational decisions, both in the arena of health care and public policy.

REFERENCES

1. US Bureau of Census (1989) *Statistical Abstract of the United States*. US Printing Officer, Washington, DC, p. 109.
2. Spencer G (1990) Projections of the population of the United States by age, sex, and race: 1988 to 2088. *1989 Current Population Report*, US Bureau of the Census Series

P-25 No. 1018, US Printing Office, Washington, DC.

3. Schneider EL, Guralnik JM (1990) The aging of America: impact on health care costs. *JAMA* **263**: 2335–2340.

4. Page LB (1987) Introductory remarks (Proceedings of the 18th Bethesda Conference on Cardiovascular Disease in the Elderly). *J Am Coll Cardiol* **10** (Suppl.): 7A–9A.

5. Elveback LR, Connolly DC, Kurland LT (1981) Coronary heart disease in residents of Rochester, Minnesota. II. Mortality, incidence, and survivorship, 1950–1975. *Mayo Clinic Proc* 665–672.

6. Wei J, Gersh BJ (1987) Heart disease in the elderly. *Curr Probl Cardiol* **12**: 7–65.

7. Hlatky MA, Greenfield JC (1990) Technologic innovation and care of elderly patients with cardiovascular disease: how will the diagnosis-related group system respond? *Am J Med* **88**: 1-1N–1-2N.

8. Wenger NK, Furberg CD, Pitt E (eds) *Coronary Heart Disease in the Elderly*. Elsevier, New York.

9. Dustan HP, Hamilton MP, McCullough L, Page LB (1987) Social, political, and ethnical considerations in the treatment of cardiovascular disease in the elderly. *J Am Coll Cardiol* **10** (Suppl.): 14A–17A.

10. Callahan D (1987) *Setting Limits*. Simon & Schuster, New York.

11. Weisfeldt ML, Lakatta EG, Gerstenblith G (1992) Aging and the heart. In *Heart Disease: A Textbook Cardiovascular Medicine*, 4th edn, Braunwald E (ed.). Saunders, Philadelphia, pp. 1656–1669.

12. Lakatta EG (1990) Heart and circulation. In *Handbook of the Biology of Aging*, 3rd edn, Schneider EL, Rowe J (eds). Academic Press, New York, pp. 181–216.

13. Lakatta EG (1991) Normal changes of aging. In *Merck Manual of Geriatrics*, Abrams WB, Berkow R (eds). Merck Sharp & Dohme Research Laboratories, Rahway, NJ, pp. 310–325.

14. Lakatta EG (1991) Excitation–contraction coupling in heart failure. *Hosp Prac* **26**: 85–98.

15. Lakatta EG (1991) Regulation of cardiac muscle function in the hypertensive heart. In *Cellular and Molecular Mechanisms of Hypertension*, Cox RH (ed.). Plenum, New York, pp. 149–173.

16. de la Bastie D, Levitsky D, Rappaport L *et al.* (1990) Function of the sarcoplasmic reticulum and expression of its Ca^{2+}-ATPase gene in pressure overload-induced cardiac hypertrophy in the rat. *Circ Res* **66**: 554–564.

17. Kozak LG (1989) Hospital inpatient surgery: United States, 1983–1987. *Advance Data from Vital and Health Statistics*, No. 169, DHHS Publication No. (PHS) 89-1250, Public Health Service, Hyattsville, MD.

18. Backes RJ, Gersh BJ (1991) The treatment of coronary artery disease in the elderly. *Cardiovasc Drug Ther* **5**: 449–456.

19. Mullany CJ, Darling GE, Pluth JR *et al.* (1990) Early and late results after isolated coronary artery bypass surgery in 159 patients aged 80 years and older. *Circulation* **82** (Suppl.): IV-229–IV-236.

20. Neunheim KS, Kern MJ, McBride LR *et al.* (1987) Coronary artery bypass surgery in patients aged 80 years or older. *Am J Cardiol* **59**: 804–807.

21. Tsai TP, Matloff JM, Chaux A *et al.* (1986) Combined valve and coronary artery bypass procedures in septuagenarians and octogenarians: results in 120 patients, *Ann Thorac Surg* **42**: 681–684.

22. Edmund LH Jr, Stephenson LW, Edie RN, Ratcliffe MB (1988) Open-heart surgery in octogenarians. *N Engl J Med* **319**: 131–136.

23. Gersh BJ, Kronmal RA, Frye RL *et al.* and participants in the Coronary Artery Surgery Study (1983) Coronary arteriography and coronary artery bypass surgery: morbidity and mortality in patients aged 65 years or older. A report from the

Coronary Artery Surgery Study. *Circulation* **67**: 483–491.

24. Gersh BJ, Califf RM, Loop FD *et al.* (1989) Coronary bypass surgery in chronic stable angina. *Circulation* **79** (Suppl.): I-46–I-59.

25. Gersh BJ, Kronmal RA, Schaff HV *et al.* (1985) Comparison of coronary artery bypass surgery and medical therapy in patients 65 years of age or older: a nonrandomized study from the Coronary Artery Surgery Study (CASS) Registry. *N Engl J Med* **313**: 217–224.

26. Califf RM, Harrell FE, Lee KL *et al.* (1989) The evolution of medical and surgical therapy for coronary artery disease: a 15-year perspective. *JAMA* **261**: 2077–2086.

27. Jerome S, Aaron D, Juanteguy J, Veltri EP (1991) Automatic implantable cardioverter–defibrillator in the elderly (Abstract). *J Am Coll Cardiol* **17** (Suppl. A): 329A.

28. Thompson RC, Holmes DR, Gersh BJ *et al.* (1991) Percutaneous transluminal coronary angioplasty in the elderly: early and long-term results. *J Am Coll Cardiol* **17**: 1245–1250.

29. Waldo DR, Sonnefeld ST, McKusick DR, Arnett R III (1989) III. Health expenditures by age group, 1977 and 1987. *Health Care Finance Rev* **10**: 111–120.

30. Gersh BJ, Kronmal RA, Schaff HV (1983) Long-term (5 year) results of coronary bypass surgery in patients 65 years old or older: a report from the Coronary Artery Surgery Study. *Circulation* **68** (Suppl. II): II-190–II-199.

31. Loop FD, Lytle VW, Gosgrove DM *et al.* (1988) Coronary artery bypass graft surgery in the elderly: indications and outcomes. *Cleve Clin J Med* **55**: 23–24.

32. Mock MB, Holmes DR Jr, Vlietstra RE *et al.* (1984) Percutaneous transluminal coronary angioplasty (PTCA) in the elderly patient: experience in the National Heart, Lung, and Blood Institute PTCA Registry. *Am J Cardiol* **53**: 89C–91C.

34 Ethical Considerations

J. J. TAYLOR

States Laboratory, St Helier, Jersey, Channel Islands

'Armchair ethicists' list a number of ethical imperatives which should govern an acceptable moral code of conduct. Most rational people agree with most of these. When treating patients the position is more complex since the doctor (who is the responsible and capable moral agent) has to decide and act as *he* thinks right. In making up his mind he must not only have a personally formulated moral code of conduct, but will need also to take account of any relevant law, general guidance (such as that issued in the UK by the General Medical Council), International Declarations (e.g. Helsinki, Tokyo), professional codes and advice of trusted colleagues.

Patients also have a conscience and may choose to follow its dictates—when, for example, rejecting medical advice or proposed therapeutic or research procedure. The right so to do, even though death may result, is recognized, both in law and in ethics under the principle of consent.

Normally the doctor makes his judgements in daily practice without the need to study philosophy or theology; his ethics are part of him and he 'does his best for the patient'. This latter contains the real truth of all doctoring for, despite the advances of science and technology, the doctor knows in his innermost heart that all such measures are secondary to helping his patient ('beneficence'). Treatment is tailored to a particular individual—taking into account all the factors mentioned above—and is not specific to the disease present irrespective of the human being in whom it is found. The proper concern of ethics is with man.

Difficulties arise, however, when one vacates the armchair for the minefields of clinical practice and research. Issues such as abortion, care of handicapped neonates, and screening for early detection all raise particular problems, and emotional tidal waves tend to drown rational debate. Important as all these matters are, increasingly they are being overtaken by the massive problems arising from the ever-increasing numbers of elderly people. Practice in this area is complicated by the multiplicity of diseases often present, altered financial and family circumstances and, of particular relevance to the problem of consent in research, the large number of patients with progressive dementia.

This chapter is not intended to be an ethical text but rather a guide to basic concepts and a brief study of their application to some research problems relating to cardiac disease in the elderly.

Geriatric Cardiology. Principles and Practice. Edited by A. Martin and A. J. Camm
© 1994 John Wiley & Sons Ltd

The following section briefly describes ethical principles and how they may guide us in the present field of study. Omissions are deliberate and personal and will not (hopefully) prove too irksome to those fully familiar with the matter in hand.

ETHICS

Ethics is the systematic study of moral conduct, the standards of right and wrong by which it may be directed and the goals toward which such conduct is directed. It is therefore concerned with choices, actions and character. It involves examination of the nature of the person as a moral being, the source and meaning of values in life and the beliefs upon which they are based. Historically ethics is a branch of philosophy which seeks the truth of moral obligation under the guidance of reason.

MEDICAL ETHICS

This term is used in at least three ways:

1. *A professional code of conduct.* This refers to those principles which guide the conduct of doctors (and other health care professionals). In the stricter application to doctors it deals with relationships to patients, families, other doctors and society.
2. *Moral issues in medicine.* This use of the term comprehensively covers the moral decisions that doctors face in dealing with patients and which are built on the principle of covenant. In this sense the morality of transplantation, care of the dying and allocation of resources would be seen as included in the field.
3. *Courses of study.* Older medical texts contain sections on medical etiquette in dealing with patients or colleagues. New horizons of technological and scientific medicine require that doctors are trained in ethical matters so that they may appreciate not only the new problems arising but learn also to deliberate and discern right courses of action. Such courses are being increasingly extended into medical student training in the UK following the publication of the Pond Report, and recognize that medicine still is an art—despite an increasingly scientific component. Medicine also is a moral undertaking since it deals with the rights of persons and the pursuit of their well-being. The ultimate aim of these deliberations is to move beyond the question of what *can* be done to the moral question of what, *for this particular patient, ought* to be done?

Many doctors find these difficult waters and are uncomfortable discussing them and their relevance to *their* clinical practice and research. The writer, for instance, was recently invited to address a national meeting and spent some time preparing his contribution for this—only to learn that both the title and the proposed contribution would be 'unacceptable' to an audience of 'scientifically trained health professionals'. The title was 'We can—but should we?' For those who wish to renew their acquaintance with these fundamental ethical concepts (or perhaps discover them for the first time) suitable introductory references are provided (1–3).

MORALITY AND ETHICAL THEORY

Medical ethics, unlike cardiovascular surgery, is not something new: 'Vita brevis, ars longa, tempus praeceps, experimentum periculosum, judicium difficile' (Hippocrates, Aphorism, i).

The occurrence of landmark cases (e.g. Bourne, Gillick, Baby Doe) and more recently the heightened general perception of new views on old problems (highlighted, for example, by the AIDS epidemic—with its voluminous literature, research and meetings dealing among other matters with testing, consent and appropriate disbursement of funds) serve to emphasize the fundamental importance of ethical approaches in medicine.

PRINCIPLES

There are four main principles to be considered in medical ethics: autonomy, beneficence, justice and non-malificence. Whilst there are many theories of ethics, there are two major schools of thought exemplified by the Kantian and the utilitarian viewpoints. These briefly state that conduct should be determined either by one's duty ('deontological')—*regardless* of what the end result may be—or alternatively that which produces (or maximizes) the greatest possible balance of value over disvalue for all persons. Now it is easy to see how the physician or surgeon will 'do his (utmost) duty' in respect of the patient sitting before him; doctors often find the application of the utilitarian viewpoint less attractive when, for example, lack of funds prevents operations being carried out on a small number of patients (one of which happens to be *their* patient) because the money has been used for some other purpose.

Case note

The lay trustees of the Massachusetts General Hospital announced on 1 February 1980 that they had voted *not* to permit heart transplants. The explanatory note stated 'there is a clear responsibility to evaluate new procedures in terms of the greatest good for the greatest number'.

Later that year the Secretary for the American Department of Health and Human Services withdrew authorization for medical cover, stating that such funding could no longer depend solely on the safety, effectiveness and acceptance of a technology by the medical community; it must also be evaluated in terms of its 'social consequences'—of which cost (especially high cost) is a factor.

This is a simple demonstration of how the utiltiarian philosophy has been translated into actual practice.

ETHICS AND RESEARCH

There is no simple absolute solution to the multiple problems posed by medical research (whether that be in children, elderly, mentally impaired, cancer sufferers or indeed any other condition). The problem is a complex balancing of all the factors in every case.

Generally speaking, doctors are no better (and no worse) at making ethical judgements than anyone else. There is a problem, however, when the doctor making moral evaluations is responsible not only for *medical* (i.e. therapeutic) decisions but wishes also to carry out some form of research on the patients under his medical care. At the heart of the Helsinki Declaration lies the kernel of informed consent; since this declaration or its implications form part of modern research protocols, the next section examines the nature of informed consent. For many research workers informed consent proves a thorn in the flesh. In elderly patients this is more likely to be so because of the frequent association of a variable degree of mental impairment.

WHAT IS INFORMED CONSENT?

Opinions expressed range from 'informed consent means telling patients everything about their condition and leaving the choice of treatment to them' to the dismissive 'informed consent is a nonsense because patients cannot understand what they are told and should not be allowed to make decisions for themselves'.

Between these extremes are the vast numbers of conscientious doctors who agonize daily about how much information they should give their patients, how it should be communicated and whether this makes things better or worse for the patient. The doctor's prime duty is always to act in the best interests of the (particular) patient. It is how those best interests are interpreted and whose opinion prevails which is the crux of the problem. Lack of informed consent has been the basis for many successful legal actions—but if the morals of the position are understood and practised legal action is not likely.

Health care and patients' rights are relatively recent entrants into the rights arena and the subject of controversy (along with euthanasia, abortion, brain death, *in vitro* fertilization, genetic engineering, etc).

Moral and legal

Rights are justified claims based on acknowledged principles which may be moral or legal. Moral rights are grounded in principles which apply universally (i.e. if you possess that right so does everyone else). Moral rights are not necessarily legally enforceable (although if enough people feel strongly enough on a moral issue they may organize legislation to protect that right).

A legal right, on the other hand, does not have to be supported by any moral principle. *Per se*, unlike a moral principle, it is not concerned with good or bad, only what is right or wrong according to the law. Bad laws can be changed, whereas the essence of a moral principle is that it is seen to be intrinsically good and therefore *not* subject to change.

Informed consent is not a legal right in the UK but it is generally accepted to be a moral right.

Enforced examinations

In a few special situations, mostly in the field of public health, medical examination can be enforced even against the wishes of the subject.

Thus persons suffering from notifiable diseases may be examined after an order from a magistrate. Immigrants may be examined at ports and airports to ensure absence of communicable diseases. Members of HM Forces and new admissions to prisons may be also so examined without consent. (This applies only with sentenced prisoners; however, those on remand remain in possession of their civil rights and *may* withhold consent.)

Court probation orders may direct psychiatric examination (Section 28, Mental Health Act 1959).

Food handlers and dairy workers may be required to submit to medical examination if suspected of, for example, salmonella infection.

School children must be medically examined by law; but where parents object to the School Medical Officer carrying out this examination they must arrange an examination by a doctor of their choice.

Courts can order blood tests in cases of disputed paternity.

In all these situations the right of the individual has been overridden by requirements of society. Thus the utilitarian approach impairs autonomy in such cases with the legal approval of society. That approval does not, however, of itself make the situations morally acceptable.

Special circumstances

Children and the mentally handicapped generally are not capable of giving fully informed consent, although this statement needs to be seen in the light of the age and mental ability of each particular case. The parents or authority *in loco parentis* are generally accepted as having the right and responsibility to give or withhold consent in relation to medical matters. With older children more involvement is possible than with youngsters. With babies some of the most difficult problems arise because of the complete inability of the baby to communicate meaningfully, and the total lack of any possibility of explaining to the infant what is proposed. There the duty of the parents in relation to their offspring, and the duty of care of the physician are particularly exposed. Recent legal cases (Dr Arthur and Baby Doe) have shown the public and professional disquiet in this area.

There is no doubt that there is great room for improvement in the handling of this issue. The large number of so-called 'consent forms' which are signed daily which purport to authorize certain tests or treatments are really nothing of the kind. In truth they are documents which are included in the patient's case-notes and whose real purpose is to answer any adversary proceedings that might be brought at some future date. Personal investigation and some in the literature shows that many are signed *without* the patient being *fully* informed.

Whilst the difficulty of obtaining as fully informed consent as is possible has been described in the context of clinical therapy and trials, another difficult area concerns 'non-clinical' research. When the research involved requires the use of normal subjects for drug testing or for psychological studies the application of fully informed consent is particularly difficult. Some believe that in this context fully informed consent can be given only by those fully identified with the research project, i.e. the researchers themselves, but here one of the basic ingredients of informed consent, namely free power of choice, may not be operative. (It may, for example, be the case that unless a researcher takes part in a project as a subject his or her future in the research team might be jeopardized and this would clearly influence his judgement.) Others have argued that the provision of payment for partaking in research similarly erodes the voluntary aspect of choice. The amount of inducement payment offered is now in some areas of research under scrutiny to try to control this variable as much as possible. This issue has gained some notoriety particularly with the use of students in research and at least two well-publicized deaths during a research programme. (One of these may well have been coincidental but these tragic events naturally colour the approach to such projects.)

A further difficulty is encountered where it is thought that some degree of deception is necessary to institute a project. Now the moral viewpoint is that deception is unacceptable. There is a problem then, for some experiments seem to require that the subjects not be told the purpose of the study, or that they be induced to hold false beliefs about the nature of the experiment during the experiment itself. (For example, they may be told they will receive a psychoactive drug or a placebo in the trial, and told which they are to receive—but in fact are given the other.)

In this area the real problem is whether such deception is ever justified. Can the knowledge be obtained in some other way without deception; is the deception being used for pragmatic purposes (i.e. to save time or money) alone? Excluding such 'deception of convenience' there still may be some degree of deception that cannot be eliminated from the project (on logistical grounds); and the paternalistic and utilitarian defences for this position are unsatisfactory. A further attempt to justify deception is that of *ex post facto*—deception justified by its acceptance by those who have already taken part in it. This, too, is at best a shaky moral position. Two further possibilities, of 'presumptive consent' and 'prior general consent', I dismiss as inadequate to justify deception, but the more complicated matter of combined proxy and prior general consent requires closer examination.

Thus far only two positions are tenable: (i) no experiments involving ineliminable deception are permissible; (ii) all such experiments are permissible. It is the latter position which seeks to reduce the significance of the 'informed' condition of the principle of informed consent.

The application of prior general consent—rejected as a valid method of its own—combined with proxy consent might be an acceptable method. Here each subject nominates a person who will inspect the experimental protocol. This person is empowered by the subject to accept or reject experiments (on the basis that they carry unacceptable risks, employ too much deception or aim to produce knowledge which might be misused). The proxy makes these judgements from the *viewpoint of the subject*, not from his own viewpoint. This method combines the concept that consent to deception *is* compatible with the principle of informed consent together with the consultation of persons other than the research subjects themselves. I am not aware that this method is in actual use yet for the obvious radical changes in practical implementation that would be involved, but suggest later that it may be a way forward in some forms of cardiac resuscitation research.

All this is difficult. What, for example, is 'adequately informed'? Who is to decide?

We cannot push aside informed consent simply because it is difficult to define or operate. Nor should we take the viewpoint that since it is difficult (and perhaps really impossible to define fully—i.e. *truly* unobtainable) all clinical research should cease. This would bring the advancement of science and improvements in medical care to future generations to a halt—itself an immoral position to hold *unless* the actual as distinct from the personally perceived risks are excessive compared with the minimal benefit.

CLINICAL TERMS

It is now widely accepted that randomized clinical trials are the most ethical approach to assess potential new treatments; but it must be remembered that this is so *only* if the probability of the efficacy of the proposed new treatment relative to the control group is about 50%. Secondly, whilst *widely* accepted this approach is not *generally* accepted. Critics of randomized trial work base their arguments on the following premises:

1. *The patient is being deceived.* If the patient is unaware that a placebo is being used, this is dishonest and carries the ethical cost of deception. This, it is argued, is a breach of trust between doctor and patient, denies the patient choice and is therefore morally unacceptable (5).
2. *One group will knowingly receive inferior treatment.* The conflict here is between medical judgement and statistical significance (6,7).

When we move into 'high-tech' areas the practical problems seem ever greater but the fundamental moral reasoning remains the same. It should, however, be possible by prior consideration to formulate an approach which will withstand criticism and allow progress in practice.

Resuscitation research

Continuing with the problem of consent let us consider the approach in resuscitation research. The principle that improvements in treatment should be sought is not at issue. Any attempt to do so, however, must be secondary to the care of the current patient (8). In countries where regulations exist to protect subjects in clinical research, the central role of informed consent is accepted; but this is not usually possible (at least in the generally accepted sense) in those who unexpectedly require resuscitation. Abramson argued that in such circumstances obtaining informed consent was not necessary (9), and later (10) proposed that informed consent for emergency treatment may be waived (under American regulations and law). The distinction between the requirements for resuscitation *research* and emergency *treatment* too blurred for practical use. They also stated that 'deferred consent' should be obtained 'at an appropriate later time from the family'; but subsequent refusal could create legal difficulties, and in any event one cannot meaningfully consent to an event which has already occurred.

Because prior individual consent to resuscitation *research* is not usually possible (since none of us knows when we may need it), and since deferred consent cannot exist, this leaves only proxy consent.

Proxy consent is nothing new with treatment and research. It has been practised for many years without being formally so entitled, particularly in the field of mental disorders. In general medical and surgical diseases when rationality or consciousness of the patient is obscured—whether temporarily or permanently—proxy consent is commonly used. Similarly, in dealing with children, who legally may not consent, parental, guardian or court proxy consent is the norm.

With patients admitted unconscious and requiring urgent *treatment*, only that which is life-saving is permissible without consent (in British law). Prospects for research under such restrictive conditions therefore seem remote since clearly informed consent, as generally understood, cannot be obtained. Moreover, in the acute situation where life is threatened it is often either physically impossible to contact the next of kin, or impractical within the time-scale needed. These difficulties can be overcome by a form of prior proxy consent.

The management of a previously unknown patient who requires resuscitation is a complex mix of the skills of a team. In the acute situation there is relatively little room for manoeuvre, and departmental protocols should be normal practice. These should have been generally agreed in advance.

Any variation to assess likely improvement will need great care and forethought since unfavourable results might lead to successful litigation later. It seems to me, however irritating it may be to the resuscitation team, that deviations from the protocol must be conducted in a scientific way if they are to provide information of value and if they are to be acceptable also on ethical grounds. It is therefore necessary for all the team to know that a comparison is being made between the 'standard' departmental approach and a modification, that nobody yet knows which is best, and that as soon as a sufficient number of patients has been compared a decision will be made on whether to revert to the standard or adopt the modified approach as the new standard. It is also crucial for the team to know that the modified regime has been considered by the Institutional Research Ethical Committee which has given approval for this approach. Whilst this will not, of course, prevent successful legal action for negligence in the way treatment is applied, it will provide a framework in which the employing authority and its employees will be seen to be acting in the public interest, and probably provide a legal safeguard against subsequent litigation.

The Research Ethical Committee therefore would have an onerous responsibility in considering such matters and requires to be fully informed on both the standard and modified approaches. It is not good enough to have a 'cosy chat' over these momentous matters. The reason for the creation of ethics committees was to safeguard patients' rights, and where for any reason patients are not able to understand what is being, or about to be done, to them this responsibility is heightened. Current discussion regarding the formation of a National Ethics Committee (UK) serves to illustrate that there is genuine disquiet in some quarters on these matters.

The variable performance of local ethical committees has been documented and leaves no doubt of the need for a firm directive in this matter.

Lay members of ethics committees (and I do not intend here to indicate how they should be selected and appointed) are extremely important, and it is always crucial to ensure that they are fully satisfied at all stages of the committee's enquiry.

A particular advantage of prior proxy consent for patients in this category could be that current debate regarding randomization and the confusion this causes patients and relatives (and the difficulties it creates for doctors) could be avoided. Similar to the proposal of Zelen (11) the research ethical committee could consider randomization and agree (or not) that the particular study would only be scientifically valid with randomization. Some argue that this removes clinical autonomy but of course it does nothing of the kind, since in conventional randomized clinical trials the randomization is not under the control of the clinician. Indeed it is undesirable that it should be; Guyatt's scheme for conducting randomized trials in individual patients could be applied in cardiac research in the elderly, and where competence is impeached (12).

Transplantation

I exclude from consideration here ethical considerations in the criteria of 'suitability', organ procurement ('required decision', 'presumed consent'), acceptable criteria of cerebral death, 'beating heart donors', and discuss only artificial hearts and transplantation in the elderly.

At the time of writing, all patients who have received an artificial heart as a permanent implant on a research basis have died of thromboembolism and/or infection. They are no longer approved by the Food and Drug Administration (FDA) for permanent use, and generally at the present time are restricted to temporary usage. The gradual adoption of mechanical supports, whether uni- or biventricular, clearly saves the lives of some patients and is unlikely to remain restricted to the under-65 age group for much longer. It exacerbates the problem, however, because it increases the number of those waiting for transplantation, and this in turn increases the need for further donor hearts; the alternative of totally implantable artificial hearts, already in use in animals, may become more widespread eventually than real heart transplantations. The costs of such a programme have been estimated to be similar to that of current renal dialysis and transplant programmes.

Carefully controlled prospective trials may be the best scientific way to evaluate these new technologies, and there is the view that this is the only ethical way to proceed. Yet new treatments are often introduced in an uncontrolled way; the decision to do so may be based on retrospective studies, anecdote, personal experience or apparent plausibility. Perhaps the latter approach more than the former recognizes the uncertainties that attend the search for knowledge. Decisions about innovations in clinical practice still remain in the realm of practical wisdom rather than of theoretical science. It was noted by Aristotle that the same degree of certainty should not be expected in areas of human activity demanding practical wisdom as in the natural sciences. This uncertainty may be the price we have to pay in order not to sacrifice other important ethical values.

REFERENCES

1. Faulder C (1985) *Whose Body Is It?* Virago Press, London.
2. Kant I (1933) *Critique of Pure Reason.* Macmillan, London.
3. Gillon R (1986) *Philosphical Medical Ethics.* Wiley, Chichester.
4. Gillick and West Norfolk and Wisbech Area Health Authority (1984) *Times Law Report* 21 December, p. 9.
5. Editorial (1979) Controlled trials; planned deception? *Lancet* i: 534.
6. Oliver MF, Heady JA, Manes JW (1978) Clofibrate in heart disease. *Br Med J* **40**: 1069.
7. Armitage P (1975) *Sequential Medical Trials.* Blackwell Scientific, Oxford, p. 70.
8. Miller BL (1988) Philosophical, ethical and legal aspects of resuscitation medicine. *Crit Care Med* **16**: 1059–1062.
9. Abramson NS, Meisel AO, Safar P (1981) Informed consent in resuscitation research. *JAMA* **246**: 2828.
10. Abramson NS, Meisel AO, Safar P (1986) A new approach for resuscitation research in comatose patients. *JAMA* **255**: 2466.
11. Zeelen M (1979) A new design for randomized clinical trials. *N Engl J Med* **300**: 1242–1245.

12. Guyatt G, Satchett D, Taylor D *et al.* (1986) Determining optional therapy randomized trials in individual patients. *N Engl J Med* **314**: 889–892.

Other helpful references

Applebaum PS, Lidz CW, Meisel A (1987) *Informed Consent, Legal Theory and Clinical Practice.* Oxford University Press, Oxford.

Devine RJ (1987) *Ethics and Regulation of Clinical Research.* Urban & Schwarzenberg, Baltimore.

Herxheimer A (1988) The rights of the patient in clinical research. *Lancet* **ii**: 1128.

Maine A (1988) Performing drug studies in the elderly: a personal view on the ethical issues. *J Clin Pharmacol Ther* **13**: 307–312.

Mill JS (1910) *Utilitarianism.* Dent, London.

Robertson GS (1983) Ethical dilemmas of brain failure in the elderly. *Br Med J* **287**: 1774–1777.

Silverman W (1985) *Human Experimentation: A Guided Step into the Unknown!* Oxford University Press, Oxford.

35 Ethical Considerations in the Conduct of Cardiovascular Research in the Elderly: An American Perspective

HENRY D. McINTOSH
University of Florida School of Medicine, Gainesville, University of South Florida School of Medicine, and St Joseph's Heart Institute, Tampa, Florida, USA

The remaining years of this decade, leading to the millennium, will witness increasing attention to the ethical considerations of cardiovascular research in the elderly. This will be so for at least five reasons:

1. The ageing segments of developed societies are the most rapidly expanding in the population (1,2).
2. Cardiovascular disease is, and most likely will continue to be, the major cause of death in this rapidly expanding ageing population (3,4)
3. The aged segments of societies have been intentionally excluded from many investigative studies of cardiovascular disease, so that the presently available knowledge of the effect of many therapies in the aged in scant (5).
4. Females significantly outnumber males at all advanced ages and, although there are deficiencies in knowledge about the ideal management of cardiovascular disease in the elderly male, even less is known about the disease and its management in the elderly female (5).
5. The increasing efforts of society to assist ageing individuals to attain and maintain autonomy (6) will require that those responsible for investigative studies involving the elderly ensure that the individual experimental subjects have given, voluntarily, a knowledgeable, thoughtfully derived, informed consent.

Each of these topics must be considered by investigators conducting research into cardiovascular disease in the elderly. If the knowledge base is deficient, serious attention must be directed towards abolishing the ignorance. But those interested in expanding the knowledge of the aetiology and management of

Geriatric Cardiology. Principles and Practice. Edited by A. Martin and A. J. Camm
© 1994 John Wiley & Sons Ltd

cardiovascular disease in the elderly must appreciate that the task will be far from simple.

Diseases in the elderly are rarely 'pure'. Several systems may be the site of declining physiological function. Because the elderly frequently have several diseases, they may take a number of drugs. Individuals less than 65 years of age purchase an average of four prescription drugs per year, whereas those over 65 purchase 11 prescription drugs per year. Individuals over 65 years of age purchase 50% of all drugs prescribed in the USA (7).

These facts may have contributed to age-related exclusions from some studies of the therapy for cardiovascular disease. It could be argued that the higher prevalence of comorbid conditions in the elderly could result in a higher frequency of endpoints not related to the study intervention, and therefore potentially causing a dilution of the beneficial effects of the therapy studied (5).

Although desirable, expanding the knowledge base of the management of cardiovascular disease in the elderly may prove difficult for other reasons. As will be seen, ethical considerations more complex than living walls, advanced directives and autonomy will require attention. The doctrine of informed consent is still being written. What appears ethical today may be unethical in years to come.

Each of these five identified facts must be faced or the medical community will do the elderly a disservice.

Expansion of the ageing population in developed societies

The year 1991 saw the end of the Cold War. Although there continues to be the most brutal of fighting among ethnic groups in a number of locations on this fragile planet Earth, not only in what should be classified as advanced societies but also in developing and Third World nations, the loss of life from such hostilities is far less than was suffered during World War II and during the other multinational conflicts, such as in Vietnam and Korea. During World War II, the combatant countries suffered more than 15 million military casualties, and the non-combatant societies suffered even more as a result of the conflict. Those casualties, for the most part, could be classified as premature deaths. They therefore reduced the life expectancy of the societies involved (8).

According to the World Health Organization, tobacco was responsible for the premature, unnecessary death of 2.5 million persons throughout the world in 1986. A large percentage of that number was in developed societies. The 15 million combat-related casualties of World War II occurred over 6 years, from 1 September 1939 to 2 September 1945. Thus, the average annual combat-related deaths were 2.5 million—the same number that died unnecessarily per year from tobacco during the last decade.

Although far too many still ignore the obvious hazards and continue to smoke, efforts in the USA to reduce the use of tobacco have been, and are continuing to be, somewhat successful. Furthermore, the incidence of unnecessary death is declining from other public health efforts on a number of fronts. With the end of the Cold War, the threat of unnecessary premature deaths from international conflicts was greatly lessened, so the present trend for an increasing life expectancy should continue.

There are more than 30 million Americans 65 years and older. This constitutes 12% of the population. In 1900, only 4% of the population in the USA was $\geqslant 65$ years. By the year 2000, it is predicted that there will be more than 50 million Americans over 65 years of age, or 13% of the total population (1,7,8). It is anticipated that half of all Americans now alive will live to be 85 years of age. As a result, persons $\geqslant 85$ years constitute the fastest-growing segment of American society. In actual numbers, in 1987 there were approximately 2.7 million citizens in the USA $\geqslant 85$ years, whereas it is predicted that in the year 2030 there will be 16 million (1,3).

Other societies have even longer life expectancies. In Japan, in 1988, the life expectancy for males was 75.9 years and, for females, 82.1 years (8).

Clearly, the outlook for long life is not as bright in many undeveloped Third World societies, but their plight is beyond the scope of this discussion.

Cardiovascular disease is the major cause of death in advanced societies in the expanding ageing populations

Ischaemic heart disease is the single most frequent cause of death in the USA, causing over 500 000 deaths per year. There are another 1.25 million non-fatal heart attacks annually. In 1987, 57% of all patients hospitalized with an acute myocardial infarction were $\geqslant 65$ years, but only 20% of the fatal heart attacks occurred in individuals $\leqslant 65$ years of age. Sixty per cent of these deaths in the older population occurred in persons $\geqslant 75$ years (8,9). It follows that, as the older population becomes a larger segment of the total population, the incidence of death due to cardiovascular disease will likely become an even larger percentage of the total deaths.

Age-based exclusions have frequently been included in the design of studies of cardiovascular disease

Gurwitz and associates (5) recently conducted a systematic search of the English literature from January 1960 to September 1991 to identify all studies of specific pharmacotherapies used in the treatment of acute myocardial infarctions. A total of 214 trials embracing 150 920 study subjects were identified. Over 60% of all the trials excluded persons $\geqslant 75$ years. It was of interest that age-based exclusions were more common in studies published after 1980 than before. Gurwitz *et al.* (5) showed that more than 60% of the clinical trials specifically devoted to drug therapy in acute myocardial infarctions had excluded the elderly, frequently using upper age cut-offs as low as 65 years. Trials of thrombolytic therapy, and those involving an invasive procedure, were more likely to exclude elderly patients compared to other studies. The GISSI-2 trial, a multicentre randomized study embracing originally 38 086 patients admitted to coronary care units for the purpose of comparing the benefits and risks of streptokinase and tissue-type plasminogen activator, excluded 25 596 (67%) from participation. Almost 80% of patients older than 70 years were excluded, whereas only 61% of patients ≤ 70 were excluded.

Gurwitz et al. (5) quite correctly stated that these limitations in patient studies 'severely limit the ability to generalize study findings to the very age that experienced the most morbidity and mortality' from cardiovascular diseases. As the useful therapeutic knowledge of the treatment of elderly people with coronary artery disease is based on smaller numbers of older subjects, who experience the largest incidence of death from coronary artery disease, efforts should be made during the coming years to correct this data deficit. Clearly, the study of specific pharmacotherapies, as well as invasive procedures, in the elderly must be given a high priority.

Age-based and sex-based exclusions in clinical investigation have compromised the therapeutic knowledge available more for females than males

Roberts (9) reported that at least 75% of males destined to experience a fatal atherosclerotic event did so before their 70th birthday. It is well known that atherosclerotic events are not common in women before the 60th birthday but, by the 70th birthday, such events are not uncommon. But women still trail the frequency of such events in men until later years.

Feinleib and Gillum (10) reported in 1986 that deaths due to coronary artery disease in men aged 65–74 years were 2.1 times higher for men than women, while at ages ≥ 85 years the rate for men was only 1.2 times higher than that in women. That women presently survive longer than men is resulting in striking demo-graphic changes in our society. In 1988, in the 55- to 64-year-old category, there were 88 men for every 100 women; whereas in the ≥ 85-year-old group there were only 42 men for every 100 females (8). Not surprisingly, the American Heart Association reports that women now surpass men in the annual number of deaths due to cardiovascular disease (11).

It should be clear, for reasons previously defined, that the therapeutic knowledge deficit is greater for elderly women than men. Thus, we can anticipate initiation of more clinical investigation involving not only elderly men but elderly females in years to come. If the deficiencies are not corrected, therapeutic practices will be based more on speculation than carefully controlled and collected and analysed scientific data. To treat large segments of society for a major disease in this age of large clinical trials, with therapies of unknown clinical value, without seeking knowledge of results of therapy, borders on the unethical.

Society's increasing desire to assist and/or encourage older citizens to attain and maintain autonomy will require investigators to compulsively ensure that elderly experimental subjects understand the risks and benefits that could result from participating in an experimental study and voluntarily agree to participate

What is autonomy? Webster defines it as: 'The quality of being self-governing'. When used medically, autonomy means the right of individuals to exercise control over the course of their lives. For the public to want the doctor to give autonomy is an expectation of relatively recent origin. Until the years that followed the Nuremburg War Trials in 1946, the public accepted that medical decision making and medical actions by the physician were guided by the principles of beneficence. The efforts of the doctor were directed primarily towards the well-being of the patient. Such a belief led to the widespread practice and acceptance of medical parentalism: the doctor was considered the devoted father; the patient, the dependent child. These two philosophical principles— beneficence and parentalism—guided for century after century the practice of medicine. They were at the core of the Hippocratic tradition. The physician carried out these responsibilities according to the belief of Francis Peabody, who stated that 'the secret of the care of the patient is in caring for the patient' (12).

But the glaring atrocities of Nazi physicians in numerous concentration camps during the war emphasized that medical acts might not always be in the best interest of the individual. After much investigation and thoughtful deliberation, the medical tribunal conducting the Nuremburg War Trials stated that 'voluntary consent of the human subject is absolutely essential, and the person involved in a treatment should have the legal capacity to give consent'. Furthermore, the Nuremburg tribunal stated that 'in order to give a bona fide consent, the individual must be legally competent'. The individual must be able to handle his or her affairs in an adequate, socially acceptable manner. Clearly, those who judged the Nazi physicians at Nuremburg intended that physicians in the future recognize that the competent patient had matured to the level of being able to give an informed consent and could no longer be treated as a 'child'. But the admonitions given to the House of Medicine, at least the American House of Medicine, by the war tribunal were, at the time, ignored. It was only due to events that occurred 15–20 years later that the need for informed consent in human experimentation and other medical practices was accepted, almost grudgingly, as a part of the practice of medicine.

Even though we have grave deficiencies in our knowledge about the treatment of an acute myocardial infarction in the elderly, especially the elderly female, we must be certain that if we incorporate an elderly subject in a randomized trial or other type of investigation, to evaluate the benefits of a specific therapy or reaction, the patient is able to comprehend the problem(s) to be investigated, the approach to be used to correct or reduce the problem, the risk(s) entailed and the benefits that could be gained from participating in the study. Furthermore, the subject must be competent at the inception of the study, and it must be anticipated that the subject will remain competent for the year(s) of follow-up required to complete the study. For, only if that be so, can an investigator, striving to be ethical, accept the individual as a study subject. But clearly, as individuals age, the competency of many—the ability to handle his or her affairs in an adequate, socially acceptable manner—becomes less certain and predictable.

Unless the individual is legally competent, the individual cannot give voluntarily an informed consent. But what the patient consents to is frequently dependent on what is presented. Furthermore, what is percevied to have been presented may vary with the presenter. The dilemma that can arise can be emphasized by a review of the reports of the Thrombolytic Therapy in the Older Patient Population (TTOPP) Study (14). This study was intended to be a large, multicentre, randomized trial evaluating thrombolytic therapy versus placebo in patients with an acute myocardial infarction who were ⩾ 75 years of age. The endpoints were to include mortality and complications of the therapy. In marked contrast to the substantial numbers of older patients in the GISSI (15) and the ISIS-2 (16) trials, reported in 1986 and 1987, respectively, Ross (14) reported in 1990 that the 25 participating TTOPP study centres managed to enrol only 70 patients over a 1-year period. The study was thus ended. The small number of enrolled elderly patients was thought to be due to physicians of large numbers of patients above 75 years of age considering that the patient had contraindications to thrombolytic therapy. The physicians of many other patients believed that, in light of the results of the earlier studies, it was unethical to recommend randomization to placebo for patients who did not have a contraindication to thrombolytic therapy. It is likely that the same physician at one time or another excluded what might appear to be similar patients for both reasons. Minor differences between patients may prompt the physician to define the problem as strikingly different. Furthermore, minor differences in patients might result in differing descriptions and/or decisions on different days by the same physician. It would not be surprising that the patient might have difficulty in giving voluntarily a meaningful informed consent to one physician but not another. Clearly, the consent might vary, depending on the 'messenger'.

To complicate the situation further, reflection on the history of the doctrine of informed consent in American medicine reveals that it is a recent addition to the practice and continues to be far from finalized. In the treatment of no segment of the population is a knowledge of the history of informed consent as important as in the elderly. For that doctrine presents to the physician most clearly the principles of medical ethics. A consideration of that doctrine prompts the author to offer the caveat: 'He who does not read history must be prepared to relive it'.

THE HISTORY OF THE DOCTRINE OF INFORMED CONSENT

Before World War II, the actions of the physician were guided by beneficence and medical parentalism. Before the war, the medical research enterprise was typically a small-scale, intimate, cottage industry. Medical researchers were few in number. They frequently worked alone. They carried out experiments on themselves, their families and their immediate neighbours. The research questions were almost always therapeutic in nature. The experimental subject usually benefited directly, if the experiments were successful; if not successful, little harm was done to the subject (17). However, the events associated with World War II had a profound effect on the American medical community, especially as regards medical ethics. A common enemy was readily identified: men, sons and/or sons of neighbours, were dying on the battlefield, dying of diseases and/or infections and/or trauma. The so-called research industry was mobilized to fight the human afflictions produced by the enemy. Individual, part-time researchers were replaced by or transformed into elaborate, complex but well-coordinated, federally funded team ventures. One hundred and thirty-five universities or major hospitals or research institutes carried out over 600 federally approved and funded research projects. Most of the studies dealt with problems common to combat and/or military life: dysentery, wound infection, venereal disease, sleep deprivation, exposure to frigid temperatures. Many studies involved the use of humans as experimental subjects. Because of the urgency of the wartime effort, investigators developed the belief that answers were the primary goal, if not the only goal; how the answers were obtained was of secondary importance (17).

When the war ended, decisions had to be made as to the future of a large, dedicated, responsive medical research capability. Vannever Bush, the Director of the Office of Scientific Research and Development, which had directed the wartime medical research programme(s), stated: 'Medicine is on the verge of its most heroic explorations. It would be foolhardy to close off the Frontiers of Science by ending Federal support' (17).

Senator John Ransdell of Louisiana, supporting Bush's claims, said: 'We have found the cause of a number of epidemic diseases and practically conquered them. May we not expect the same kind of success against the so-called degenerative diseases if we work hard enough?'

The *New York Times*, in 1945, wrote: 'It is sad to realize that, had it not been for the war, penicillin might not have been put in the hands of physicians. We need something more than the natural curiosity of the research scientist to speed discovery that means so much to mankind' (17).

It was with similar widespread support that the National Institutes of Health (NIH) were established in 1947 with an annual budget of $700 000. Because of the enthusiastic support by society, by 1970 the budget had risen to $1.5 billion. Superficially, the design, or at least the name, of the research programme was shifted from wartime efforts to peacetime pursuits. However, the day-to-day efforts of the individual investigators appeared unchanged. Results remained the primary goal. How the results were obtained appeared to be of little importance, particularly if the results were publishable. 'Publish or perish' became the watchword of the young academician, who usually was a young, enthusiastic physician scientist of the postwar generation, trained by mentors matured by wartime pressures and goals (18). In retrospect, it is clear that the wartime mentality had been carried over into the peacetime academic laboratory (17,18). It was these academic investigators who constituted the major segments of the faculties that taught the medical students of the nation.

The Nuremburg War Trials, with the resulting Nuremburg Code, published in 1947, had little effect on the American House of Medicine (13,18). Few gave the proclamation a passing thought, if they had even heard of or read it. The Nuremburg Proclamation stated that 'the voluntary consent of the human subject is absolutely essential. This means that the person involved should have legal capacity to give consent.' Nor were the members of the American House of Medicine impressed that the subject 'should be so situated as to be able to exercise free power of choice' and 'should have knowledge and comprehension of the elements of the subject matter involved, so as to make an understanding and enlightened decision'. The author attended medical school after 4 years of combat in the late 1940s and cannot recall a single mention of the Nuremburg Code being made in a formal teaching session (18).

By 1965, the NIH had funded between 1500 and 2000 research projects which, by title, indicated that the research would be done on humans. Yet, the NIH had no requirement to assure that the investigator would obtain an informed consent from each experimental subject.

But from the ranks of a profession that outwardly showed little concern whether experimental subjects were given the protection dictated by the Nuremburg Code, a whistle-blower arose. On 16 June 1966, Henry K. Beecher, the Door Professor of Research Anesthesiology at the Massachusetts General Hospital, Boston, Massachusetts, published in the *New England Journal of Medicine* (20) an article listing 22 abstracts describing studies of investigators in the most prestigious institutions in America. Each of these investigators had used, according to Beecher, 'participants as experimental subjects when it must be apparent that they would not have been available if they had been truly aware of the uses that would have been made of them'. Beecher concluded that 'the ethical approach to experimentation in man has several components: two are more important than the others: the first being informed consent. The second is the more reliable safeguard provided by the presence of an intelligent, informed, conscientious, compassionate, responsible investigator.'

But even that article did not get the attention of the leaders, much less the followers, in the American House of Medicine. As Professor of Medicine and Director of the Cardiovascular Division of a prestigious medical school at the time the article was published, the author cannot recall any discussion of Beecher's article in his institution or at medical meeetings. (18).

The Food and Drug Administration (FDA), fearing congressional sanctions, did publish, on 30 August 1966, a statement concerning the use of investigational new drugs on humans (21). But the members of the American House of Medicine, for the most part, continued 'business as usual' (18).

Finally, in 1973, Edward Kennedy, US Senator from Massachusetts, stated: 'The question is whether we can tolerate a system where the individual physician is the sole determinant of the safety of the experimental procedure. After all, it is the patient who must live with the consequences of the decision' (22).

With that statement, Congress established the National Commission for the Protection of Human Subjects. There followed the birth of the Doctrine of Informed Consent. Shortly thereafter, the policy for institutional review committees to oversee human investigation was established. What doctors of the American House of Medicine had failed to do voluntarily was now mandated.

Another protection of the right of the individual patient is now gaining increasing publicity and even congressional support (23). The patient, especially the elderly, is being encouraged to attain and maintain autonomy. In November 1991, the Patient Self-Determination Act was established. That Act ensured that hospitals, nursing homes, health care maintenance organizations, hospices and health care companies that participated in Medicare and Medicaid not only must inform patients of their rights, but also note in the patient's medical record whether the patient has, in writing, rejected life support.

Thus far, members of the American House of Medicine and its leaders have paid little more attention to this action than they did to the Nuremburg Code or the whistle-blowing efforts of Henry K. Beecher. It would appear that American physicians have not learned that 'he who does not read history must be prepared to relive it'. Physicians did not recognize the right of the individual to be informed by the physician, nor did physicians assume the responsibility for establishing and monitoring the elements of the Doctrine of Informed Consent. It was formulated and is monitored by lawyers, clergymen, ethicists and others from the non-medical community. Such were referred to by Rothman as 'strangers at the bedside' (13).

There is still much to be written about the Doctrine of Informed Consent. How can fetal tissue be used therapeutically? Already, forces favouring euthanasia and doctor-assisted suicide and attitudes for and/or against abortion are gaining strength. Will national policies regarding these issues be thoughtfully developed by physicians motivated by beneficence and parentalism, or mandated for physicians to carry out, by 'strangers at the bedside'?

Similarly, attitudes are being developed regarding the Doctrine of Attaining and Maintaining Autonomy. Will the American House of Medicine wait to be told by the legislators and other 'strangers at the bedside' what will be done, or will doctors thoughtfully develop a philosophy, acceptable to society, for the attainment and management of individual autonomy? For example, what policies will guide decisions regarding an 80-year-old, mentally sound widower with limited financial resources who, despite his objections, would be 'better protected from potentially serious physical harm' by confinement, even if involuntary, to a nursing home? Such a commitment would require this 'independent soul' to conform to the heinous (to the patient) routines of nursing home life. Will the individual be confined involuntarily? Or should the elderly individual be told that 'you are autonomous', 'you are free to refuse treatment', 'you are free to live even on the streets'—even though it would likely be an entrée to unsolicited suicide.

Such are the problems of the present decade confronting members of the American House of Medicine. By the time we reach the millennium, hopefully, doctors will have returned to their roots and, whether in the research laboratory or at the bedside, demonstrate that they 'care for the patient by caring for the patient'. May we learn again the value of 'pneumonia, the old man's friend', and that many prefer quality of life to quantity of life. May we as physicians never be forced overtly to give life to one patient and death to the next. Furthermore, may we have the wisdom to learn from our past complacency and accept, as a member of the House of Medicine, the responsibility to help individuals of society 'attain and maintain autonomy'.

REFERENCES

1. McIntosh HD (1992) Who will pay for the aging? *Am J Geriatr Cardiol* **1**: 27–28.
2. US Public Health Service (1990) *National Health Promotion and Disease Prevention Objectives. Healthy People 2000.* US Department of Health and Human Services, Washington, D.C.
3. Page LB (1987) Introductory Remarks II. 18th Bethesda Conference: Cardiovascular Disease in the Elderly. Wenger NK, chairperson. *J Am Coll Cardiol* **10**: 7A.
4. National Center for Health Statistics (1987) *National Hospital Discharge Survey. Advance Data from Vital and Health Statistics.* DHHS Publication 88-1250, **159**: 1–16.
5. Gurwitz JH, Col NF, Avorn J (1992) The exclusion of the elderly and women from clinical trials in acute myocardial infarction. *JAMA* **268**: 1417–1422.
6. Gamble ER, McDonald PJ, Lichstein PR (1991) Knowledge, attitudes, and behavior of elderly persons regarding living wills. *Arch Intern Med* **151**: 277–280.
7. Montamat SC, Cusack BJ, Vestal RE (1989) Management of drug therapy in the elderly. *N Engl J Med* **321**: 303.
8. McIntosh HD (1990) Geriatric cardiology: a subspecialty ... or mainstream for the twenty-first century? *Prog Cardiol* **3**: 117–125.
9. Roberts WC (1989) Atherosclerotic risk factors: are there ten or is there only one? *Am J Cardiol* **64**: 552–560.
10. Feinleib M, Gillum RF (1986) Coronary heart disease in the elderly: the magnitude of the problem in the United States. In *Coronary Heart Disease in the Elderly*, Wenger NK, Furberg CD, Pitt E (eds). Elsevier, New York, pp. 29–59.
11. American Heart Association (1992) *Heart and Stroke Facts.* American Heart Association, Dallas.
12. Peabody FW (1927) The care of the patient. *JAMA* **88**: 877–882.
13. Rothman DJ (1991) *Strangers at the Bedside.* Basic Books, New York, p. 62.
14. Ross AM (1990) The TTOPP Study: lessons from an aborted trial. *J Myocard Ischemia* **2**: 65–69.
15. Gruppo Italio per lo Studio della Streptochenasi nell' Infarto Miocardico (GISSI) (1986) Effectiveness of intravenous thrombolytic treatment in acute myocardial infarction. *Lancet* **i**: 397–401.
16. ISIS-2 (Second Collaborative Study of Infarct Survival) Collaborative Group (1987) Randomized trial of intravenous streptokinase, oral aspirin, both, or neither among 17 187 cases of suspected acute myocardial infarction: ISIS-2. *Lancet* **i**: 349–360.
17. Rothman DJ (1991) *Strangers at the Bedside.* Basic Books, New York, pp. 18–27.

18. McIntosh HD. Personal observation.
19. Rothman DJ (1991) *Strangers at the Bedside*. Basic Books, New York, p. 59.
20. Beecher HK (1966) Ethics and clinical research. *New Engl J Med* **274**: 1354–1360.
21. Rothman DJ (1991) *Strangers at the Bedside*. Basic Books, New York, pp. 88–90.
22. Rothman DJ (1991) *Strangers at the Bedside*. Basic Books, New York, pp. 168–190.
23. Charnow JA (1991) Law spurs upfront talk with patients about advanced directives. *ACP Observer* December: 4.

Index

Index compiled by Liza Weinkove